WORKBOOK

Emergency Care

12th Edition

WORKBOOK

Bob Elling

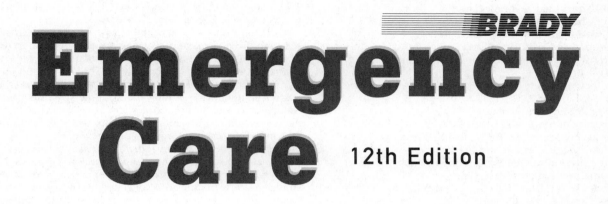

Emergency Care

BRADY

12th Edition

DANIEL LIMMER | MICHAEL F. O'KEEFE

MEDICAL EDITOR
EDWARD T. DICKINSON, MD, FACEP

LEGACY AUTHORS
Harvey D. Grant | Robert H. Murray, Jr. | J. David Bergeron

Brady is an imprint of Pearson

Boston   Columbus   Indianapolis   New York   San Francisco   Upper Saddle River
Amsterdam   Cape Town   Dubai   London   Madrid   Milan   Munich   Paris   Montreal   Toronto
Delhi   Mexico City   São Paulo   Sydney   Hong Kong   Seoul   Singapore   Taipei   Tokyo

Dedicated to my two beautiful daughters: Laura and Caitlin. And to my lovely wife, Kirsten. May you always maintain humility as your accomplishments meet the stars!

B.E.

Publisher: Julie Levin Alexander
Publisher's Assistant: Regina Bruno
Editor-in-Chief: Marlene McHugh Pratt
Acquisitions Editor: Sladjana Repic
Senior Managing Editor for Development: Lois Berlowitz
Project Manager: iD8-Triple SSS Press Media Development, LLC
Assistant Editor: Jonathan Cheung
Director of Marketing: David Gesell
Marketing Manager: Brian Hoehl
Marketing Specialist: Michael Sirinides
Managing Editor for Production: Patrick Walsh
Production Liaison: Faye Gemmellaro
Production Editor: Kannan Poojli Vadivelu, S4Carlisle Publishing Services
Manufacturing Manager: Alan Fischer
Manager of Design Development: John Christiana
Cover Design: John Christiana
Cover Photography: foreground image, Michal Heron for Pearson Education; background image, © Daniel Limmer
Printer/Binder: Bind-Rite Graphics
Cover Printer: Lehigh-Phoenix Color/Hagerstown
Composition: S4Carlisle Publishing Services

NOTICE ON CARE PROCEDURES

This workbook reflects current EMS practices based on the 2010 U.S. Department of Transportation's National Emergency Medical Services Educational Standards: Emergency Medical Technician Instructional Guidelines. It is the intent of the authors and publisher that this workbook be used as part of a formal Emergency Medical Technician education program taught by qualified instructors and supervised by a licensed physician. The procedures described in this workbook are based upon consultation with EMS and medical authorities. The authors and publisher have taken care to make certain that these procedures reflect currently accepted clinical practice; however, they cannot be considered absolute recommendations.

The material in this workbook contains the most current information available at the time of publication. However, federal, state, and local guidelines concerning clinical practices, including, without limitation, those governing infection control and Standard Precautions, change rapidly. The reader should note, therefore, that new regulations may require changes in some procedures.

It is the responsibility of the reader to familiarize himself with the policies and procedures set by federal, state, and local agencies as well as the institution or agency where the reader may be employed. The author and the publisher of this workbook disclaim any liability, loss, or risk resulting directly or indirectly from the suggested procedures and theory, from any undetected errors, or from the reader's misunderstanding of the text. It is the reader's responsibility to stay informed of any new changes or recommendations made by any federal, state, and local agency as well as by his or her employing institution or agency.

If, when reading this workbook, you find an error, have an idea for how to improve it, or simply want to share your comments with us, please send your letter to the address below.

Managing Editor
Brady/Pearson Health Science
Pearson Education
One Lake Street
Upper Saddle River, New Jersey 07458

Or send comments directly to the author at:

bobelling@usa.net

NOTICE ON BLS PROCEDURES

The national standards for BLS are reviewed and revised every five years and may change slightly after this book is printed. It is important that you know the most current procedures for CPR, both for the classroom and your patients. The most current information may always be downloaded from www.bradybooks.com or obtained from your instructor.

Brady
is an imprint of

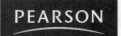

Pearson Health Science
Upper Saddle River, NJ 07458
www.bradybooks.com

10 9 8 7 6 5 4 3 2 1

ISBN 10: 0-13-237534-6
ISBN 13: 978-0-13-237534-4

Contents

©2012 Pearson Education, Inc.
Emergency Care, 12th Ed.

Introduction

▶ OVERVIEW

This workbook is designed to accompany the textbook *Emergency Care,* 12th Edition. The workbook covers the course knowledge and National Highway Transportation Safety Administration (NHTSA) Education Standards to which all standardized testing instruments will be referenced. In all areas where the textbook goes beyond the national core standards to present current trends in medical care, this workbook also follows along very closely. It is neither meant to replace the text nor to be a substitute for a well-designed course in emergency care.

This is a self-instructional workbook. It has been designed to allow you to work at your own pace and evaluate your own progress. To benefit from this workbook, follow the procedures in this introduction. Thousands of EMT students before you have used prior editions of this workbook as part of their emergency medical training. The system works, having helped them to learn and excel on state and national certification and registration examinations. By doing your best on each chapter, you, as well as those patients to whom you deliver emergency care, will benefit.

This edition continues the emphasis of the Education Standards on patient assessment. In addition, there are a number of updated sections and new features in this workbook. Additional Case Studies have been added and the EMT Performance Checklists have been updated.

▶ FEATURES

Each chapter in this workbook contains these elements:

- **Match Terminology/Definitions**—In this section, you are asked to match chapter terminology with appropriate definitions, which appear in the chapter's running text or in the chapter glossary, or both. The terms have been placed in alphabetical order so that, after reading the definitions, you can quickly select the appropriate term.
- **Multiple-Choice Review**—This section provides, on average, 25 to 45 questions. Emphasis is placed on multiple-choice questions because this is the format of state and national exams used for certification or registration. Practice in answering multiple-choice questions can help improve your understanding of the material as well as your course grades. These multiple-choice questions generally appear in the sequential order that the topics appear in the textbook, enabling you to build on prior knowledge. When similar questions appear in the three Interim Exams, the order is scrambled, as is done on state and national exams.

- **Complete the Following**—This section focuses on your recalling and listing specific information on chapter objectives, such as the signs and symptoms of shock or the five stages of grief.
- **Label the Diagram/Photograph and Complete the Chart**—In some chapters, you are asked to study a visual and to identify its content or to complete a partially filled-in chart. These diagrams, photographs, and charts correspond to those in the textbook.
- **Inside/Outside**—Many chapters have questions that are based on this feature found in the text. It specifically delves into the physiology of trauma or diseases so that the reader can reflect on what is happening "inside" the body and "outside" the body.
- **Street Scenes Discussion**—Each chapter of the textbook has a section called Street Scenes. These scenarios are designed to apply what you have learned in the respective chapter to a situation that can easily be found in your work as an EMT. In the workbook, you are asked to reread the Street Scenes and then use the knowledge you have obtained thus far in your course to answer a few more questions.
- **Case Study**—After every few chapters, a case study requires you to synthesize information that you have learned up to that particular point in the course and to apply this knowledge to a real-life situation. As each step of the case is presented, you are asked a series of questions that build on the facts of the case.
- **Answer Key**—The Answer Key at the back of the workbook provides answers for all of the workbook elements. For the Street Scenes Discussion questions, rationales appear for each answer. For the Multiple-Choice Review questions, rationales are provided where appropriate, along with the textbook page reference(s) where each topic is discussed.
- **EMT Skills Performance Checklists**—Most workbook chapters include a list of the EMT skills that incorporate national standards, the

most current American Heart Association guidelines, or the National EMS: EMT Education Standard description of a method of doing each skill.

▶ STEPS FOR SUCCESS

To get the most out of this workbook, you should complete the following eight steps:

Step 1—Learn the Course Objectives

Each chapter of the textbook begins with objectives that were developed as part of the NHTSA's National Education Standard Instructional Guidelines. Most state and national certifying examinations are based on these objectives. To score well on those exams, you must learn the objectives of the course. Use the objectives in the textbook in the following way:

1. Read them over.
2. Read the text.
3. Reread the objective in the form of a question.
4. Write down your answer to each question on a blank piece of paper.
5. Perform a self-assessment or ask your instructor to assess how well you understand the material in the chapter.

Step 2—Learn the Language of the EMT

Emergency Medical Services (EMS) is clearly a medical field and, as such, it is necessary for the EMT to learn and understand the language of medicine. This will help you communicate with the other members of the health care team in a clear, concise, and accurate manner. In addition, learning the language of medicine will facilitate your understanding of medical and trade journal articles as you work to keep current in the constantly changing EMS field.

First, review the medical terminology in the text and then put aside the text. Next, test your understanding of the terminology by completing the Match Terminology/Definitions exercise in each workbook chapter. Complete the entire matching exercise before checking your answers against the Answer Key. For those terms that you were unable to match, write down the word on one side of a 3″ × 5″ card and write the definition on the other side of the card. Carry these cards in your pocket and refer to them frequently to help you learn the terms.

Step 3—Learn the Structure of the Body

The language of medicine also includes learning the names and locations of the structures of the human body. Imagine being unable to take a peripheral pulse because you could not find the radial artery in the wrist! To help you learn the structures of the body, in workbook chapters in which it is appropriate, anatomical drawings and diagrams are provided. For example, the drawing of the respiratory system in the workbook has blank numbered lines that point to each of the system's different structures. Label each structure as requested and check your answers in the answer key at the back of the workbook. For those body structures that you miss, go to the textbook page suggested and study the body structure again.

Step 4—Answer the Multiple-Choice Questions

For each Multiple-Choice Review, complete the entire exercise at one sitting. Read each question and all the answer choices before you mark your answer. If you jump to a conclusion without fully reading the question, you could answer incorrectly. Also, watch out for questions with negative expressions or the word *except*. You will notice that the author has minimized the use of "all of the above" as an answer to questions in this edition. This was done to ensure that exam items mirror those used in standardized tests. Once you have completed the exercise, refer to the Answer Key to check your performance. A textbook page reference has been provided for the theory or principle tested in each question. Many answers have an author comment whenever it is appropriate to clarify the answer to a question.

You will need to practice reading, and not reading into, multiple-choice questions. If it has been many years since you took a standardized test, leave extra time to review this section of each workbook chapter. If you notice any trends in your performance on these questions, you may wish to consult your instructor for test-taking assistance.

Step 5—Use the Inside/Outside and Street Scenes Discussion

These features are written to enrich your understanding of the content of the chapter.

Step 6—Review the EMT Skill Performance Checklists

Whenever a skill is introduced in the chapter, a checklist has been included in the workbook. Work in pairs and use these checklists to test each other.

Step 7—Take the Interim Exams

Once you have completed each individual workbook chapter, move on to the next chapter and repeat steps one to six. Three full-length Interim Exams are spread throughout the workbook and are similar to the interim exams your instructor may use in the EMT course. Each exam covers material in the chapters that precede it. Therefore,

©2012 Pearson Education, Inc.
Emergency Care, 12th Ed.

when you have completed all of the material in the chapters preceding an exam, it's time to take the Interim Exam.

Also be sure to review the extra materials in the Appendix at the end of the workbook because many state and national exams have a section on BLS and CPR.

Step 8—Pay Close Attention to the Case Studies

The case studies integrated in the workbook help you synthesize your knowledge and apply it to real-life situations. They actually put you at a scene and require you to think quickly and accurately. Answers at the back of the workbook will help you sort out any problems you confront.

So that's it: *eight* simple steps. It will take your time and commitment to work through each of the steps. This is a self-instructional workbook, so it will be up to you to reward yourself for doing well on chapters. At the same time, you need to be honest with yourself. If you are having difficulty with a chapter, let your instructor know immediately so he or she can offer additional assistance.

It is the hope of the *Emergency Care* authors and development team that using this workbook as an integral part of your EMT training package will help you improve your understanding of the material and enhance your performance in the field. After all, isn't quality patient care what EMS is all about? See you in the streets!

▶ **ACKNOWLEDGMENTS**

The author of the *Emergency Care Workbook*, 12th Edition, would like to thank the publishing team led by Julie Alexander, Sladjana Repic, Marlene Pratt, and Lois Berlowitz for all their hard work and support on the Emergency Care series. Appreciation is extended to Dan Limmer and Mike O'Keefe for their friendship and confidence and the opportunity to partake in this important project. Gratitude is extended to Triple SSS Press Media Development for excellent developmental guidance. And last, but not least, a special thanks to a dear friend and mentor, J. David Bergeron.

▶ **ABOUT THE AUTHOR**

Bob Elling, MPA, EMT-P, has been passionately involved in EMS for three and a half decades. He is an active paramedic with the Town of Colonie (New York), the Times Union Center, and Whiteface Mountain Medical Services. He is a Clinical Instructor with Albany Medical Center, teaching in the Capital District as well as the Adirondacks. He is a dedicated advocate for the American Heart Association, having served in many leadership roles: from BLS/ACLS/PALS Instructor to National Faculty, to Guidelines 2005 Editor. He is also Regional Faculty for the NYS Bureau of EMS. Bob has served as a paramedic and lieutenant for NYC EMS, Program Director for Hudson Valley Community College's Paramedic Program, Associate Director of the NYS EMS Program, and the Education Coordinator for PULSE: Emergency Medical Update. Bob enjoys writing and is the author/coauthor/editor of over twenty EMS publications, including these popular Brady books: *Pocket Reference for BLS Providers, MedReview for the EMT-B, Essentials of Emergency Care, Paramedic Care: Principles & Practice Workbook Volume 5, EMT Achieve: Basic Test Preparation,* and *EMT Achieve: Online First Responder Test Preparation.*

He lives in Colonie and Lake Placid, where he enjoys distance running (he has completed 25 marathons), skiing, cycling, hiking, photography, and spending time with his family.

You can reach him at his e-mail address: bobelling@usa.net.

1

Introduction to Emergency Medical Care

Standard: Preparatory (EMS Systems, Research); Public Health

Competency: Applies fundamental knowledge of the EMS system, safety/well-being of the EMT, medical/legal and ethical issues to the provision of emergency care.

OBJECTIVES

After reading this chapter you should be able to:

1.1 Define key terms introduced in this chapter.

1.2 Give an overview of the historical events leading to the development of modern emergency medical services (EMS).

1.3 Describe the importance of each of the National Highway Traffic Safety Administration standards for assessing EMS systems.

1.4 Describe the components of an EMS system that must be in place for a patient to receive emergency medical care.

1.5 Compare and contrast the training and responsibilities of EMRs, EMTs, AEMTs, and paramedics.

1.6 Explain each of the specific areas of responsibility for the EMT.

1.7 Give examples of the physical and personality traits that are desirable for EMTs.

1.8 Discuss various job settings that may be available to EMTs.

1.9 Describe the purpose of the National Registry of Emergency Medical Technicians.

1.10 Explain the purpose of quality improvement programs in EMS programs.

1.11 Explain EMTs' role in the quality improvement process.

1.12 Explain medical direction as it relates to EMS systems.

1.13 List ways in which research may influence EMT practice.

1.14 Give examples of how EMS providers can play a role in public health.

1.15 Given scenarios, decide how an EMT may demonstrate professional behavior.

MATCH TERMINOLOGY/ DEFINITIONS

A. A system for telephone access to report emergencies

B. A process of continuous self-review with the purpose of identifying and correcting aspects of the system that require improvement

C. The oversight of the patient-care aspects of an EMS system by the Medical Director

D. A physician who assumes ultimate responsibility for the patient-care aspects of the EMS system

E. Consists of standing orders issued by the Medical Director that allow EMTs to give certain medications or perform certain procedures without speaking to the Medical Director or another physician

F. Lists of steps, such as assessments and interventions, to be taken in different situations

G. A policy or protocol issued by a Medical Director that authorizes EMTs and others to perform particular skills in certain situations

H. Orders from the on-duty physician given directly to an EMT in the field by radio or telephone

I. An EMT or other person authorized by a Medical Director to give medications and provide emergency care

_I_ 1. Designated agent

_E_ 2. Off-line medical direction

_H_ 3. On-line medical direction

_A_ 4. 911 system

_C_ 5. Medical direction

_D_ 6. Medical Director

_B_ 7. Quality improvement

_F_ 8. Protocols

_G_ 9. Standing order

MULTIPLE-CHOICE REVIEW

_B_ 1. The earliest documented emergency medical service was in:
   A. England in the 1890s.
   B. France in the 1790s.
   C. Seattle in the 1970s.
   D. Miami in the 1960s.

_C_ 2. In 1966, the _____ charged the United States _____ with developing EMS standards.
   A. Uniform Traffic Act; Department of Transportation
   B. president; Fire Academy
   C. National Highway Safety Act; Department of Transportation
   D. American Medical Association; Department of Health and Human Services

_B_ 3. Of the following, which is *not* a major component in the National Highway Traffic Safety Administration's EMS system assessment standards?
   A. Transportation
   B. Computerization
   C. Communications
   D. Evaluation

_A_ 4. An example of a specialty hospital in the EMS system is a(n):
   A. emergency department.
   B. correctional facility.
   C. poison control center.
   D. primary care center.

_A_ 5. National levels of EMS training include all of the following *except*:
   A. advanced first aid.
   B. emergency medical responder.
   C. advanced EMT.
   D. EMT-paramedic.

_C_ **6.** The major emphasis of the curriculum for the EMT deals with _____
of the ill or injured patient in the prehospital setting.
   A. immediate life-threatening care
   B. interpretation of electrocardiograms
   C. assessment and care
   D. techniques of advanced airway care

_B_ **7.** Patient care provided by the EMT should be:
   A. delayed until transportation.
   B. based on assessment findings.
   C. guided by the service's attorney.
   D. based upon the diagnosis of the patient.

_A_ **8.** An example of ensuring continuity during the transfer of care of the patient
would be:
   A. providing pertinent patient information to the hospital staff.
   B. performing more hospital procedures in the field.
   C. only giving a report directly to a physician.
   D. none of these.

_D_ **9.** Patient advocacy is:
   A. assessing your patient.
   B. abandoning your patient.
   C. executing your primary responsibility as an EMT.
   D. speaking up for your patient.

_A_ **10.** Good personality traits are very important to the EMT. You should be:
   A. cooperative and resourceful.
   B. respectful and condescending.
   C. cunning and inventive.
   D. emotionally stable and shy.

_D_ **11.** If an EMT is *not* in control of personal habits, he or she might:
   A. contaminate the patient's wounds.
   B. make inappropriate decisions.
   C. render improper care.
   D. do all of the above.

_C_ **12.** To prevent violating patient confidentiality, the EMT should:
   A. communicate with medical direction.
   B. perform an accurate interview.
   C. avoid inappropriate conversation.
   D. develop the ability to listen to others.

_C_ **13.** An EMT may further his or her EMS education by:
   A. rereading the EMT textbook.   **C.** attending EMS conferences.
   B. repeating the EMT course.   **D.** all of these.

_C_ **14.** A process of continuous self-review of all aspects of an EMS system for the
purpose of identifying and correcting aspects of the system that require
improvement is called:
   A. off-line medical direction.   **C.** quality improvement.
   B. patient advocacy.   **D.** continuing education.

_B_ **15.** Obtaining feedback from patients and the hospital staff is a means of:
   A. obtaining on-line medical direction.
   B. providing quality improvement.
   C. determining what is wrong with patients.
   D. avoiding charges of negligence.

_C_ **16.** Participation in continuing education and keeping carefully written documentation are examples of the EMT's role in:
  A. patient advocacy.
  B. medical direction.
  C. quality improvement.
  D. transfer of care.

_D_ **17.** Every EMS system should have a:
  A. minimum of three EMTs on each vehicle.
  B. call review on a monthly basis.
  C. contract with the local hospital.
  D. Medical Director.

_C_ **18.** An EMT is operating as the Medical Director's:
  A. employee.
  B. replacement.
  C. designated agent.
  D. peer.

_D_ **19.** The difference between on-line and off-line medical direction is that:
  A. off-line medical direction does not need protocols.
  B. off-line orders are given by the on-duty physician, usually over the radio or phone.
  C. on-line medical direction uses standing orders.
  D. on-line orders are given by the on-duty physician, usually over the radio or phone.

_A_ **20.** An example of a medication carried by EMTs that may require a physician consultation to administer is:
  A. lidocaine.
  B. oral glucose.
  C. oxygen.
  D. aspirin.

_A_ **21.** As a new EMT, you will witness many changes in the EMS system and patient care, moving from practices that have been based on _____ to those that are based on _____.
  A. in-hospital; prehospital
  B. tradition; research
  C. gut instincts; traditions
  D. research; tradition

_A_ **22.** It is the responsibility of the EMT to treat patients:
  A. as quickly as possible.
  B. in their community or district.
  C. in a nonjudgmental and fair manner.
  D. who are insured or injured at work.

_D_ **23.** A general procedure involved in making evidence-based patient care decisions includes:
  A. reviewing the literature.
  B. an evaluation of evidence.
  C. forming a hypothesis.
  D. all of these.

_B_ **24.** Injury prevention for geriatric patients and campaigns to reduce tobacco use are examples of:
  A. hospital responsibilities.
  B. an EMT's role in public health.
  C. the nursing domain.
  D. off-line medical direction.

COMPLETE THE FOLLOWING

1. List at least six of the categories and standards of an EMS system established by the National Highway Traffic Safety Administration.

A. _Regulation and Policy_

B. _RESOURCES MANAGEMENT_

C. _HUMAN RESOURCES and TRAINING_

D. TRANSPORTATION

E. FACILITES

F. COMMUNICATIONS

2. List the six types of specialty hospitals.

A. Burn Centers

B. Trauma Centers

C. Cardiac centers

D. Poison Control Centers

E. stroke centers

F. pediatric centers

3. List the four levels of EMS certification.

A. Emergency Medical Responder (EMR)

B. Emergency Medical Technician (EMT)

C. Advanced Emergency Medical Technician (AEMT)

D. PARAMEDIC

STREET SCENES DISCUSSION

Review the Street Scene on page 20 in the textbook. Then answer the following question.

What responsibilities of the EMT are illustrated in this scenario?

Checking the equipment on the ambulance
Being respectful when dealing with a patient
while transporting the patient, being reassureing
Having good technical skills
and must ~~act~~ act as a professional
Safety scene, patient assessment, (first) (and then)
patient care, lifting and moving patients, and patient
transport.

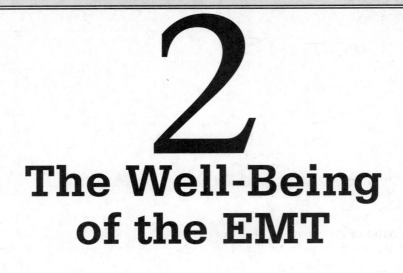

The Well-Being of the EMT

Standard: Preparatory (Workforce Safety and Wellness)

Competency: Applies fundamental knowledge of the EMS system, safety/well-being of the EMT, medical/legal and ethical issues to the provision of emergency care.

OBJECTIVES

After reading this chapter you should be able to:

2.1   Define key terms introduced in this chapter.

2.2   Describe health habits that promote physical and mental well-being.

2.3   Given an example of a patient-care situation, determine the appropriate personal protective equipment to prevent exposure to infectious disease.

2.4   Describe proper procedures for hand washing and using alcohol-based hand cleaners.

2.5   Discuss the health concerns related to exposure to hepatitis B, hepatitis C, tuberculosis, and AIDS.

2.6   Access the Centers for Disease Control web site to obtain the latest information on diseases of concern to EMS providers.

2.7   Explain the essential provisions of OSHA, the CDC, and the Ryan White CARE Act as they relate to infection control in EMS.

2.8   Describe the indications for use of an N-95 or HEPA respirator.

2.9   Describe the purpose of the tuberculin skin test (TST).

2.10 Give examples of common stressors in EMS work.

2.11 Describe the stages of the stress response, including the effects of each stage on the body.

2.12 Differentiate among acute, delayed, and cumulative stress reactions.

©2012 Pearson Education, Inc.
Emergency Care, 12th Ed.

2.13 List lifestyle changes that can be used to manage stress.

2.14 Explain the purpose of critical incident stress management (CISM).

2.15 Given a scenario, recognize a patient's or family member's reaction to death and dying.

2.16 Given a scenario involving death or dying, use effective techniques for interacting with the patient and family members.

2.17 List indications of the potential for danger to yourself or others at the scene of an EMS call.

2.18 Outline proper responses to incidents, including:

    a. Hazardous materials incidents
    b. Terrorist incidents
    c. Rescue operations
    d. Violence

2.19 Given a scenario of an emergency response involving a safety threat, describe actions you should take to protect yourself and other EMS providers.

2.20 Identify with the feelings of a patient who has a communicable disease.

2.21 Promote the importance of safety on EMS calls.

MATCH TERMINOLOGY/ DEFINITIONS

A. A strict form of infection control based on the assumption that all blood and other body fluids are infectious

B. A comprehensive system that includes education and resources to both prevent stress and to deal with stress appropriately when it occurs

C. The introduction of dangerous chemicals, disease, or infectious materials

D. Equipment that protects the EMS worker from infection and/or exposure to the dangers of rescue operations

E. The organisms that cause infection, such as viruses and bacteria

F. An emergency involving multiple patients

G. The removal or cleaning of dangerous chemicals and other dangerous or infectious materials

H. The release of a harmful substance into the environment

I. A state of physical and/or psychological arousal to a stimulus

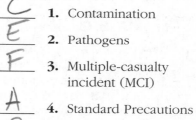

C **1.** Contamination

E **2.** Pathogens

F **3.** Multiple-casualty incident (MCI)

A **4.** Standard Precautions

B **5.** Critical incident stress management (CISM)

G **6.** Decontamination

H **7.** Hazardous-material incident

I **8.** Stress

D **9.** Personal protective equipment (PPE)

MULTIPLE-CHOICE REVIEW

_D_ **1.** Each of the following is a good tip for the EMT to maintain a healthy lifestyle *except*:
  A. maintaining solid personal relationships.
  B. participating in an exercise program to improve strength, flexibility, and fitness.
  C. being careful not to sleep more than 6 hours a day.
  D. limiting alcohol and caffeine intake.

_D_ **2.** An organism that causes infection is referred to as a(n):
  A. airborne.   **C.** allergen.
  B. bloodborne.   **D.** pathogen.

_A_ **3.** Some of the most important decisions EMTs make in routinely dealing with patients in the field involve:
  A. universal precautions.   **C.** Standard Precautions.
  B. general isolation.   **D.** quarantine isolation.

_C_ **4.** To provide the appropriate level of precautions used to protect from infectious disease in the field, the EMT may need to use:
  A. hand washing and SCBA.
  B. a HEPA mask and shoe covers.
  C. disposable gloves and eye protection.
  D. a paper gown and leather gloves.

_D_ **5.** An EMT should routinely wear a mask when treating a patient with:
  A. hepatitis B or C.   **C.** AIDS.
  B. potential for blood or fluid spatter.   **D.** all of these.

_D_ **6.** When an EMT covers a patient's mouth and nose with a mask to prevent the spread of an airborne disease, he or she should:
  A. monitor the respirations and airway closely.
  B. write "TB alert" on the patient's prehospital care report.
  C. wear a surgical mask to reduce the spread of TB.
  D. notify his or her supervisor prior to transporting the patient.

_B_ **7.** All of the following are ways the EMT can plan safety precautions in advance of the call *except*:
  A. keeping his or her tetanus immunization current.
  B. maintaining a list of communicable patients.
  C. verifying immune status.
  D. obtaining the hepatitis B vaccine.

_C_ **8.** It is suggested that all EMTs who work or volunteer for an ambulance service be immunized with all of the following vaccines *except*:
  A. tetanus.   **C.** purified protein derivative.
  B. hepatitis B.   **D.** influenza.

_C_ **9.** A federal organization responsible for issuing guidelines for employee safety around biohazards is called the:
  A. Food and Drug Administration.
  B. Federal Communications Commission.
  C. Occupational Safety and Health Administration.
  D. Public Health Service.

_C_ **10.** Every employer of EMTs must provide, free of charge:
  A. a yearly physical examination.
  B. a life insurance policy.
  C. a hepatitis B vaccination.
  D. universal health insurance.

B **11.** A federal act that establishes procedures by which emergency response workers can find out if they have been exposed to life-threatening infectious diseases is:
  A. OSHA 1910.1030.
  B. the Ryan White CARE Act.
  C. NFPA 1207.
  D. OSHA 1910.1200.

A **12.** After contact with the blood or body fluids of a patient, an EMT may submit a request for a determination of exposure to his or her:
  A. employer.
  B. Medical Director.
  C. designated officer.
  D. local hospital.

B **13.** Always assume that any person with:
  A. a cold has a bloodborne disease.
  B. a productive cough has TB.
  C. a fever has typhoid.
  D. dehydration and sores has AIDS.

C **14.** From an EMT's perspective, what do the diseases H1N1, chicken pox, German measles, and whooping cough have in common?
  A. They are all caused by bloodborne pathogens.
  B. They are all spread by exposure to oral secretions during suctioning.
  C. They are all spread by the airborne route.
  D. They all can be prevented by eating the right foods.

D **15.** The EMT can safeguard his or her well-being by:
  A. understanding and dealing with job stress.
  B. ensuring scene safety.
  C. practicing Standard Precautions.
  D. all of these.

C **16.** Each of the following is an example of a call that has a high potential for causing excess stress on EMS providers *except*:
  A. trauma to infants and children.
  B. an adult cardiac arrest.
  C. elder abuse.
  D. death or serious injury of a coworker.

C **17.** Some warning signs that an EMT is being affected by stress include:
  A. overeating and ringing in the ears.
  B. rapid urination and sweating.
  C. indecisiveness and guilt.
  D. increased sexual activity and sleep.

D **18.** All of the following are lifestyle changes that may benefit an EMT in preventing and dealing with EMS job stress *except*:
  A. developing more healthful and positive dietary habits.
  B. devoting time to relaxing.
  C. exercising.
  D. avoiding talking about his or her feelings.

C **19.** After the crash of a van carrying six children who were severely injured, the EMS Director conferred with the Medical Director and they decided to set up a meeting of all the providers who were involved in the call. A meeting held by a team of peer counselors and mental health professionals within 24 to 72 hours after an incident like this is called a(n):
  A. incident critique.
  B. MCI critique.
  C. critical incident stress debriefing.
  D. quality circle.

D **20.** It is thought by some psychologists that, for CISM to be effective:
  A. it must not be an investigation of the events of the call.
  B. information discussed must remain confidential.
  C. an EMT must feel open to discuss feelings, fears, and reactions.
  D. all of these.

_A_ **21.** Most medical professionals and EMS leaders agree that the best course of action for an EMT who is experiencing significant stress from a serious call that involved multiple deaths is to:
   A. seek help from a mental health professional who is experienced in these issues.
   B. give the EMT a week off from work.
   C. encourage the EMT to exercise vigorously.
   D. assign other EMTs to go talk with the EMT.

_C_ **22.** When a patient finds out that he is dying, he may go through which of the following emotional stages?
   A. Anger and laughter
   B. Denial and empathy
   C. Depression and acceptance
   D. Bargaining and elation

_B_ **23.** As an EMT, you have been assigned to take a terminally ill patient back and forth to radiation therapy on multiple trips for the past few weeks. You have come to know the patient and realize that he has been going through emotional stages in the following order:
   A. acceptance, rage, depression, acceptance, bargaining.
   B. denial, anger, bargaining, depression, acceptance.
   C. bargaining, acceptance, denial, anger, depression.
   D. depression, bargaining, denial, acceptance, anger.

_B_ **24.** An EMT will occasionally need to assist the patient who has a terminal illness. Experts suggest all of the following *except*:
   A. listen empathetically to the patient.
   B. tell the patient that everything will be fine.
   C. be tolerant of angry reactions from the patient or family members.
   D. try to recognize the patient's needs.

_C_ **25.** All of the following are part of the three Rs of reacting to danger *except*:
   A. retreat.
   B. respond.
   C. radio.
   D. reevaluate.

_D_ **26.** Stressors affecting the EMT may include:
   A. unpleasant dealings with people.
   B. environmental factors.
   C. performance expectations.
   D. all of these.

_B_ **27.** The body's response to stress was studied by Dr. Hans Selye, who found there is a(n):
   A. resistance syndrome.
   B. excess of the chemical cortisone.
   C. general adaptation syndrome.
   D. exhaustion syndrome.

_D_ **28.** The phases of adaptation to stress include alarm, exhaustion, and:
   A. reaction.
   B. distress.
   C. resistance.
   D. rest.

_C_ **29.** A stress reaction that involves either physical or psychological behavior manifested days or weeks after an incident is called a(n):
   A. acute stress reaction.
   B. post-traumatic stress disorder.
   C. cumulative stress reaction.
   D. burnout.

_D_ **30.** The Centers for Disease Control and Prevention recommends the use of _____ when soap and water are not immediately available to help kill microorganisms on a rescuer's hands.
   A. liquid Cydex II solution
   B. hydrogen peroxide solution
   C. dry powder application
   D. alcohol-based hand cleaners

©2012 Pearson Education, Inc.
Emergency Care, 12th Ed.

C **31.** The normal mode of transmission of the disease chicken pox (varicella) is thought to be through:

    A. blood or stool.
    C. airborne droplets.
    B. accidental needlesticks.
    D. ventilation systems.

A **32.** Each of the following diseases is thought to be spread by respiratory secretions or oral or nasal secretions *except*:

    A. hepatitis.
    C. pneumonia.
    B. bacterial meningitis.
    D. tuberculosis.

D **33.** A disease that mothers are thought to be able to pass to their unborn children is:

    A. chicken pox (varicella).
    C. tuberculosis.
    B. AIDS.
    D. mumps.

B **34.** The stress triad, which Selye described as occurring during the exhaustion stage of stress, includes all of the following clinical signs *except*:

    A. enlargement of the adrenal glands.
    B. excessive weight gain.
    C. bleeding gastric ulcers.
    D. wasting of the lymph nodes.

COMPLETE THE FOLLOWING

1. List five types of calls with a high potential of stress for EMS personnel.

    A. Multiple-Casuality incidents
    B. Calls involving infants and children
    C. Severe injuries
    D. Abuse and neglect
    E. Death of a co-worker

2. List five signs or symptoms of stress.

    A. Irritability with family, friends and co-workers
    B. Inability to concentrate
    C. Changes in daily activities, ie, difficult sleeping
    D. guilt
    E. loss of interest in work

3. List at least five of the critical elements of the infection control plan required by Title 29 Code of Federal Regulations 1910.1030.

    A. Infection exposure Control plan
    B. Education and training
    C. Hepatitis B vaccination
    D. Personal protective equipment
    E. Methods of control

STREET SCENES DISCUSSION

Review the Street Scene on page 47 in the textbook. Then answer the following questions.

1. Because the EMT had an open cut on his hands and was exposed to the patient's blood from the facial laceration, what are some of the diseases he may have been exposed to?

   AIDS, Hepatitis,

2. Due to the potential exposure to HIV, what medication, tests, and instructions would you expect the ED physician to prescribe for the EMT?

   TO DETERMIND IF you've been EXPOSED

3. Aside from wearing PPE, could the EMT have prevented contracting any of the bloodborne diseases listed in your answer to question 1? Explain your answer.

   NOT Really because of wearing the PPE

4. Of the diseases the EMT may have been exposed to, which one would he have the greatest chance of catching and how serious is the disease?

   Hepatitis, it can cause Death

EMT SKILLS PERFORMANCE CHECKLIST

▶ **HAND WASHING PROCEDURE (P. 26)**

❑ Remove watch and rings. Roll up sleeves.

❑ Adjust water flow and temperature.

❑ Wet hands and distal forearms.

❑ Dispense soap into hands.

❑ Scrub lower arms and hands. Clean around and under the nails.

❑ Rinse thoroughly under running water to remove all soap. Do not touch the sink!

❑ Use a paper towel to shut off the faucet to avoid recontaminating hands.

NOTE: Even though you wear protective gloves with your patients, hand washing must still be performed immediately after each call.

3

Lifting and Moving Patients

Standard: Preparatory (Workforce Safety and Wellness)

Competency: Applies fundamental knowledge of the EMS system, safety/well-being of the EMT, medical/legal and ethical issues to the provision of emergency care.

OBJECTIVES

After reading this chapter you should be able to:

3.1 Define key terms introduced in this chapter.

3.2 Describe the factors that you must consider before lifting any patient.

3.3 Use principles of proper body mechanics when lifting and moving patients and other heavy objects.

3.4 Demonstrate the power lift and power grip when lifting a patient-carrying device.

3.5 Follow principles of good body mechanics when reaching, pushing, and pulling.

3.6 Give examples of situations that require emergency, urgent, and nonurgent patient moves.

3.7 Demonstrate emergency, urgent, and nonurgent moves.

3.8 Given several scenarios, select the best patient-lifting and moving devices for each situation.

3.9 Demonstrate proper use of patient-lifting and carrying devices.

3.10 Differentiate between devices to be used to lift and carry patients with and without suspected spinal injuries.

3.11 Identify with the feelings of a patient whom EMS personnel are lifting or carrying.

©2012 Pearson Education, Inc.
Emergency Care, 12th Ed.

MATCH TERMINOLOGY/ DEFINITIONS

A. Stretcher, made of steel wire mesh and tubular steel rim or plastic and steel rim, used to transport patients from one level to another or over rough terrain

B. Portable folding chair with wheels used to transport patient in a sitting position up or down stairs

C. Stretcher that splits into halves, which can be pushed together under the patient

D. Method of transferring a patient from bed to stretcher in which two or more rescuers curl the patient to their chests, then reverse the process to lower the patient to the stretcher

E. Patient move that may be made if speed is not a priority

F. Method of lifting and carrying a patient in which one rescuer slips hands under the patient's armpits and grasps the wrists, while another rescuer grasps the patient's knees

G. A lift from a squatting position with weight to be lifted close to the body; feet apart and flat on the ground, body weight on or just behind balls of feet, back locked in; the upper body is raised before the hips

H. Proper use of the body to facilitate lifting and moving and to prevent injury

I. Gripping with as much hand surface as possible in contact with the object being lifted, with all fingers bent at the same angle

J. Patient move that should be done quickly yet without any compromise of spinal integrity

K. Method of transferring a patient from bed to stretcher by grasping and pulling the loosened bottom sheet of the bed

L. Line that runs down the center of the body from the top of the head and along the spine

M. Method of lifting and carrying a patient from ground level to a stretcher during which two or more rescuers kneel, curl the patient to their chests, stand, then reverse the process to lower the patient to the stretcher

N. Removal of a patient from a hazardous environment in which safety is the first priority and spinal integrity is the second priority

O. Procedure done by three or four rescuers that is designed to move a patient onto a long backboard without compromising spinal integrity

_____ **1.** Basket stretcher

_____ **2.** Body mechanics

_____ **3.** Direct carry

_____ **4.** Direct ground lift

_____ **5.** Draw-sheet method

_____ **6.** Emergency move

_____ **7.** Extremity lift

_____ **8.** Log roll

_____ **9.** Long axis

_____ **10.** Nonurgent move

_____ **11.** Power grip

_____ **12.** Power lift

_____ **13.** Scoop (orthopedic) stretcher

_____ **14.** Stair chair

_____ **15.** Urgent move

MULTIPLE-CHOICE REVIEW

_____ 1. To ensure your own safety when lifting an adult patient, it is important to:
   A. always wear a back brace.
   B. keep the weight as far away from your body as possible.
   C. use your legs, not your back, to lift.
   D. avoid lifting a patient who weighs more than you do.

_____ 2. When lifting a patient, you should do all of the following *except*:
   A. communicate clearly with your partner.
   B. twist while you lift the patient.
   C. know your physical ability and limitations.
   D. communicate frequently with your partner.

_____ 3. When lifting a cot or stretcher,
   A. use an even number of people so that balance is maintained.
   B. keep both of your feet together and flat on the ground.
   C. use a third person positioned on the heaviest side.
   D. and if you must use one hand only, compensate by using your back.

_____ 4. When you place all fingers and the palm in contact with the object being lifted, you are using a:
   A. power grip.   C. lock grip.
   B. power lift.   D. grip lift.

_____ 5. When you must push an object:
   A. keep the line of pull through the center of your body by bending your knees.
   B. push from an overhead position, keeping your knees locked.
   C. keep the weight you are pushing at least 20 inches away from your body.
   D. keep the elbows straight with arms close to your sides.

_____ 6. The situations in which an emergency move would be used include all of the following *except*:
   A. fire or immediate danger of fire.
   B. explosives or other hazardous chemicals.
   C. inability to protect the patient from other hazards at the scene.
   D. dispatcher is holding another, more serious, call.

_____ 7. You are assigned to move as many patients as possible from the hall of a nursing home because there is a fire in another wing of the building. The next patient you come to is on the floor, and you have decided to use an emergency move. This patient can be moved by:
   A. rolling her like a log.
   B. using a spine board and strapping her down.
   C. pulling on her clothing in the neck and shoulder area.
   D. using one rescuer on each extremity.

_____ 8. If the patient has an altered mental status, the EMT should consider a(n) _____ move.
   A. emergency   C. nonurgent
   B. urgent   D. immediate

_____ 9. When doing a log roll, lean from your hips and:
   A. keep your back curved only while leaning over the patient.
   B. position yourself at least 10 inches from the patient.
   C. use your shoulder muscles to help with the roll.
   D. roll the patient as fast as possible.

_____ **10.** The final step in packaging a patient on a wheeled stretcher is:
  A. securing the patient to the stretcher.
  B. placing a towel under the patient's head.
  C. covering the patient with a top sheet.
  D. adjusting the position of the back rest.

_____ **11.** If you are carrying a patient down stairs, when possible:
  A. flex at the waist with bent knees.
  B. keep your lower back muscles loose.
  C. place one hand on the railing for balance.
  D. use a stair chair instead of a stretcher.

_____ **12.** Your patient is approximately 400 pounds and experiencing breathing difficulty. While providing initial assessment and care, it would be helpful for you to call for:
  A. ALS providers if they are available. **C.** additional crew members.
  B. a bariatric stretcher.   **D.** all of these.

_____ **13.** You have a patient who was injured on the rooftop of a three-story structure. He is currently positioned on a scoop-style stretcher, and the fire department will be lowering him down a ladder bed to the ground. You should:
  A. place the stretcher and patient in a plastic basket stretcher.
  B. transfer the patient to a Reeves stretcher.
  C. place the patient on a short spine board.
  D. lower the patient in the scoop stretcher.

_____ **14.** To avoid trauma to a patient with an injured spine, the best patient-carrying device would be the:
  A. long spine board.   **C.** Stokes basket.
  B. wheeled stretcher.   **D.** portable ambulance stretcher.

_____ **15.** The direct ground lift is an example of a(n) _____ move for a patient who has no spine injury.
  A. emergency   **C.** immediate
  B. urgent   **D.** nonurgent

_____ **16.** Another name for the squat-lift used by weight lifters and EMTs is:
  A. leg lift.   **C.** thigh thrust.
  B. power lift.   **D.** power grip.

_____ **17.** How should the EMT's feet be positioned when lifting?
  A. Shoulder-width apart   **C.** On flat ground
  B. On firm ground   **D.** All of these

_____ **18.** When the EMT has to lift with one hand, as in a litter carry, he must be careful *not* to:
  A. lift with the legs.
  B. compensate by leaning.
  C. lift with the weight close to the body.
  D. take breaks if they are needed.

_____ **19.** A comfortable device that can be used to transport a patient in the supine position who has sustained a spinal injury is a:
  A. scoop stretcher.   **C.** vacuum mattress.
  B. stair chair with tracks.   **D.** KED.

_____ **20.** When using an air mattress (vacuum mattress) the patient is placed on the device and the air is _____ by a pump. Then the mattress will form a _____ and conforming surface around the patient.
  A. inflated; rigid   **C.** inflated; soft
  B. withdrawn; rigid   **D.** withdrawn; soft

COMPLETE THE FOLLOWING

1. List five patient-carrying devices.

   A. _____

   B. _____

   C. _____

   D. _____

   E. _____

2. List four principles that will help you lift efficiently and prevent injury.

   A. _____

   B. _____

   C. _____

   D. _____

3. List the two types of stretchers.

   A. _____

   B. _____

LABEL THE PHOTOGRAPHS

Fill in the name of each lift, move, or drag on the line provided.

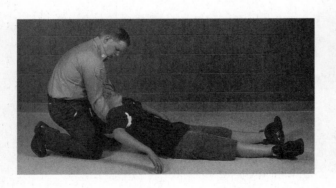

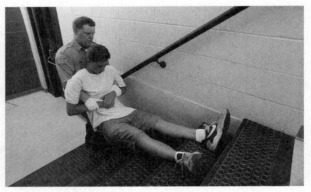

1. _____   2. _____

©2012 Pearson Education, Inc.
Emergency Care, 12th Ed.

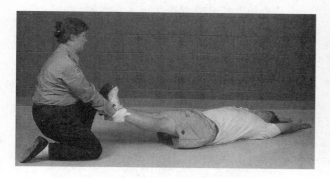

3. _____

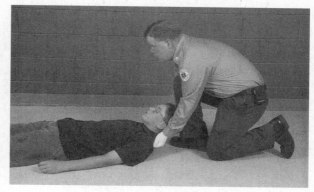

4. _____

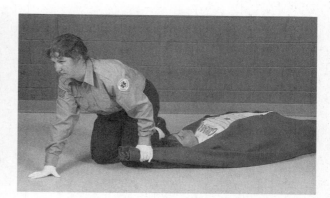

5. _____

6. _____

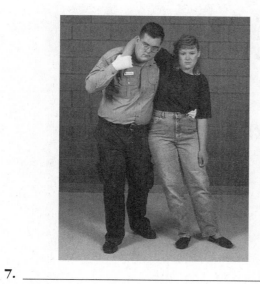

7. _____

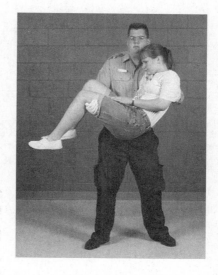

8. _____

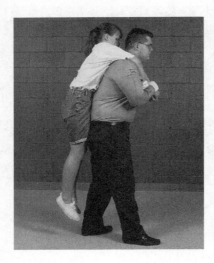

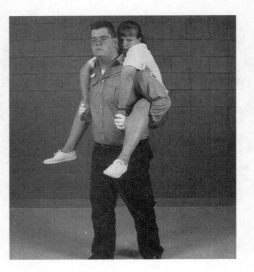

9. _____   10. _____

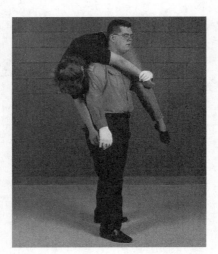

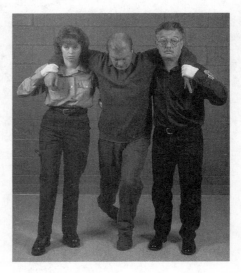

11. _____   12. _____

STREET SCENES DISCUSSION

Review the Street Scene on page 72 in the textbook. Then answer the following questions.

1. In the call, the patient's weight was not discussed. Suppose the patient weighed 350 lb. Should you consider using a different device to immobilize her?

©2012 Pearson Education, Inc.
Emergency Care, 12th Ed.

2. When it is time to remove the patient from the automobile, suppose that the vest-type immobilization device does not go entirely around her and the leg straps are too short. What should you do?

3. After getting the patient out of the car with some extra help, she lies supine in the vest-type immobilization device on a long backboard. She complains that the vest is making it difficult for her to breathe. What can you do?

CASE STUDY

This case study is designed to help you apply the concepts presented in this textbook. The case study describes a situation you might encounter in the field and is followed by questions about the situation. The questions require you to explain and apply key concepts from your reading.

▶ **More Than the Average Patient**

Your unit is on the scene of a patient whose daughter called EMS because her father cannot get out of bed. Apparently he has continued to gain weight over the past few years, and he is so obese at this point that he can barely get out of bed. She states that she gives him a bedpan and/or a urinal to relieve himself. Today he has been complaining of back pain and needs to go to the hospital.

After donning protective gloves, mask, goggles, and a disposable gown because the patient has feces on him, you decide to call the dispatcher to have the fire department dispatched to the scene. You conduct a primary assessment and find a 50-year-old male who you estimate at some 500 lbs. He states that his back hurts and he cannot roll on his side any more.

1. Normally a stair chair is used to remove patients on the second floor. Would it be appropriate in this case?

2. What type of lift would be more appropriate for this patient: a direct ground lift or a draw-sheet method?

3. Why was the decision to call the fire department made?

Once the fire department arrives, you work together to devise a plan to get the patient out of the bed, down the stairs, and into the ambulance. With your supervisor now on the scene, the special bariatric unit is dispatched to the scene. The patient is visibly embarrassed but does answer all of your questions appropriately about his medical history.

4. What is a bariatric unit, and how might that be different from your ambulance?

5. Which would be a safer device to get the patient down the stairs: the Reeves stretcher or the scoop stretcher?

It takes five EMTs and rescue workers to carefully roll the patient onto the Reeves stretcher and then to drag the patient and stretcher down the steps and exit the house. Fortunately the special stretcher is rated for obese patients and has a lift to make it possible to get into the ambulance. On the way to the hospital, you call ahead and alert the ED you will need extra assistance upon arrival.

6. If you were unable to get the patient down the stairs in the Reeves, what may have been another useful device to consider?

7. After the call, you and your partner discuss the call and decide there may have been a lot of rescuers involved but everyone was absolutely necessary. What is the highest priority in these calls?

EMT SKILLS PERFORMANCE CHECKLISTS

▶ FIREFIGHTER'S DRAG (P. 53)

❑ Place the patient in the supine position.

❑ Secure the patient's hands together with something that will not cut into the skin.

❑ Straddle the patient, facing his head.

❑ Crouch and pass your head through the patient's trussed arms and then raise your body to lift the patient's head, neck, and upper trunk.

❑ Crawl on your hands and knees, dragging the patient and keeping the patient's head low to the ground.

▶ BLANKET DRAG (P. 53)

❑ Gather half of the blanket up against the patient's side.

❑ Roll the patient toward your knees.

❑ Gently roll the patient back onto the blanket.

❑ Roll up the blanket by the patient's head, neck, and shoulders and drag this rolled material, keeping the patient's head as low to the ground as possible.

▶ ONE-RESCUER ASSIST (P. 54)

❑ Place the patient's arm around your neck.

❑ Grasp the patient's hand in your hand.

❑ Place your other arm around the patient's waist.

❑ Help the patient walk to safety, communicating with him about obstacles or uneven terrain.

▶ CRADLE CARRY (P. 54)

❑ Place one arm across the patient's back with your hand under his arm.

❑ Place your other arm under his knees and lift.

❑ If the patient is conscious, have him place his nearest arm over your shoulder.

▶ PACK STRAP CARRY (P. 54)

❑ Have the patient stand.

❑ Turn your back to the patient, bringing his arms over your shoulders to cross your chest.

©2012 Pearson Education, Inc.
Emergency Care, 12th Ed.

❑ Keep the patient's arms as straight as possible and armpits over your shoulders.

❑ Hold the patient's wrists, bend, and pull the patient onto your back.

▶ PIGGYBACK CARRY (P. 54)

❑ Assist the patient to a standing position.

❑ Turn your back to the patient, placing the patient's arms over you so the arms cross your chest.

❑ While the patient holds on with his arms, crouch and grasp the patient's thighs.

❑ Use a lifting motion to move the patient onto your back.

❑ Pass your forearms under the patient's knees and grasp his wrists.

▶ FIREFIGHTER'S CARRY (P. 54)

❑ Place your toes against the patient's toes and pull the patient toward you.

❑ Bend at the waist and flex your knees.

❑ Duck and pull the patient across your shoulder, keeping hold of one of his wrists.

❑ Use your free arm to reach between his legs and grasp his thigh.

❑ Let the weight of the patient fall onto your shoulders.

❑ Stand up, transferring your grip on the patient's thigh to his wrist.

▶ TWO-RESCUER ASSIST (P. 55)

❑ An EMT stands at each side of the patient.

❑ Each EMT places a patient's arm around his shoulder and grips the patient's hand.

❑ Each EMT then places his own free arm around the patient's waist.

❑ Both EMTs then help the patient walk to safety.

▶ LOADING THE WHEELED STRETCHER INTO THE AMBULANCE (PP. 59–60)

❑ Lift the rear step of the ambulance if necessary.

❑ Move the stretcher as close to the ambulance as possible.

❑ Make sure the stretcher is locked in its lowest level before lifting (depends on local procedure and type of stretcher).

❑ Position EMTs on opposite sides of the stretcher, bend at the knees, and grasp the lower bar of the stretcher frame.

❑ Both EMTs should come to a full standing position with their backs straight.

❑ Use sideways stepping movements to move the stretcher into the ambulance.

❑ Secure the stretcher in the ambulance, using the appropriate securing device.

❑ Engage both forward and rear catches to hold the stretcher in place.

▶ EXTREMITY CARRY (P. 66)

❏ EMT #1 places the patient on his back with his knees flexed.

❏ EMT #1 kneels at the patient's head and places his hands under the patient's shoulders.

❏ EMT #2 kneels at the patient's feet and grasps the patient's wrists.

❏ EMT #2 lifts the patient forward while EMT #1 slips his arms under the patient's armpits and grasps the patient's wrists.

❏ EMT #2 grasps the patient's knees while facing him or turns and grasps the patient's knees while facing away from him.

❏ EMT #1 and EMT #2 both crouch, then stand at the same time and move as a unit when carrying the patient.

▶ DIRECT GROUND LIFT (P. 67)

❏ Set the stretcher in its lowest position and place opposite the patient.

❏ Two EMTs get in position along one side of the patient. EMT #1 is at the head, and EMT #2 is at the feet.

❏ The EMTs drop to one knee facing the patient.

❏ Place the patient's arms on his chest.

❏ EMT #1 at the head-end cradles the patient's head and neck by sliding one arm under the patient's neck to grasp the patient's shoulder; the other arm is placed under the patient's lower back.

❏ EMT #2 at the foot-end slides one arm under the patient's knees and the other under the patient above the buttocks.

❏ If a third rescuer is available, he should place both arms under the patient's waist while the two EMTs slide their arms up to the mid-back or down to the buttocks.

❏ On a signal, the EMTs lift the patient to their knees.

❏ On a signal, the EMTs stand and carry the patient to the stretcher. They drop to one knee and roll forward to place the patient onto the mattress.

▶ DRAW-SHEET METHOD (P. 65)

❏ Loosen the bottom sheet of the bed and roll it from both sides toward the patient.

❏ Ensure that the stretcher is at the same height as the bed and the side rail is down.

❏ Push the stretcher and the bed tightly together.

❏ Firmly grasp the rolled sheet, holding it taut, with an underhand grasp in the area of the head/chest and hip/knee.

❏ On the count of three, EMTs carefully slide the patient onto the stretcher.

▶ DIRECT CARRY (P. 65)

❏ EMTs #1 and #2: Get in position along one side of the patient. EMT #1 is at the head-end; EMT #2 is at the foot-end.

❏ EMT #1 cradles the patient's head and neck by sliding one arm under the patient's neck to grasp the patient's shoulder.

©2012 Pearson Education, Inc.
Emergency Care, 12th Ed.

- ❑ EMT #2 slides a hand under the patient's hip and lifts slightly.

- ❑ EMT #1 slides his other arm under the patient's back.

- ❑ EMT #2 places his arms under the patient's hips and calves.

- ❑ Both EMTs slide the patient to the edge of the bed and bend toward him with their knees slightly bent.

- ❑ They lift and curl the patient to their chests and return to a standing position.

- ❑ They rotate and then slide the patient gently onto the stretcher.

4

Medical/Legal and Ethical Issues

Standard: Preparatory (Medical/Legal and Ethics)

Competency: Applies fundamental knowledge of the EMS system, safety/well-being of the EMT, medical/legal and ethical issues to the provision of emergency care.

OBJECTIVES

After reading this chapter you should be able to:

4.1   Define key terms introduced in this chapter.

4.2   Describe your scope of practice as an EMT.

4.3   Differentiate between scope of practice and standard of care.

4.4   Given a variety of scenarios, determine which type of patient consent applies.

4.5   Given a variety of ethical dilemmas, discuss the issues that must be considered in each situation.

4.6   Explain legal and ethical considerations in situations where patients refuse care.

4.7   Discuss the EMT's obligations with respect to advance directives, including do not resuscitate orders.

4.8   Given a variety of scenarios, identify circumstances that may allow a claim of negligence to be established.

4.9   Explain the purpose of Good Samaritan laws.

4.10 Identify situations that would constitute a breach of patient confidentiality.

4.11 Identify situations that would constitute libel or slander.

4.12 Recognize medical identification devices and organ donor status.

4.13 List items that may be considered evidence at a crime scene.

4.14 Describe ways in which you can minimize your impact on evidence while meeting your obligations to care for your patient.

4.15 Recognize situations that may legally require reporting to authorities.

4.16 Given a scenario involving an ethical challenge, decide the most appropriate response for an EMT.

MATCH TERMINOLOGY/ DEFINITIONS

A. The consent that is presumed a patient or patient's parent or guardian would give if they could, such as for an unconscious patient or a parent who cannot be contacted when care is needed

B. A DNR order

C. Being held legally responsible

D. An obligation to provide care to a patient

E. Consent given by adults who are of legal age and mentally competent to make a rational decision in regard to their medical well-being

F. Permission from the patient for care or other action by the EMT

G. A series of laws, varying in each state, designed to provide limited legal protection for citizens and some health care personnel who are administering emergency care

H. A set of regulations and ethical considerations that define the scope, or extent and limits, of the EMT's job

I. The location where a crime has been committed or any place that evidence relating to a crime may be found

J. A finding of failure to act properly in a situation in which there was a duty to act, that needed care as would reasonably be expected of the EMT was not provided, and that harm was caused to the patient as a result

K. A legal document, usually signed by the patient and his or her physician, stating that the patient has a terminal illness and does not wish to prolong life through resuscitative efforts

L. The obligation not to reveal information obtained about a patient except to other health care professionals involved in the patient's care, or under subpoena, or in a court of law, or when the patient has signed a release of confidentiality

M. Leaving a patient after care has been initiated and before the patient has been transferred to someone with equal or greater medical training

N. A person who has completed a legal document that allows for donation of organs and tissues in the event of death

O. A federal law protecting the privacy of patient-specific health care information and providing the patient with control over how this information is used and distributed

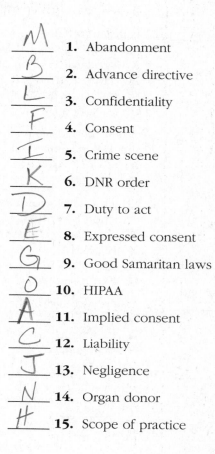

_M_ **1.** Abandonment

_B_ **2.** Advance directive

_L_ **3.** Confidentiality

_F_ **4.** Consent

_I_ **5.** Crime scene

_K_ **6.** DNR order

_D_ **7.** Duty to act

_E_ **8.** Expressed consent

_G_ **9.** Good Samaritan laws

_O_ **10.** HIPAA

_A_ **11.** Implied consent

_C_ **12.** Liability

_J_ **13.** Negligence

_N_ **14.** Organ donor

_H_ **15.** Scope of practice

MULTIPLE-CHOICE REVIEW

_B_   **1.** The collective set of regulations and ethical considerations governing the EMT is called:
- **A.** duty to act.
- **B.** scope of practice.
- **C.** advance directives.
- **D.** Good Samaritan laws.

_B_   **2.** Legislation that governs the skills and medical interventions that may be performed by an EMT is:
- **A.** standardized (uniform) throughout the country.
- **B.** different from state to state.
- **C.** standardized (uniform) for regions within a state.
- **D.** governed by the U.S. Department of Transportation.

_C_   **3.** When the EMT-B makes the physical/emotional needs of the patient a priority, this is considered a(n) _____ of the EMT.
- **A.** advance directive
- **B.** protocol
- **C.** ethical responsibility
- **D.** legal responsibility

_C_   **4.** Which one of the following is *not* a type of consent required for any treatment or action by an EMT?
- **A.** Child and mentally incompetent adult
- **B.** Implied
- **C.** Applied
- **D.** Expressed

_A_   **5.** When you inform the adult patient of a procedure you are about to perform and its associated risks, you are asking for her or his:
- **A.** expressed consent.
- **B.** negligence.
- **C.** implied consent.
- **D.** applied consent.

_C_   **6.** You are treating a patient who was found unconscious at the bottom of a stairwell. Consent that is based on the assumption that an unconscious patient would approve the EMT's life-saving interventions is called:
- **A.** expressed.
- **B.** negligence.
- **C.** implied.
- **D.** applied.

_C_   **7.** Your record of a patient's refusal of medical care (aid) or transport should include all of the following *except*:
- **A.** informing the patient of the risks and consequences of refusal.
- **B.** documenting the steps you took.
- **C.** signing of the form by the Medical Director.
- **D.** obtaining a release form with the patient's witnessed signature.

_B_   **8.** Forcing a competent adult patient to go to the hospital against his or her will may result in _____ charges against the EMT.
- **A.** abandonment
- **B.** assault and battery
- **C.** implied consent
- **D.** negligence

_B_   **9.** Which one of the following is an action you should *not* take if a patient refuses care?
- **A.** Leave phone stickers with emergency numbers.
- **B.** Recommend that a relative call the family physician to report the incident.
- **C.** Tell the patient to call his or her family physician if the problem reoccurs.
- **D.** Call a relative or neighbor who can stay with the patient.

_D_   **10.** Another name for a DNR order is:
- **A.** deviated nervous response.
- **B.** duty not to react.
- **C.** refusal of treatment.
- **D.** advance directive.

©2012 Pearson Education, Inc.
Emergency Care, 12th Ed.

_A_ **11.** There are varying degrees of DNR orders, expressed through a variety of detailed instructions that may be part of the order, such as:
  A. allowing CPR only if cardiac or respiratory arrest was observed.
  B. allowing comfort-care measures such as intravenous feeding.
  C. disallowing the use of long-term life-support measures.
  D. specifying that only 5 minutes of artificial respiration will be attempted.

_B_ **12.** In a hospital, long-term life-support and comfort-care measures would consist of intravenous feeding and:
  A. routine inoculations.
  B. the use of a respirator.
  C. infection control by the health care providers.
  D. hourly patient documentation.

_B_ **13.** If an EMT with a duty to act fails to provide the standard of care, and if this failure causes harm or injury to the patient, the EMT may be accused of:
  A. *res ipsa loquitur.*   **C.** abandonment.
  B. negligence.   **D.** assault.

_C_ **14.** Leaving a patient on the hallway stretcher in a busy ED and leaving without giving a report to a health care professional is an example of:
  A. liability infraction.   **C.** abandonment.
  B. battery.   **D.** breach of duty.

_D_ **15.** The EMT should not discuss information about a patient except to relay pertinent information to the physician at the emergency department. Information considered confidential includes:
  A. patient history gained through interview.
  B. assessment findings.
  C. treatment rendered.
  D. all of these.

_D_ **16.** The EMT can release confidential patient information in all of the following circumstances *except* to:
  A. inform other health care professionals who need to know information to continue care.
  B. report incidents required by state law, such as rape or abuse.
  C. comply with a legal subpoena.
  D. protect the other victims of a motor vehicle collision.

_C_ **17.** A medical identification device that indicates serious patient medical conditions comes in the form of each of the following *except*:
  A. bracelets.   **C.** cards.
  B. necklaces.   **D.** patches.

_D_ **18.** You responded to a high-speed collision involving a motorcycle and an automobile. The 22-year-old male cyclist has severe head injuries and is not likely to live through the evening. When treating this critical patient, who happens to have an organ donor card, the EMT should:
  A. transport without delay and document a DNR.
  B. treat the patient the same as any other patient and inform the ED physician.
  C. withhold oxygen therapy from the patient to keep the organ hypoxic.
  D. all of these.

_A_ **19.** You are at the scene of a home invasion where the homeowner was shot to death by the perpetrators. At this crime scene, you should:
  A. avoid disturbing any evidence at the scene unless emergency care requires.
  B. immediately remove the patient from the scene.
  C. move all obstacles from around the patient to make more room to work.
  D. search the house for clues to the cause of the crime.

B **20.** Commonly required reporting situations include all of the following *except*:
  A. child and elder abuse.
  B. crimes in public places.
  C. sexual assault.
  D. domestic abuse.

C **21.** The extent of limits of the EMT's job is called the:
  A. ethical dilemma.
  B. national curriculum.
  C. scope of practice.
  D. regional protocol.

B **22.** You were called to the scene of an incident where a 21-year-old male was knocked unconscious (out) in a bar fight. Upon your arrival, the patient is awake and has a broken nose but no life threats. He admits to drinking six beers in the last hour. He wants to refuse medical attention. Why should you discourage a refusal (RMA)?
  A. He is not legally old enough to consent.
  B. He may not be mentally competent at this time.
  C. Patients die from broken noses all the time.
  D. He is unable to actually sign the release.

C **23.** The federal law designed to protect the patient's private medical information is the:
  A. NHTSA.   **C.** HIPAA.
  B. ANSI.   **D.** OSHA.

A **24.** You are on the scene of a call where a patient barricaded himself and his wife in their home and is threatening to do harm. The police have been at the scene for hours and, after the wife escaped, they rushed in. It is now your responsibility to transport this now-restrained patient to the local ED. What should be your highest priority?
  A. Monitoring the patient's mental status and vital signs
  B. Making sure your documentation shows you did not apply handcuffs
  C. Restraining the patient so he is not able to move
  D. Explaining to the patient that he no longer has any rights to refuse care

B **25.** The police are concerned about the presence of microscopic evidence at the scene of a violent assault. Your crew was asked to be careful and limit their involvement in the scene to essential patient care. What are examples of microscopic evidence?
  A. The position the patient was initially found in
  B. Any dirt and carpet fibers
  C. Fingerprints that were found at the scene
  D. The condition of the scene

COMPLETE THE FOLLOWING

1. What are four criteria and/or conditions that must be fulfilled for a patient to refuse care or transport?

  A. _Patient must be legally able to consent_
  B. _Patient must be mentally competent and oriented_
  C. _Patient must be legally informed_
  D. _Patient will be asked to sign a "release" from._

©2012 Pearson Education, Inc.
Emergency Care, 12th Ed.

2. A finding of negligence, or failure to act properly, requires that all of the following circumstances be proven:

A. _The EMT had a duty to the patient (duty to act)_

B. _The EMT did not provide the standard of care (committed a breach of duty)_

C. _There was proximate causation_

3. Four types of medical conditions that may be listed on a medical identification device (such as a necklace, bracelet, or card) include:

A. _Heart Conditions_

B. _Allergies_

C. _Diabetes_

D. _Epilepsy_

STREET SCENES DISCUSSION

Review the Street Scene on page 91 in the textbook. Then answer the following questions.

1. Suppose you observed that the patient's home was filthy. Would it be a violation of patient confidentiality to discuss the "roach house" with fellow workers? Explain.

Yes, because you're in violation of Patient Care information

2. Is it appropriate to write that the patient has AIDS on the prehospital care report? Explain your answer.

No, it's not. Because you don't have the proof that this person has AIDS.

3. Is a patient's vomitus a hazard to your health? If so, what equipment would be appropriate for Standard Precautions?

a Gown and mask

CASE STUDY

This case study is designed to help you apply the concepts presented in this textbook. The case study describes a situation you might encounter in the field and is followed by questions about the situation. The questions require you to explain and apply key concepts from your reading.

▶ A WITNESSED COLLISION: FIRST ON THE SCENE

It's a summer morning and you are traveling on the interstate highway with your family to the lake. Although the speed is posted at 55 mph, traffic has been moving along at least 10 mph faster. All of a sudden, you observe the SUV a few cars in front of you going from the center lane to the passing lane, cutting off a car, and then veering off the center of the road down a ravine and rolling over numerous times. The vehicle comes to rest on its roof.

1. If you are an off-duty EMT, are you legally required to stop and offer assistance? *No, You're not legally required to stop but morally you could be.*

2. Are you protected from a lawsuit? Explain your answer. *No, because .*

3. Are you protected from a liability suit provided your treatment is appropriate?

As you secure your vehicle off the shoulder and assign another helper to set out some flares, your spouse uses a cellular phone to call for emergency assistance.

4. In most communities, what is the universal emergency phone number?

5. What types of questions would you expect the dispatcher to ask about the collision?

6. What emergency response agencies would you expect to be sent?

©2012 Pearson Education, Inc.
Emergency Care, 12th Ed.

As you carefully climb down through the brush to the car, you notice there are two patients who were ejected from the vehicle. Another citizen arrives and she identifies herself as an EMT. You ask her to check the two ejected patients while you check the car for additional patients. She reports that one ejected patient is dead, and the other is unconscious and has an obvious head injury.

7. As additional help arrives, how can they help with this patient?

8. What types of injuries could the patient have?

9. Do you need permission to treat the patient?

Inside the car is a conscious male patient approximately 40 years old who appears to have been injured by the steering wheel in the left upper quadrant of his abdomen. He also has a broken upper left leg. You also notice that the car continues to leak gasoline from the dented fuel tank. After obtaining some additional help, you decide to carefully move this patient out of the car.

10. What additional potential injuries might this patient have?

11. How can you help minimize further injury to the leg?

12. Do you need permission to treat this patient? Explain.

Once the patient is out of the car, two ambulances arrive, as does the fire department, with a paramedic engine and a heavy rescue truck. Meanwhile the police have arrived and are dealing with the traffic congestion that has developed.

13. Because plenty of help is now on the scene, can you leave?

14. What would be the problem if you left prior to help arriving?

EMT SKILLS PERFORMANCE CHECKLIST

▶ PATIENT REFUSAL PROCEDURE (PP. 77–79)

❑ Spend time effectively communicating with the patient (includes reasoning, persistence, and strategies to convince the patient to go to the hospital).

❑ Clearly inform the patient of the consequences of not going to the hospital.

❑ Consult with medical direction.

❑ Contact family to help convince the patient.

❑ Call law enforcement, who may be able to order or "arrest" the serious patient in order to force the patient to go to the hospital.

❑ Try to determine why the patient is refusing care.

❑ Thoroughly document the refusal. Have both the patient and a witness (e.g., bystander, police officer) sign the refusal release.

NOTE: Procedures may differ by state and jurisdiction. Always follow your Medical Director's advice.

5

Medical Terminology and Anatomy and Physiology

Standard: Anatomy and Physiology; Medical Terminology

Competency: Applies fundamental knowledge of the anatomy and function of all human systems to the practice of EMS.

Uses foundational anatomical and medical terms and abbreviations in written and oral communication with colleagues and other health care professionals.

OBJECTIVES

After reading this chapter you should be able to:

5.1   Define key terms introduced in this chapter.

5.2   Describe the importance of the proper use of medical terminology.

5.3   Apply definitions of common prefixes, suffixes, and roots to determine the meaning of medical terms.

5.4   Recognize the meaning of acronyms and abbreviations commonly used in EMS.

5.5   Give examples of when it is better to use a common or lay term to describe something than it is to use a medical term.

5.6   Use anatomical terms of position and direction to describe the location of body structures and position of the body.

5.7   Utilize topographical anatomical landmarks as points of reference.

5.8   Describe the structures and functions of each of the following body systems:
   a. Musculoskeletal
   b. Respiratory
   c. Cardiovascular
   d. Nervous
   e. Digestive

f. Integumentary
g. Endocrine
h. Renal
i. Male and female reproductive

5.9 Given a series of models or diagrams, label the anatomical structures of each of the following body systems:
a. Skeletal
b. Respiratory
c. Cardiovascular
d. Nervous
e. Skin
f. Endocrine
g. Renal/urinary
h. Male and female reproductive

5.10 Describe differences in the reproductive anatomy of children compared to adults.

5.11 Apply understanding of anatomy and physiology to explain the function of the life support chain.

MATCH TERMINOLOGY/DEFINITIONS

▶ **PART A**

A. The front of the body or body part

B. The standard reference position for the body in the study of anatomy; in this position, the body is standing erect, facing the observer, with arms down at the sides and the palms of the hands forward

C. A small tube located near the junction of the small and large intestines in the right lower quadrant of the abdomen, the function of which is not well understood

D. The microscopic sacs of the lungs where gas exchange with the bloodstream takes place

E. The study of body structure

F. The largest artery in the body; it transports blood from the left ventricle to begin systemic circulation

G. The ability of the heart to generate and conduct electrical impulses on its own

H. The highest portion of the shoulder

I. Any blood vessel carrying blood away from the heart

J. The conversion of glucose into energy without the use of oxygen

K. Four divisions of the abdomen used to pinpoint the location of a pain or injury

L. The two upper chambers of the heart; the right chamber receives unoxygenated blood returning from the body, and the left chamber receives oxygenated blood returning from the lungs

M. The conversion of glucose into energy by the use of oxygen

K	**1.** Abdominal quadrants
N	**2.** Acetabulum
P	**3.** Acromioclavicular joint
H	**4.** Acromion process
M	**5.** Aerobic metabolism
D	**6.** Alveoli
J	**7.** Anaerobic metabolism
B	**8.** Anatomical position
E	**9.** Anatomy
A	**10.** Anterior
F	**11.** Aorta
C	**12.** Appendix
O	**13.** Arteriole
I	**14.** Artery
L	**15.** Atria
G	**16.** Automaticity

N. The pelvic socket into which the ball of the proximal end of the femur fits to form the hip joint

O. The smallest kind of artery

P. The joint where the acromion and the clavicle meet

▶ PART B

A. The system made up of the heart and the blood vessels

B. Blood vessels that supply the muscle of the heart

C. The ring-shaped structure that forms the lower portion of the larynx

D. The carotid and femoral pulses, which can be felt in the central part of the body

E. The top, back, and sides of the skull

F. The brain and spinal cord

G. The wrist bones

H. Specialized involuntary muscle found only in the heart

I. The collarbone

J. The cardiovascular system

K. A system of specialized muscle tissue that conducts electrical impulses that, in turn, stimulate the heart to beat

L. The large neck arteries, one on each side of the neck, that carry blood from the heart to the head

M. A thin-walled, microscopic blood vessel where the oxygen/carbon dioxide and nutrient/waste exchange with the body's cells takes place

N. Artery of the upper arm; the site of the pulse checked during infant CPR

O. The division of the peripheral nervous system that controls involuntary motor functions

P. The heel bone

Q. The two large sets of branches that come off the trachea and enter the lungs

R. On both sides

S. The pressure caused by blood exerting force against the walls of the blood vessels

T. The round saclike organ of the renal system used as a reservoir for urine

_O_	**1.** Autonomic nervous system
_R_	**2.** Bilateral
_T_	**3.** Bladder
_S_	**4.** Blood pressure
_N_	**5.** Brachial artery
_Q_	**6.** Bronchi
_P_	**7.** Calcaneus
_M_	**8.** Capillary
_K_	**9.** Cardiac conduction system
_B_	**10.** Cardiac muscle
_A_	**11.** Cardiovascular system
_L_	**12.** Carotid arteries
_G_	**13.** Carpals
_F_	**14.** Central nervous system (CNS)
_D_	**15.** Central pulses
_J_	**16.** Circulatory system
_I_	**17.** Clavicle
_H_	**18.** Coronary arteries
_E_	**19.** Cranium
_C_	**20.** Cricoid cartilage

▶ PART C

A. The bone of the upper arm, between the shoulder and the elbow

B. The proximal opening of the trachea

C. A sitting position

D. Further away from the torso

E. Inadequate perfusion of the cells and tissues of the body caused by insufficient flow of blood through the capillaries

_G_	**1.** Dermis
_I_	**2.** Diaphragm
_N_	**3.** Diastolic blood pressure
_J_	**4.** Digestive system

F. A sac on the underside of the liver that stores bile produced by the liver

G. The inner layer of the skin, rich in blood vessels and nerves, found beneath the epidermis

H. A hormone produced by the body; as a medication, it dilates respiratory passages and is used to relieve severe allergic reaction

I. The muscular structure that divides the chest cavity from the abdominal cavity

J. System by which food travels through the body and is broken down into absorbable forms

K. Artery supplying the foot, lateral to the large tendon of the big toe

L. Referring to the back of the body or the back of the hand or foot

M. The outer layer of the skin

N. The pressure in the arteries when the left ventricle is refilling

O. The large bone of the thigh

P. System of glands that produce chemicals called hormones that help to regulate many body activities and functions

Q. A leaf-shaped structure that prevents food and foreign matter from entering the trachea

R. A passive process in which the intercostal muscles and the diaphragm relax, causing the chest cavity to decrease in size and air to flow out of the lungs

S. The lateral and smaller bone of the lower leg

T. The major artery supplying the leg

D	5. Distal
L	6. Dorsal
K	7. Dorsalis pedis artery
P	8. Endocrine system
M	9. Epidermis
Q	10. Epiglottis
H	11. Epinephrine
R	12. Exhalation
T	13. Femoral artery
O	14. Femur
S	15. Fibula
C	16. Fowler's position
F	17. Gall bladder
B	18. Glottic opening
A	19. Humerus
E	20. Hypoperfusion

▶ **PART D**

A. The lower, posterior portions of the pelvis

B. The voicebox

C. The two fused bones forming the upper jaw

D. To the side, away from the midline of the body

E. Toward the midline of the body

F. The free-floating bone in the neck that provides structure to the larynx

G. The lower jaw bone

H. The superior and widest portion of the pelvis

I. Organs of the renal system used to filter blood and regulate fluid levels in the body

J. Away from the head; usually compared with another structure that is closer to the head

K. The largest organ of the body; produces bile to assist in breakdown of fats and assists in the metabolism of various substances in the body

	1. Hyoid bone
H	2. Ilium
	3. Inferior
	4. Inhalation
	5. Insulin
	6. Involuntary muscle
A	7. Ischium
	8. Joint
	9. Kidney
	10. Large intestine

©2012 Pearson Education, Inc.
Emergency Care, 12th Ed.

L. An active process in which the intercostal muscles and the diaphragm contract, expanding the size of the chest cavity and causing air to flow into the lungs

M. The superior portion of the sternum

N. A hormone produced by the pancreas or taken as a medication by many diabetics

O. Protrusion on the side of the ankle

P. Muscle that responds automatically to brain signals but cannot be consciously controlled

Q. The point where two bones come together

R. The muscular tube that removes water from waste products received from the small intestine and removes anything absorbed by the body toward excretion from the body

S. The organs where exchange of atmospheric oxygen and waste carbon dioxide take place

T. Tissue that connects bone to bone

_B_ **11.** Larynx

_D_ **12.** Lateral

_____ **13.** Ligament

_____ **14.** Liver

_____ **15.** Lungs

_____ **16.** Malleolus

_G_ **17.** Mandible

_____ **18.** Manubrium

_C_ **19.** Maxillae

_E_ **20.** Medial

▶ **PART E**

A. The basin-shaped bony structure that supports the spine and is the point of proximal attachment for the lower extremities

B. The kneecap

C. Referring to the palm of the hand

D. The area directly posterior to the mouth

E. The bony structures around the eyes; the eye sockets

F. The nose bones

G. The radial, brachial, posterior tibial, and dorsalis pedis pulses, which can be felt at peripheral points of the body

H. A gland located behind the stomach that produces insulin and juices that assist in digestion of food in the duodenum of the small intestine

I. The hand bones

J. A line drawn vertically from the middle of the armpit to the ankle

K. The supply of oxygen to and removal of wastes from the cells and tissue of the body as a result of the flow of blood through the capillaries

L. The nerves that enter and leave the spinal cord and travel between the brain and organs without passing through the spinal cord

M. An imaginary line drawn down the center of the body, dividing it into right and left halves

N. The foot bones

O. Tissue that can contract to allow movement of a body part

P. The line through the center of each clavicle

Q. The system of brain, spinal cord, and nerves that governs sensation, movement, and thought

_____ **1.** Metacarpals

_____ **2.** Metatarsals

_____ **3.** Mid-axillary line

_____ **4.** Mid-clavicular line

_____ **5.** Midline

_____ **6.** Muscle

_____ **7.** Musculoskeletal system

_____ **8.** Nasal bones

_____ **9.** Nasopharynx

_____ **10.** Nervous system

_____ **11.** Orbits

_____ **12.** Oropharynx

_____ **13.** Palmar

_____ **14.** Pancreas

_____ **15.** Patella

_____ **16.** Pelvis

_____ **17.** Penis

_____ **18.** Perfusion

_____ **19.** Peripheral nervous system

_____ **20.** Peripheral pulses

R. The system of bones and skeletal muscles that supports and protects the body and permits movement

S. The organ of male reproduction responsible for sexual intercourse and the transfer of sperm

T. The area directly posterior to the nose

▶ PART F

A. Lying on the side

B. The body system that regulates fluid balance and filtration of blood

C. The lateral bone of the forearm

D. A flat surface formed when slicing through a solid object

E. Components of the blood that carry oxygen to and carbon dioxide away from the cells

F. Artery of the lower arm; it is felt when taking the pulse at the wrist

G. The toe bones and finger bones

H. Lying face down

I. The area directly posterior to the mouth and nose; it is made up of the oropharynx and the nasopharynx

J. Referring to the sole of the foot

K. The back of the body or body part

L. The fluid portion of the blood

M. Artery supplying the foot, behind the medial ankle

N. The study of body function

O. The rhythmic beats caused as waves of blood move through and expand the arteries

P. Components of the blood; membrane-enclosed fragments of specialized cells

Q. Closer to the torso

R. The vessels that carry blood from the right ventricle of the heart to the lungs

S. The vessels that carry oxygenated blood from the lungs to the left atrium of the heart

T. The medial anterior portion of the pelvis

_____ **1.** Phalanges

_____ **2.** Pharynx

_____ **3.** Physiology

_____ **4.** Plane

_____ **5.** Plantar

_____ **6.** Plasma

_____ **7.** Platelets

_____ **8.** Posterior

_____ **9.** Posterior tibial artery

_____ **10.** Prone

_____ **11.** Proximal

_____ **12.** Pubis

_____ **13.** Pulmonary artery

_____ **14.** Pulmonary vein

_____ **15.** Pulse

_____ **16.** Radial artery

_____ **17.** Radius

_____ **18.** Recovery position

_____ **19.** Red blood cells

_____ **20.** Renal system

▶ PART G

A. An organ located in the left upper quadrant of the abdomen that acts as a blood filtration system and a reservoir for reserves of blood

B. Muscular sac between the esophagus and the small intestine where digestion of food begins

C. Toward the head

D. The pressure created in the arteries when the left ventricle contracts and forces blood out into the circulation

_____ **1.** Reproductive system

_____ **2.** Respiration

_____ **3.** Respiratory system

_____ **4.** Scapula

_____ **5.** Shock

_____ **6.** Skeleton

E. Tissue that connects muscle to bone

F. The wing-shaped plate of cartilage that sits anterior to the larynx and forms the adams apple

G. The bony structure of the head

H. The bones of the body

I. The shoulder blade

J. The process of moving oxygen and carbon dioxide between circulating blood and the cells

K. The system of nose, mouth, throat, lungs, and muscles that brings oxygen into the body and expels carbon dioxide

L. The body system that is responsible for human reproduction

M. The layer of tissue between the body and the external environment

N. Hypoperfusion

O. The muscular tube between the stomach and the large intestine, divided into the duodenum, the jejunum, and the ileum, which receives partially digested food from the stomach and continues digestion

P. The breastbone

Q. The layers of fat and soft tissue found below the dermis

R. The ankle bones

S. Lying on the back

T. The chest

_____ 7. Skin

_____ 8. Skull

_____ 9. Small intestine

_____ 10. Spleen

_____ 11. Sternum

_____ 12. Stomach

_____ 13. Subcutaneous layers

_____ 14. Superior

_____ 15. Supine

_____ 16. Systolic blood pressure

_____ 17. Tarsals

_____ 18. Tendon

_____ 19. Thorax

_____ 20. Thyroid cartilage

▶ PART H

A. The female organ of reproduction used for both sexual intercourse and as an exit from the uterus for the fetus

B. Any blood vessel returning blood to the heart

C. The tubes connecting the bladder to the ureter or penis for excretion of urine

D. The process of moving gasses (oxygen and carbon dioxide) between inhaled air and the pulmonary circulation of the blood

E. A position in which the patient's feet and legs are higher than the head

F. The two lower chambers of the heart

G. The trunk of the body; the body without the head and the extremities

H. The 33 bones of the spinal column

I. Components of the blood; they produce substances that help the body fight infection

J. Form the structure of the cheeks

K. The medial and larger bone of the lower leg

_____ 1. Tibia

_____ 2. Torso

_____ 3. Trachea

_____ 4. Trendelenburg position

_____ 5. Ulna

_____ 6. Urethra

_____ 7. Uterus

_____ 8. Vagina

_____ 9. Valve

_____ 10. Vein

_____ 11. Vena cava

_____ 12. Ventilation

_____ 13. Ventral

L. The windpipe; the structure that connects the pharynx to the lungs

M. The medial bone of the forearm

N. Female organ of reproduction used to house the developing fetus

O. A structure that opens and closes to permit the flow of a fluid in only one direction

P. The superior vena cava and the inferior vena cava, which return blood from the body to the right atrium

Q. Referring to the front of the body

R. The smallest kind of vein

S. Muscle that can be consciously controlled

T. The inferior portion of the sternum

U. The male organ that produces sperm

V. Word endings that form nouns, adjectives, or verbs

W. The foundation of a word

X. Roots that are combined in medical terms

Y. Two or more whole words combined to form another term

Z. Used to modify or qualify a root word

_____ **14.** Ventricles

_____ **15.** Venule

_____ **16.** Vertebrae

_____ **17.** Voluntary muscle

_____ **18.** White blood cells

_____ **19.** Xiphoid process

_____ **20.** Zygomatic arches

_____ **21.** Combining form

_____ **22.** Compound

_____ **23.** Prefix

_____ **24.** Root

_____ **25.** Suffix

_____ **26.** Testes

MULTIPLE-CHOICE REVIEW

_____ **1.** All the following are body systems *except*:
   A. respiratory.
   B. cardiovascular.
   C. abdominal.
   D. musculoskeletal.

_____ **2.** If a patient is lying on his or her left side, the patient is said to be in the _____ position.
   A. Fowler's
   B. recovery
   C. left supine
   D. left prone

_____ **3.** When a patient who has been having difficulty breathing is placed in a sitting-up position on a stretcher, this position is called:
   A. prone.
   B. supine.
   C. Fowler's.
   D. Trendelenburg.

_____ **4.** When treating a patient who is dizzy and passing out, the EMT should place the patient lying flat with her or his head lower than her or his legs. This position is called:
   A. prone.
   B. supine.
   C. Fowler's.
   D. Trendelenburg.

_____ **5.** The musculoskeletal system has three main functions. It gives the body shape, provides for body movements, and:
   A. gives the body sensation.
   B. protects vital internal organs.
   C. provides for the body's outer covering.
   D. allows transport of oxygen into the cells.

_____ 6. Your patient was involved in a fight in a bar. You suspect he may have broken his upper jaw. What is the name of the bone involved?
   A. Mandible
   B. Orbit
   C. Maxillae
   D. Nasal bone

_____ 7. The spinal column includes the _____ vertebrae.
   A. thoracic and coccyx
   B. cervical and orbit
   C. lumbar and sternal
   D. sacrum and pelvic

_____ 8. An injury to the spinal cord at the _____ level may be fatal because control of the muscles of breathing arise from the spinal cord at this level.
   A. lumbar
   B. sacral
   C. cervical
   D. thoracic

_____ 9. Your patient was standing on the street corner when suddenly a truck cut the corner too close and ran over his legs. The bones in the lower extremities that he may have broken include the:
   A. femur, calcaneus, and phalanges.
   B. ischium, tibia, and ulna.
   C. orbit, lumbar, and shin.
   D. radius, fibula, and metatarsals.

_____ 10. Bones in the upper extremities include the:
   A. humerus and radius.
   B. humerus and calcaneus.
   C. phalanges and tibia.
   D. ulna and cervical.

_____ 11. The types of muscle tissue include:
   A. striated.
   B. involuntary.
   C. cardiac.
   D. all of these.

_____ 12. When a patient is walking, she is using which type of muscle?
   A. Voluntary
   B. Involuntary
   C. Cardiac
   D. Smooth

_____ 13. Involuntary, or smooth, muscle is found in the:
   A. trachea.
   B. walls of the blood vessels.
   C. heart.
   D. quadriceps and biceps.

_____ 14. The structure in the throat that is described as the voicebox is called the:
   A. pharynx.
   B. larynx.
   C. trachea.
   D. sternum.

_____ 15. A leaf-shaped valve that prevents food and foreign objects from entering the trachea is called the:
   A. pharynx.
   B. epiglottis.
   C. larynx.
   D. bronchi.

_____ **16.** Oxygen passes from the environment to the lungs in what order?
  A. Nose, bronchi, larynx, trachea, lung
  B. Larynx, esophagus, trachea, bronchi, alveoli
  C. Mouth, pharynx, trachea, bronchi, alveoli
  D. Epiglottis, trachea, cricoid, bronchi, alveoli

_____ **17.** When the diaphragm and intercostal muscles relax, the size of the chest cavity:
  A. increases, causing inhalation.
  B. increases, causing exhalation.
  C. decreases, causing exhalation.
  D. decreases, causing inhalation.

_____ **18.** The difference between the adult airway and the pediatric airway is that:
  A. the adult's tongue takes up proportionately more space in the mouth than the child's.
  B. the trachea is softer and more flexible in an adult.
  C. the cricoid cartilage is softer in an adult.
  D. all structures are smaller and more easily obstructed in a child.

_____ **19.** The body system that is responsible for the breakdown of food into absorbable forms is called the _____ system.
  A. nervous
  B. digestive
  C. endocrine
  D. integumentary

_____ **20.** An organ containing acidic gastric juices that begin the breakdown of food into components that the body will be able to convert to energy is the:
  A. large intestine.
  B. small intestine.
  C. stomach.
  D. liver.

_____ **21.** The major artery in the thigh is called the:
  A. carotid.
  B. femoral.
  C. radial.
  D. brachial.

_____ **22.** The vessel that carries oxygen-poor blood from the portions of the body below the heart and back to the right atrium is called the:
  A. posterior tibial.
  B. internal jugular.
  C. inferior vena cava.
  D. aorta.

_____ **23.** The heart has a right and left side as well as upper and lower chambers. The left atrium:
  A. receives blood from the veins of the body.
  B. receives blood from the pulmonary veins.
  C. pumps blood to the lungs.
  D. pumps blood to the body.

_____ **24.** The fluid that carries the blood cells and nutrients is called:
  A. platelets.
  B. urine.
  C. plasma.
  D. none of these.

_____ **25.** The blood component that is essential to the formation of blood clots is called:
  A. plasma.
  B. platelets.
  C. white blood cells.
  D. red blood cells.

©2012 Pearson Education, Inc.
Emergency Care, 12th Ed.

_____ 26. The pressure on the walls of an artery when the left ventricle contracts is called the _____ pressure.
- **A.** systolic
- **B.** arterial
- **C.** diastolic
- **D.** residual

_____ 27. The two main divisions of the nervous system are:
- **A.** central and peripheral.
- **B.** bones and muscles.
- **C.** brain and skin.
- **D.** spinal cord and brain.

_____ 28. Patients have many different types of nerves. Nerves that carry information from throughout the body to the brain are _____ nerves.
- **A.** motor
- **B.** cardiac
- **C.** spinal
- **D.** sensory

_____ 29. One of the functions of the integumentary system is to:
- **A.** eliminate excess oxygen into the atmosphere.
- **B.** regulate the diameter of the blood vessels in the circulation.
- **C.** protect the body from the environment, bacteria, and other organisms.
- **D.** allow environmental water to carefully enter the body.

_____ 30. The system that secretes hormones, such as insulin and adrenaline, and that is responsible for regulating many body activities, is called the _____ system.
- **A.** integumentary
- **B.** nervous
- **C.** endocrine
- **D.** gastrointestinal

_____ 31. Your patient was in a car wreck, and on assessment you note he has no sensation and movement in both of his legs. When documenting this on the prehospital care report, you should note that the patient:
- **A.** demonstrated quadriplegia.
- **B.** demonstrated paraplegia.
- **C.** had extreme pain in his extremities.
- **D.** was completely paralyzed.

_____ 32. Your patient is being treated for lung disease and was referred to a specialist for further treatment. The type of physician he is going to see is most likely a(n):
- **A.** cardiologist.
- **B.** internist.
- **C.** asthmatologist
- **D.** pulmonologist.

COMPLETE THE FOLLOWING

1. List the names of nine arteries in the body.

A. _____   F. _____

B. _____   G. _____

C. _____   H. _____

D. _____   I. _____

E. _____

2. List five functions of the skin.

A. _____

B. _____

C. _____

D. _____

E. _____

3. Define the following directional terms:

A. lateral _____

B. medial _____

C. proximal _____

D. distal _____

E. superior _____

F. inferior _____

INSIDE/OUTSIDE: RECOGNIZING SYMPATHETIC NERVOUS SYSTEM REPONSE

The 62-year-old male patient discussed on page 122 of the book is having a "silent-MI," which is an MI that is painless.

Elderly patients, females, and what other group of patients have silent MIs? _____

When the brain signals to the adrenal glands that the body is undergoing severe stress, such as that which occurs during an MI, the adrenal glands secrete two chemicals: adrenalin (epinephrine) and norepinephrine. What do these two chemicals cause the body to do? _____

What body system is the adrenal gland a component of? _____

What body system is the heart a component of? _____

LABEL THE DIAGRAMS

Fill in the name of each anatomical position on the line provided.

▶ **ANATOMICAL POSITIONS**

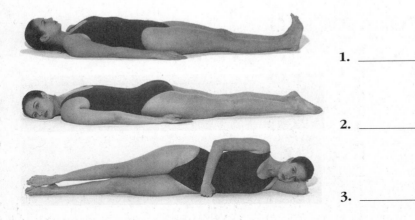

1. _____

2. _____

3. _____

Fill in the appropriate directional term or landmark on the line provided.

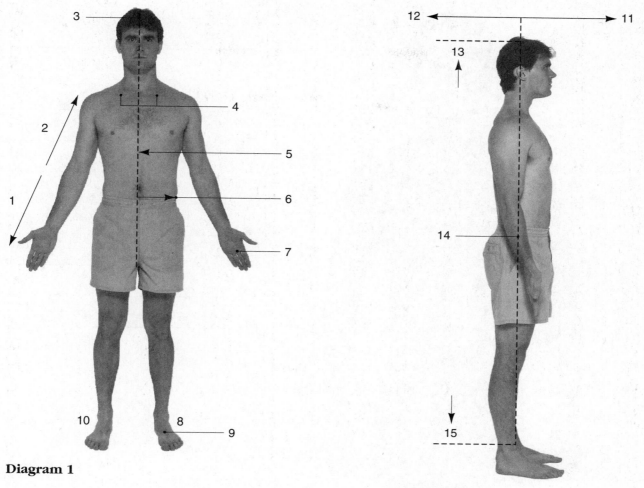

Diagram 1

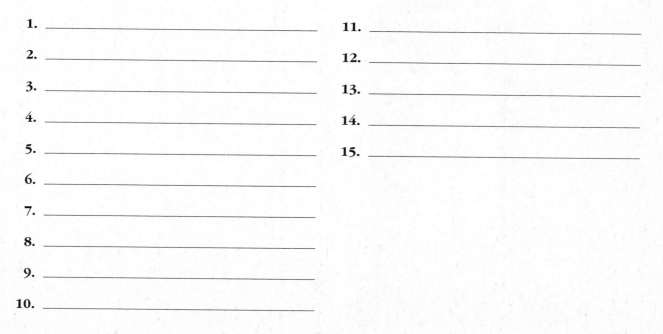

Diagram 2

1. _____   11. _____

2. _____   12. _____

3. _____   13. _____

4. _____   14. _____

5. _____   15. _____

6. _____

7. _____

8. _____

9. _____

10. _____

Fill in the name of each body region or structure on the line provided.

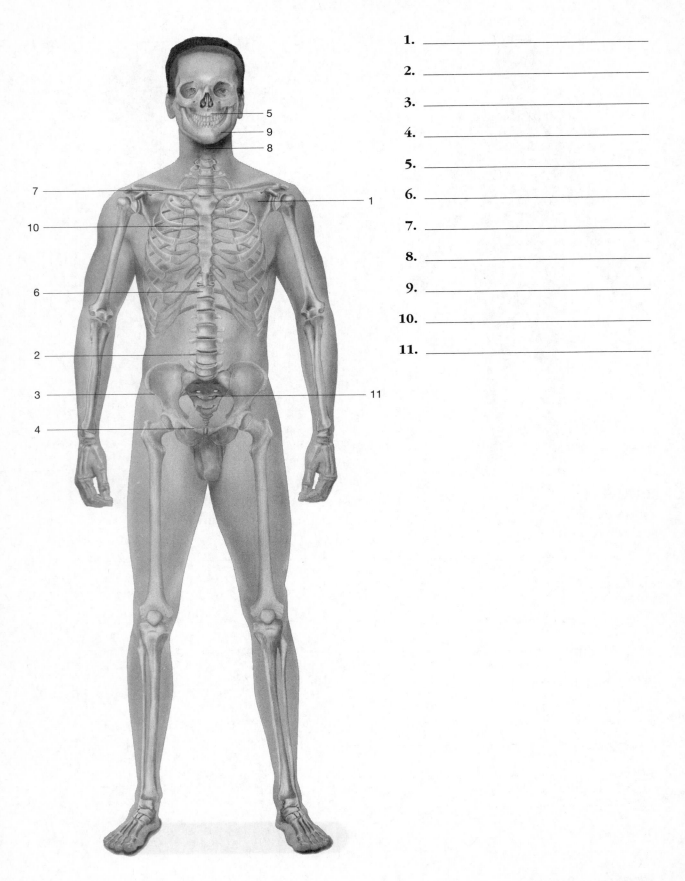

1. _____

2. _____

3. _____

4. _____

5. _____

6. _____

7. _____

8. _____

9. _____

10. _____

11. _____

STREET SCENES DISCUSSION

Review the Street Scene on page 134 of the textbook. Then answer the following questions.

1. Why was it necessary to stabilize the child's head and neck when you got into the car?

2. Because the driver of the truck was walking around, was he still a patient in need of evaluation? Explain your answer.

6

Principles of Pathophysiology

Standard: Pathophysiology

Competency: Applies fundamental knowledge of the pathophysiology of respiration and perfusion to patient assessment and management.

OBJECTIVES

After reading this chapter you should be able to:

6.1 Define key terms introduced in this chapter.

6.2 Describe the basic roles and structures of body cells.

6.3 Describe the roles of water, glucose, and oxygen in the cell.

6.4 Describe conditions that can threaten cardiopulmonary function.

6.5 Explain how impaired cardiopulmonary function affects the body.

6.6 Discuss the mechanisms the body uses to compensate for impaired cardiopulmonary function.

6.7 Explain the pathophysiology of shock.

6.8 Identify signs and symptoms that indicate the body is attempting to compensate for impaired cardiopulmonary function.

6.9 Describe ways in which the body's fluid balance can become disrupted.

6.10 Recognize indications that the body's fluid balance has been disrupted.

6.11 Describe ways in which the nervous system may be impaired.

6.12 Recognize indications that the nervous system may be impaired.

6.13 Describe the effects on the body of:

   a. Endocrine dysfunction
   b. Digestive system dysfunction
   c. Immune system dysfunction

MATCH TERMINOLOGY/ DEFINITIONS

A. The amount of blood ejected from the heart in one contraction

B. The amount of blood ejected from the heart in 1 minute (HR × SV)

C. A substance that, when dissolved in water, separates into charged particles

D. Fraction of inspired oxygen; the concentration of oxygen in the air we breathe

E. The volume of air moved in 1 minute by the lungs

F. Swelling associated with the movement of water into the interstitial space

G. An abnormally low amount of water in the body

H. An exaggerated response by the immune system to a particular substance

I. The constant supply of oxygen and nutrients to the cells by the flow of blood

J. The study of how disease processes affect the function of the body

K. The push of water out of the bloodstream as a result of the pressure within the vessel

L. Sensors in the blood vessels designed to identify internal pressure

M. The pressure in the peripheral blood vessels that the heart must overcome to pump blood

N. The volume of air moved in or out during one cycle of breathing

O. Open, clear, and free from obstruction

P. The cellular process where oxygen is used to metabolize glucose

Q. Air that occupies the space between the mouth and alveoli but does not actually reach the area of gas exchange

R. The cellular function of converting nutrients to energy necessary for cell function

S. Chemical sensors in the brain and blood vessels that identify changing levels of oxygen and carbon dioxide

T. The cellular process where glucose is metabolized into energy without oxygen

U. The pull exerted on water in and around the body cells into the bloodstream by large proteins in the plasma portion of the blood

V. Ventilation/perfusion match

_____ **1.** Pathophysiology

_____ **2.** Electrolyte

_____ **3.** Metabolism

_____ **4.** Aerobic metabolism

_____ **5.** Anaerobic metabolism

_____ **6.** Patent

_____ **7.** Tidal volume

_____ **8.** Dead air space

_____ **9.** Chemoreceptors

_____ **10.** Plasma oncotic pressure

_____ **11.** Hydrostatic pressure

_____ **12.** Cardiac output

_____ **13.** Systemic vascular resistance

_____ **14.** V/Q match

_____ **15.** Perfusion

_____ **16.** Dehydration

_____ **17.** Edema

_____ **18.** Hypersensitivity

_____ **19.** Stretch receptors

_____ **20.** FiO_2

_____ **21.** Minute volume

_____ **22.** Stroke volume

MULTIPLE-CHOICE REVIEW

_____ 1. It is very useful for EMTs to understand how common illnesses and injuries affect the body and how the body reacts. The study of how disease processes affect the function of the body is called:
   A. anatomy.
   B. physiology.
   C. pathophysiology.
   D. kinetics.

_____ 2. The cell structure that contains the DNA, which is the genetic blueprint, is called the:
   A. endoplasmic reticulum.
   B. nucleus.
   C. mitochondria.
   D. golgi apparatus.

_____ 3. Water management by the cells of the body is important because:
   A. it influences the concentrations of electrolytes.
   B. too much water leads to hypernatremia.
   C. too little water stops basic cell function.
   D. all of these are true.

_____ 4. When the legs are crushed under a slab of concrete, the blood supply is diminished to the cells in the legs. This condition often results in:
   A. carbon dioxide being produced.
   B. lactic acid being produced.
   C. aerobic metabolism.
   D. all of these.

_____ 5. Movement of air in and out of the chest requires:
   A. a patent airway.
   B. an alert mental status.
   C. a large tidal volume to overcome the dead space.
   D. all of these.

_____ 6. The best assessment of the amount of air that gets into and out of the lungs each minute is the:
   A. end-tidal CO_2.
   B. tidal volume.
   C. minute volume.
   D. SPO_2.

_____ 7. An example of a patient whose minute volume is likely to have diminished considerably would be:
   A. a 35-year-old female experiencing an asthma attack.
   B. a 22-year-old male who has overdosed on a narcotic.
   C. a 16-year-old who just broke three ribs.
   D. all of these.

_____ 8. The seat of the brain's respiratory control is a section called the:
   A. medulla.
   B. foramen magnum.
   C. cerebellum.
   D. cerebrum.

_____ 9. Respiration is activated by changing pressure within the thorax. _____ is a(n) _____ process, and _____ is a(n) _____ process.
   A. Exhalation; active; inhalation; passive
   B. Inhalation; active; exhalation; passive
   C. Exhalation; active; inhalation; voluntary
   D. Inhalation; passive; exhalation; involuntary

_____ 10. The brain stimulation to the respiratory system to increase the rate and/or tidal volume originates with the:
   A. ribs and chest vault.
   B. nervous system and spinal cord.
   C. chemoreceptors in the brain and vascular system.
   D. pressure sensors located in the aortic arch and carotids.

©2012 Pearson Education, Inc.
Emergency Care, 12th Ed.

_____ 11. The force exerted by large proteins in the blood that tends to attract water away from the area around body cells and into the bloodstream is called the:

A. gravitational pull.
B. inertia.
C. hydrostatic pressure.
D. plasma oncotic pressure.

_____ 12. Your patient is dehydrated, yet also has massive edema. This could be due to:

A. blood loss from injury.
B. a dysfunctioning liver.
C. an excessive amount of eating.
D. all of these.

_____ 13. When a patient's blood vessels constrict due to external blood loss, this process was originated by the brain due to messages received from the:

A. chemoreceptors in the aortic arch.
B. stretch receptors in certain blood vessels.
C. marrow in the long bones.
D. endocrine system.

_____ 14. A major risk factor in heart disease and stroke is due to:

A. low blood pressure.
B. low blood sugar.
C. constriction of peripheral vessels.
D. all of these.

_____ 15. Patients who develop sepsis are prone to problems with:

A. capillary permeability.
B. lack of insulin.
C. blood vessel constriction.
D. all of these.

_____ 16. The average person ejects approximately 60 ml of blood with each contraction of the heart. This is known as:

A. afterload.
B. vascular resistance.
C. preload.
D. stroke volume.

_____ 17. The more forceful the squeezing of the heart, the greater the stroke volume. This concept refers to the _____ of the heart.

A. resistance
B. contractility
C. preload
D. afterload

_____ 18. The patient's stroke volume depends on the patient's:

A. afterload.
B. contractility.
C. preload.
D. all of these.

_____ 19. An elderly patient is experiencing a fight-or-flight situation, and her body is attempting to compensate by increasing her cardiac output. How will the body do this on a moment's notice?

A. By decreasing her pulse rate
B. By increasing the stroke volume
C. By increasing the heart rate
D. By decreasing the respiratory rate

_____ 20. When a cardiac patient has another heart attack and his cardiac output drops, this is often due to:

A. ventricular irritability.
B. a decrease in the tidal volume.
C. a decrease in the strength of contractions.
D. an increase in the heart rate.

_____ 21. Fluid distribution is determined by:

A. the brain and kidneys regulating thirst and eliminating excess fluid.
B. the large proteins in our blood plasma pulling fluid into the bloodstream.
C. the permeability of both cell membranes and the walls of the capillaries helping to determine how much water can be held in and pushed out of cells and blood vessels.
D. all of these.

_____ **22.** A patient who has severe vomiting and diarrhea may have:
  A. an excess of body fluids.
  B. a condition call dehydration.
  C. edema in the extremities.
  D. all of these.

_____ **23.** Signs of neurological impairment include:
  A. inability or difficulty speaking.
  B. visual or hearing disturbance.
  C. weakness (sometimes limited to one side).
  D. all of these.

_____ **24.** A example of a condition where glands of the body are producing too much of a hormone is:
  A. Graves disease.
  B. diabetes.
  C. meningitis.
  D. a stroke.

_____ **25.** The most common disorder of the digestive system is:
  A. dizziness.
  B. nausea and/or vomiting.
  C. severe thirst.
  D. chills and fever.

COMPLETE THE FOLLOWING

1. For the "air to go in and air to go out and blood to go round and round," the system must be working! List what needs to be functioning properly:

  A. In the respiratory system: _____

  B. In the cardiovascular system: _____

2. A ventilation/perfusion match involves:

  A. _____

  B. _____

3. Shock is commonly defined as:

  _____

INSIDE/OUTSIDE: RECOGNIZING COMPENSATION

Based on the discussion of recognizing compensation in the text, list five (5) things that happen to the body during a fight-or-flight situation.

1. _____

2. _____

3. _____

4. _____

5. _____

©2012 Pearson Education, Inc.
Emergency Care, 12th Ed.

STREET SCENES DISCUSSION

Review the Street Scene on page 155 in the textbook. Then answer the following questions.

1. Was it in the patient's best interest to let him stand up? What will you do the next time?

2. What is the relevance of the history of days of diarrhea and not eating much?

3. What is a severe gastrointestinal bleed, and how serious is this condition?

7

Life Span Development

Standard: Life Span Development

Competency: Applies fundamental knowledge of life span development to patient assessment and management.

OBJECTIVES

After reading this chapter you should be able to:

7.1 Define key terms introduced in this chapter.

7.2 Describe the physical and physiological characteristics, including normal vital signs, for individuals in each of the following age groups:

   a. Infant
   b. Toddler
   c. Preschool age
   d. School age
   e. Adolescent
   f. Early adult
   g. Middle adult
   h. Late adult

7.3 Describe the typical psychosocial characteristics and concerns of individuals at each stage during the life span.

7.4 Use knowledge of physical, physiological, and psychosocial development to anticipate the needs and concerns of patients of all ages.

MATCH TERMINOLOGY/ DEFINITIONS

A. When you stroke a hungry infant's lips, he will start sucking

B. When you touch a hungry infant's cheek, he will turn his head toward the side touched

C. The infant's reaction to his environment

D. Stage of life from 12 to 36 months

E. Stage of life from 13 to 18 years

F. Stage of life from 20 to 40 years

G. Stage of life from 61 years and older

H. Stage of life from birth to 1 year of age

I. When you place your finger in an infant's palm, he will grasp it

J. Concept developed from an orderly, predictable environment versus a disorderly, irregular environment

K. Stage of life from 6 to 12 years

L. Stage of life from 41 to 60 years

M. Building on what one already knows

N. Stage of life from 3 to 5 years

O. The sense that needs will be met

P. When startled, an infant throws his arms out, spreads his fingers, then grabs with his fingers and arms

_____ 1. Infancy

_____ 2. Moro reflex

_____ 3. Palmar reflex

_____ 4. Rooting reflex

_____ 5. Sucking reflex

_____ 6. Bonding

_____ 7. Trust versus mistrust

_____ 8. Scaffolding

_____ 9. Temperament

_____ 10. Toddler phase

_____ 11. Preschool age

_____ 12. School age

_____ 13. Adolescent

_____ 14. Early adulthood

_____ 15. Middle adulthood

_____ 16. Late adulthood

MULTIPLE-CHOICE REVIEW

_____ 1. Your patient is a nose breather and her head is equal to 25 percent of her total body weight. What age group is she in?
   A. Toddler
   B. Infancy
   C. School age
   D. Preschool age

_____ 2. Why can nasal congestion be a major problem in the first few months of life?
   A. Because these children breathe with their diaphragm.
   B. Because the liver is so large in a patient of this age.
   C. Because children of this age are primarily nasal breathers.
   D. Because it is an indication of life-threatening airway compromise.

_____ 3. Infants get their immunity and antibodies from:
   A. breastfeeding by their mother.
   B. the vaccinations they receive.
   C. beginning to produce their own.
   D. all of these.

_____ 4. Which of the following nervous system reflexes is *not* normally found in an infant?
   A. The Cushing reflex
   B. The Moro reflex
   C. The rooting reflex
   D. None of these

_____ 5. When the mother strokes the infant's lips and the baby starts sucking, this is a nervous system reflex known as the:
A. Moro reflex.
B. sucking reflex.
C. palmar reflex.
D. rooting reflex.

_____ 6. When a mother states that her baby daughter is developing her reactions to the environment, this is also known as the psychosocial characteristic referred to as:
A. trust versus mistrust.
B. temperament.
C. bonding.
D. scaffolding.

_____ 7. When an infant develops anxiety and insecurity, this is often due to the psychosocial characteristic referred to as:
A. trust versus mistrust
B. temperament.
C. bonding.
D. scaffolding.

_____ 8. A toddler has continuing developments and improvements from infancy. Examples include each of the following _except_:
A. the brain is now 90 percent of an adult's brain weight.
B. the alveoli increase in numbers.
C. the child is less susceptible to illness.
D. all of the primary teeth should be in place.

_____ 9. The adolescent years are the beginning of:
A. self-destructive behaviors.
B. excellent decision-making skills.
C. nasal breathing.
D. the replacement of primary teeth.

_____ 10. The peak physical condition occurs between the ages of _____ and _____.
A. 12; 16
B. 19; 26
C. 30; 40
D. 35; 45

_____ 11. You have been called to the home of a woman who fell in the kitchen. When you get a medical history, you find she is taking medicine for control of high cholesterol, and she states that she has been dieting this week and was a little dizzy. What is her most likely age (age group)?
A. School age
B. Adolescent
C. Young adulthood
D. Middle adulthood

_____ 12. Examples of the psychosocial challenges a person in late adulthood has to deal with include:
A. financial burdens.
B. self-worth.
C. living environment.
D. all of these.

_____ 13. How might the age of the patient affect your assessment?
A. The parent or caregiver will need to help you when assessing an infant.
B. The patient who is in late adulthood is likely to have cardiovascular disorders.
C. The adolescent often experiments with alcohol and tobacco.
D. All of these are challenges you might come across.

_____ 14. All of the following are examples of how an EMT's ability to communicate with a young patient can be complicated _except_:
A. fear of strangers.
B. fear of death and dying.
C. separation anxiety.
D. embarrassment during adolescence.

_____ 15. During the adolescent years of development, both males and females:
A. begin to develop self-esteem.
B. reach reproductive maturity.
C. replace their primary teeth.
D. all of these are correct.

_____ **16.** Girls are usually finished growing by the age of:

      A. 14.   **C.** 18.

      B. 16.   **D.** 20.

_____ **17.** Boys are usually finished growing by the age of:

      A. 14.

      B. 16.

      C. 18.

      D. 20.

_____ **18.** Serious family conflicts occur in some _____ as the children strive for _____ and the parents strive for _____ .

      A. school-age children; freedom; control

      B. adolescents; independence; control

      C. early adults; control; independence

      D. preschoolers; independence; control

_____ **19.** The leading cause of death in the young adulthood age group is (are):

      A. overdose.

      B. heart attacks.

      C. accidents.

      D. strokes.

_____ **20.** The experts believe that the highest levels of job stress occur in which age group?

      A. Adolescent

      B. School-age

      C. Middle adult

      D. Young adult

COMPLETE THE FOLLOWING

1. List the eight life stages discussed in Chapter 7 of the textbook.

      A. _____

      B. _____

      C. _____

      D. _____

      E. _____

      F. _____

      G. _____

      H. _____

2. List examples of characteristics for each of the following age groups:

      A. 2 months: _____

      B. 3 months: _____

      C. 4 months: _____

      D. 5 months: _____

STREET SCENES DISCUSSION

Review the Street Scene on page 169 of your textbook. Then answer the following questions.

1. What age group does the patient fit into?

2. If the patient had been unconscious and had a pulse, what would have been the highest management priority (airway, breathing, or circulation)?

3. Assume that your second set of vital signs revealed the following: a pulse of 140, a respiratory rate of 34, and a systolic BP of 72 mmHg. Would you react differently? If so, how?

8

Airway Management

Standard: Airway Management, Respiration, and Artificial Ventilation (Airway Management)

Competency: Applies knowledge (fundamental depth, foundational breadth) of general anatomy and physiology to patient assessment and management in order to ensure a patent airway, adequate mechanical ventilation, and respiration for patients of all ages.

OBJECTIVES

After reading this chapter you should be able to:

8.1 Define key terms introduced in this chapter.

8.2 Describe the anatomy and physiology of the upper and lower airways.

8.3 Given a diagram or model, identify the structures of the upper and lower airways.

8.4 Describe common pathophysiologic problems leading to airway obstruction.

8.5 Demonstrate assessment of the airway in a variety of patient scenarios.

8.6 Associate abnormal airway sounds with likely pathophysiologic causes.

8.7 Identify patients who have an open airway but who are at risk for airway compromise.

8.8 Recognize patients who have an inadequate airway.

8.9 Demonstrate manually opening the airway in pediatric and adult medical and trauma patients.

    a. Head-tilt, chin-lift maneuver
    b. Jaw-thrust maneuver

8.10 Describe the indications, contraindications, use, and potential complications of airway adjuncts, including:

    a. Oropharyngeal airway
    b. Nasopharyngeal airway

8.11 Recognize the indications for suctioning of the mouth and oropharynx.

8.12 Describe risks and limitations associated with suctioning the mouth and oropharynx.

8.13 Demonstrate the following airway management skills:

    a. Inserting an oropharyngeal airway
    b. Inserting a nasopharyngeal airway
    c. Suctioning the mouth and oropharynx

8.14 Describe modifications in airway management for pediatric patients, patients with facial trauma, and patients with airway obstruction.

MATCH TERMINOLOGY/ DEFINITIONS

A. A method for (means of) correcting blockage of the airway by moving the jaw forward without tilting the head or neck; this method is indicated when trauma, or injury, is suspected to open the airway without causing further injury to the spinal cord in the neck

B. A curved device inserted through the patient's mouth into the pharynx to help maintain an open airway

C. An airway that is open and clear and will remain open and clear, without interference to the passage of air into and out of the lungs

D. Vomiting or retching that may result when something is placed in the back of the pharynx; this is tied to the swallow reflex

E. The passageway by which air enters or leaves the body; the structures of the airway are the nose, mouth, pharynx, larynx, trachea, bronchi, bronchioles, and alveoli

F. A method of correcting blockage of the airway by the tongue by tilting the head back and lifting the chin; this method is indicated when no trauma, or injury, is suspected.

G. Use of a vacuum device to remove blood, vomitus, and other secretions or foreign materials from the airway

H. A flexible breathing tube inserted through the patient's nose into the pharynx to help maintain an open airway

_____ **1.** Airway

_____ **2.** Patent airway

_____ **3.** Head-tilt, chin-lift

_____ **4.** Jaw-thrust maneuver

_____ **5.** Oropharyngeal airway

_____ **6.** Nasopharyngeal airway

_____ **7.** Gag reflex

_____ **8.** Suctioning

MULTIPLE-CHOICE REVIEW

_____ **1.** During respiration, the movement of air into and out of the lungs requires that:
    A. oxygen exits on the exhalation phase.
    B. carbon dioxide enters on the inhalation phase.
    C. air flow be unobstructed and move freely.
    D. the mouth be open at all times that the patient is breathing.

_____ **2.** When a patient inhales, air enters the throat, which is divided into the:
    A. nasopharynx.   **C.** laryngopharynx.
    B. oropharynx.   **D.** all of these.

_____ 3. The hypopharynx is also called the:
   A. nares.
   B. laryngopharynx.
   C. trachea.
   D. glottis.

_____ 4. The large leaf-life structure that protects the opening to the trachea is called the:
   A. oropharynx.
   B. xiphoid process.
   C. epiglottis.
   D. cricoid cartilage.

_____ 5. When we say that a patient is experiencing lower airway obstruction, it is likely that:
   A. he or she is choking on a foreign object.
   B. his or her bronchial passages or alveoli are congested.
   C. his or her tongue is swollen.
   D. none of these.

_____ 6. Signs of a potentially inadequate airway include all of the following *except*:
   A. absent air movement.
   B. air that can be felt at the nose or mouth on expiration.
   C. unusual hoarse or raspy sound quality to the voice.
   D. abnormal noises such as wheezing, crowing, or stridor.

_____ 7. An inadequate airway in a child is defined as:
   A. less than 15 breaths per minute.
   B. retractions above the clavicles and between and below the ribs.
   C. breathing that is primarily from the nose in infants.
   D. none of these.

_____ 8. When you question an elderly woman with a respiratory complaint, she speaks in short, two- or three-word sentences. Is this significant?
   A. No, she is probably always like that.
   B. Yes, she must have a complete airway obstruction.
   C. No, elderly people always talk slowly.
   D. Yes, she is probably very short of breath.

_____ 9. Your patient was the driver of a car that stopped suddenly when she hit a pole. She was not wearing her seatbelt and has a bruise on her neck. When you question her, she speaks very softly and seems to have a raspy voice. Is this significant or just a sign of nervousness about the collision?
   A. No, many patients get quiet after a motor vehicle crash.
   B. Yes, if she were nervous, she would be more excited.
   C. No, but the bruise could mean that she has significant bleeding.
   D. Yes, low volume and raspy tone could be due to airway swelling from neck or laryngeal trauma.

_____ 10. One indication that a child is experiencing inadequate breathing is that she:
   A. has a headache.
   B. complains of nausea.
   C. has nasal flaring when breathing.
   D. is dizzy when standing.

_____ 11. The very first step to aid a patient who is not breathing is to:
   A. clear the mouth.
   B. administer oxygen.
   C. apply positive ventilation.
   D. open the airway.

_____ 12. What is the importance of mechanism of injury (MOI) to airway care?
   A. An injured patient will need more oxygen.
   B. The procedure for opening the patient's airway is different in trauma.
   C. Patients without a mechanism of injury will have an open airway.
   D. An injury can make airway care easier to manage than a medical emergency.

_____ 13. To open the airway of a patient with a suspected head, neck, or spine injury, the EMT should use a _____ maneuver.
   A. jaw-thrust
   B. head-tilt, chin-lift
   C. head-tilt, neck-lift
   D. modified chin-thrust

_____ 14. When performing the head-tilt, chin-lift maneuver, the EMT should:
   A. not allow the patient's mouth to close.
   B. position himself at the top of the patient's head.
   C. tilt the head by applying pressure to the patient's chin.
   D. use fingertips to lift the neck.

_____ 15. When performing the jaw-thrust maneuver, the EMT should do each one of the following _except_:
   A. kneel at the top of the patient's head.
   B. stabilize the patient's head with the forearms.
   C. use the index fingers to push the angles of the patient's lower jaw forward.
   D. tilt the head by applying gentle pressure to the patient's forehead.

_____ 16. The main purpose of the jaw-thrust maneuver is to:
   A. open the mouth with only one hand.
   B. open the airway without moving the head or neck.
   C. create an airway for the medical patient.
   D. create an airway when it is not possible to jut the jaw.

_____ 17. An oral or nasal airway should be:
   A. cleaned for reuse after the call.
   B. inserted in all critically injured patients.
   C. used to keep the tongue from blocking the airway.
   D. used in order to prevent the need for suctioning.

_____ 18. If something is placed in the patient's throat, the gag reflex causes the patient to:
   A. take deep breaths.
   B. pass out.
   C. vomit or retch.
   D. all of these.

_____ 19. An oropharyngeal airway of proper size extends from the:
   A. corner of the patient's mouth to the tip of the earlobe.
   B. lips to the larynx.
   C. nose to the angle of the jaw.
   D. none of these.

_____ 20. An oral airway should be inserted:
   A. upside down, with the tip toward the roof of the mouth, then flipped 180 degrees over the tongue.
   B. right side up, using a tongue depressor to press the tongue down and forward to keep it from obstructing the airway.
   C. either of these.
   D. neither of these.

_____ 21. A nasopharyngeal airway should be:
   A. inserted with the bevel on the lateral side of the nostril.
   B. measured from the patient's nostril to the earlobe.
   C. inserted in the left nostril when possible.
   D. turned 180 degrees with the tip facing the roof of the mouth.

_____ 22. When inserting a nasopharyngeal airway, lubricate the outside of the tube with:
   A. petroleum jelly.
   B. an oil-based lubricant.
   C. a silicone-based gel.
   D. a water-based lubricant.

_____ 23. The purposes of suctioning may include removal of:
   A. teeth and large pieces of solid material.
   B. excess oxygen from the patient.
   C. blood, vomitus, and other secretions.
   D. all of these.

64 Section 2 • _Airway Management, Respiration, and Artificial Ventilation_

©2012 Pearson Education, Inc.
Emergency Care, 12th Ed.

24. When a patient begins to vomit, it is essential that you have a(n) _____ ready to go at the patient's side.
  A. suction unit
  C. blood pressure cuff
  B. oxygen tank
  D. pocket mask

25. You are treating a 29-year-old female who has major airway problems. She has thick secretions and blood in her upper airway that needs to be suctioned with a Yankauer. Which of the following is *not* true of the Yankauer suction tip?
  A. It has a rigid tip.
  B. It allows for excellent control over the distal end of the device.
  C. It is used most successfully with responsive patients.
  D. It has a larger bore than flexible catheters.

INSIDE/OUTSIDE: THE SOUNDS OF A PARTIALLY OBSTRUCTED AIRWAY

1. Of the abnormal sounds that patients make when the airway is partially obstructed, which sound is typically high-pitched?

_____

2. Which sound may be due to a swelling airway or a developing respiratory burn?

_____

3. Which primarily soft tissue can create impedance to the flow of air?

_____

4. Which sound is usually due to liquid in the airway?

_____

COMPLETE THE FOLLOWING

1. Identify and list at least six signs of an inadequate airway.

  A. _____

  B. _____

  C. _____

  D. _____

  E. _____

  F. _____

2. Identify five indications for using airway adjuncts.

  A. _____

  B. _____

C. _____

D. _____

E. _____

STREET SCENES DISCUSSION

Review the Street Scene on page 195 of your textbook. Then answer the following questions.

1. If the patient had no gag reflex, what airway adjunct would you consider using? How would you insert it?

2. If the patient vomits during ventilation with a bag mask device, what should you do?

3. If the patient's pulse had not rapidly increased, should you have called for an ALS intercept? Why or why not?

CASE STUDY

This case study is designed to help you apply the concepts presented in this textbook. The case study describes a situation you might encounter in the field and is followed by questions about the situation. The questions require you to explain and apply key concepts from your reading.

▶ THE RAPIDLY CHANGING AIRWAY

Your BLS unit and the police are dispatched to the scene of a call for a woman who is having difficulty breathing. The call was made by a family member who came home and found his 45-year-old mother wheezing and struggling. The police arrive before you and advise that the scene is secure (safe) and that you should respond directly to the scene of a private home in a suburban community 2 minutes from your station. As you enter the house, you can hear a woman wheezing and the sound gets louder as you go up the stairs. She is in the rear upper bedroom. After donning your protective gloves, mask, and goggles, you begin to question the patient as your partner obtains a set of baseline vital signs. The patient talks in short, choppy sentences, and it is clear she is having a very severe asthma attack.

1. Does this patient have an upper or lower airway obstruction?

_____

2. What is the significance of the patient being able to speak only in short choppy sentences?

_____

3. If this patient were to become unconscious while you are providing care, what type of airway would be used first?

_____

4. Once the patient is unconscious and placed on your stretcher, how would you manually open the airway?

_____

5. You are assisting the patient, who is now unconscious on your stretcher. ALS has been called for, and you are preparing to carry her out the front door to the ambulance. The patient starts to make a snoring noise. What is that, and what should you do?

_____

6. After dealing with the airway noise, you now notice that there is a gurgling sound. What causes this sound and how do you take care of it?

_____

EMT SKILLS PERFORMANCE CHECKLISTS

▶ **POSITIONING THE ADULT PATIENT FOR BASIC LIFE SUPPORT (P. 181)**

❑ Take Standard Precautions.

❑ Straighten the patient's legs and position the arm closest to you above his head.

❑ Cradle the patient's head and neck. Grasp under the distant armpit.

❑ Move the patient as a unit onto his side.

❑ Move the patient onto his back and reposition the extended arm.

NOTE: This maneuver is used to initiate airway evaluation, artificial ventilation, or CPR when the EMT must act alone. When trauma is suspected, the four-rescuer log roll is the preferred technique.

► HEAD-TILT, CHIN-LIFT MANEUVER (P. 181)

❑ Take Standard Precautions.

❑ Once the patient is supine, place one hand on the forehead. Place the fingertips of your other hand under the bony area at the center of the patient's lower jaw.

❑ Tilt the head by applying gentle pressure to the patient's forehead.

❑ Use your fingertips to lift the chin and to support the lower jaw. Move the jaw forward to a point where the lower teeth are almost touching the upper teeth. Do not compress the soft tissues under the lower jaw.

❑ Do not close the patient's mouth. It is best to insert an oral airway if the patient has no gag reflex.

► JAW-THRUST MANEUVER (P. 182)

❑ Take Standard Precautions.

❑ Carefully keep the patient's head, neck, and spine aligned, moving him as a unit as you place him in the supine position.

❑ Kneel approximately 18 inches above the head of the supine patient.

❑ Reach forward and gently place one hand on each side of the patient's lower jaw. Run your fingers along the jaw until you just pass the angle of the jaw.

❑ Stabilize the patient's head with your palms and forearms.

❑ Using your index fingers, push the angles of the patient's lower jaw forward.

❑ To keep the mouth open, use an oropharyngeal airway on a patient with no gag reflex.

❑ Do not tilt or rotate the patient's head.

NOTE: Remember that the purpose of the jaw-thrust maneuver is to open the airway without moving the head or neck from the neutral position.

► OROPHARYNGEAL (ORAL) AIRWAY INSERTION (OPA) (P. 185)

❑ Take Standard Precautions.

❑ Select appropriate-size airway.

❑ Measure airway (center of mouth to angle of jaw, or corner of mouth to tip of earlobe).

❑ Insert airway without pushing the tongue back into the throat. Insert upside down and rotate (flip) 180 degrees over the tongue, or insert straight in with a tongue blade holding tongue forward.

❑ Remove oropharyngeal airway quickly if patient gags.

► NASOPHARYNGEAL (NASAL) AIRWAY INSERTION (NPA) (P. 187)

❑ Take Standard Precautions.

❑ Select appropriate-size airway (diameter of patient's little finger). An alternative method is to measure length from patient's nostril to earlobe or to angle of jaw.

❑ Measure airway (nostril to earlobe).

©2012 Pearson Education, Inc.
Emergency Care, 12th Ed.

❏ Lubricate nasopharyngeal airway with water-soluble gel.

❏ Fully insert the airway with the bevel facing the nasal septum.

▶ OROPHARYNGEAL SUCTIONING (P. 191)

❏ Take Standard Precautions.

❏ Position yourself at the patient's head, and turn the patient onto his or her side.*

❏ A rigid tip (Yankauer) is preferred. When inserting, never lose sight of the tip.

❏ Measure a flexible suction catheter (distance between the patient's earlobe and corner of mouth, or center of mouth to angle of jaw).

❏ Turn suction unit on. Attach the catheter and test for suction.

❏ Open and clear the patient's mouth.

❏ Place the rigid pharyngeal tip so that the convex (bulging-out) side is against the roof of the patient's mouth. Insert tip just to the base of the tongue. Do not push the tip down into the throat or larynx.

❏ Apply suction only after the tip of the catheter or rigid tip is in place, suctioning intermittently on the way out, moving tip from side to side. Suction for no longer than 15 seconds. (As per U.S. DOT, suction toddlers for no longer than 10 seconds and infants for no longer than 5 seconds.†) If the patient continues to vomit, you must still continue to suction.

❏ Ventilate the patient with 100 percent oxygen.

*If trauma is suspected, leave the patient supine.

†AHA Guidelines say that EMTs must limit any interruptions in chest compressions during CPR to 10 seconds.

©2012 Pearson Education, Inc.
Emergency Care, 12th Ed.

9

Respiration and Artificial Ventilation

Standard: Airway Management, Respiration, and Artificial Ventilation (Respiration, Artificial Ventilation)

Competency: Applies knowledge (fundamental depth, foundational breadth) of general anatomy and physiology to patient assessment and management in order to ensure a patent airway, adequate mechanical ventilation, and respiration for patients of all ages.

OBJECTIVES

After reading this chapter you should be able to:

9.1 Define key terms introduced in this chapter.

9.2 Explain the physiological relationship between assessing and maintaining an open airway, assessing and ensuring adequate ventilation, and assessing and maintaining adequate circulation.

9.3 Describe the mechanics of ventilation.

9.4 Explain mechanisms that control the depth and rate of ventilation.

9.5 Explain the relationships among tidal volume, respiratory rate, minute volume, dead space air, and alveolar ventilation.

9.6 Describe the physiology of external and internal respiration.

9.7 Recognize patients at risk for failure of the cardiopulmonary system.

9.8 Differentiate among adequate and inadequate breathing (respiratory failure) and respiratory arrest.

9.9 Use information from the scene size-up and patient assessment to anticipate hypoxia.

9.10 Given a variety of scenarios, differentiate between patients who require artificial ventilation and those who do not.

9.11 Identify patients who require administration of supplemental oxygen.

9.12 Discuss the potential negative effects of positive pressure ventilation and how to minimize complications from positive pressure ventilation.

9.13 Demonstrate the following techniques of artificial respiration for pediatric (as applicable) and adult medical and trauma patients:

  a. Mouth-to-mask
  b. Two-rescuer bag-valve-mask (BVM)
  c. One-rescuer BVM
  d. Flow-restricted, oxygen-powered ventilation device
  e. Automatic transport ventilator (as permitted by local protocol)

9.14 Assess the adequacy of artificial ventilations.

9.15 Demonstrate the application of cricoid pressure.

9.16 Modify artificial ventilation and oxygen techniques for patients with stomas.

9.17 Discuss considerations for selecting the best device for delivering oxygen for a variety of patient scenarios.

9.18 Demonstrate administration of oxygen by:

  a. Nonrebreather mask
  b. Nasal cannula

9.19 Describe the purpose and use of partial rebreather masks, Venturi masks, and tracheostomy masks.

9.20 Demonstrate safe transport, storage, and use of oxygen.

9.21 Describe the purpose of each part of an oxygen delivery system.

9.22 Describe the use of humidified oxygen.

MATCH TERMINOLOGY/DEFINITIONS

▶ PART A

A. When breathing completely stops

B. The reduction of breathing to the point where oxygen intake is not sufficient to support life

C. A blue or gray color resulting from lack of oxygen in the body

D. The passageway by which air enters or leaves the body; the structures of the airway are the nose, mouth, pharynx, larynx, trachea, bronchi, and lungs

E. A means of correcting blockage of the airway by the tongue by tilting the head back and lifting the chin; used when no trauma, or injury, is suspected

F. An airway (passage from nose or mouth to lungs) that is open and clear and will remain open and clear, without interference to the passage of air into and out of the body

G. The amount of air breathed in during each respiration multiplied by the number of breaths per minute

H. Areas of the respiratory tract outside the alveoli where gas exchange with the blood does not take place

I. Breathing

J. Increased work of breathing; a sensation of shortness of breath

_____ **1.** Respiration

_____ **2.** Respiratory distress

_____ **3.** Respiratory failure

_____ **4.** Respiratory arrest

_____ **5.** Minute volume

_____ **6.** Dead space

_____ **7.** Cyanosis

_____ **8.** Airway

_____ **9.** Patent airway

_____ **10.** Head-tilt, chin-lift maneuver

▶ **PART B**

A. A device, usually with a one-way valve, to aid in artificial ventilation. A rescuer breathes through the valve when the mask is placed over the patient's face. It also acts as a barrier to prevent contact with a patient's breath or body fluids. It can be used with supplemental oxygen when fitted with an oxygen inlet.

B. Forcing air or oxygen into the lungs when a patient has stopped breathing or has inadequate breathing.

C. A device that uses oxygen under pressure to deliver artificial ventilations. Its trigger is placed so that the rescuer can operate it while still using both hands to maintain a seal on the face mask. It has automatic flow restriction to prevent overdelivery of oxygen to the patient.

D. A device that provides positive pressure ventilations. It includes settings designed to adjust ventilation rate and volume, is portable, and is easily carried on an ambulance.

E. A flexible breathing tube inserted through the patient's nose into the pharynx to help maintain an open airway.

F. A curved device inserted through the patient's mouth into the pharynx to help maintain an open airway.

G. A handheld device with a face mask and self-refilling bag that can be squeezed to provide artificial ventilations to a patient. It can deliver air from the atmosphere or oxygen from a supplemental oxygen supply system.

H. A permanent surgical opening in the neck through which the patient breathes.

I. A means of correcting blockage of the airway by moving the jaw forward without tilting the head or neck. Used when trauma, or injury, is suspected to open the airway without causing further injury to the spinal cord in the neck.

J. The breathing in of air or oxygen or providing breaths artificially.

_____ **1.** Jaw-thrust maneuver

_____ **2.** Ventilation

_____ **3.** Artificial ventilation

_____ **4.** Pocket face mask

_____ **5.** Bag-valve mask

_____ **6.** Stoma

_____ **7.** Flow-restricted, oxygen-powered ventilation device (FROPVD)

_____ **8.** Automatic transport ventilator (ATV)

_____ **9.** Oropharyngeal

_____ **10.** Nasopharyngeal

▶ **PART C**

A. A device connected to an oxygen cylinder to reduce cylinder pressure to a safe level for delivery of oxygen to a patient

B. A cylinder filled with oxygen under pressure

C. A valve that indicates the flow of oxygen in liters per minute

D. An insufficiency of oxygen in the body's tissues

E. A device connected to the flowmeter to add moisture to the dry oxygen coming from an oxygen cylinder

F. Use of a vacuum device to remove blood, vomitus, and other secretions or foreign materials from the airway

G. A face mask and reservoir bag device that delivers high concentrations of oxygen; the patient's exhaled air escapes through a valve and is not rebreathed

_____ **1.** Gag reflex

_____ **2.** Suctioning

_____ **3.** Hypoxia

_____ **4.** Oxygen cylinder

_____ **5.** Pressure regulator

_____ **6.** Flowmeter

_____ **7.** Humidifier

_____ **8.** Nonrebreather mask

_____ **9.** Nasal cannula

_____ **10.** Venturi mask

H. Vomiting or retching that results when something is placed in the back of the pharynx; it is tied to the swallow reflex

I. A device that delivers low concentrations of oxygen through two prongs that rest in the patient's nostrils

J. A face mask and reservoir bag device that delivers specific concentrations of oxygen by mixing oxygen with inhaled air

MULTIPLE-CHOICE REVIEW

_____ **1.** During the process of ventilation:
  A. the intercostal muscles expand, causing the air to be forced out of the chest.
  B. carbon dioxide enters the body during each expiration.
  C. oxygen enters the body during each expiration.
  D. the diaphragm and chest muscles contract and relax to change the pressure in the chest.

_____ **2.** The EMT needs to recognize respiratory distress and manage it so it does not proceed to respiratory failure. Respiratory failure is:
  A. the complete cessation of inspiration.
  B. inadequate breathing, which is a precursor to respiratory arrest.
  C. another term for respiratory arrest.
  D. caused by electrocution in young children.

_____ **3.** Which of the following is a sign that your patient may not be breathing adequately?
  A. Air moving out of the nose and mouth
  B. Equal expansion of both sides of the chest
  C. Breathing limited to abdominal movement
  D. Absence of blue or gray skin coloration

_____ **4.** You are assessing a 6-year-old male who is having difficulty breathing. Signs of inadequate breathing in a child this age may include:
  A. cyanotic skin, lips, tongue, or earlobes.
  B. retractions between and below the ribs.
  C. nasal flaring.
  D. all of these.

_____ **5.** Each of the following is a sign of inadequate breathing in an adult patient _except_:
  A. inspirations or expirations that are prolonged.
  B. breathing rate in an adult of 14–18 breaths per minute.
  C. breathing is very shallow, very deep, or appears labored.
  D. the patient is unable to speak in full sentences.

_____ **6.** You are treating a patient who has signs of inadequate breathing. These signs could include all of the following _except_:
  A. absent or minimal chest movement.
  B. air that can be felt at the nose or mouth on exhalation.
  C. diminished or absent breath sounds.
  D. noises such as wheezing, gurgling, stridor, or crowing.

_____ **7.** Your patient is a child approximately 4 years old and is in respiratory distress, which may be leading to respiratory failure. Inadequate breathing in a child this age is defined as:
  A. less than 12 breaths per minute.
  B. more than 36 breaths per minute.
  C. cyanosis of the lips and earlobes.
  D. any of these.

_____ 8. A difference between a patient with respiratory distress and a patient with respiratory failure includes:
   A. respiratory failure shows mottled or blotchy skin color.
   B. respiratory failure shows an alert mental status.
   C. respiratory distress shows blue skin.
   D. respiratory distress results in a comatose patient.

_____ 9. Cyanosis can be checked by observing the patient's:
   A. tongue.
   B. earlobes.
   C. nail beds.
   D. tongue, nail beds, and earlobes.

_____ 10. One indication that a patient is experiencing inadequate breathing is that she:
   A. has a headache.
   B. complains of nausea.
   C. talks in short, choppy sentences.
   D. is dizzy when standing.

_____ 11. The very first step to aid a patient who is not breathing is to:
   A. clear the mouth.
   B. administer oxygen.
   C. apply positive ventilation.
   D. open the airway.

_____ 12. Your patient has overdosed on a narcotic medication that was prescribed for pain after a surgical procedure. This medicine has been known to depress respirations and lead to:
   A. cyanosis.
   B. hypoxia.
   C. tachycardia.
   D. delayed capillary refill.

_____ 13. The normal or adequate breathing rate for an adult should be:
   A. 6 to 10 breaths per minute
   B. 12 to 20 breaths per minute.
   C. 15 to 30 breaths per minute
   D. 25 to 50 breaths per minute.

_____ 14. When the EMT determines that the patient is not breathing or breathing is inadequate, it will be necessary to provide:
   A. positive pressure ventilation.
   B. artificial ventilation.
   C. assistance with a BVM device.
   D. any of these.

_____ 15. The negative side effects of positive pressure ventilation include each of the following *except*:
   A. hypothermia.
   B. gastric distension.
   C. decreasing cardiac output.
   D. dropping blood pressure.

_____ 16. You have been ventilating a patient with a BVM device. Your partner states you should be careful not to hyperventilate the patient because it causes:
   A. hypoxia in the heart tissue.
   B. vasoconstriction and limited blood flow to the brain.
   C. the blood pressure to increase excessively.
   D. all of these.

_____ 17. Various techniques can be used by the EMT to provide artificial ventilation in the field. Given plenty of trained helpers, which would be the *least* effective?
   A. One-rescuer using a bag-valve mask
   B. A flow-restricted, oxygen-powered ventilation device
   C. Two rescuers using a bag-valve mask with high-concentration supplemental oxygen at 15 lpm
   D. Mouth-to-mask with high-concentration supplemental oxygen at 15 lpm

©2012 Pearson Education, Inc.
Emergency Care, 12th Ed.

_____ 18. Which of the following indicates adequate artificial ventilations?
  A. Chest does not rise and fall with ventilation.
  B. Rate of ventilation is too slow or too fast.
  C. Patient's color changes from cyanotic to pink.
  D. Patient's heart rate does not return to normal with ventilations.

_____ 19. When performing mouth-to-mask ventilation on an adult patient, ventilations should be delivered over _____ second(s).
  A. ½   **C.** 2
  B. 1   **D.** 3

_____ 20. The bag-valve mask on your EMS unit should have:
  A. a nonrefilling shell that is easily cleaned.
  B. a nonjam valve with an oxygen inlet.
  C. a standard 9/12-mm fitting.
  D. manual disabling pop-off valve.

_____ 21. The bag-valve mask should be capable of:
  A. withstanding cold temperatures.
  B. providing a high pressure in the chest and airway.
  C. blowing off at pressures above 40 mm of water pressure.
  D. receiving an oxygen inlet flow of 25 liters per minute.

_____ 22. When ventilating a 35-year-old male head trauma patient with a bag-valve mask, it is most effective to do all of the following _except_:
  A. use a device with a volume of 1,000 to 1,600 mL.
  B. use two EMTs to perform the procedure.
  C. position the EMT who is maintaining the mask seal at the patient's head.
  D. maintain the head-tilt, chin-lift maneuver.

_____ 23. When ventilating an unconscious patient, a bag-valve mask is complete if it is used with:
  A. a reservoir bag.
  B. an oral airway.
  C. an oxygen tank and liter flow regulator.
  D. all of these.

_____ 24. If the patient's chest does not rise and fall when using a bag-valve mask, the EMT should do all of the following _except_:
  A. reposition the head and reattempt ventilations.
  B. check for escape of air around the mask.
  C. use an alternative method of artificial ventilation.
  D. increase the rate at which the bag is squeezed.

_____ 25. If the patient has a _____ and needs ventilatory assistance, the best device to use is a _____.
  A. stoma; pocket mask
  B. tracheotomy; positive pressure ventilator
  C. stoma; bag-valve mask
  D. tracheotomy; nasal airway

_____ 26. The flow-restricted, oxygen-powered ventilation device should:
  A. operate in both ordinary and extreme environmental conditions.
  B. have an audible alarm when the relief valve is activated.
  C. have a trigger so two hands can be used to seal the mask.
  D. do all of these.

_____ 27. A technique that is designed to reduce the entry of air into the esophagus during ventilation is the:
  A. jaw-thrust maneuver.   **C.** Sellick maneuver.
  B. hyperventilation technique.   **D.** chest-thrust technique.

_____ 28. When prolonged ventilations need to be done on a patient and there is only one EMT on the airway, you should consider using a(n):
A. nonrebreather mask.
B. automatic transport ventilator.
C. pocket face mask.
D. BVM device.

_____ 29. A fully pressurized oxygen tank should have approximately _____ psi.
A. 1,000
B. 1,500
C. 2,000
D. 2,500

_____ 30. Which *portable* oxygen cylinder, when full, lasts the longest when delivering oxygen?
A. D
B. E
C. A
D. M

_____ 31. Before connecting a regulator to an oxygen supply cylinder, the EMT should:
A. remove the protective seal and then open the valve.
B. stand to the side of the main valve opening and crack the cylinder valve slightly.
C. attach the nonrebreather mask to the flowmeter, then attach to the tank.
D. do all of these.

_____ 32. Humidified oxygen is:
A. not possible in an ambulance.
B. not used for patients on chronic oxygen therapy.
C. not needed in adult patients being transported for short distances.
D. habit forming.

_____ 33. Concerns about the dangers of giving too much oxygen to elderly patients with COPD:
A. are invalid in the out-of-hospital setting of a patient in respiratory distress.
B. have been understated and proven to be a major problem.
C. are invalid when the patient is over the age of 60.
D. are dealt with by using a nonrebreather mask at low flow rates.

_____ 34. Your patient may be having a heart attack. The best method for an EMT to use when giving a high concentration of oxygen to this breathing patient is a:
A. nasal cannula.
B. venturi mask.
C. simple face mask.
D. nonrebreather mask.

_____ 35. The oxygen concentration of a nonrebreather mask is between:
A. 50 and 60 percent.
B. 60 and 70 percent.
C. 70 and 80 percent.
D. 80 and 90 percent.

_____ 36. The flow rate of a nonrebreather mask should be:
A. adjusted so that when the patient inhales, the bag deflates by two-thirds.
B. 12 to 15 liters per minute.
C. adjusted to 6 liters per minute.
D. all of these.

_____ 37. The oxygen concentration of a nasal cannula is between:
A. 4 and 6 percent.
B. 8 and 20 percent.
C. 24 and 44 percent.
D. 50 and 65 percent.

_____ 38. You are treating an elderly patient who fell and injured her ribs. She was found breathing at a rate of 44 and shallowly, yet she is starting to turn cyanotic. Why is this a serious threat to her life?
A. She is inhaling too much oxygen.
B. Her minute volume may be diminished.
C. Her minute volume is excessive.
D. She is exceeding her dead space.

©2012 Pearson Education, Inc.
Emergency Care, 12th Ed.

_____ **39.** What is meant by anatomical dead space?
   A. The maximum amount of room for dying cells in the body
   B. The compartment where tissue swells like edema
   C. Hollow chambers like the sinus
   D. The area in the lungs outside the alveoli

_____ **40.** What is the most important consideration when assessing and managing the breathing of a child?
   A. The chest wall is more rigid and harder to ventilate.
   B. Children use a lot less oxygen than an adult uses.
   C. The trachea is softer and more flexible.
   D. All of these are equally important.

COMPLETE THE FOLLOWING

1. To determine the signs of adequate breathing, the EMT should:

   A. _____

   B. _____

   C. _____

   D. _____

   E. _____

2. To determine the signs of adequate artificial ventilation, the EMT should:

   A. _____

   B. _____

3. The patient may have inadequate artificial ventilation when the EMT notices:

   A. _____

   B. _____

INSIDE/OUTSIDE: RESPIRATORY DISTRESS TO RESPIRATORY FAILURE

1. When a patient is having an asthma attack and the respiratory system is trying to compensate, what happens to the respiratory rate?

2. When the fight-or-flight response is stimulated, what happens to the blood vessels in the arms and legs?

3. Why does the patient have wheezes when you listen with your stethoscope?

4. When the patient starts to get very anxious, what is the likely cause?

5. When the asthmatic patient starts to get tired, what is the potential result?

STREET SCENES DISCUSSION

Review the Street Scene on page 241 of your textbook. Then answer the following questions.

1. If the patient had no gag reflex, what airway adjunct would you consider using? How would you insert it?

2. If the patient vomits during BVM ventilation, what should you do?

3. If the patient's pulse had not increased so quickly, should you have called for an ALS intercept? Why or why not?

CASE STUDY

This case study is designed to help you apply the concepts presented in this textbook. The case study describes a situation you might encounter in the field and is followed by questions about the situation. The questions require you to explain and apply key concepts from your reading.

▶ **THE COMPLICATED AIRWAY: THE SELF-INFLICTED SHOOTING**

Your unit and the police are dispatched to the scene of an attempted suicide with shots fired. Apparently the call was placed by a family member, who was called by the patient threatening to do harm to himself with a handgun. The police arrive before you and advise that the scene is secure (safe) and that you should respond directly to the scene, which is a private home in a suburban community. Upon arrival, you find a 45-year-old male lying with his face covered with blood. He is moaning, and his chest and abdomen appear to be moving as he breathes. After donning protective gloves, mask, and goggles, both you and your partners carefully provide manual stabilization of the neck and log roll the patient onto a long backboard. What is revealed is a mandible and tongue that are severely lacerated, and the mouth and nose are bubbling with blood as the patient attempts to breathe.

1. How should you open the airway of this patient?

©2012 Pearson Education, Inc.
Emergency Care, 12th Ed.

2. (A) Does this patient need to be suctioned? (B) If so, what is the maximum amount of time to accomplish this procedure?

   A.

   B.

3. Should an airway adjunct be used on this patient?

Once the patient's airway is opened and cleared, you need to oxygenate this patient. He has no other obvious injuries, yet you are treating him for a possible spinal injury due to the impact of the bullet and his backward fall from his desk chair during the incident. The police think that this is why he shot his chin instead of his brain during the suicide attempt. You evaluate the patient's breathing rate as 28, shallow, and labored, and his pulse as 120, weak, and regular.

4. What device should be used to administer oxygen to this patient?

5. (A) What is the proper liter flow to set the regulator for the device you chose in question number 4? (B) If your unit has a pulse oximeter, should it be used?

   A.

   B.

6. Your portable D cylinder was full at the beginning of the shift and this is your first call. (A) How many liters are in the tank? (B) How much pressure is in the tank? (C) How much time can you expect to get out of the tank, considering your service's policy is to refill tanks at 200 psi?

   A.

   B.

   C.

7. As you prepare to transport the patient, you continue to suction him, making sure not to exceed (A) _____ seconds per attempt because, as you suction, you are also removing (B) _____.
(C) Which would be better to use: a rigid-tip or a flexible catheter?

A.

B.

C.

8. The patient has a blood pressure of 100/70 mmHg and his oxygen saturation is 95 percent, so you decide his priority is (A) [high, low]. The major problem with this patient is his (B) _____. He should be transported (C) [right away, in a few minutes] to the (D) [local hospital, trauma center].

A.

B.

C.

D.

9. From your knowledge of your EMS system, what ALS (advanced life support) treatment(s) might be helpful to this patient if you can arrange for an ALS intercept?

10. What should you do if you hear hissing or bubbling around the mask as you ventilate?

EMT SKILL PERFORMANCE CHECKLISTS

▶ **MOUTH-TO-MASK VENTILATION (P. 210)**

❑ Take Standard Precautions.

❑ Connect one-way valve to mask.

©2012 Pearson Education, Inc.
Emergency Care, 12th Ed.

❏ Connect oxygen to inlet on face mask. Oxygen should be run at 15 lpm.

❏ Kneel about 18 inches above the head of the supine patient.

❏ Open the airway (manually or with adjunct).

❏ Position mask on patient's face so that the apex is over bridge of nose and the base is between lower lip and prominence of chin.

❏ Position thumbs over top half of mask, index and middle fingers over the bottom half.

❏ Use ring and middle fingers to bring the patient's jaw up to the mask and maintain head-tilt, chin-lift. *Tilt the head back as if you were trying to stand the patient on his or her head!*

❏ Ventilate over 1 second to achieve visible chest rise.

❏ Remove your mouth from the port to allow for passive exhalation.

NOTE: Do not delay mouth-to-mask ventilation if oxygen is not immediately available.

▶ **TWO-RESCUER BAG-VALVE MASK VENTILATION (P. 214)**

❏ Take Standard Precautions.

❏ Open the medical patient's airway using head-tilt, chin-lift maneuver.

❏ Suction and insert an oropharyngeal airway.

❏ Select correct bag-valve-mask size (adult, child, or infant). A pop-off valve is not acceptable!

❏ Kneel approximately 18 inches above the head of the supine patient.

❏ Position mask on the patient's face so that the apex is over bridge of nose and the base is between the lower lip and prominence of chin.

❏ Position thumbs over top half of mask, index and middle fingers over bottom half.

❏ Use ring and middle fingers to bring the patient's jaw up to mask and maintain head-tilt, chin-lift. *Tilt the head back as if you were trying to stand patient on his or her head!*

❏ The second rescuer should connect bag to mask, if this is not already done. While you maintain mask seal, the second rescuer should squeeze the bag with two hands, providing a ventilation over 1 second to achieve visible chest rise.

❏ The second rescuer should release pressure on the bag and let the patient exhale passively. While this occurs, the oxygen reservoir is refilling.

NOTE: This technique may be used for a trauma patient by combining a jaw-thrust maneuver with manual stabilization of the head and neck.

▶ **PREPARING THE OXYGEN DELIVERY SYSTEM (P. 216)**

❏ Select desired cylinder. Check label and hydrostat date.

❏ Place the cylinder in an upright position and stand to one side.

❏ Remove the plastic wrapper or cap protecting the cylinder outlet.

❏ Keep the plastic washer (true for some setups).

❏ Crack the main valve for 1 second to clean it out.

❏ Select the correct pressure regulator and flowmeter.

❏ Place cylinder valve gasket on regulator oxygen port.

- ❏ Make certain that the pressure regulator is closed.
- ❏ Align pins or thread by hand.
- ❏ Tighten T-screw for pin yoke.
- ❏ Tighten with a wrench for a threaded outlet.
- ❏ Attach tubing and delivery device.

▶ OXYGEN ADMINISTRATION—NONREBREATHER MASK (P. 229)

- ❏ Take Standard Precautions.
- ❏ Assemble regulator onto tank.
- ❏ Open main valve on tank.
- ❏ Check for leaks.
- ❏ Check tank pressure.
- ❏ Attach nonrebreather mask.
- ❏ Adjust liter flow to 12 to 15 liters per minute.
- ❏ Prefill reservoir.
- ❏ Apply and adjust mask to the patient's face, explaining the need for oxygen.
- ❏ Secure tank during transport.

▶ OXYGEN ADMINISTRATION—NASAL CANNULA (P. 230)

- ❏ Take Standard Precautions.
- ❏ Assemble regulator onto tank.
- ❏ Open main valve on tank.
- ❏ Check for leaks.
- ❏ Check tank pressure.
- ❏ Attach nasal cannula to regulator.
- ❏ Place nasal prongs into the patient's nose, and adjust tubing for comfort.
- ❏ Adjust liter flow to 1 to 6 liters per minute.
- ❏ Secure tank during transport.

▶ DISCONTINUING OXYGEN ADMINISTRATION (P. 228)

- ❏ Remove delivery device from patient.
- ❏ Turn off the liter flow rate.
- ❏ Close the main valve.
- ❏ Remove the delivery tubing.
- ❏ Bleed the flowmeter.
- ❏ Change the tank before the volume reaches 200 psi or less (or change per your service policy).

Interim Exam 1

Use the answer sheet on pp. 94–95 to complete this exam. It is perforated, so it can be removed easily from this workbook.

1. Most EMT training programs are based on standards developed by the:
   A. American Red Cross (ARC).
   B. American Heart Association (AHA).
   C. National Highway Transportation Safety Administration (NHTSA).
   D. National Institutes of Health (NIH).

2. An EMT can inspire patient confidence and cooperation by:
   A. transporting the patient from the scene to a hospital.
   B. providing patient care without regard for her own personal safety.
   C. telling the patient that everything will be all right.
   D. being pleasant, cooperative, and sincere, and a good listener.

3. If an on-duty EMT fails to provide the standard of care and if this failure causes harm or injury to the patient, the EMT may be accused of:
   A. assault.
   B. abandonment.
   C. negligence.
   D. breach of promise.

4. You are treating a conscious and mentally competent adult patient who wants to refuse your care and transport to the hospital. This refusal must be _____ and documented.
   A. implied   C. involuntary
   B. actual   D. informed

5. The EMT is authorized to treat and transport an unconscious patient because of the legal consideration known as _____ consent.
   A. applied   C. triage
   B. implied   D. immunity

6. A child falls off a trampoline at an elementary school and twists her ankle. Because the parents are not present, the child's consent is:
   A. not needed.
   B. actual.
   C. implied.
   D. meaningless.

7. In some states, _____ help protect the off-duty EMT from lawsuits when stopping at the scene of a collision to offer assistance.
   A. professional associations
   B. blanket insurance policies
   C. Good Samaritan laws
   D. abandonment laws

8. Each of the following is the responsibility of an EMT at a hazardous-materials (hazmat) incident *except*:
   A. entering hazmat scenes with SCBA.
   B. protecting yourself and others.
   C. recognizing potential problems.
   D. notifying the hazardous-materials response team.

9. The form of infection control that assumes that all body fluids should be considered potentially infectious is:
   A. infectious disease.
   B. Standard Precautions.
   C. immunity.
   D. universal precautions.

10. When planning to lift a patient, all of the following are important considerations for the EMT *except*:
    A. the weight of the patient.
    B. one's physical characteristics.
    C. communicating with one's partner.
    D. the distance the patient needs to be carried.

11. When lifting an injured patient, the EMT should:
    A. keep the back loose and knees locked.
    B. twist or attempt to make moves other than the lift.
    C. use the leg muscles to do the lift.
    D. try not to talk to her or his partner.

12. You are treating a 45-year-old male who twisted his ankle in the upstairs bathroom. To carry this patient on the stairs, you should:
    A. keep the stretcher as level as possible.
    B. use a long backboard at all times.
    C. use a stair chair whenever possible.
    D. do all of these.

13. Ways an EMT can avoid a potential back injury include all the following *except*:
    A. push, rather than pull, a load.
    B. keep the back locked in while lifting.
    C. keep arms straight when pulling.
    D. push or pull from a kneeling position if the weight is below waist level.

14. An emergency move is required in each of the following situations *except* when:
    A. the scene is hazardous.
    B. care of life-threatening conditions requires repositioning.
    C. other patients who have life threats must be reached.
    D. the patient is unconscious.

15. Which of the following is the greatest danger to the patient in an emergency move?
    A. A spinal injury may be aggravated.
    B. Bleeding may increase after movement.
    C. The airway may become obstructed.
    D. There is no danger associated with an emergency move.

16. A method of lifting and carrying a patient in which one EMT slips hands under the patient's armpits and grasps the wrists while another EMT grasps the patient's knees is called the:
    A. direct ground lift.
    B. extremity lift.
    C. draw-sheet method.
    D. direct carry method.

17. Your patient is a medical patient with a suspected drug overdose. He is lying supine on your stretcher, and you have been maintaining his airway. When moving him from the ambulance stretcher to the hospital stretcher, you probably will use the:
    A. cradle carry.
    B. modified draw-sheet method.
    C. direct ground lift.
    D. extremity lift.

18. To load the wheeled ambulance stretcher into the ambulance, the two EMTs should position themselves on _____ of the stretcher.
    A. opposite sides
    B. opposite ends
    C. the same side
    D. one end and one side

19. You are treating a 28-year-old conscious diabetic who has an altered level of consciousness. She is lying on the floor at the moment. To move her from the floor to a stair chair, use the:
    A. indirect carry.   C. slide transfer.
    B. extremity lift.   D. chair lift.

20. Drags are used only in emergencies because they:
    A. do not protect the patient's neck and spine.
    B. require excessive energy from the EMT.
    C. may injure the EMT's back.
    D. provide full immobilization.

21. To maintain balance when lifting a patient-carrying device, it is best to use _____ rescuers to carry the device.
    A. three
    B. an even number of
    C. an odd number of
    D. bystanders and

22. You are treating the driver of a vehicle involved in a collision. He is a 22-year-old male who requires immediate airway and bleeding control. You are unable to provide this treatment in the vehicle. You should:
    A. check the patient's vital signs.
    B. make an urgent move.
    C. remove the patient on a short backboard.
    D. do all of these.

23. Your patient is an unconscious adult female stroke patient. Which carry is considered very difficult to use with an unconscious person?
    A. Cradle   C. Shoulder
    B. Three-rescuer   D. Piggyback

24. The _____ carry must be performed in one unbroken sweep.
    A. pack strap   C. firefighter's
    B. front piggyback   D. four-rescuer

25. A canvas or rubberized stretcher that can be used to move a patient through a narrow hallway or restricted area is called a _____ stretcher.
    A. basket
    B. portable
    C. flexible
    D. wheeled-ambulance

26. A patient with obvious spinal injuries is found on the floor of a burning building. The EMT rates the situation hazardous but not yet dire. Alone and without special equipment, the EMT should use the:
    A. cradle carry.
    B. clothes drag.
    C. firefighter's carry.
    D. pack-strap method.

27. The patient-carrying device of choice for the 20-year-old male who is dizzy but not injured is the _____ stretcher.
    A. portable ambulance
    B. wire basket
    C. wheeled ambulance
    D. slat

28. If you are an EMT with a service that does not provide the appropriate personal protective equipment, why should you serve as an advocate for this equipment?
   A. Your crew members could be injured unnecessarily.
   B. You could be seriously injured.
   C. An injured EMT is of little help to the patient.
   D. All of these are reasons to serve as an advocate.

29. During an EMS call, a lethal threat is made by the 24-year-old intoxicated male. The EMT should first:
   A. retreat to a safe area.
   B. radio for assistance.
   C. reevaluate the situation.
   D. remedy the situation.

30. Of the different types of stress, which is a positive form that helps the EMT work under pressure and respond effectively?
   A. Eumulative stress
   B. Eustress
   C. Distress
   D. Critical incident stress

31. When responding to a violent situation, observation begins when you:
   A. enter the scene.
   B. exit the ambulance.
   C. enter the neighborhood.
   D. arrive at the patient's side.

32. To ensure crew safety, one member of the crew should always:
   A. remain in the ambulance.
   B. carry a portable radio.
   C. wear a bulletproof vest.
   D. carry a canister of pepper gas.

33. While you are treating a patient with a severely bleeding forearm, the patient's pet dog appears. The patient states, "He won't hurt you. He's very friendly." Your best course of action would be to:
   A. have your partner observe the dog closely while you treat the patient.
   B. quickly control the bleeding; then have the dog locked in another room.
   C. ignore the dog because the patient assures you it is friendly and will not harm you.
   D. do all of these.

34. If a patient refuses care and then becomes unconscious, it is best for the EMT to:
   A. refuse to treat or transport the patient.
   B. ask a family member for permission to treat.

35. An advantage of the advance directive is that:
   A. the patient is not involved in making a decision about her treatment.
   B. the patient's expressed wishes may be followed.
   C. no matter what the family says, CPR is not given.
   D. it protects the EMT from charges of negligence.

36. In most cases, the oral wishes of the patient's family to withhold care are:
   A. all that is needed to stop CPR from being initiated.
   B. all that is needed to stop CPR once it is initiated.
   C. not a reason to withhold medical care.
   D. not sufficient unless they are given in writing.

37. Some EMTs participate in activities that attract legal actions, while most EMTs are rarely involved in legal entanglements. You can prevent most lawsuits if you:
   A. provide care within the scope of your practice.
   B. properly document your care.
   C. are courteous and respectful to all your patients.
   D. do all of these.

38. The negligent EMT may be required to pay for all of the following *except* the patient's:
   A. lost wages.
   B. medical expenses.
   C. pain and suffering.
   D. health insurance costs.

39. Which of the following is *not* a function of the musculoskeletal system?
   A. It gives the body shape.
   B. It protects the internal organs.
   C. It provides for body movement.
   D. It regulates body temperature.

40. The superior portion of the sternum is called the:
   A. xiphoid process.   C. manubrium.
   B. sternal body.   D. clavicle.

41. A young girl fell while ice skating and injured the protrusion on the inside of the ankle. The medical term for this location is the:
   A. acromion.
   B. medial malleolus.
   C. lateral malleolus.
   D. calcaneus.

42. The heart muscle has a property called
_____. This means that the heart
has the ability to generate and conduct electrical impulses on its own.
   A. contractility
   B. automaticity
   C. involuntary contraction
   D. conductibility

43. A division of the peripheral nervous system
that controls involuntary motor functions is
called the _____ nervous system.
   A. autonomic   C. sensory
   B. central   D. motor

44. When in the anatomical position, a person is
facing:
   A. away from you.   C. face down.
   B. the observer.   D. face up.

45. In the anatomical position, the person's
palms will be facing:
   A. forward.   C. upward.
   B. backward.   D. downward.

46. An anatomical term that is occasionally used
to refer to the sole of the foot is:
   A. calcaneus.   C. dorsal.
   B. ventral.   D. plantar.

47. The bones of the cheek are called the
_____ bones.
   A. orbit
   B. maxillae
   C. zygomatic
   D. mandible

48. The heart is _____ to the
stomach.
   A. distal
   B. medial
   C. proximal
   D. superior

49. When comparing body structure positions,
the knees are said to be _____ to
the toes, and the toes are _____
to the knees.
   A. inferior; superior
   B. proximal; distal
   C. distal; dorsal
   D. anterior; posterior

50. A patient found lying on her back is in the
_____ position.
   A. anatomical
   B. prone
   C. supine
   D. lateral recumbent

51. To assist in describing the location of abdominal organs, we divide the abdomen
into _____ parts.
   A. two
   B. three
   C. four
   D. five

52. Your 18-year-old male patient has severe
burns of the entire front (anterior) surface of
the torso. The torso of the body is composed of the abdomen, pelvis, and:
   A. thorax.
   B. upper arms and legs.
   C. extremities.
   D. head.

53. The heart is located in the center of the
_____ cavity.
   A. thoracic
   B. cranial
   C. pelvic
   D. cardiac

54. The structure that divides the chest cavity
from the abdominal cavity is the:
   A. meninges.
   B. duodenum.
   C. diaphragm.
   D. spinal column.

55. The anatomical name for the kneecap is the:
   A. ilium.
   B. malleolus.
   C. patella.
   D. phalange.

56. The cranium consists of the:
   A. facial bones.
   B. mandible and maxillae.
   C. top, back, and sides of the skull.
   D. zygomatic bones.

57. The highest point in the shoulder is the:
   A. acromion process.
   B. humerus.
   C. metatarsal.
   D. clavicle.

58. At the scene of a collision, an off-duty EMT
provides care to the patient, acting in good
faith and to the best of her abilities. In many
states, this EMT is protected from care-related lawsuits by _____ laws.
   A. applied consent
   B. total immunity
   C. Good Samaritan
   D. jeopardy

©2012 Pearson Education, Inc.
Emergency Care, 12th Ed.

59. When confronted with an unconscious minor without parents or a legal guardian present, the EMT should:
   A. seek a physician's approval before beginning care.
   B. consider consent for care to be implied and begin care.
   C. ask the child for consent and begin care.
   D. consider consent to be applied and begin care.

60. The legal concept of negligence requires that three circumstances must be demonstrated. Which of the following is *not* one of the three circumstances?
   A. The EMT had a duty to act.
   B. The EMT committed a breach of duty.
   C. The EMT had a local duty.
   D. The breach of duty caused harm.

61. A person lying on his stomach with his face down is in the _____ position.
   A. supine
   B. prone
   C. coma
   D. recovery

62. As an EMT, you have been assigned to take a terminally ill patient back and forth to chemotherapy multiple times a week for the next few weeks. You realize that the patient has been going through emotional stages in the following order:
   A. depression, bargaining, denial, acceptance, anger.
   B. acceptance, rage, depression, acceptance, bargaining.
   C. denial, anger, bargaining, depression, acceptance.
   D. bargaining, acceptance, denial, anger, depression.

63. In 1970, the _____ was founded to establish professional standards for EMS personnel.
   A. American Medical Association
   B. National Registry of Emergency Medical Technicians
   C. National Highway Traffic Safety Administration
   D. U.S. Department of Transportation

64. Safe, reliable transportation is a critical component of an EMS system. Most patients can be transported effectively by:
   A. airplane.
   B. helicopter.
   C. rescue vehicle.
   D. ambulance.

65. An _____ is a national-level EMT who has been trained to start IVs, perform advanced airway techniques, and administer some medicines beyond the EMT.
   A. EMT-First Responder
   B. EMT-Intermediate
   C. EMT-Critical Care
   D. EMT-Paramedic

66. A continuous self-review with the purpose of identifying and correcting aspects of the EMS system that require improvement is called:
   A. standing orders.
   B. quality improvement.
   C. protocols.
   D. medical direction.

67. A physician who assumes the ultimate responsibility for the patient-care aspects of the EMS system is called the:
   A. Designated Agent.
   B. Medical Director.
   C. Off-line Director.
   D. Primary Care Physician.

68. Situations that are higher risks of a lawsuit against an EMS agency are:
   A. patients who refuse care.
   B. on-scene deaths.
   C. cardiac arrest cases.
   D. pedestrians struck by cars.

69. The legal extent or limits of the EMT's job are formally defined by the:
   A. patient.
   B. DOT curriculum.
   C. state.
   D. scope of practice.

70. Which is *not* generally considered a sign or symptom of stress?
   A. Decisiveness
   B. Guilt
   C. Loss of interest in work
   D. Difficulty sleeping

71. All the following are types of calls that have a high potential for causing excessive stress *except*:
   A. calls involving infants and children.
   B. patients with severe injuries.
   C. cases of abuse and neglect.
   D. motor vehicle collisions.

72. Lifestyle changes that can help the EMT deal with stress include all of the following *except*:
   A. exercise to burn off tension.
   B. increased consumption of fatty foods.
   C. decreased consumption of caffeine.
   D. decreased consumption of alcohol.

73. Changes in your professional life to reduce and prevent stress can include:
   A. requesting a change of shift or location.
   B. taking on another part-time position.
   C. working additional overtime shifts.
   D. requesting a busier location.

74. One of the functions of the integumentary system is to:
   A. regulate the diameter of the blood vessels in the circulation.
   B. eliminate excess oxygen into the atmosphere.
   C. allow environmental water to carefully enter the body.
   D. protect the body from the environment, bacteria, and other organisms.

75. Stress after a major EMS incident is:
   A. unusual and unexpected.
   B. a sign of weakness.
   C. normal and to be expected.
   D. part of the grieving process.

76. Retreating to a world of one's own after hearing one is going to die is a result of the stage of grief called:
   A. bargaining.   C. denial.
   B. depression.   D. anxiety.

77. When a patient's lower extremities are trapped under a farm tractor, the blood supply is diminished to the cells in the legs. This injury can result in:
   A. no lactic acids being produced.
   B. anaerobic metabolism.
   C. no carbon dioxide being produced.
   D. none of these.

78. A disease that is spread by exposure to an open wound or sore of an infected individual is caused by a(n) _____ pathogen.
   A. universal   C. bloodborne
   B. airborne   D. infectious

79. An infection that causes inflammation of the liver is called:
   A. meningitis.   C. typhoid.
   B. tuberculosis.   D. hepatitis.

80. A disease spread by inhaling or absorbing droplets from the air through the eyes, nose, or mouth is considered:
   A. bloodborne.
   B. noncommunicable.
   C. airborne.
   D. viral.

81. The communicable disease that kills the most health workers every year in the United States is:
   A. tuberculosis.
   B. HIV/AIDS.
   C. meningitis.
   D. hepatitis B virus.

82. Always assume that any patient with a:
   A. cold has a bloodborne disease.
   B. productive cough has TB.
   C. fever has typhoid.
   D. rash has measles.

83. Which of the following is *not* true about the human immunodeficiency virus (HIV)?
   A. It attacks the immune system.
   B. It doesn't survive well outside the human body.
   C. It can be introduced through puncture wounds.
   D. It is an airborne pathogen.

84. Your patient has hepatitis B. You are accidentally stuck with a needle that has some of this patient's infected blood on it. Your chance of contracting the disease is about:
   A. 10 percent.
   B. 20 percent.
   C. 30 percent.
   D. 40 percent.

85. Your patient has HIV. You are accidentally stuck with a needle that has some infected blood on it. Your chance of contracting the disease is about:
   A. 0.5 percent.
   B. 5 percent.
   C. 10 percent.
   D. 15 percent.

86. If you think your patient has TB, you should wear the usual personal protective equipment plus a:
   A. surgeon's mask.
   B. gown.
   C. HEPA or N-95 respirator.
   D. Tyvek suit.

87. Instead of providing mouth-to-mouth ventilations on the nonbreathing patient, the EMT, when acting alone, should use a(n):
   A. pocket mask with a one-way valve.
   B. one-way valve.
   C. bag-valve mask.
   D. endotracheal tube.

©2012 Pearson Education, Inc.
Emergency Care, 12th Ed.

88. Which method of infection control reduces exposure to yourself, your crew, and your next patient?
   A. Wearing a HEPA or N-95 respirator
   B. Taking universal precautions
   C. Hand washing after each patient contact
   D. None of these

89. An act that establishes procedures through which emergency response workers can find out if they have been exposed to life-threatening infectious diseases is called:
   A. OSHA 1910.1030.
   B. the Ryan White CARE Act.
   C. AIDS Protection Act.
   D. OSHA 1910.120.

90. Each emergency response employer must develop a plan that identifies and documents job classifications and tasks in which there is the possibility of exposure to potentially infectious body fluids. This is required by:
   A. OSHA 1910.1030.
   B. the Ryan White CARE Act.
   C. the AIDS Protection Act.
   D. OSHA 1910.120.

91. Every employer of EMTs must provide free of charge:
   A. a yearly physical examination.
   B. a life insurance policy.
   C. universal health insurance.
   D. hepatitis B vaccination.

92. Engineering controls that prevent the spread of bloodborne diseases include:
   A. pocket masks.
   B. needle containers.
   C. disposable airway equipment.
   D. all of these.

93. Which of the following is *not* required by the OSHA bloodborne pathogen standard?
   A. Postexposure evaluation and follow-up
   B. Personal protective equipment
   C. HEPA or N-95 respirator
   D. Housekeeping controls and labeling

94. Which of the following is *not* considered a high-risk area for TB?
   A. Correctional facilities
   B. Daycare centers
   C. Homeless shelters
   D. Nursing homes

95. As you near an emergency scene, you should:
   A. sound your siren to broadcast your arrival.
   B. go straight to the front door.
   C. secure the scene as quickly as possible.
   D. turn off your lights and siren.

96. If anyone at the scene is in possession of a weapon, the EMT should:
   A. notify the police immediately.
   B. ask the person to give it to you.
   C. ignore the person with the weapon.
   D. advise the person to leave the scene.

97. The reduction of breathing to the point where oxygen intake is not sufficient to support life is called:
   A. respiratory failure.
   B. anoxic metabolism.
   C. respiratory arrest.
   D. respiratory support.

98. Adequate signs of breathing include all of the following *except*:
   A. equal expansion of both sides of the chest.
   B. air moving in and out of the nose.
   C. blue or gray skin coloration.
   D. present and equal breath sounds.

99. The widening of the nostrils of the nose with respirations is called:
   A. hyperventilating.
   B. nasal flaring.
   C. nasal gurgling.
   D. wheezing.

100. The condition in which a patient's skin or lips are blue or gray is called:
   A. stridor.   C. pallor.
   B. cyanosis.   D. anemia.

101. If a patient is unable to speak in full sentences, this could be a sign of:
   A. complete airway blockage.
   B. snoring.
   C. shortness of breath.
   D. respiratory arrest.

102. The procedures by which life-threatening respiratory problems are initially treated by the EMT include all of the following *except*:
   A. opening and maintaining the airway.
   B. inserting an endotracheal tube immediately.
   C. providing supplemental oxygen to the breathing patient.
   D. ensuring a clear airway with frequent suctioning.

103. You are assessing the airway of an unconscious male patient. You recall that most airway problems are caused by:
   A. the tongue.
   B. asthma.
   C. shock.
   D. the epiglottis.

104. You are treating a patient who fell down a flight of metal stairs. Which maneuver is most appropriate for an unconscious patient found lying at the bottom of a stairwell?
- **A.** Head-tilt, chin-lift
- **B.** Head-tilt, neck-lift
- **C.** Jaw-pull lift
- **D.** Jaw-thrust

105. You are managing a 34-year-old male who you suspect has had a narcotic overdose. His respirations are very slow and shallow, and you will need to assist them. When choosing a means of ventilating a patient, your *last* choice would be:
- **A.** flow-restricted, oxygen-powered ventilation device.
- **B.** one-rescuer bag-valve mask.
- **C.** two-rescuer bag-valve mask.
- **D.** mouth-to-mask with high-flow supplemental oxygen.

106. Artificial ventilation may be inadequate if the:
- **A.** chest rises with each ventilation.
- **B.** heart rate returns to normal.
- **C.** rate of ventilation is too fast or too slow.
- **D.** skin becomes warm and dry.

107. The standard respiratory fitting on a bag-valve mask that ensures a proper fit with other respiratory equipment is:
- **A.** 15/22 mm.
- **B.** 10/14 mm.
- **C.** 5/20 mm.
- **D.** 20/26 mm.

108. A bag-valve mask should have or be all of the following *except*:
- **A.** a self-refilling shell.
- **B.** a clear face mask.
- **C.** easily cleared and sterilized.
- **D.** a pop-off valve.

109. The proper oxygen flow rate when ventilating a patient with a BVM is _____ liters per minute.
- **A.** 5
- **B.** 10
- **C.** 15
- **D.** 20

110. According to the American Heart Association guidelines, when ventilating a patient with a bag mask that has supplementary oxygen, the volume administered should be:
- **A.** 400 milliliters.
- **B.** sufficient to achieve visible chest rise.
- **C.** 800 milliliters.
- **D.** as much as possible during the 1-second time frame.

111. The first step in providing artificial ventilation of a stoma breather is to:
- **A.** leave the head and neck in a neutral position.
- **B.** ventilate at the appropriate rate for the patient's age.
- **C.** clear any mucus or secretions obstructing the stoma.
- **D.** establish a seal using a pediatric-sized mask.

112. A flow-restricted, oxygen-powered ventilation device should have all of the following features *except*:
- **A.** an audible alarm when ventilation is activated.
- **B.** a trigger that enables the rescuer to use both hands.
- **C.** a peak flow rate of up to 40 liters per minute.
- **D.** a rugged design and construction.

113. The two most common airway adjuncts for the EMT to use are the oropharyngeal airway and the:
- **A.** nasal cannula.
- **B.** nasopharyngeal airway.
- **C.** endotracheal tube.
- **D.** Yankauer.

114. An oropharyngeal airway should be inserted in:
- **A.** all patients with inadequate breathing.
- **B.** trauma patients with a gag reflex.
- **C.** medical patients with a gag reflex.
- **D.** all unconscious patients with no gag reflex.

115. When suctioning a 19-year-old patient who you suspect has bleeding into his throat, you should:
- **A.** suction on the way in and the way out.
- **B.** avoid using eyewear or a mask.
- **C.** never suction for longer than 15 seconds.
- **D.** hypoventilate prior to suctioning.

116. The emergency situation in which there is a failure of the cardiovascular system to provide sufficient blood to all the vital tissues is called:
- **A.** respiratory arrest.
- **B.** respiratory failure.
- **C.** shock.
- **D.** cardiac arrest.

117. An insufficiency in the supply of oxygen to the body's tissues is called:
- **A.** anoxia.
- **B.** no-oxia.
- **C.** hypoxia.
- **D.** cyanosis.

118. Before the oxygen cylinder's pressure gauge reads a minimum of _____ psi, you must switch to a fresh cylinder.
   A. 200
   B. 400
   C. 800
   D. 1,000

119. When handling oxygen cylinders, the EMT should do all of the following *except*:
   A. have the cylinders hydrostatically tested every 5 years.
   B. ensure that valve seat inserts and gaskets are in good condition.
   C. store reserve cylinders in a warm, humid room.
   D. use medical-grade oxygen in all cylinders.

120. The best way to deliver high-concentration oxygen to a breathing patient is to use a:
   A. nonrebreather mask.
   B. partial rebreather mask.
   C. bag-valve mask.
   D. nasal cannula.

121. A nasal cannula provides between _____ percent and _____ percent oxygen concentrations.
   A. 10; 21
   B. 24; 44
   C. 36; 58
   D. 72; 96

122. You are assessing a 54-year-old woman who is unconscious and has a noisy upper airway. If she has dentures, during airway procedures the EMT should:
   A. remove them right away.
   B. leave them in unless they are loose.
   C. remove the teeth one at a time.
   D. hold them in place with a free hand.

123. When managing the airway of a child, an airway consideration you should remember is that:
   A. the mouth and nose are smaller and more easily obstructed.
   B. the chest wall is firmer in a child.
   C. the trachea is wider and less easily obstructed.
   D. all of these are airway considerations in a child.

124. You are dealing with a patient who is in severe distress from a life-threatening asthma attack. If breathing stops completely, the patient is in:
   A. respiratory arrest.
   B. ventilatory reduction.
   C. artificial ventilation.
   D. respiratory failure.

125. Which ventilation device is contraindicated in infants and children?
   A. Bag-valve mask
   B. Pediatric pocket mask
   C. Flow-restricted, oxygen-powered ventilation device
   D. Nonrebreather mask

126. A device that allows the control of oxygen in liters per minute is called a:
   A. flowmeter.
   B. G tank.
   C. humidifier.
   D. reservoir.

127. A type of flowmeter that has no gauge and allows for the adjustment of flow in liters per minute and in stepped increments is called a:
   A. Bourdon gauge flowmeter.
   B. constant flow selector valve.
   C. humidifier.
   D. pressure compensated flowmeter.

128. Why do some EMS systems use humidified oxygen?
   A. Lack of humidity can dry out the patient's mucous membranes.
   B. It provides a reservoir for the oxygen.
   C. It limits the risk of infection.
   D. It is helpful when transporting patients short distances.

129. A patient in the end stage of a respiratory disease may have switched over to:
   A. hyperventilation syndrome.
   B. hyperbaric therapy.
   C. hypoxic drive.
   D. carbon dioxide drive.

130. You are talking with a patient and he states that he has had COPD for the past 10 years. What is COPD?
   A. A type of shock
   B. A type of ventilation
   C. A mechanism of breathing
   D. Chronic pulmonary disease

131. When using an air mattress, the patient is placed on the device and the air is _____ by a pump. The mattress will then form a _____ and conforming surface around the patient.
   A. inflated; rigid
   B. withdrawn; soft
   C. inflated; soft
   D. withdrawn; rigid

132. The body system that is responsible for the breakdown of food into absorbable forms is called the _____ system.
   A. urinary
   C. digestive
   B. nervous
   D. integumentary

133. A stress reaction that involves either physical or psychological behavior manifested days or weeks after an incident is called a(n):
   A. cumulative stress disorder.
   B. burnout.
   C. post-traumatic stress disorder.
   D. acute stress reaction.

134. An agency privacy officer is required by the:
   A. Ryan White Law.
   B. Health Insurance Portability and Accountability Act.
   C. National Fire Protection Association Standards.
   D. Privacy Control Act of 2002.

135. When an adult patient is breathing at a respiratory rate of 12 times a minute, you would expect that the minute volume would be approximately _____ mL per minute.
   A. 3,000
   C. 5,000
   B. 4,500
   D. 6,000

136. Your patient is a 45-year-old female who has been vomiting and has had diarrhea for the past week. There is a danger that she may have a condition called:
   A. extremity edema.
   B. an excess of body fluid.
   C. dehydration.
   D. all of these.

137. You question an elderly man sitting on a bench in the park. He has a respiratory complaint, and he speaks in short, two- or three-word sentences. Is this significant?
   A. Yes, he is probably very short of breath.
   B. No, elderly patients always talk slowly.
   C. No, he is probably always like that.
   D. Yes, he probably has a complete airway obstruction.

138. Why can nasal congestion be a major problem in the first few months of life?
   A. Because the liver is so large in patients in this age group.
   B. Because children in this age group are primarily nasal breathers.
   C. Because it is an indication of life-threatening airway compromise.
   D. Because children in this age group breathe with their diaphragm.

139. When the mother strokes the infant's lips and the baby starts sucking, this is a nervous system reflex known as the _____ reflex.
   A. Moro
   B. sucking
   C. palmar
   D. rooting

140. The adolescent years are the beginning of:
   A. better decision-making skills.
   B. nasal breathing.
   C. self-destructive behaviors.
   D. all of these.

141. You are treating a patient who was involved in a serious accident. Based on the leading causes of death, what age group is this patient most likely to be in?
   A. Infant
   B. School age
   C. Adolescent
   D. Young adult

142. Serious conflicts occur in families as the issues of control and independence collide with children in which age group?
   A. Toddler
   B. Preschool
   C. School age
   D. Adolescent

143. Girls are usually finished growing by the age of:
   A. 14.
   C. 18.
   B. 16.
   D. 20.

144. You are examining an elderly woman sitting on a park bench. She is sitting forward with her elbows outward and speaking in short, choppy sentences. Is this significant in her history?
   A. No, she is probably always like that.
   B. Yes, she is probably short of breath.
   C. No, elderly patients like to sit forward like that.
   D. Yes, she probably has a spine injury.

145. You have been called to a restaurant for a patient who collapsed at the dinner table. According to a family member, she did not strike her head as she slid out of the chair when she went unconscious. To open her airway, the EMT should use a _____ maneuver.
   A. modified jaw-thrust
   B. head-tilt, chin-lift
   C. head-tilt, neck-lift
   D. modified chin-lift

©2012 Pearson Education, Inc.
Emergency Care, 12th Ed.

146. A nasopharyngeal airway should be:
   A. turned 180 degrees with the tip facing the roof of the mouth.
   B. inserted with the bevel on the lateral side of the nostril.
   C. measured from the patient's nostril to the earlobe.
   D. inserted in the left nostril when possible.

147. You are treating a patient who initially had a chief complaint of severe difficulty breathing. You have concerns that this may be leading to respiratory failure, which is:
   A. caused by electrocution in young adults.
   B. another term used to describe respiratory arrest.
   C. inadequate breathing and is a precursor to respiratory arrest.
   D. the complete cessation of expiration.

148. The patient described in multiple-choice question 147 has inadequate breathing. She could have any of the following signs *except*:
   A. absent or minimal chest movement.
   B. noises such as wheezing, gurgling, stridor, or crowing.
   C. diminished or absent breath sounds.
   D. air that can be felt at the nose or mouth on exhalation.

149. You are treating a patient who your partner states has a normal breathing rate for an adult. The patient's breathing rate is most likely:
   A. 6 to 10 per minute.
   B. 12 to 20 per minute.
   C. 15 to 30 per minute.
   D. 25 to 50 per minute.

150. As you assess and manage the patient in multiple-choice question 147, you decide she is either not breathing or her breathing is inadequate. Thus, it will be necessary to provide:
   A. artificial ventilation.
   B. positive pressure ventilation.
   C. assistance with a bag-valve mask device.
   D. all of these are correct.

Interim Exam 1 Answer Sheet

Fill in the correct answer for each item. For scoring purposes, note that there are 150 questions valued at 0.667 points each.

1. [ ] A	[ ] B	[ ] C	[ ] D		36. [ ] A	[ ] B	[ ] C	[ ] D
2. [ ] A	[ ] B	[ ] C	[ ] D		37. [ ] A	[ ] B	[ ] C	[ ] D
3. [ ] A	[ ] B	[ ] C	[ ] D		38. [ ] A	[ ] B	[ ] C	[ ] D
4. [ ] A	[ ] B	[ ] C	[ ] D		39. [ ] A	[ ] B	[ ] C	[ ] D
5. [ ] A	[ ] B	[ ] C	[ ] D		40. [ ] A	[ ] B	[ ] C	[ ] D
6. [ ] A	[ ] B	[ ] C	[ ] D		41. [ ] A	[ ] B	[ ] C	[ ] D
7. [ ] A	[ ] B	[ ] C	[ ] D		42. [ ] A	[ ] B	[ ] C	[ ] D
8. [ ] A	[ ] B	[ ] C	[ ] D		43. [ ] A	[ ] B	[ ] C	[ ] D
9. [ ] A	[ ] B	[ ] C	[ ] D		44. [ ] A	[ ] B	[ ] C	[ ] D
10. [ ] A	[ ] B	[ ] C	[ ] D		45. [ ] A	[ ] B	[ ] C	[ ] D
11. [ ] A	[ ] B	[ ] C	[ ] D		46. [ ] A	[ ] B	[ ] C	[ ] D
12. [ ] A	[ ] B	[ ] C	[ ] D		47. [ ] A	[ ] B	[ ] C	[ ] D
13. [ ] A	[ ] B	[ ] C	[ ] D		48. [ ] A	[ ] B	[ ] C	[ ] D
14. [ ] A	[ ] B	[ ] C	[ ] D		49. [ ] A	[ ] B	[ ] C	[ ] D
15. [ ] A	[ ] B	[ ] C	[ ] D		50. [ ] A	[ ] B	[ ] C	[ ] D
16. [ ] A	[ ] B	[ ] C	[ ] D		51. [ ] A	[ ] B	[ ] C	[ ] D
17. [ ] A	[ ] B	[ ] C	[ ] D		52. [ ] A	[ ] B	[ ] C	[ ] D
18. [ ] A	[ ] B	[ ] C	[ ] D		53. [ ] A	[ ] B	[ ] C	[ ] D
19. [ ] A	[ ] B	[ ] C	[ ] D		54. [ ] A	[ ] B	[ ] C	[ ] D
20. [ ] A	[ ] B	[ ] C	[ ] D		55. [ ] A	[ ] B	[ ] C	[ ] D
21. [ ] A	[ ] B	[ ] C	[ ] D		56. [ ] A	[ ] B	[ ] C	[ ] D
22. [ ] A	[ ] B	[ ] C	[ ] D		57. [ ] A	[ ] B	[ ] C	[ ] D
23. [ ] A	[ ] B	[ ] C	[ ] D		58. [ ] A	[ ] B	[ ] C	[ ] D
24. [ ] A	[ ] B	[ ] C	[ ] D		59. [ ] A	[ ] B	[ ] C	[ ] D
25. [ ] A	[ ] B	[ ] C	[ ] D		60. [ ] A	[ ] B	[ ] C	[ ] D
26. [ ] A	[ ] B	[ ] C	[ ] D		61. [ ] A	[ ] B	[ ] C	[ ] D
27. [ ] A	[ ] B	[ ] C	[ ] D		62. [ ] A	[ ] B	[ ] C	[ ] D
28. [ ] A	[ ] B	[ ] C	[ ] D		63. [ ] A	[ ] B	[ ] C	[ ] D
29. [ ] A	[ ] B	[ ] C	[ ] D		64. [ ] A	[ ] B	[ ] C	[ ] D
30. [ ] A	[ ] B	[ ] C	[ ] D		65. [ ] A	[ ] B	[ ] C	[ ] D
31. [ ] A	[ ] B	[ ] C	[ ] D		66. [ ] A	[ ] B	[ ] C	[ ] D
32. [ ] A	[ ] B	[ ] C	[ ] D		67. [ ] A	[ ] B	[ ] C	[ ] D
33. [ ] A	[ ] B	[ ] C	[ ] D		68. [ ] A	[ ] B	[ ] C	[ ] D
34. [ ] A	[ ] B	[ ] C	[ ] D		69. [ ] A	[ ] B	[ ] C	[ ] D
35. [ ] A	[ ] B	[ ] C	[ ] D		70. [ ] A	[ ] B	[ ] C	[ ] D

©2012 Pearson Education, Inc.
Emergency Care, 12th Ed.

71. [ ] A	[ ] B	[ ] C	[ ] D		111. [ ] A	[ ] B	[ ] C	[ ] D
72. [ ] A	[ ] B	[ ] C	[ ] D		112. [ ] A	[ ] B	[ ] C	[ ] D
73. [ ] A	[ ] B	[ ] C	[ ] D		113. [ ] A	[ ] B	[ ] C	[ ] D
74. [ ] A	[ ] B	[ ] C	[ ] D		114. [ ] A	[ ] B	[ ] C	[ ] D
75. [ ] A	[ ] B	[ ] C	[ ] D		115. [ ] A	[ ] B	[ ] C	[ ] D
76. [ ] A	[ ] B	[ ] C	[ ] D		116. [ ] A	[ ] B	[ ] C	[ ] D
77. [ ] A	[ ] B	[ ] C	[ ] D		117. [ ] A	[ ] B	[ ] C	[ ] D
78. [ ] A	[ ] B	[ ] C	[ ] D		118. [ ] A	[ ] B	[ ] C	[ ] D
79. [ ] A	[ ] B	[ ] C	[ ] D		119. [ ] A	[ ] B	[ ] C	[ ] D
80. [ ] A	[ ] B	[ ] C	[ ] D ·		120. [ ] A	[ ] B	[ ] C	[ ] D
81. [ ] A	[ ] B	[ ] C	[ ] D		121. [ ] A	[ ] B	[ ] C	[ ] D
82. [ ] A	[ ] B	[ ] C	[ ] D		122. [ ] A	[ ] B	[ ] C	[ ] D
83. [ ] A	[ ] B	[ ] C	[ ] D		123. [ ] A	[ ] B	[ ] C	[ ] D
84. [ ] A	[ ] B	[ ] C	[ ] D		124. [ ] A	[ ] B	[ ] C	[ ] D
85. [ ] A	[ ] B	[ ] C	[ ] D		125. [ ] A	[ ] B	[ ] C	[ ] D
86. [ ] A	[ ] B	[ ] C	[ ] D		126. [ ] A	[ ] B	[ ] C	[ ] D
87. [ ] A	[ ] B	[ ] C	[ ] D		127. [ ] A	[ ] B	[ ] C	[ ] D
88. [ ] A	[ ] B	[ ] C	[ ] D		128. [ ] A	[ ] B	[ ] C	[ ] D
89. [ ] A	[ ] B	[ ] C	[ ] D		129. [ ] A	[ ] B	[ ] C	[ ] D
90. [ ] A	[ ] B	[ ] C	[ ] D		130. [ ] A	[ ] B	[ ] C	[ ] D
91. [ ] A	[ ] B	[ ] C	[ ] D		131. [ ] A	[ ] B	[ ] C	[ ] D
92. [ ] A	[ ] B	[ ] C	[ ] D		132. [ ] A	[ ] B	[ ] C	[ ] D
93. [ ] A	[ ] B	[ ] C	[ ] D		133. [ ] A	[ ] B	[ ] C	[ ] D
94. [ ] A	[ ] B	[ ] C	[ ] D		134. [ ] A	[ ] B	[ ] C	[ ] D
95. [ ] A	[ ] B	[ ] C	[ ] D		135. [ ] A	[ ] B	[ ] C	[ ] D
96. [ ] A	[ ] B	[ ] C	[ ] D		136. [ ] A	[ ] B	[ ] C	[ ] D
97. [ ] A	[ ] B	[ ] C	[ ] D		137. [ ] A	[ ] B	[ ] C	[ ] D
98. [ ] A	[ ] B	[ ] C	[ ] D		138. [ ] A	[ ] B	[ ] C	[ ] D
99. [ ] A	[ ] B	[ ] C	[ ] D		139. [ ] A	[ ] B	[ ] C	[ ] D
100. [ ] A	[ ] B	[ ] C	[ ] D		140. [ ] A	[ ] B	[ ] C	[ ] D
101. [ ] A	[ ] B	[ ] C	[ ] D		141. [ ] A	[ ] B	[ ] C	[ ] D
102. [ ] A	[ ] B	[ ] C	[ ] D		142. [ ] A	[ ] B	[ ] C	[ ] D
103. [ ] A	[ ] B	[ ] C	[ ] D		143. [ ] A	[ ] B	[ ] C	[ ] D
104. [ ] A	[ ] B	[ ] C	[ ] D		144. [ ] A	[ ] B	[ ] C	[ ] D
105. [ ] A	[ ] B	[ ] C	[ ] D		145. [ ] A	[ ] B	[ ] C	[ ] D
106. [ ] A	[ ] B	[ ] C	[ ] D		146. [ ] A	[ ] B	[ ] C	[ ] D
107. [ ] A	[ ] B	[ ] C	[ ] D		147. [ ] A	[ ] B	[ ] C	[ ] D
108. [ ] A	[ ] B	[ ] C	[ ] D		148. [ ] A	[ ] B	[ ] C	[ ] D
109. [ ] A	[ ] B	[ ] C	[ ] D		149. [ ] A	[ ] B	[ ] C	[ ] D
110. [ ] A	[ ] B	[ ] C	[ ] D		150. [ ] A	[ ] B	[ ] C	[ ] D

10

Scene Size-Up

Standard: Assessment (Scene Size-Up)

Competency: Applies scene information and patient assessment findings (scene size-up, primary and secondary assessment, patient history, and reassessment) to guide emergency management.

OBJECTIVES

After reading this chapter you should be able to:

10.1   Define key terms introduced in this chapter.

10.2   Explain the ongoing nature of scene size-up beyond the initial moments at the scene.

10.3   Given a scene-arrival scenario, list several examples of potential hazards for which the EMT should actively search.

10.4   Describe considerations in establishing a danger zone at the scene of a vehicle collision.

10.5   Recognize indications of possible crime scenes and the potential for violence.

10.6   Use information from the scene size-up to make decisions about the use of Standard Precautions to protect against disease exposure.

10.7   Use information from the scene size-up to determine the mechanism of injury or nature of the illness.

10.8   Explain the importance of determining the number of patients and the need for additional resources in the scene size-up.

10.9   Given a number of scenarios, perform a scene size-up, including:

  a. Recognizing potential dangers
  b. Making decisions about body substance isolation
  c. Determining the nature of the illness or mechanism of injury
  d. Determining the number of patients
  e. Determining the need for additional resources

©2012 Pearson Education, Inc.
Emergency Care, 12th Ed.

MATCH TERMINOLOGY/ DEFINITIONS

A. Injury caused by an object that passes through the skin or other body tissues

B. Injury caused by a blow that does not penetrate the skin or other body tissues

C. A force or forces that may have caused injury

D. The area around the wreckage of a vehicle collision or other incident within which special safety precautions should be taken

E. Awareness that there may be injuries

F. What is medically wrong with a patient

G. Steps taken by an ambulance crew when approaching the scene of an emergency call: checking scene safety; taking Standard Precautions; noting the mechanism of injury or nature of the patient's illness; determining the number of patients; and deciding what, if any, additional resources to call for

G **1.** Scene size-up

D **2.** Danger zone

C **3.** Mechanism of injury

A **4.** Penetrating trauma

B **5.** Blunt-force trauma

E **6.** Index of suspicion

F **7.** Nature of the illness

MULTIPLE-CHOICE REVIEW

A **1.** The scene size-up is the first part of the patient assessment process. It begins as you approach the scene, surveying it to determine:
A. if there are any threats to your patient's safety.
B. the number of injured.
C. personal safety of all those involved in the call.
D. the mechanism of injury (MOI).

D **2.** Which of the following is the most accurate statement about scene size-up?
A. It takes place as you are approaching the scene.
B. It is replaced by patient care once you arrive at the scene.
C. It occurs during the first part of the assessment process.
D. It continues throughout the call.

B **3.** If you arrive at a collision scene where there are police, fire vehicles, and other ambulances already present, you should:
A. immediately begin patient care.
B. conduct your own scene size-up.
C. ensure that no bystanders are injured.
D. all of these.

D **4.** Which of the following is *not* an appropriate action when you near the scene of a traffic collision?
A. Look and listen for other EMS units as you near intersections.
B. Look for signs of collision-related power outages.
C. Observe traffic flow to anticipate blockage at the scene.
D. Attempt to park your vehicle downhill from the scene.

A **5.** When you are in sight of the collision scene, you should watch for the signals of police officers and other emergency service personnel because:
A. they may have information about hazards or the location of injured persons.
B. the first ones on the scene are considered to be in charge.
C. federal law requires you to follow the command of other responders.
D. they are considered the medical-care experts on the scene.

_B_ **6.** When there are no apparent hazards, consider the danger zone to extend at least _____ feet in all directions from the wreckage.
   A. 25   **C.** 100
   B. 50   **D.** 200

_C_ **7.** When a collision vehicle is on fire, consider the danger zone to extend at least _____ feet in all directions, even if the fire appears small and limited to the engine compartment.
   A. 25   **C.** 100
   B. 50   **D.** 200

_D_
_A_ **8.** It is essential that the EMT do a good scene size-up. Your scene size-up should identify:
   A. the potential for a violent situation.
   B. the name and amount of toxic substances.
   C. the number of patients and their diagnoses.
   D. all of these.

_D_ **9.** The EMT's Standard Precautions equipment during the scene size-up may include all of the following *except*:
   A. eye protection.
   B. disposable gloves.
   C. face mask or eyeshield.
   D. nonrebreather mask.

_B_ **10.** Standard Precautions should be taken with all patients. The key element of Standard Precautions is to:
   A. always wear all the protective clothing.
   B. always have personal protective equipment readily available.
   C. place equipment on the patient as well as the rescuer.
   D. determine which body fluids are a danger to the EMT.

_B_ **11.** Certain injuries are common to particular situations. Injuries to bones and joints are usually associated with:
   A. fights and drug usage.
   B. falls and vehicle collisions.
   C. fires and explosions.
   D. bullet wounds.

_C_ **12.** Knowing the mechanism of injury assists the EMT in:
   A. immobilizing the patient's spine.
   B. determining which Standard Precautions to use.
   C. predicting various injury patterns.
   D. all of these.

_C_ **13.** The physical forces and energy that impinge on the patient are influenced by the laws of physics. One of those laws, the law of inertia, states that:
   A. the faster you enter a turn, the more your vehicle will be pulled straight.
   B. the slower the speed, the greater the energy loss.
   C. a body in motion will remain in motion unless acted upon by an outside force.
   D. the mass or weight of an object is the most important contributor to an injury.

_A_ **14.** You are treating a patient who was involved in a head-on collision. She was the unrestrained driver who took the "up-and-over" pathway. To which part of her body was she most likely to have sustained injuries?
   A. Skull   **C.** Knees
   B. Fibula   **D.** Femur

_C_ **15.** Which of the following is *least* likely to be considered a mechanism of injury for the patient who was in the crash described in multiple-choice question 14?
   A. Steering wheel   **C.** Brake pedal
   B. Windshield   **D.** Dashboard

_B_ **16.** You are on the scene of a car crash. Your patient has stable vital signs and is complaining of knee, leg, and hip pain. He also states that he was in the front seat of the car and did not have his seat belt on. What type of collision did he most likely experience?
- **A.** Head-on, up-and-over
- **B.** Rear-end
- **C.** Head-on, down-and-under
- **D.** Rotational impact

_D_ **17.** Which type of collision is most serious when the occupant is not restrained because it has the potential for multiple impacts?
- **A.** Side impact
- **B.** Rear-end impact
- **C.** Head-on, up-and-over
- **D.** Roll-over

_A_ **18.** You are walking around a vehicle that was involved in a collision. All of the following are examples of mechanisms of injury *except* a:
- **A.** patient who fell three times her height.
- **B.** spiderweb crack in the windshield.
- **C.** broken steering column in a collision.
- **D.** flat rear tire.

_A_ **19.** A severe fall for an adult is:
- **A.** over 15 feet.
- **B.** often accompanied by an amputation.
- **C.** less than 10 feet.
- **D.** always fatal.

_C_ **20.** You are evaluating a patient who sustained a penetrating injury. The injury is usually limited to the penetrated area in a _____ injury.
- **A.** low-velocity
- **B.** medium-velocity
- **C.** high-velocity
- **D.** super-velocity

_C_ **21.** The pressure wave around the bullet's tract through the body is called:
- **A.** exsanguination.
- **B.** gas penetration.
- **C.** cavitation.
- **D.** pressure damage.

_C_ **22.** You are evaluating a patient who sustained an injury caused by a blow that hit the body but did not penetrate the skin. This type of injury is called a(n):
- **A.** inertia trauma.
- **B.** cavitation.
- **C.** blunt-force trauma.
- **D.** rotational impact.

_B_ **23.** In which of the following situations would it be necessary for you and your partner to call for additional assistance?
- **A.** You are treating a patient who has flulike symptoms and also has a toddler with similar symptoms.
- **B.** Your patient is a 350-pound male who fell down the stairs and has a broken leg.
- **C.** You are treating a patient with a deep laceration in his right forearm.
- **D.** Your patient loses consciousness while you are carrying her to the ambulance.

_A_ **24.** While in the living room of a private home and treating a patient for nausea, headache, and general body weakness, your eyes begin to tear. Three family members have the same symptoms. You should immediately:
- **A.** evacuate all people from the building.
- **B.** call for three additional ambulances.
- **C.** notify the police department.
- **D.** begin to flush out everyone's eyes.

_B_ **25.** If the number of patients is more than the responding units can effectively handle, the EMT should:
- **A.** involve bystanders in care of the injured.
- **B.** call for additional EMS resources immediately.
- **C.** advise medical direction that assistance is needed.
- **D.** do all of these.

_C_ **26.** When arriving at the scene of a collision, the EMT should:

_B_
    A. start placing flares across the road.
    B. don head protection, bunker coat, and a reflective vest.
    C. immediately start additional units.
    D. contact medical direction on the radio.

_B_ **27.** A significant danger faced by the EMT is violence. On arriving at the scene of a

_C_
    private home, you hear screaming from inside; there are beer cans piled up on
    the front porch; and, as you knock on the door, it suddenly gets very quiet
    inside. What should you do next?
    A. Enter the residence and search for weapons.
    B. Contact the dispatcher to inquire if they have ever had violence at this location.
    C. Retreat to a safe location and ask for the police to respond to secure the scene.
    D. Yell into the house that you are EMS and not the police.

_A_ **28.** You arrive on the scene of a large fire. If the personnel at the scene are using
    the incident command/management system, you should:
    A. follow the instructions of the person in charge.
    B. drive past the scene and park off the road.
    C. transport the first patient you come across.
    D. tag all of the patients.

COMPLETE THE FOLLOWING

1. List the five signals that violence may be a danger on your call.

    A. _____

    B. _____

    C. _____

    D. _____

    E. _____

2. List the guidelines for establishing a danger zone.

    A. _____

    B. _____

    C. _____

    D. _____

    E. _____

3. List five types of motor vehicle collisions and the common injury pattern
    for each.

    A. _____

    B. _____

    C. _____

©2012 Pearson Education, Inc.
Emergency Care, 12th Ed.

D. _____

E. _____

STREET SCENES DISCUSSION

Review the Street Scene on page 263 of the textbook. Then answer the following questions.

1. Suppose the situation played out in a different way. On arrival at the scene, the driver of the truck comes running up to your ambulance and says, "My truck is overturned and leaking toxic chemicals all over the place." What should you do next?

2. Suppose upon arrival you find the driver of the truck is acting as if he is intoxicated. He also is holding a rifle in his lap, with his right hand in position for firing. What should you do?

11

The Primary Assessment

Standard: Assessment (Primary Assessment)

Competency: Applies scene information and patient assessment findings (scene size-up, primary and secondary assessment, patient history, and reassessment) to guide emergency management.

OBJECTIVES

After reading this chapter you should be able to:

11.1 Define key terms introduced in this chapter.

11.2 Explain the purpose of the primary assessment.

11.3 Discuss the difference in first steps to assessment if the patient is apparently lifeless (C-A-B approach) or if the patient has signs of life, including a pulse (A-B-C approach).

11.4 Given several scenarios, perform the following:

    a. Form a general impression
    b. Determine the chief complaint
    c. Determine the patient's mental status
    d. Assess the airway
    e. Assess breathing
    f. Assess circulation
    g. Determine the patient's priority for transport

11.5 Recognize findings in the primary assessment that require immediate intervention.

11.6 Differentiate the approach to the primary assessment based on the following:

    a. Mechanism of injury/nature of the illness and level of responsiveness
    b. Patient's age (adult, child, or infant)

MATCH TERMINOLOGY/DEFINITIONS

A. Impression of the patient's condition that is formed on first approaching the patient, based on the patient's environment, chief complaint, and appearance

B. Level of responsiveness

C. Airway, breathing, and circulation

D. In emergency medicine, the reason EMS was called, usually in the patient's own words

E. The first element in assessment of a patient: steps taken for the purpose of discovering and dealing with any life-threatening problems

F. A memory aid for classifying a patient's levels of responsiveness, or mental status

G. Actions taken to correct a patient's problem

H. The decision regarding the need for immediate transport of the patient versus further assessment and care at the scene

_C_ **1.** ABCs

_F_ **2.** AVPU

_D_ **3.** Chief complaint

_A_ **4.** General impression

_G_ **5.** Interventions

_B_ **6.** Mental status

_E_ **7.** Primary assessment

_H_ **8.** Priority

MULTIPLE-CHOICE REVIEW

_D_ **1.** Which of the following steps is *not* part of the primary assessment of a responsive patient with a medical problem?
   A. Assess the patient's mental status.
   B. Assess the adequacy of breathing.
   C. Determine the patient's priority.
   D. Obtain the patient's blood pressure.

_D_ **2.** The general impression is an evaluation of all of the following *except*:
   A. the patient's chief complaint.
   B. appearance.
   C. the environment.
   D. past medical history.

_B_ **3.** You are assessing a patient and making observations about the scene. Finding drug-use paraphernalia at the scene of an emergency is an example of:
   A. an indication of the patient's chief complaint.
   B. the environment part of the general impression.
   C. an assessment of the scene safety.
   D. a medical history of drug addiction.

_B_ **4.** When the patient tells you, in his own words, why he requested that an ambulance be called, this is referred to as the:
   A. general impression.
   B. chief complaint.
   C. primary assessment.
   D. secondary assessment.

_D_ **5.** During the general impression, the EMT should:
   A. look.
   B. listen.
   C. smell.
   D. do all of these.

_B_ **6.** One way to determine the patient's level of responsiveness is to:
   A. put ammonia inhalants into each nostril.
   B. rub the patient's sternum briskly.
   C. place the patient's hands in water.
   D. press on the patient's nail beds.

_D_ **7.** You are assessing a patient who fell off his bike and landed on his right shoulder. First you determine his mental status using AVPU. What does the "A" in AVPU stand for?
   A. Action
   B. Airway
   C. Assess
   D. Alert

_C_ **8.** You have determined that your patient is a V as far as mental status is concerned. What does the "V" in AVPU stand for?
   A. Violent
   B. Very painful
   C. Verbal
   D. Venous

_B_ **9.** You are concerned because your patient may have a depressed mental status. What does the "P" in AVPU stand for?
   A. Priority
   B. Painful
   C. Position
   D. Patient

_B_ **10.** One major difference between the primary assessment of a responsive trauma patient and the primary assessment of an unresponsive trauma patient is:
   A. the assessment is done more quickly on the responsive patient.
   B. the unresponsive patient is a higher priority for immediate transport.
   C. there is no difference between the two assessments.
   D. a jaw-thrust maneuver should always be used on the responsive patient.

_D_ **11.** You are assessing a patient who was involved in a serious motor vehicle collision. She is not alert and her breathing rate is slower than 8. As the EMT in charge, you should:
   A. give high-concentration oxygen via nonrebreather mask.
   B. quickly evaluate the patient's circulation and treat for shock.
   C. suction the patient and perform rescue breathing.
   D. provide positive pressure ventilations with 100 percent oxygen.

_B_ **12.** During your primary assessment of a patient who is alert and has a breathing rate that is greater than 24, you should provide the patient with:
   A. positive pressure ventilations with 100 percent oxygen.
   B. high-concentration oxygen via nonrebreather mask.
   C. low-concentration oxygen via bag-valve mask.
   D. medium-concentration oxygen via nasal cannula.

_D_ **13.** In the primary assessment, the circulation assessment includes evaluating all of the following *except*:
   A. pulse.
   B. skin.
   C. severity of bleeding.
   D. blood pressure.

_D_ **14.** If a patient's skin is warm, dry, and a normal color, it indicates:
   A. a serious sunburn.
   B. heat exposure.
   C. alcohol abuse.
   D. good circulation.

©2012 Pearson Education, Inc.
Emergency Care, 12th Ed.

_C_ 15. Your patient has no life-threatening external hemorrhage but has skin that is cool, pale, and moist. This could be an indication of:
   A. increased perfusion.
   B. high blood pressure.
   C. poor circulation.
   D. cold exposure.

_D_ 16. To evaluate skin color in a dark-skinned patient, the EMT should also:
   A. evaluate the tissues of the lips or nail beds.
   B. evaluate the tissues of the heels of the feet.
   C. check the pupils of the eyes.
   D. do all of these.

_C_ 17. When assessing the circulation during the primary assessment, the EMT should check for and control severe bleeding. This is important to do because:
   A. open wounds can become infected.
   B. it may lead to long-term complications.
   C. a patient can bleed to death in minutes.
   D. the blood pressure may drop over time.

_B_ 18. When a life threat is observed in the primary assessment, the EMT should:
   A. complete the assessment, then treat.
   B. treat it immediately.
   C. determine the patient's priority, then treat.
   D. package the patient for transport.

_D_ 19. High-priority conditions include:
   A. poor general impression.
   B. unresponsiveness.
   C. shock (hypoperfusion).
   D. all of these.

_C_ 20. All of the following would be considered high-priority conditions *except*:
   A. difficulty breathing.
   B. responsive but not following commands.
   C. an uncomplicated childbirth.
   D. chest pain with systolic pressure less than 100.

_C_ 21. During the primary assessment of an adult medical patient with a chief complaint of chest pain, you note that the breathing rate is 28. You should consider:
   A. oxygen by a nasal cannula.
   B. providing bag-valve mask ventilations.
   C. administering oxygen by nonrebreather mask.
   D. using a paper bag to slow down the rate.

_A_ 22. In the adult trauma patient, why is the capillary refill no longer used to assess the circulation?
   A. It is not a good indicator.
   B. Only children have capillary refill.
   C. It is still a very important step.
   D. Because EMTs have difficulty remembering to use it.

_C_ 23. The steps of the primary assessment:
   A. are patient dependent.
   B. depend on the baseline vital signs.
   C. must be followed in order.
   D. depend on the age and sex of the patient.

_B_ **24.** When doing an assessment on a patient who is apparently lifeless, the approach is adapted to include:
   A. the pulse check for at least 20 seconds.
   B. the C-A-B approach per AHA Guidelines.
   C. the routine A-B-C approach per AHA Guidelines.
   D. none of these are appropriate.

COMPLETE THE FOLLOWING

1. The primary assessment is the first element in the total assessment of the patient. List the six steps of the primary assessment.

   A. _____

   B. _____

   C. _____

   D. _____

   E. _____

   F. _____

2. State what the letters in AVPU stand for.

   A. _____

   V. _____

   P. _____

   U. _____

3. List five high-priority conditions.

   A. _____

   B. _____

   C. _____

   D. _____

   E. _____

STREET SCENES DISCUSSION

Review the Street Scene on page 223 of the textbook. Then answer the following questions.

1. Imagine that your 78-year-old patient, who fell to the floor, does not wake up, and his respirations continue with gurgling sounds due to blood in the back of his throat. What should you do?

2. What priority would this patient be? Would it be appropriate to call for ALS?

3. Look again at the third patient encounter. Is it necessary to take this patient to the hospital? Explain.

CASE STUDY

This case study is designed to help you apply the concepts presented in this textbook. The case study describes a situation you might encounter in the field and is followed by questions about the situation. The questions require you to explain and apply key concepts from your reading.

▶ CAR-BIKE COLLISION ON MAIN STREET USA

Your unit has been dispatched to a call for a car-versus-bike collision on Main Street. The report from the scene from bystanders is that the patient is awake and in a lot of pain. The police have also been dispatched and they arrive as you are arriving at the scene.

1. With the police available to attend to the traffic control, what is the EMT's initial responsibility?

_____

As you turn to start attending to the patient, a bystander tells you that the cyclist was "tooling right along with the traffic when the guy in the car parked at the curb suddenly opened his driver's door." He continues to describe that the cyclist hit the door and flew off the bike into the air.

2. The first actual patient survey you obtain is called the _____.

3. What do we call the description of the incident that you received from the bystander?

_____

4. How can this information sometimes be invaluable?

_____

You introduce yourself to the patient. He says that his name is Tony and he was in a rush on the way to work. Tony goes on to say, "That guy did not even look. He just opened his door in front of me and I could not stop." You notice that Tony was wearing a heavy coat and a bright reflective vest as well as a helmet. You also note that Tony seems to be protecting his right arm and shoulder and looks like he is in pain.

5. Now that you know Tony's name, why is it also important to quickly ask if he knows where he is and the day of the week?

_____

6. Tony states, "I am on Main Street and it is a Friday. I was looking forward to the weekend." What would you decide his mental status is?

_____

7. His airway is open and he is talking but in pain. He has nothing in his mouth, so you ask him to take a deep breath to see if his pain is worsened by his breathing. Why do this now?

_____

8. Tony's breathing is a little faster than normal, but he is able to talk in full sentences and the pain is not from his chest. Next you check his radial pulse. It is strong and fast because his heart must be pumping from fright right now. What else should you check as part of your circulation assessment?

_____

9. You decide that Tony would be a high priority. Why?

_____

Moving Tony to the ambulance will involve a backboard and collar because your partner has been maintaining cervical spine immobilization throughout your primary assessment. Before moving Tony, you do a quick head-to-toe exam to see what other injuries he may have. Fortunately, in this case, he did not injure his head. He has some bumps, bruises, scratches, and a broken clavicle. Your partner reminds you that that is a very common injury for a cyclist, so Tony was pretty lucky!

EMT SKILL PERFORMANCE CHECKLIST

▶ **PRIMARY ASSESSMENT (PP. 210–213)**

❏ Take Standard Precautions.

❏ Form a general impression based on assessment of the environment and the patient's chief complaint and appearance.

❏ Assess mental status. Determine level of responsiveness using AVPU (alert, verbal, painful, unresponsive).

❏ Assess the airway. If it is not open or if it is endangered, take measures to open it.

❏ Assess breathing. If needed, initiate any appropriate oxygen therapy and ensure adequate ventilation.

❏ Assess circulation (assess for and control major bleeding; assess pulse; assess skin color, temperature, and condition).

❏ Determine patient's treatment priority (high/low, stable/unstable) and make a transport decision.

NOTE: Apply manual stabilization upon first contact with any patient who you suspect may have an injury to the spine.

©2012 Pearson Education, Inc.
Emergency Care, 12th Ed.

Vital Signs and Monitoring Devices

Standard: Assessment (Monitoring Devices)

Competency: Applies scene information and patient assessment findings (scene size-up, primary and secondary assessment, patient history, and reassessment) to guide emergency management.

OBJECTIVES

After reading this chapter you should be able to:

12.1 Define key terms introduced in this chapter.

12.2 Identify the vital signs used in prehospital patient assessment.

12.3 Explain the use of vital signs in patient-care decision making.

12.4 Integrate assessment of vital signs into the patient assessment process, according to the patient's condition and the situation.

12.5 Discuss the importance of documenting vital signs and the times they were obtained in the patient-care record.

12.6 Demonstrate assessment of:

    a. Pulse
    b. Respirations
    c. Blood pressure
    d. Skin
    e. Pupils
    f. Oxygen saturation
    g. Blood glucose

12.7 Integrate assessment of mental status and ongoing attention to the primary assessment while obtaining vital signs.

12.8 Demonstrate alternative approaches to obtaining patients' vital signs.

12.9 Differentiate between vital signs that are within expected ranges for a given patient and those that are not.

Emergency Care, 12th Ed.

12.10 Compare and contrast the techniques of assessment and expected vital sign values for pediatric and adult patients.

12.11 Explain the importance of communicating your actions to patients when assessing vital signs.

12.12 Recognize actions that must be taken based on vital sign values.

12.13 Discuss limitations in the interpretation of patients' conditions based on vital sign values.

MATCH TERMINOLOGY/ DEFINITIONS

▶ **PART A**

A. The pressure remaining in the arteries when the left ventricle of the heart is relaxed and refilling

B. A slow pulse; any pulse rate below 60 beats per minute

C. Force of blood against the walls of the blood vessels

D. The pulse felt along the large artery on either side of the neck

E. Touching or feeling; a pulse or blood pressure may be palpated with the fingertips

F. The number of pulse beats per minute

G. In the pupils of the eyes, reacting to light by changing size

H. The rhythmic beats felt as the heart pumps blood through the arteries

I. The rhythm (regular or irregular) and force (strong or weak) of the pulse

J. Major artery of the arm

K. The black center of the eye

L. When a stethoscope is used to listen for characteristic sounds

M. Get larger

N. Get smaller

O. The pulse felt at the wrist

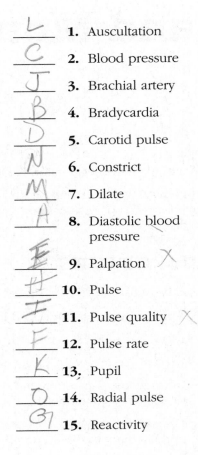

_L_ **1.** Auscultation

_C_ **2.** Blood pressure

_J_ **3.** Brachial artery

_B_ **4.** Bradycardia

_D_ **5.** Carotid pulse

_N_ **6.** Constrict

_M_ **7.** Dilate

_A_ **8.** Diastolic blood pressure

_E_ **9.** Palpation X

_H_ **10.** Pulse

_I_ **11.** Pulse quality X

_F_ **12.** Pulse rate

_K_ **13.** Pupil

_O_ **14.** Radial pulse

_G/_ **15.** Reactivity

▶ **PART B**

A. The number of breaths taken in 1 minute

B. Normal or abnormal (shallow, labored, noisy) character of breathing

C. A rapid pulse; any pulse rate above 100 beats per minute

D. The pressure created when the heart contracts and forces blood into the arteries

E. The regular or irregular spacing of breaths

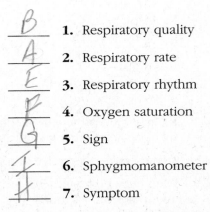

_B_ **1.** Respiratory quality

_A_ **2.** Respiratory rate

_E_ **3.** Respiratory rhythm

_F_ **4.** Oxygen saturation

_G_ **5.** Sign

_I_ **6.** Sphygmomanometer

_H_ **7.** Symptom

F. The ratio of the amount of oxygen present in the blood to the amount that could be carried, expressed in a percentage

G. An indication of a patient's condition that is objective, or can be observed by another person; an indication that can be seen, heard, smelled, or felt by the EMT or others

H. An indication of a patient's condition that cannot be observed by another person but rather is subjective or something felt and reported by the patient

I. The cuff and gauge used to measure blood pressure

J. Outward signs of what is going on inside the body, including respiration; pulse; skin color, temperature, and condition (plus capillary refill in infants and children); pupils; and blood pressure

K. The pulse felt in the upper arm

L. An electronic device for determining the amount of oxygen carried in the blood, known as the oxygen saturation or SpO_2

M. Machine that automatically inflates a blood pressure cuff and measures blood pressure

___D___ **8.** Systolic pressure

___C___ **9.** Tachycardia

___M___ **10.** Blood pressure monitor

___L___ **11.** Pulse oximeter

___J___ **12.** Vital signs

___K___ **13.** Brachial pulse

MULTIPLE-CHOICE REVIEW

___D___ **1.** You are treating a 35-year-old male who was involved in a fall. The components of the vital signs you will assess include all of the following *except*:
A. respiratory rate and quality.
B. skin color and condition.
C. pulse rate and quality.
D. pulse oximetry.

___B___ **2.** A sign that gives important information about the patient's condition but is *not* considered a vital sign is:
A. blood pressure.
B. mental status.
C. pulse rate.
D. respiratory rhythm.

___D___ **3.** Why is it essential that vital signs be recorded as they are obtained?
A. To avoid having to take them more than once
B. To prevent forgetting them and to note the time they were taken
C. To give the patient a chance to calm down
D. Because they will always change quickly

___D___ **4.** You are assessing a 24-year-old female who was involved in a car crash. You take her pulse, and the rate exceeds 100 beats per minute. This is called:
A. normal.
B. regular.
C. bradycardia.
D. tachycardia.

___D___ **5.** Based upon the pulse alone, a sign that something may be seriously wrong with a patient could be:

    A. a sustained rate below 48 beats per minute.
    B. a sustained rate above 126 beats per minute.
    C. a rate above 150 beats per minute.
    D. all of these.

___B___ **6.** In addition to the answer to multiple-choice question 5, another serious indicator found in the pulse may be a(n):

    A. regular strong rhythm.
    B. irregular rhythm.
    C. athlete with a pulse of 54.
    D. an increase in rate during exercise.

___C___ **7.** Assessing the quality of the pulse includes determining the:

    A. rhythm and rate.
    B. rate and force.
    C. rhythm and force.
    D. presence and balance.

___C___ **8.** A patient who sustained serious trauma is described as having a thready pulse. This patient most likely has a(n) _____ pulse.

    A. strong
    B. irregular
    C. weak
    D. infrequent

___C___ **9.** The normal pulse rate for a school-age child (6–10 years) is:

    A. 120 to 160.
    B. 60 to 100.
    C. 70 to 110.
    D. 80 to 120.

___A___ **10.** When assessing the pulse rate of a typical adult who is not in distress, you would expect to obtain a rate of:

    A. 60 to 100.
    B. 70 to 110.
    C. 80 to 120.
    D. 90 to 140.

___B___ **11.** The pulse at the thumb side of the wrist is referred to as the _____ pulse.

    A. femoral
    B. radial
    C. carotid
    D. brachial

___D___ **12.** When assessing the carotid pulse, the EMT should:

    A. palpate the artery as hard as he can.
    B. assess both sides at exactly the same time.
    C. be aware that excessive pressure can slow the heart.
    D. apply pressure until he feels the pulse rate rise.

___C___ **13.** The number of breaths a patient takes in 1 minute is called the:

    A. minute volume.
    B. minute pressure.
    C. respiratory rate.
    D. all of these.

_____A___ **14.** The respiratory rate is classified as:
- **A.** normal, slow, or rapid.
- **B.** noisy, shallow, or normal.
- **C.** labored, quick, or noisy.
- **D.** weak, thready, or full.

_____C___ **15.** If the EMT is treating a patient with a sustained respiratory rate above _____ or below _____ breaths per minute, high-concentration oxygen must be administered.
- **A.** 20; 10
- **B.** 20; 12
- **C.** 24; 8
- **D.** 24; 10

_____B___ **16.** Your partner obtains a set of vitals and tells you his 45-year-old male patient has a normal respiratory rate. The patient's rate at rest should be:
- **A.** 12 to 24.
- **B.** 12 to 20.
- **C.** 20 to 30.
- **D.** 20 to 40.

_____C___ **17.** The normal respiration rate for a toddler (1–3 years) is:
- **A.** 12 to 24.
- **B.** 12 to 20.
- **C.** 20 to 30.
- **D.** 20 to 40.

_____A___ **18.** Shallow breathing occurs when:
- **A.** there is only slight movement of the chest or abdomen.
- **B.** there is stridor or grunting on expiration.
- **C.** there is a complete obstruction.
- **D.** the chest muscles fully expand with each breath.

_____ **19.** Many resting people breathe more with their _____ than with their _____ muscles.
- **A.** diaphragm; pelvic
- **B.** diaphragm; chest
- **C.** chest; abdominal
- **D.** chest; pelvic

_____D___ **20.** Signs of labored breathing include all of the following *except*:
- **A.** increase in the work of breathing.
- **B.** use of accessory muscles.
- **C.** retractions above the collarbones.
- **D.** delayed capillary refill.

_____C___ **21.** A noisy, harsh sound when the patient is breathing in is called:
- **A.** nasal flaring.
- **B.** grunting.
- **C.** crowing.
- **D.** gurgling.

_____C___ **22.** When the quality of a patient's respirations is abnormal due to something blocking the flow of air, this is referred to as _____ breathing.
- **A.** normal
- **B.** shallow
- **C.** noisy
- **D.** labored

_____A___ 23. You are treating a patient who was found unconscious in an alley. During your primary survey, you hear an airway sound that usually indicates the need for suction. This sound is called:
   A. gurgling.
   B. crowing.
   C. stridor.
   D. wheezing.

_____ 24. The best places to assess skin color in adults are:
   A. under the chin and the nostrils.
   B. the inside of the cheek and the nail beds.
   C. the nail beds and the upper chest.
   D. the toes and the earlobes.

_____ 25. Your patient may have sustained a significant blood loss from an injury. This condition may result in skin that is:
   A. flushed.
   B. gray.
   C. pale.
   D. jaundiced.

_____ 26. A patient with a lack of oxygen in the red blood cells resulting from inadequate breathing or inadequate heart function will exhibit _____ skin.
   A. pink
   B. pale
   C. flushed
   D. cyanotic

_____ 27. On interviewing your 45-year-old male patient, you are told he has a liver abnormality. This may help explain why his skin appears:
   A. flushed.
   B. mottled.
   C. pale.
   D. jaundiced.

_____ 28. A passerby called the ambulance for a homeless patient you are now assessing because she thought he was unconscious. He has cold, dry skin, which is frequently associated with:
   A. high fever and/or heat exposure.
   B. exposure to cold.
   C. shock and anxiety.
   D. a body that is losing heat.

_____ 29. Hot, dry skin is frequently associated with:
   A. high fever and heat exposure.
   B. exposure to cold.
   C. shock and anxiety.
   D. heat loss.

_____ 30. Patients with diabetes routinely test the level of sugar in their blood using a device called a(n):
   A. capnograph.
   B. glucose meter.
   C. end-tidal CO_2 monitor.
   D. oximeter.

©2012 Pearson Education, Inc.
Emergency Care, 12th Ed.

_____ **31.** The reading on the device in multiple-choice question 30 is reported in:
  A. percentage of oxygen in the hemoglobin.
  B. percentage of CO_2 in the exhaled air.
  C. milligrams of glucose per deciliter of blood.
  D. none of these.

_____ **32.** It is a bright sunny day and you are treating a woman who fell off her bike.
  She is lying supine on the sidewalk. When you assess her pupils, you should:
  A. use a very bright light that is similar to the environmental light.
  B. cover the patient's eyes for a few moments, then uncover one eye at a time.
  C. apply a cold towel to the patient's eyelids for 10 seconds.
  D. move the patient indoors to an area that has dimmer light.

_____ **33.** The pupils may be unequal due to any of the following conditions _except_:
  A. stroke.
  B. head injury.
  C. eye injury.
  D. shock.

_____ **34.** Fright, blood loss, drugs, and treatment with eye drops may cause the patient's
  pupils to become:
  A. constricted.
  B. dilated.
  C. unequal.
  D. unreactive.

_____ **35.** When the left ventricle of the heart relaxes and refills, the pressure in the
  arteries is called the _____ pressure.
  A. diastolic
  B. carotid
  C. ventricular
  D. systolic

_____ **36.** The pulse oximeter should be used routinely with:
  A. patients who have carbon monoxide poisoning.
  B. patients complaining of respiratory problems.
  C. any patient who is hypothermic.
  D. any patient suffering from severe shock.

_____ **37.** The pulse oximeter is helpful because it:
  A. encourages you to be more aggressive with oxygen therapy.
  B. helps you decide when you should withhold oxygen.
  C. indicates when a patient is about to become hypothermic.
  D. indicates that the patient is a heavy smoker.

_____ **38.** You are treating a firefighter in the rehab sector at a house fire. Your partner
  reminds you that the oximeter produces falsely high readings in patients with:
  A. hypoxia.
  B. barbiturate poisoning.
  C. carbon monoxide poisoning.
  D. croup.

_____ **39.** Chronic smokers may have a pulse oximeter reading that is:
  A. lower than normal.
  B. higher than it actually is.
  C. 20 to 25 percent off.
  D. difficult to read.

_____ **40.** In a normal healthy person, one would expect the oximeter reading to be:
  A. 86 to 90 percent.
  B. 91 to 94 percent.
  C. 95 to 99 percent.
  D. none of these.

_____ **41.** To determine a patient's skin temperature, the EMT should:
  A. hold a thermometer in the axilla for 30 seconds.
  B. have the patient exhale onto a warming device.
  C. feel the patient's skin with the back of the hand.
  D. listen carefully with a stethoscope.

_____ **42.** The normal blood glucose meter reading should be:
  A. 40 to 60 mg/dl.
  B. 60 to 80 mg/dl.
  C. 80 to 100 mg/dl.
  D. 100 to 120 mg/dl.

_____ **43.** The systolic blood pressure is:
  A. created when the heart contracts.
  B. listed as the lower number in the BP fraction.
  C. created when the heart relaxes.
  D. seldom used in prehospital care.

_____ **44.** You are treating a patient who was assaulted, and the bar where the fight occurred is still noisy. In a situation like this, it makes sense to take the patient's BP by _____, revealing only the _____ pressure.
  A. auscultation; systolic
  B. auscultation; diastolic
  C. palpation; systolic
  D. palpation; diastolic

_____ **45.** Serious hypotension in an adult patient is normally defined as a systolic below _____ mmHg.
  A. 200
  B. 140
  C. 90
  D. 60

_____ **46.** When assessing a patient who has an altered mental status, it is not uncommon for the EMT to utilize:
  A. a glucose meter.
  B. a BP cuff and stethoscope.
  C. a pulse oximeter.
  D. all of these.

COMPLETE THE FOLLOWING

1. List five of the vital signs assessed in the prehospital setting.

  A. _____

  B. _____

©2012 Pearson Education, Inc.
Emergency Care, 12th Ed.

C. _____

D. _____

E. _____

2. List the potential causes of the following:

   A. High blood pressure: _____

   B. Low blood pressure: _____

   C. Cool, clammy skin: _____

   D. Cold, moist skin: _____

   E. Cold, dry skin: _____

   F. Hot, dry skin: _____

   G. Hot, moist skin: _____

3. List the different location where you can find the patient's pulse.

   A. _____

   B. _____

   C. _____

   D. _____

   E. _____

STREET SCENES DISCUSSION

Review the Street Scene on page 314 of the textbook. Then answer the following questions.

1. This patient's vital signs were not normal, which helped make it clear that she should go to the hospital. If her vital signs had been normal, would a refusal of transport have been acceptable? (*Hint:* Review Table 12–1.)

2. What would be considered the "normal" range of vital signs for this patient? Would an SpO_2 of 97 percent be acceptable?

3. Would you include in your prehospital care report the fact that the patient was having "black, tarry stools." Why or why not?

CASE STUDY

Call for a "Man Down"

You are dispatched to a call for a "man down" in the alleyway behind an auto repair shop in the downtown district. This location has seen trouble before, so the police are automatically dispatched also. As you arrive on the scene, the patrol car pulls up in front of you.

There is a male patient in his thirties lying by the dumpster, and everyone recognizes him as an alcoholic whom you have transported many times in the past. Although you know his name and a lot of his "history," you remember that your EMT instructor said always to begin with the primary survey and not to cut any corners until you are sure the ABCs are properly assessed and managed!

1. What must be assessed in the primary survey?

   _____

2. If the patient sounds like he is gurgling when he breathes, what piece of equipment should you have at the patient's side?

   _____

You attempt to place an OPA and he gags and then wakes up. He is a bit drowsy and you decide to assess his mental status. He seems to know his name, but he has no idea of the day of the week. He does know he is in the alley behind the auto repair shop, where he drinks antifreeze occasionally.

3. What would you say his mental status is?

   _____

You decide that the primary survey does not reveal any life threats, so you move on to obtain some baseline vital signs.

4. What would be considered a normal set of vital signs for an adult patient in his thirties?

   _____

©2012 Pearson Education, Inc.
Emergency Care, 12th Ed.

5. You recall that this patient has a history of hypertension and diabetes. Given his altered mental status, what additional testing would you consider?

_____

The patient says that he has been eating and actually just had some bread with his "fine" wine. The reading on the glucometer is 60 mg/dl.

6. In your EMS system, you have authorization to administer oral glucose to diabetic patients with low blood sugar as long as they have a gag reflex. Would this patient be a candidate for the oral glucose?

_____

7. How often should you reassess the patient's vital signs on the way to the hospital?

_____

This patient is actually quite the jolly guy, and he has you laughing all the way to the hospital. On arrival, you give your report to the ED nurse and know they will take good care of him tonight.

EMT SKILLS PERFORMANCE CHECKLISTS

▶ BLOOD PRESSURE BY AUSCULTATION (P. 302)

❑ Place the stethoscope around your neck.

❑ The patient should be seated or lying down.

❑ If the patient has not been injured, support his arm at the level of his heart.

❑ Place the cuff snugly around the upper arm so that the bottom of the cuff is about 1 inch above the crease of the elbow.

❑ With your fingertips, palpate the brachial artery at the crease of the elbow.

❑ Place the tips of the stethoscope arms in your ears.

❑ Position the diaphragm of the stethoscope directly over the brachial pulse or over the medial anterior elbow (front of the elbow) if no brachial pulse can be felt. Listen for the brachial pulse.

❑ Inflate the cuff with the bulb valve closed.

❑ Once you no longer hear the brachial pulse, continue to inflate the cuff until the gauge reads 30 mmHg higher than the point where the sound of the pulse disappeared.

❑ Slowly release air from the cuff by opening the bulb valve, allowing the pressure to fall smoothly at the rate of approximately 10 mm per second.

- ❑ When you hear the first clicking or tapping sounds, note the reading on the gauge. This is the systolic pressure.

- ❑ Continue to deflate the cuff and listen for the point at which these distinctive sounds fade. When the sounds turn to dull, muffled thuds, the reading on the gauge is the diastolic pressure.

- ❑ After obtaining the diastolic pressure, let the cuff deflate rapidly.

▶ **BLOOD PRESSURE BY PALPATION (P. 304)**

- ❑ Find the radial pulse on the arm to which the blood pressure cuff is applied.

- ❑ With the bulb valve closed, inflate the cuff to a point where you can no longer feel the radial pulse.

- ❑ Note this point on the gauge and continue to inflate the cuff until the gauge reads 30 mmHg higher than the point where the pulse disappeared.

- ❑ Slowly deflate the cuff, noting the reading at which the radial pulse returns. This reading is the systolic pressure.

- ❑ After obtaining the systolic reading, let the cuff deflate.

NOTE: You cannot determine a diastolic reading by palpation.

▶ **USING THE PULSE OXIMETER (P. 309)**

- ❑ Review the manufacturer's instruction manual for the specific unit you are using.

- ❑ Properly assemble the finger-clip sensor and extension to pulse oximeter.

- ❑ Properly affix the finger-clip sensor to a finger. (It may be necessary to quickly remove the patient's fingernail polish.)

- ❑ Turn on the pulse oximeter, and record heart and oxygen readings.

- ❑ When you are done using the oximeter, shut off the unit. After each use, disassemble and store wiring and accessories in the pouch provided.

- ❑ Review operation of all display indicators, pulse amplitude, low battery, pulse search, oxygen saturation, and pulse rate.

- ❑ Review all controls (i.e., measure button, battery check button, printer on/off, printer paper advance).

- ❑ Change battery and paper printout as needed.

▶ **USING A BLOOD GLUCOSE METER (EMT SKILL WITH MEDICAL DIRECTION AUTHORIZATION) (PP. 310–311)**

- ❑ Take Standard Precautions.

- ❑ Prepare the blood glucose meter and supplies (i.e., lancet, test strip, Band-aid, sharps container, alcohol prep).

- ❑ Cleanse the skin with an alcohol prep. Allow the alcohol to dry before performing the stick.

- ❑ Use the lancet to perform a stick. Wipe away the first drop of blood that appears. Squeeze the puncture wound to get a second drop of blood.

- ❑ Apply the blood to the test strip. This may be done by holding the strip to the finger to draw the blood into the strip.

- ❑ Dispose of the lancet in a sharps container.

©2012 Pearson Education, Inc.
Emergency Care, 12th Ed.

❑ Read the blood glucose level displayed on the glucose meter. It may take from 15 to 30 seconds for the device to provide a reading. (Newer devices take 5 seconds and use less blood.)

❑ Assess the puncture site and apply direct pressure or a Band-aid to control the bleeding.

The reading is in mg/dl (milligrams of glucose per deciliter of blood). Normal "fasting" blood sugar values are 70–110 mg/dl. If the patient has a value less than 60–80 mg/dl and is symptomatic, treatment should be provided following local medical control.

13

Assessment of the Trauma Patient

Standard: Assessment (Secondary Assessment)

Competency: Applies scene information and patient assessment findings (scene size-up, primary and secondary assessment, patient history, and reassessment) to guide emergency management.

OBJECTIVES

After reading this chapter you should be able to:

13.1 Define key terms introduced in this chapter.

13.2 Differentiate between trauma patients with a significant mechanism of injury and those without a significant mechanism of injury.

13.3 Conduct a systematic secondary assessment of the trauma patient with no significant mechanism of injury.

13.4 Select the appropriate physical examination for a patient with no significant mechanism of injury.

13.5 Recognize patients for whom manual stabilization of the cervical spine and application of a cervical collar are indicated.

13.6 Conduct a systematic secondary assessment of an unstable or potentially unstable trauma patient, or patient with a significant mechanism of injury.

13.7 Explain the purpose of the rapid trauma assessment.

13.8 Recognize significant findings in the rapid trauma assessment.

13.9 Recognize situations in which you should consider requesting advanced life support personnel to assist with the management of a trauma patient.

13.10 Incorporate a detailed physical examination of the unstable or potentially unstable trauma patient at the appropriate time for a given scenario.

13.11 Integrate the secondary assessment of trauma patients with the primary assessment and reassessment portions of the patient assessment process.

©2012 Pearson Education, Inc.
Emergency Care, 12th Ed.

MATCH TERMINOLOGY/ DEFINITIONS

A. The grating sensation or sound or feeling of broken bones rubbing together

B. Movement of part of the chest in the opposite direction to the rest of the chest during respiration

C. Persistent erection of the penis that can result from spinal cord injury and some medical problems

D. Quick assessment of the head, neck, chest, abdomen, pelvis, extremities, and posterior body to detect signs and symptoms of injury

E. A surgical opening in the wall of the abdomen with a bag in place to collect excretions from the digestive system

F. A memory aid to remember deformities, contusions, abrasions, punctures/penetrations, burns, tenderness, lacerations, and swelling—symptoms of injury found by inspection or palpation during patient assessment

G. A surgical incision in the neck held open by a metal or plastic tube

H. Bulging of the neck veins

I. The step of patient assessment that follows the primary assessment

J. See colostomy

K. A condition of being stretched, inflated, or larger than normal

L. An assessment of the head, neck, chest, abdomen, pelvis, extremities, and posterior of the body to detect signs and symptoms of injury

M. A permanent surgical opening in the neck through which the patient breathes

N. A patient suffering from one or more physical injuries

_____ **1.** Colostomy

_____ **2.** Crepitation

_____ **3.** DCAP-BTLS

_____ **4.** Detailed physical exam

_____ **5.** Distention

_____ **6.** Focused history and physical exam

_____ **7.** Ileostomy

_____ **8.** Jugular vein distention

_____ **9.** Paradoxical motion

_____ **10.** Priapism

_____ **11.** Rapid trauma assessment

_____ **12.** Stoma

_____ **13.** Tracheostomy

_____ **14.** Trauma patient

MULTIPLE-CHOICE REVIEW

_____ **1.** When evaluating a patient during the focused physical exam, the EMT needs to _____ each body part.
   A. auscultate and visualize
   B. percuss and palpate
   C. inspect and palpate
   D. visualize and percuss

_____ **2.** When a patient tells you that he called because he cut his wrist with a razor, this is called the:
   A. primary assessment.
   B. chief complaint.
   C. SAMPLE history.
   D. secondary assessment.

_____ 3. The history of the present illness or injury for a trauma patient includes:
   A. the direction and strength of the force.
   B. actions taken to prevent or minimize injury.
   C. equipment used to protect the patient.
   D. all of these.

_____ 4. The physical exam includes the basics of inspection, auscultation, and:
   A. interaction.   C. palpation.
   B. intuition.   D. observation.

_____ 5. The "P" in DCAP-BTLS refers to:
   A. punctures/penetrations.
   B. palpation/pulse.
   C. priapism/penetrations.
   D. paradoxical motion/punctures.

_____ 6. The "S" in DCAP-BTLS refers to:
   A. soft tissue.   C. swelling.
   B. stable.   D. stomach.

_____ 7. Your patient was thrown from his motorcycle when he stopped suddenly. His thighs are very painful and a strange shape. When a body part is injured and it no longer has its normal shape, this is referred to as a:
   A. hematoma.   C. fracture.
   B. deformity.   D. crepitation.

_____ 8. Your patient has been outdoors in the sun most of the day. He has reddened and blistered areas on his shoulders and neck called:
   A. abrasions.   C. lacerations.
   B. burns.   D. contusions.

_____ 9. In the secondary assessment, you will be checking the patient from head to foot for pain and tenderness. The difference between pain and tenderness is:
   A. pain occurs only when you squeeze an injury site, whereas tender areas hurt all the time.
   B. pain is considered unbearable, whereas tenderness is usually bearable.
   C. tenderness may not hurt unless the area is palpated, whereas pain is evident without palpation.
   D. pain hurts only for the first 10 minutes, whereas tenderness doesn't go away.

_____ 10. A common result of injured capillaries bleeding under the skin is called:
   A. swelling.   C. laceration.
   B. puncture.   D. abrasion.

_____ 11. When is it appropriate to apply a cervical collar?
   A. If the mechanism of injury exerts great force on the upper body
   B. If there is any pain in the abdomen
   C. If there is any burn injury to the neck
   D. If the patient has experienced any trauma

_____ 12. You are treating a pitcher who was hit in the face with a ball that was hit by the batter. You remember from your EMT training that any blow above the _____ may damage the cervical spine.
   A. clavicles   C. femur
   B. diaphragm   D. pelvis

_____ 13. Experienced EMTs often refer to a soft cervical collar as:
   A. the device of choice for a neck injury.
   B. a "neck warmer."
   C. the requirement for all auto collision patients.
   D. the preferred extrication collar.

©2012 Pearson Education, Inc.
Emergency Care, 12th Ed.

_____ **14.** If a cervical collar is the wrong size, it may:
   A. cause additional injury to the spine.
   B. make breathing more difficult or obstruct the airway.
   C. prevent the patient from moving her neck.
   D. take too much time to adjust and apply correctly.

_____ **15.** The need for cervical immobilization should be based on:
   A. the trauma patient's level of responsiveness.
   B. the location of injuries to the patient.
   C. the mechanism of injury.
   D. all of these.

_____ **16.** When assessing and interviewing a patient, we ask about and look for signs and symptoms. What is a sign?
   A. A photograph of the patient's wrecked vehicle
   B. The patient's description of how the injury occurred
   C. An objective finding you can see, hear, or feel when examining the patient
   D. A subjective finding that the patient tells you about his current condition

_____ **17.** When considering the mechanism of injury (MOI), which of the following would *not* be considered a significant MOI in an adult?
   A. High-speed motorcycle crash
   B. Vehicle–pedestrian collision
   C. A 10-foot fall
   D. Rollover vehicle collision

_____ **18.** You are treating a patient who was in the front seat of an automobile involved in a collision. You observe a spider-web crack in the windshield and the facial lacerations on the patient. Most likely the patient:
   A. will have a life-threatening head injury.
   B. did not wear a seat belt or three-point harness.
   C. will also complain of leg injuries.
   D. was involved in a rollover collision.

_____ **19.** The EMT should lift and look under the airbag after the patient has been removed from the vehicle in order to:
   A. obtain the serial number of the airbag.
   B. see if a hazardous chemical has been released.
   C. note any visible damage to the steering wheel.
   D. determine if it deployed properly.

_____ **20.** When assessing the head of an adult male critical trauma patient, the EMT should inspect/palpate for _____ in addition to wounds and deformities.
   A. hematoma   **C.** crepitation
   B. scalp lacerations   **D.** abrasions

_____ **21.** When assessing the neck of an adult female critical trauma patient, the EMT should inspect/palpate for _____ in addition to wounds and deformities.
   A. jugular vein distention   **C.** lacerations
   B. swelling   **D.** burns

_____ **22.** The neck veins are usually not visible when the patient is:
   A. lying flat.   **C.** supine.
   B. sitting up.   **D.** prone.

_____ **23.** When assessing the chest of an adult female critical trauma patient, the EMT should inspect/palpate for _____ in addition to crepitations and deformities.
   A. hematoma   **C.** hemothorax
   B. paradoxical motion   **D.** jugular vein distention

_____ 24. When assessing the abdomen of an adult male critical trauma patient, the EMT should inspect/palpate for _____ in addition to wounds and deformities.
   A. distention of the kidneys
   B. colostomy and/or ileostomy
   C. crepitation
   D. paradoxical motion

_____ 25. When assessing the pelvis of an adult male critical trauma patient, the EMT should inspect/palpate for _____ in addition to wounds, deformities, and tenderness.
   A. paradoxical motion
   B. burns
   C. priapism
   D. rectal bleeding

_____ 26. An important principle to remember when examining a patient is to:
   A. tell the patient what you are going to do.
   B. assume spinal injury.
   C. try to maintain eye contact.
   D. all of these are correct.

_____ 27. If you are treating a severely injured trauma patient, it may be appropriate to skip the:
   A. initial physical exam.
   B. detailed physical exam.
   C. baseline vital signs.
   D. primary assessment.

_____ 28. A difference between the detailed physical exam and the rapid trauma exam includes:
   A. skipping the face, ears, eyes, nose, and mouth in the detailed exam.
   B. the detailed exam is usually done en route to the ED.
   C. the lungs are not listened to in a detailed exam.
   D. the extremities and posterior are not assessed in the rapid exam.

_____ 29. The final step of the detailed physical exam is to:
   A. complete the examination of airway, breathing, and circulation.
   B. make sure you have notified the ED.
   C. remove the collar and recheck the neck.
   D. roll the patient to examine the posterior of the body.

_____ 30. You are examining a patient who was struck on the head last night. His mental status is altered, and he has a bruise behind the ear. This is referred to as:
   A. raccoon's eyes.
   B. orbital hematoma.
   C. Battle's sign.
   D. Cushing reflex.

_____ 31. When performing the detailed physical exam, you note blood in the anterior chamber of the eye. This tells you that the:
   A. patient was wearing contact lenses.
   B. patient has a serious brain injury.
   C. patient's eye is bleeding inside.
   D. all of these.

_____ 32. Clear fluid that is draining from the ears and nose is called _____ fluid.
   A. lymphatic
   B. cerebrospinal
   C. mucous
   D. synovial

©2012 Pearson Education, Inc.
Emergency Care, 12th Ed.

_____ **33.** In addition to looking for deformities, you should look for all of the following *except* _____ when examining the mouth.
   A. possible airway obstructions
   B. loose or broken teeth
   C. tongue lacerations or swelling
   D. crepitation

_____ **34.** The detailed physical exam is *not* designed for the:
   A. trauma patient with a significant mechanism of injury (MOI).
   B. trauma patient with an unclear mechanism of injury (MOI).
   C. medical patient with very few signs and symptoms.
   D. critical trauma patient who could have a medical cause in addition to being involved in a car crash.

_____ **35.** If you are treating a patient who could be either medical or trauma, it is always best to assess for:
   A. the medical problem first.
   B. both problems at once.
   C. the trauma problem first.
   D. primary survey problems first.

COMPLETE THE FOLLOWING

1. List the components of the focused history and physical exam for a trauma patient.

   A. _____

   B. _____

   C. _____

   D. _____

   E. _____

   F. _____

   G. _____

2. Describe the areas assessed and what you are looking for in the rapid trauma assessment.

   A. _____

   B. _____

   C. _____

   D. _____

   E. _____

   F. _____

   G. _____

3. List five examples of significant injuries or signs of significant injuries.

A. _____

B. _____

C. _____

D. _____

E. _____

LABEL THE PHOTOGRAPHS

Fill in the name of area assessed in the physical exam of the trauma patient.

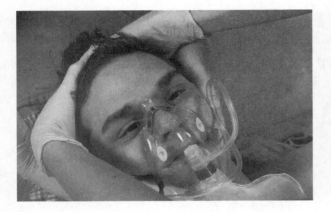

1. _____

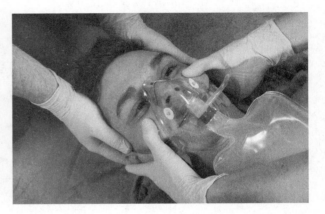

2. _____

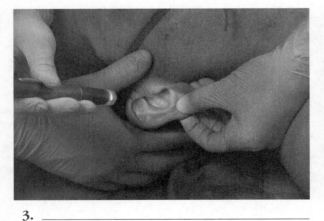

3. _____

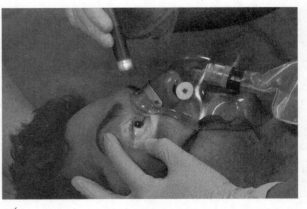

4. _____

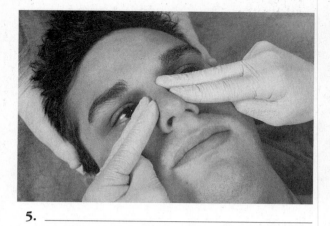

5. _____

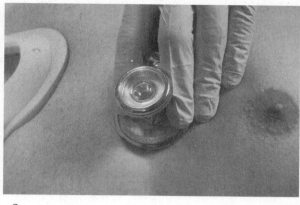

9. _____

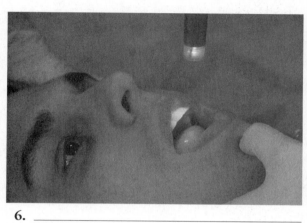

6. _____

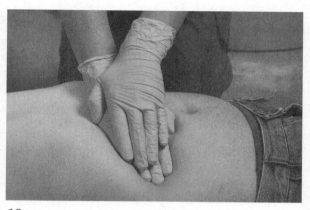

10. _____

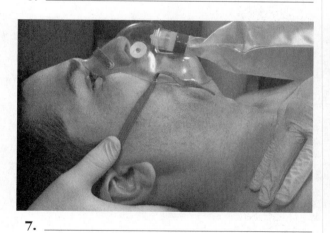

7. _____

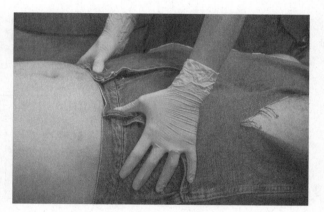

11. _____

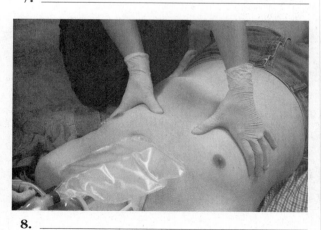

8. _____

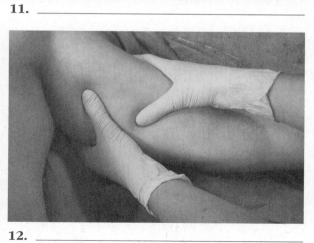

12. _____

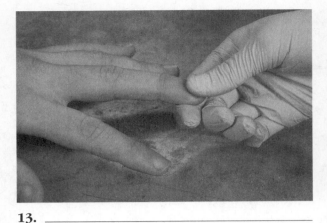

13. _____

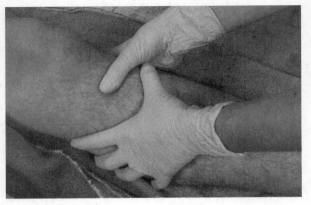

14. _____

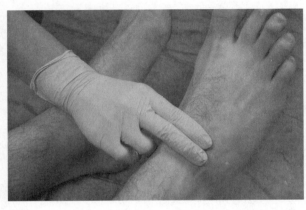

15. _____

COMPLETE THE CHART

Fill in the additional things to assess in each area of the body during the physical exam/trauma assessment.

Body Part	Wounds, Deformities, Tenderness	Plus
Head	Yes	1.
Neck	Yes	2. 3.
Chest	Yes	4. 5. 6.
Abdomen	Yes	7. 8. 9.
Pelvis	Yes	10. 11.
Extremities	Yes	12. 13. 14.
Posterior	Yes	15.

STREET SCENES DISCUSSION

Review the Street Scene on page 349 of the textbook. Then answer the following questions.

1. This patient has a wound to the chest. At what point should you consider ventilating him?

2. Should ALS be called?

3. If the patient had lost consciousness, what would have been your priorities for emergency care?

4. If the patient is injured on the left side of the chest at the mid-clavicular line and at nipple level, what organs may be injured?

CASE STUDY

▶ **MOTORCYCLE MISHAP**

You are dispatched to a motorcycle collision in an intersection in your community. Apparently, a car made a right turn on red without stopping and the motorcycle, which had the green light, collided with the left side of the car. On arrival, you conduct a scene size-up.

What four things should you be concerned about in the scene size-up of this collision?

1. _____

2. _____

3. _____

4. _____

You find out from a witness who was standing on the corner at the bus stop that the vehicles were probably traveling 40 mph and the cyclist crashed into the rear left door of the car. He was thrown off the motorcycle onto the roof of the car and then landed on his back in the street. The witness immediately rushed to aid the cyclist and at the same time motioned people in another vehicle to stop traffic and to call 911. The witness stated that the patient was in a lot of pain but never hit his head or lost consciousness. The cyclist was wearing a helmet, which he removed after the collision.

5. How does forming a general impression help you provide emergency care to the patient? On what is the general impression based?

Your general impression reveals a 20-year-old responsive male trauma patient with severe external blood loss. The patient is able to talk with you, although he is experiencing considerable pain in both his thighs and lower back. He is able to describe what happened in the collision, knows the day of the week, and is concerned about his new Sportster. His name is Tony, and he was on his way to the beach, which explains why he was wearing shorts and a T-shirt.

6. As you question Tony, what should one of your partners be doing?

7. What is Tony's mental status on the AVPU scale?

Tony keeps crying out, "It's my legs!" They are obviously broken but no longer seriously bleeding. You proceed with the primary assessment beginning with an assessment of Tony's airway.

8. Explain why it would be wrong to be distracted by Tony's pain and begin to treat his broken legs.

9. What should your primary assessment of Tony consist of?

Based on your primary assessment of Tony, you have determined he is a high-priority patient, and an ALS unit should be requested if it is not en route already. You found his airway is open and clear, his breathing is present and adequate, he is moving air into both sides of his chest equally, but he has a weak, rapid radial pulse and his skin is pale, cool, and clammy to the touch—possible signs of shock. One of your crew members has controlled the bleeding from Tony's thighs.

10. Why is Tony a high-priority patient?

11. How long should you wait for an ALS unit to arrive before transporting Tony?

As one of your crew members attends to Tony's injured legs and then places him onto a long backboard, you continue with the focused history and physical exam. Because you have reconsidered the mechanism of injury (MOI), you have decided to provide early transport for Tony as soon as he is packaged.

12. What would you be looking for as you examine the patient?

13. What would you be asking about for the SAMPLE history?

14. What vital signs should you assess?

En route to the hospital, you have time to conduct a detailed physical exam. Tony is immobilized and receiving oxygen via nonrebreather mask, the backboard is in the Trendelenburg position, and you are keeping him warm with a blanket. His vitals are a respiration rate of 20—good quality; a pulse rate of 120—weak and regular; a blood pressure of 110/70 mmHg; SpO$_2$ 90 percent; and pale, cool, and clammy skin.

15. What would the detailed physical exam include?

EMT SKILLS PERFORMANCE CHECKLISTS

▶ SIZING A CERVICAL COLLAR (P. 323)

❑ Measure the patient's neck.

❑ Measure the collar. Make sure it is not too small or tight, which would make the collar act as a constricting band.

▶ APPLYING AN ADJUSTABLE COLLAR TO A SEATED PATIENT (P. 324)

❑ Stabilize the head and neck from the rear.

❑ Properly angle the collar for placement.

❑ Position the collar bottom.

❑ Set the collar in place around the neck.

❑ Secure the collar.

❑ Maintain manual stabilization of the head and neck.

▶ APPLYING AN ADJUSTABLE COLLAR TO A SUPINE PATIENT (P. 325)

❑ Measure the patient's neck.

❑ Measure the collar. The chin piece should not lift the patient's chin and hyperextend the neck.

❑ Kneel at the patient's head and stabilize the head and neck.

❑ Set the collar in place.

❑ Secure the collar.

❑ Continue to stabilize the head and neck manually.

▶ PHYSICAL EXAMINATION—TRAUMA PATIENT (PP. 327–330)

❑ Take Standard Precautions.

❑ Reassess the MOI. If it is not significant, focus on the physical exam of only the injured part. If the MOI is significant:

- Continue manual stabilization of the head and neck.
- Consider requesting ALS personnel.
- Reconsider transport decision.
- Reassess mental status.
- Perform rapid trauma assessment.
- Transport.

©2012 Pearson Education, Inc.
Emergency Care, 12th Ed.

► HISTORY OF PRESENT ILLNESS

❑ Rapidly determine what happened to the patient to cause injury.

❑ Rapid trauma assessment:

- Rapidly assess each part of the body:
  - Head: wounds, deformities, tenderness, plus crepitation.
  - Neck: wounds, deformities, tenderness, plus jugular vein distension and crepitation.
  - Chest: wounds; deformities; tenderness; plus crepitation, paradoxical motion, and breath sounds (absent, present, equal).
  - Abdomen: wounds; deformities; tenderness; plus firm, soft, or distended.
  - Pelvis: wounds, deformities, tenderness with gentle compression for tenderness or motion.
  - Extremities: wounds; deformities; tenderness; plus distal circulation, sensation, and motor function.
  - Posterior: wounds, deformities, tenderness. (To examine posterior, roll patient using spinal precautions.)

► VITAL SIGNS

❑ Assess the patient's baseline vital signs:

- Respiration
- Pulse
- Skin color, temperature, condition (capillary refill in infants and children)
- Pupils
- Blood pressure
- Oxygen saturation (if directed by local protocol)

► PAST MEDICAL HISTORY

❑ Interview patient or (if patient is unresponsive) interview family and bystanders to get as much information as possible about the patient's problem. Ask about:

- Signs and symptoms
- Allergies
- Medications
- Pertinent past history
- Last oral intake
- Events leading up to problem

► INTERVENTIONS AND TRANSPORT

❑ Contact on-line medical directory and perform interventions as needed.

❑ Package and transport the patient.

► DETAILED PHYSICAL EXAM IN THE SEQUENCE OF ASSESSMENT PRIORITIES

❑ Scene size-up.

❑ Pprimary assessment and critical interventions for immediately life-threatening problems.

❑ History of the present illness, rapid physical exam, vital signs, plus interventions as needed.

❑ Repeat primary assessment for immediately life-threatening problems. Provide critical interventions as needed.

❑ Detailed physical exam (time and critical-care needs permitting).

❑ Reassessment for life-threatening problems, plus reassessment of vital signs. Provide critical interventions as needed.

14
Assessment of the Medical Patient

Standard: Assessment (Secondary Assessment)

Competency: Applies scene information and patient assessment findings (scene size-up, primary and secondary assessment, patient history, and reassessment) to guide emergency management.

OBJECTIVES

After reading this chapter you should be able to:

14.1 Define key terms introduced in this chapter.

14.2 Adapt the secondary assessment process to both responsive and unresponsive medical patients.

14.3 Collect a systematic history of the present illness.

14.4 Collect a relevant past medical history.

14.5 Adapt the secondary assessment process to specific patient complaints.

14.6 Adapt your approach to secondary assessment of the medical patient to overcome challenges, according to the circumstances.

14.7 Conduct a rapid physical examination for the unresponsive medical patient.

14.8 Explain the importance of checking the pupils and baseline vital signs in the unresponsive medical patient.

14.9 Recognize situations in which you should consider requesting the assistance of advanced life support personnel for a medical patient.

14.10 Identify other sources of patient information for the unresponsive or uncooperative medical patient.

©2012 Pearson Education, Inc.
Emergency Care, 12th Ed.

MATCH TERMINOLOGY/ DEFINITIONS

A. Description of where pain is located and where it spreads to

B. Description of the pain, such as stabbing, crampy, dull, or sharp

C. Description of what makes the pain worse, such as sitting, standing, eating certain foods

D. Description of how bad the pain is, often described on a scale of 1 to 10

E. A memory device for the questions asked to get a description of the present illness

F. History relating to the patient's chief complaint

G. A patient with one or more medical diseases or conditions

H. Description of how fast or slow the pain came on and what the patient was doing when the pain started

I. The reason why EMS was called, usually in the patient's own words

_____ 1. Chief complaint

_____ 2. Medical patient

_____ 3. Onset of pain

_____ 4. OPQRST

_____ 5. Pertinent past history

_____ 6. Provocation of pain

_____ 7. Quality of pain

_____ 8. Radiation of pain

_____ 9. Severity of pain

MULTIPLE-CHOICE REVIEW

_____ 1. Your patient is an alert 58-year-old male who is complaining of chest pain. The components of the secondary assessment for a responsive medical patient include all of the following *except:*
   A. history of the present illness.
   B. SAMPLE history.
   C. baseline vital signs.
   D. rapid trauma exam.

_____ 2. Many memory aids are used during the assessment process. OPQRST is a memory aid to help the EMT remember the:
   A. questions to ask about the past medical history.
   B. questions that expand on the history of the present illness.
   C. status of the patient's condition.
   D. levels of the patient's mental status.

_____ 3. When you ask a 65-year-old woman with chest pain, "Can you think of anything that might have triggered or caused this pain?" you are questioning her about the _____ of her pain.
   A. onset.
   B. provocation.
   C. quality.
   D. radiation.

_____ 4. When you ask a male patient with back pain, "How bad is the pain?" you are questioning him about:
   A. quality.
   B. severity.
   C. time.
   D. radiation.

_____ **5.** Why is it important for the EMT to determine the T in OPQRST when questioning the 58-year-old male with a chief complaint of chest pain?
A. The patient's temperature could be a contributing factor.
B. The patient may have fell and injured his tibia.
C. It is helpful to determine the time when the pain began.
D. The patient may have sustained a tension pneumothorax.

_____ **6.** The 55-year-old male continues to discuss his condition with you. His chief complaint is chest pain and when you ask, "Do you have nausea or have you been vomiting?" you are questioning him about his:
A. signs and symptoms.
B. medication history.
C. allergies.
D. pertinent past history.

_____ **7.** The alert 58-year-old male who is complaining of chest pain goes on to describe other recent hospitalizations and the medical condition his doctor is treating him for. This information is considered:
A. unnecessary information.
B. pertinent past history.
C. the cause of today's event.
D. the reason the ambulance was called.

_____ **8.** When you ask an elderly female patient "How have you been feeling today?" you are asking her about the:
A. pertinent past history.
B. signs and symptoms.
C. events leading to the illness.
D. last oral intake.

_____ **9.** When interviewing a patient with a specific chief complaint and a known history, the EMT may need to:
A. contact medical direction for additional interview questions.
B. ask additional questions pertinent to the complaint.
C. immediately administer medications.
D. any one of these.

_____ **10.** You are treating a 62-year-old female who is complaining of difficulty breathing. This medical patient does not take any prescribed medication for her condition, so you should generally:
A. look for a medical identification device.
B. consult with the patient's personal physician.
C. transport the patient to the hospital.
D. do all of these.

_____ **11.** In terms of your initial approach to the focused history and physical exam of a middle-aged male patient, the biggest difference between a responsive and an unresponsive patient is that:
A. the responsive patient gets the OPQRST questions last.
B. the unresponsive patient will be given a rapid physical exam first.
C. bystanders become more important if the patient is responsive.
D. a rapid trauma exam is not done on an unconscious patient.

_____ **12.** You will be conducting a rapid physical exam on an unresponsive 54-year-old female medical patient. You should include all of the following steps _except_:
A. look for jugular vein distention.
B. determine firmness or rigidity of abdomen.
C. check for incontinence of urine or feces.
D. ask the SAMPLE history questions.

©2012 Pearson Education, Inc.
Emergency Care, 12th Ed.

13. When assessing a 28-year-old female patient who has a medical complaint, be sure to check the extremities for:
   A. central cyanosis.
   B. sensation and motor function.
   C. edema and discoloration.
   D. capillary refill in all adult patients.

14. When conducting a physical exam of an unconscious adult patient with a suspected medical problem, you remember there was a "Vial of Life" sticker on the front door of the residence. This is important because it may:
   A. reveal the patient's name.
   B. give clues to the patient's home address.
   C. reveal that additional medical identification is in the refrigerator.
   D. be the cause of the emergency.

15. In most regions, in addition to taking the pulse and respirations, the baseline vital signs of adult medical patients include:
   A. determining what they last ate.
   B. assessing the CO_2 in their blood.
   C. determining their capillary refill time.
   D. the oxygen saturation.

16. When you are deciding which steps to follow in assessing your patient, what should you consider first and why?
   A. The past medical history of the patient because it predicts today's problem.
   B. The primary assessment because that identifies the life threats.
   C. The physical exam because subtle injuries are often severe.
   D. The vital signs reveal all the serious medical conditions the patient may have.

COMPLETE THE FOLLOWING

1. List the components of a focused history and physical exam for an unresponsive medical patient.

   A. _____

   B. _____

   C. _____

   D. _____

2. List the seven areas you assess in the medical patient during your rapid physical exam.

   A. _____

   B. _____

   C. _____

   D. _____

   E. _____

   F. _____

   G. _____

COMPLETE THE CHART

Complete the chart by writing the remainder of the word that follows each letter in the acronyms SAMPLE and OPQRST.

1. S	
2. A	
3. M	
4. P	
5. L	
6. E	
7. O	
8. P	
9. Q	
10. R	
11. S	
12. T	

STREET SCENES DISCUSSION

Review the Street Scene on page 69 of the textbook. Then answer the following questions.

1. What would it have suggested to you if the patient had been talking in short, choppy sentences?

2. You found the patient's lung sounds "equal, but noisy, like a whistling sound." If you had found that this patient's chest was silent, would that have been a good sign?

3. What is the term for the lung sounds heard in this patient's chest?

4. If the patient had her Albuterol inhaler with her, would it have been appropriate to contact medical direction for permission to assist in the administration of the medication?

5. You assess the patient with a pulse oximeter. What does an SpO_2 of 96 percent mean?

EMT SKILLS PERFORMANCE CHECKLIST

▶ **FOCUSED HISTORY AND PHYSICAL EXAM—RESPONSIVE MEDICAL PATIENT (P. 355)**

❑ Take Standard Precautions.

❑ Gather a history of the present illness from patient by asking OPQRST questions.

❑ Gather a past medical history by asking the SAMPLE questions.

❑ Conduct a focused physical exam (focusing on the affected body part or system).

❑ Obtain baseline vital signs.

❑ Perform interventions and transport (contact on-line medical direction as needed).

▶ **FOCUSED HISTORY AND PHYSICAL EXAM—UNRESPONSIVE MEDICAL PATIENT (P. 363)**

❑ Take Standard Precautions.

❑ Conduct a rapid physical exam by assessing:

- Head
- Neck
- Chest
- Abdomen
- Pelvis
- Extremities
- Posterior

❏ Obtain baseline vital signs:

- Respiration
- Pulse
- Skin CTC (capillary refill in infants and children)
- Pupils
- Blood pressure
- Oxygen saturation (if directed by local protocol)

❏ Past medical history (interview family and bystanders for present illness [OPQRST] and the SAMPLE history):

- Signs and symptoms
- Allergies
- Medications
- Pertinent past history
- Last oral intake
- Events leading to the illness

❏ Interventions and transport. Contact on-line medical direction as needed. Perform interventions as needed and transport the patient.

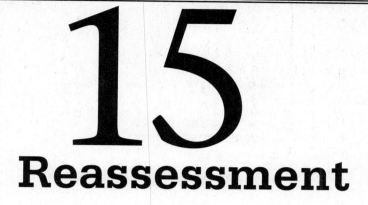

15
Reassessment

Standard: Assessment (Reassessment)

Competency: Applies scene information and patient assessment findings (scene size-up, primary and secondary assessment, patient history, and reassessment) to guide emergency management.

OBJECTIVES

After reading this chapter you should be able to:

15.1 Define key terms introduced in this chapter.

15.2 Explain the importance of reassessment.

15.3 Identify the proper points in the patient-care process at which reassessment should be performed.

15.4 Discuss the purpose of each of the components of reassessment.

15.5 Adapt the reassessment process based on patients' conditions.

15.6 Recognize both obvious and subtle changes in the patient's condition.

15.7 Assign meaning to trends in the patient's condition over time.

15.8 Discuss the importance of sharing your findings with the patient.

15.9 Document reassessment findings in the patient-care record.

15.10 Recognize when changes in patient care are needed, based on reassessment findings.

MATCH TERMINOLOGY/ DEFINITIONS

A. Changes in a patient's condition over time, such as slowing respirations or rising pulse rate, that may show improvement or deterioration, and that can be shown by documenting repeated assessments

B. A procedure for detecting changes in a patient's condition; it involves four steps: repeating the primary assessment, repeating and recording vital signs, repeating the focused assessment, and checking interventions

_____ 1. Reassessment

_____ 2. Trending

MULTIPLE-CHOICE REVIEW

_____ 1. You will need to conduct a reassessment on each of your patients. Which one of the following statements is most accurate for describing the purpose of performing the reassessment?
   A. To stabilize the patient's condition or to treat any life threats
   B. To detect and treat life threats and to evaluate the EMS system's effectiveness
   C. To evaluate the EMS system's effectiveness and to detect changes in patient condition
   D. To repeat key elements of assessment procedures already performed in order to detect changes in patient condition

_____ 2. Reassessment is done on all patients. In a few instances, the reassessment may be omitted. This is appropriate only if:
   A. the PCR is not completed.
   B. you do not want to interrupt patient conversation.
   C. life-saving interventions prevent doing it.
   D. a short transport time prevents completion.

_____ 3. Your patient is a young child who was suddenly injured. During the reassessment of a child, the EMT should do which of the following and why?
   A. Be sure to avoid eye contact at all times because it will scare the child.
   B. Try to stand above the patient so he can look up at you and see you at all times.
   C. Speak in a loud voice so the patient can hear every one of your instructions.
   D. Use a reassuring voice to help calm the patient.

_____ 4. You are treating a 45-year-old male who sustained multiple injuries in a fall. En route to the hospital, you will be conducting a reassessment, which includes all the following steps *except*:
   A. reassess vital signs.
   B. repeat the primary assessment for life threats.
   C. repeat the focused assessment.
   D. repeat all interventions.

_____ 5. You have just conducted the reassessment of a 35-year-old male patient who was struck by a vehicle. Which of the following is the last step in the reassessment?
   A. Reassess the vital signs.
   B. Check interventions.
   C. Repeat the primary assessment.
   D. Repeat the focused assessment.

©2012 Pearson Education, Inc.
Emergency Care, 12th Ed.

_____ **6.** En route to the hospital, you will be reassessing your 25-year-old male patient, who sustained a rib fracture. Which of the following is *not* a step you should do when repeating the reassessment?
   A. Reestablish patient priorities.
   B. Monitor skin color, temperature, and condition.
   C. Maintain an open airway.
   D. Apply a cervical collar.

_____ **7.** During your reassessment of a 22-year-old female who is complaining of abdominal cramps, you note that her pulse is rapid and her skin is cool, pale, and clammy. This may indicate:
   A. deterioration in mental status.
   B. an occluded airway.
   C. heat exhaustion.
   D. the onset of shock.

_____ **8.** The mental status of an unresponsive child or infant can be checked by:
   A. a sternal rub.
   B. assessing the capillaries for refill.
   C. shouting or by flicking the feet.
   D. asking the parent to stick a pin in the child's foot.

_____ **9.** An example of checking interventions during the reassessment of a medical patient is:
   A. taking an initial blood pressure.
   B. ensuring adequacy of oxygen delivery.
   C. applying a tourniquet.
   D. bandaging a severe laceration.

_____ **10.** Your patient is a 15-year-old male who fell off his bike and struck his head. Frequently reassessing this patient establishes _____; which is (are) _____ for quality patient care.
   A. a paper trail; helpful
   B. trends; essential
   C. legal evidence; required
   D. a reason for treatment; needed

_____ **11.** You are treating a 37-year-old male patient who has a chief complaint of breathing difficulty. The best way to determine if the patient is improving or deteriorating en route to the hospital is to:
   A. ask the hospital what needs to be done next.
   B. contact medical direction by radio.
   C. do frequent reassessments of the patient.
   D. keep repeating the primary assessment.

_____ **12.** You are treating a patient who fell and sustained a laceration to his right arm. The bleeding is controlled and there are no other injuries. If the patient has normal vital signs, you would consider his condition to be _____ and the recommended interval for reassessment is every _____ minutes.
   A. stable; 5
   B. stable; 15
   C. unstable; 10
   D. unstable; 20

_____ 13. You are treating a 22-year-old male patient who sustained a closed head injury when he was thrown off his bike. He is breathing adequately yet is confused about the day of the week and his location. The recommended interval for reassessment is every _____ minutes because this patient's status is _____.
   A. 5; unstable
   B. 15; stable
   C. 10; unstable
   D. 20; stable

_____ 14. You are treating a 22-year-old female who has a chief complaint of back pain from a fall. You should repeat the reassessment en route to the hospital:
   A. after you have noticed and documented trends.
   B. whenever you or your partner has the time and opportunity to do so.
   C. whenever you believe there may have been a change in the patient's condition.
   D. when directed to do so by medical direction.

_____ 15. During your reassessment of an unresponsive 45-year-old female patient whom you are treating for a suspected stroke. you hear gurgling airway sounds. What intervention is the most appropriate for you to take?
   A. Sit the patient up.
   B. Suction the patient.
   C. Check the oxygen tubing.
   D. All of these are most appropriate.

_____ 16. Of the following, which is an example of a patient who requires reassessment of your interventions en route to the hospital?
   A. A patient with a minor respiratory complaint
   B. A patient who had multiple fractures and to which you applied splints
   C. A patient whose airway you have spent the entire call attempting to clear
   D. A patient who was stable and had minor injuries

COMPLETE THE FOLLOWING

1. List the six steps involved in repeating the primary assessment.

   A. _____

   B. _____

   C. _____

   D. _____

   E. _____

   F. _____

2. List the three steps you should always do when checking interventions.

   A. _____

   B. _____

   C. _____

©2012 Pearson Education, Inc.
Emergency Care, 12th Ed.

STREET SCENES DISCUSSION

Review the Street Scene on page 380 of the textbook. Then answer the following questions.

1. Why do you think it is so important to monitor and maintain the airway of a stroke patient?

2. Many times a patient experiencing a stroke can hear but not speak. Why do you think this is something you should be aware of?

EMT-BASIC SKILLS PERFORMANCE CHECKLIST

▶ **REASSESSMENT (P. 373)**

❑ Take Standard Precautions.

❑ Repeat the primary assessment for life threats:

- Reassess mental status.
- Maintain an open airway.
- Monitor breathing rate and quality.
- Reassess pulse rate and quality.
- Monitor skin color, temperature, and condition.
- Reestablish patient treatment priorities.

❑ Reassess and record vital signs.

❑ Repeat focused assessment related to chief complaint or injuries.

❑ Check interventions:

- Ensure adequacy of oxygen delivery and ventilation support.
- Ensure management of bleeding.
- Ensure adequacy of other interventions.

NOTE: Repeat the reassessment every 15 minutes for a stable patient and every 5 minutes for an unstable patient.

16

Critical Thinking and Decision Making

Standard: Clinical Behavior/Judgment (Decision Making)

Competency: Initiates basic interventions based on assessment findings intended to mitigate the emergency and provide limited symptom relief while providing access to definitive care.

OBJECTIVES

After reading this chapter you should be able to:

16.1 Define key terms introduced in this chapter.

16.2 Compare and contrast EMTs' and physicians' diagnoses.

16.3 Explain the relationship between critical thinking and diagnosis.

16.4 Explain typical steps used in the basic approach to reaching diagnoses.

16.5 Explain how diagnosis in emergency situations may differ from traditional approaches to diagnosis.

16.6 Identify some of the special challenges to EMS providers in the diagnostic process.

16.7 Discuss the relationship between diagnosis and treatment in emergency situations.

16.8 Discuss the benefits and pitfalls of diagnostic shortcuts (heuristics).

16.9 Identify heuristics commonly used in EMS.

16.10 Describe ways in which EMTs can improve their critical-thinking processes.

MATCH TERMINOLOGY/ DEFINITIONS

A. A description or label for a patient's condition, based on the patient's history, physical exam, and vital signs, that assists the EMT in further evaluation and treatment; an EMS diagnosis is often less specific than a traditional medical diagnosis

B. A list of potential diagnoses compiled early in the assessment of the patient

C. A sign or symptom that suggests the possibility of a particular problem that is very serious

D. A description or label for a patient's condition that assists a clinician in further evaluation and treatment

E. An analytical process that can help someone think through a problem in an organized and efficient manner

_____ **1.** Critical thinking

_____ **2.** Diagnosis

_____ **3.** Differential diagnosis

_____ **4.** EMS diagnosis/EMT diagnosis

_____ **5.** Red flag

MULTIPLE-CHOICE REVIEW

_____ **1.** The term used to describe the conclusion that an EMT makes about a patient's condition after assessing that patient is called the:
- **A.** presumptive diagnosis.
- **B.** EMT diagnosis.
- **C.** EMS diagnosis.
- **D.** all of these are correct.

_____ **2.** The analytical process that assists the EMT in reaching a field diagnosis is referred to as:
- **A.** active assessment.
- **B.** passive assessment.
- **C.** critical thinking.
- **D.** detailed assessment.

_____ **3.** The basic approach that clinicians use to arrive at a diagnosis includes each of the following _except_:
- **A.** gather information.
- **B.** administer many lab tests.
- **C.** consider the possibilities.
- **D.** reach a conclusion.

_____ **4.** When a clinician draws up a list of conditions that may be the cause of the patient's condition today, this is referred to as the:
- **A.** admission diagnosis.
- **B.** presenting problem.
- **C.** differential diagnosis.
- **D.** assessment finding.

_____ **5.** The signs or symptoms that suggest the possibility of a particular problem that is very serious is referred to as a(n):
- **A.** red flag.
- **B.** black triage tag.
- **C.** unstable situation.
- **D.** none of these.

_____ 6. When a highly experienced physician comes to a diagnosis, he or she most likely used:
  A. heuristics.
  B. pattern recognition.
  C. shortcuts.
  D. all of these.

_____ 7. The traditional approach to diagnosis involves:
  A. narrowing down a long list.
  B. jumping to conclusions.
  C. taking lots of shortcuts.
  D. eliminating similar conditions.

_____ 8. Each of the following are considered common heuristics or biases *except*:
  A. illusory correlation.
  B. availability.
  C. representativeness.
  D. underconfidence.

_____ 9. When a clinician is specifically looking for evidence that supports the diagnosis he or she already has in mind, he or she is committing a(n) _____ bias.
  A. anchoring
  B. confirmation
  C. satisfying
  D. illusionary

_____ 10. When a patient does not fit the classic pattern, such as a cardiac patient without crushing chest pain, the EMT has to be careful not to make a(n) _____ error or bias.
  A. confirmation
  B. representativeness
  C. overconfidence
  D. availability

_____ 11. An EMT recently had a patient with heat stroke. The next time he or she has a patient in a warm environment, the EMT is more likely to think of this as the diagnosis as opposed to more common problems, such as dehydration. This bias is referred to as:
  A. overconfidence.
  B. illusory correlation.
  C. confirmation.
  D. availability.

_____ 12. The EMT should be skeptical about one condition being the actual cause of another condition a patient presents with. Drawing conclusions about the cause of a diagnosis can lead to a(n):
  A. anchoring adjustment.
  B. illusory correlation.
  C. search satisfying bias.
  D. availability bias.

_____ 13. You are treating a patient who was found on the floor in the nursing home. It seems evident that he has a fractured hip as he lies on the floor in pain. If you stop the search for a diagnosis as soon as you come up with the cause of today's problem, this can lead to:
  A. missing out on the secondary diagnosis.
  B. overconfidence and misdiagnosis.
  C. overestimating the frequency of the problem.
  D. all of these.

©2012 Pearson Education, Inc.
Emergency Care, 12th Ed.

_____ **14.** If you are an EMT who wants to think like a highly experienced physician in your assessment of patients, you should try to:

    A. learn to hate ambiguity.

    B. utilize a single strategy in all cases.

    C. understand the limitations of technology and people.

    D. reflect on what others have learned.

_____ **15.** The EMT who wants to think like a highly experienced physician tries to do each of the following techniques *except*:

    A. organize data in her or his head.

    B. reflect on what he or she has learned.

    C. realize that no one strategy works for everything.

    D. try not to learn from others.

_____ **16.** You are an EMT treating a patient who has developed a rash and uticaria on her chest and face. If you were to begin treating this patient as a victim of a severe allergic reaction rather than questioning her about previous development of a similar rash, you would be exhibiting an example of:

    A. an availability bias.

    B. an illusionary correlation.

    C. having overconfidence in your judgment.

    D. an appropriate shortcut to take.

COMPLETE THE FOLLOWING

1. List eight ways in which an EMT can learn to think like a highly experienced physician.

    A. _____

    B. _____

    C. _____

    D. _____

    E. _____

    F. _____

    G. _____

    H. _____

STREET SCENES DISCUSSION

Review the Street Scene on page 392 of the textbook. Then answer the following questions.

1. If the patient had a normal blood sugar test, what else could have contributed to his condition today?

2. If Mr. Ronson had a cardiac and stroke history but no signs of stroke on the Cincinnati Prehospital Stroke Scale and no complaint of chest pain, could he still be having a heart attack or stroke?

3. How might your care change if Mr. Ronson became unconscious?

4. If Mr. Ronson had a good gag reflex and no trouble swallowing, would your care have been different?

©2012 Pearson Education, Inc.
Emergency Care, 12th Ed.

17

Communication and Documentation

Standard: Preparatory (Documentation; EMS System Communication)

Competency: Applies fundamental knowledge of the EMS system, safety/well-being of the EMT, medical/legal and ethical issues to the provision of emergency care.

| OBJECTIVES

After reading this chapter you should be able to:

17.1 Define key terms introduced in this chapter.

17.2 Describe the role of communication technology in EMS systems.

17.3 Describe various types of communication devices and equipment used in EMS system communication.

17.4 Explain the role of the Federal Communications Commission as it relates to EMS system communication.

17.5 Communicate effectively by radio with dispatch and hospital personnel.

17.6 Provide a thorough, organized, concise report of pertinent patient information when giving a radio report or requesting orders.

17.7 Explain the importance of asking for information to be repeated for confirmation and clarification.

17.8 Deliver an organized, complete, concise report of pertinent patient information when giving a verbal report to receiving hospital personnel.

17.9 Demonstrate principles and techniques of effective verbal and nonverbal interpersonal communication.

17.10 Adapt communication principles for effective interaction with patients of various ages and cultures.

17.11 Complete a prehospital care report in the format or formats required by your service.

17.12 Understand legal issues associated with documentation.

MATCH TERMINOLOGY/ DEFINITIONS

A. An abbreviated form of the PCR that an EMS crew can leave at the hospital when there is not enough time to complete the PCR before leaving

B. A device that picks up signals from lower-power radio units, such as mobile and portable radios, and retransmits them at a higher power; it allows low-power radio signals to be transmitted over longer distances

C. A phone that transmits through the air instead of over wires so that the phone can be transported and used over a wide area

D. A two-way radio that is used or affixed in a vehicle

E. A two-way radio at a fixed site such as a hospital or dispatch center

F. A handheld two-way radio

G. The unit of measurement of the output of a radio

E **1.** Base station

C **2.** Cell phone

D **3.** Mobile radio

F **4.** Portable radio

B **5.** Repeater

G **6.** Watt

A **7.** Drop report (or transfer report)

MULTIPLE-CHOICE REVIEW

B **1.** One of the key contributions to improvement in EMS over the years has been:
  A. the type II, van-style ambulance vehicle.
  B. development of radio links among dispatcher, mobile units, and hospitals.
  C. the military antishock trousers.
  D. air conditioning in the transport vehicles.

D **2.** Components of a communications system include:
  A. base stations.
  B. mobile units.
  C. portable radios.
  D. all of these.

C **3.** You will need to be alerting the trauma center of the patient's condition directly from the scene. Because your portable radio does not have the power to reach the hospital ED from the scene, you will need to rely on a device that picks up radio signals from lower-powered units and retransmits them at a higher power. This device is called a:
  A. mobile.
  B. cellular.
  C. repeater.
  D. portable.

A **4.** The government agency that maintains order on the airwaves is called the:
  A. FCC.
  B. FAA.
  C. FEMA.
  D. DOT.

_C_ 5. The purposes of always following the general principles of radio transmission are to allow all persons to use the frequencies and to:
   A. avoid having to repeat orders from medical direction.
   B. enable the EMT to talk in code language.
   C. prevent delays.
   D. do all of these.

_C_ 6. Of the following components of a medical radio report, which is in the correct order?
   1. Major past illness
   2. Chief complaint
   3. Unit identification and level of provider
   4. Emergency medical care given
   A. 4, 1, 2, 3
   B. 3, 4, 1, 2
   C. 3, 2, 1, 4
   D. 1, 2, 4, 3

_B_ 7. You arrive on the scene that includes a 58-year-old male patient. The ambulance was called because has had chest pain for the past hour. The "chest pain" in this situation is called the:
   A. major past illness.
   B. chief complaint.
   C. presenting diagnosis.
   D. call type.

_D_ 8. You are en route to the hospital with a 27-year-old female who is pain. During your radio report, you say, "The patient's abdomen feels rigid." You are actually advising the hospital of:
   A. the baseline vital signs.
   B. the emergency medical care given.
   C. the response of the patient to the emergency medical care.
   D. pertinent findings of the physical exam.

_C_ 9. During your radio report, you state, "The patient's mental status has not changed during our care." You are attempting to advise the hospital of the:
   A. baseline vital signs.
   B. emergency medical care you have given so far.
   C. the response of the patient to the emergency medical care you have provided.
   D. pertinent findings of the physical exam.

_A_ 10. Your local protocols require a direct medical order to allow you to assist the patient with her bronchodilator device. Whenever you request an order for medical direction over the radio, it is good practice to:
   A. repeat the physician's order word for word back to the physician.
   B. question all verbal orders that are given.
   C. speak quickly because the physician is busy.
   D. call the physician back to verify.

_B_ 11. If you receive an order from the on-line physician for ten times the normal dose of a medication (i.e., 1,500 mg of ASA instead of 150 mg), what should you do?
   A. Switch to another frequency to find another physician.
   B. Question the physician about the order.
   C. Follow the physician's order as stated.
   D. Ignore the order and do what you believe is correct.

_B_ **12.** It is three in the morning and your partner is interviewing a patient with a minor complaint. You notice that he is standing with arms crossed looking down at the patient. What nonverbal message could he be sending to the patient?

A. "I am here to help you."
B. "I am not really interested."
C. "I can empathize with your problem."
D. "I am afraid of catching your disease."

_D_ **13.** You are treating a patient who was struck by an automobile. It is obvious that the patient has a broken leg because a bone is protruding through the skin. The patient asks you, "Is my leg broken?" What would be the most appropriate response?

A. "Relax and stay calm. You will be all right."
B. "I am not qualified to make that determination."
C. "No, it's a bad cut, and I'll control the bleeding with a bandage."
D. "Yes it is, and I will be as gentle as possible splinting it."

_A_ **14.** When treating a toddler who is sitting on the couch complaining of stomach pain, the best approach is to:

A. kneel down so you are at the child's level.
B. speak louder so the child can hear you above all the crying.
C. stare directly into the child's eyes.
D. tell the child you are a friend of his parents.

_C_ **15.** The prehospital care report (PCR) serves as a legal document as well as a(n):

A. press release form for your EMS agency.
B. receipt for the patient.
C. aid to research, education, and administrative efforts.
D. form to report all calls to the local police department.

_D_ **16.** Why is it necessary to complete a prehospital care report (PCR) if, on each call, you give the emergency department staff a good oral report?

A. The QI committee needs something to hold you to.
B. It provides a means for the ED staff to review the patient's prehospital care.
C. The ED usually does not listen to oral reports.
D. Duplication is helpful in emergency call documentation.

_C_ **17.** The copy of the prehospital care report (PCR) left at the hospital:

A. is returned to the state for quality review and follow-up.
B. is thrown out once it is key-punched and added to computer file.
C. should become part of the patient's permanent hospital record.
D. is sent to the regional Emergency Medical Services agency.

_C_ **18.** You are called to court to testify about a civil matter when a patient sues the city for an injury that occurred in a public place. Which of the following will best help you recall the events of the call?

A. The questioning by the defense's attorney
B. The questioning by the plaintiff's attorney
C. A complete and accurate prehospital care report (PCR)
D. Your tape recording of the call dispatch

_D_ **19.** The person who completed a prehospital care report (PCR) may be called to court to testify about:

A. the call in a criminal proceeding.
B. the care provided to the patient.
C. the call in a civil proceeding.
D. all of these.

_B_ **20.** The routine review of prehospital care reports (PCRs) for conformity to current medical and organizational standards is a process called:
  A. initial feedback.
  B. quality improvement.
  C. stress debriefing.
  D. system research.

_B_ **21.** Each individual box on a prehospital care report (PCR) is called a(n):
  A. narrative.
  B. data element.
  C. key punch.
  D. assessment.

_C_ **22.** According to the NHTSA, in addition to other data elements, the minimum data set on a prehospital care report (PCR) should include all of the following *except*:
  A. respiratory rate and effort and skin color and temperature.
  B. times of incident, dispatch, and arrival at the patient.
  C. patient's Social Security number.
  D. capillary refill for patients less than 6 years old.

_B_ **23.** The time of dispatch is an example of _____ data on the prehospital care report (PCR).
  A. assessment
  B. run
  C. patient
  D. narrative

_A_ **24.** Examples of patient data on a prehospital care report (PCR) would be:
  A. date of birth and age.
  B. time of arrival at the hospital.
  C. ambulance identification number.
  D. the hospital transported to.

_C_ **25.** Experienced EMTs consider a good prehospital care report (PCR) as one that:
  A. protects them against a QA review.
  B. is vague enough to prevent lawsuits.
  C. paints a picture of the patient.
  D. identifies symptoms overlooked by the patient.

_B_ **26.** A statement such as "The patient has a swollen, deformed extremity" on the narrative portion of the prehospital care report (PCR) is an example of:
  A. subjective information.
  B. objective information.
  C. pertinent negative information.
  D. nonstandard abbreviations.

_A_ **27.** All the following are examples of information that should be put in quotation marks on the prehospital care report (PCR) *except*:
  A. bystander statements.
  B. chief complaint.
  C. objective information.
  D. police officer's statements.

_B_ **28.** In the narrative section of a prehospital care report (PCR), the EMT should:
  A. list his or her conclusions about the situation.
  B. include pertinent negatives.
  C. use the radio codes for each treatment.
  D. list the vital signs and times obtained.

C **29.** Medical abbreviations should be used on a prehospital care report (PCR):
   A. to save space in the narrative section.
   B. to replace all words you cannot spell.
   C. only if they are standardized.
   D. to ensure correct interpretation by physicians.

D **30.** You are treating a 22-year-old who fell off his motorcycle. He has some road rash and no major injuries and is mostly concerned about his bike. He does not want to go to the hospital and has a friend who can drive him home and take care of him. Before the leaving the scene, you should:
   A. document assessment findings and care given.
   B. try again to persuade the patient to go to a hospital.
   C. ensure the patient is able to make a rational, informed decision.
   D. do all of these.

A **31.** When completing a prehospital care report (PCR) on a patient refusal, the EMT should document all of the following *except*:
   A. that he or she was willing to return if the patient changed his or her mind.
   B. the complete patient assessment.
   C. that alternative methods of care were offered.
   D. the patient's definitive diagnosis.

B **32.** If the EMT forgot to administer a treatment that is required by the state treatment protocols, he or she should:
   A. document on the PCR only treatment actually given.
   B. be sure to document an excuse for why the treatment was skipped.
   C. record that the patient was given the forgotten treatment.
   D. do none of these.

A **33.** You are in a rush during a call and did not have time to take a second set of vital signs. Your partner says, "Just write in another set ten minutes after the first one." Falsification of information on a prehospital care report (PCR) may lead to:
   A. suspension or revocation of your license or certification.
   B. better EMT education.
   C. longer response times.
   D. none of these.

B **34.** To correct an error discovered while writing the prehospital care report, the EMT should:
   A. scribble out the error so it cannot be seen.
   B. draw a line through the error, initial it, and write the correct information.
   C. place his or her initials over the error.
   D. erase the error completely, and then write the correction.

C **35.** On returning to the station after a call, you have the chance to reread your prehospital care report (PCR). If information was omitted by mistake, you should:
   A. prepare another report and substitute that for the earlier one.
   B. notify the service Medical Director immediately.
   C. add a note with the correct information, the date, and initial it.
   D. do nothing because information should never be added after the call.

A **36.** Occasionally, EMTs may have only a limited amount of information about the patient to document on the PCR. An example of an instance in which it would *not* be unusual for the EMT to obtain only a limited amount of information is:
   A. during a multiple-casualty incident.
   B. during an interhospital transfer.
   C. while performing a nonemergency run.
   D. when encountering a child abuse case.

©2012 Pearson Education, Inc.
Emergency Care, 12th Ed.

A **37.** You were just on a call about which your agency medical director requires you to complete a special incident report. Special situation (incident) reports:
   A. document events that should be reported to local regulatory authorities.
   B. can be submitted at any time after the call.
   C. need not be accurate and/or objective.
   D. are required on each call.

B **38.** Ambulance services and EMS personnel are required by _____ to take steps to safeguard patient confidentiality.
   A. OSHA law
   B. HIPAA
   C. the NHTSA
   D. the U.S. DOT

A **39.** There are laws, both state and federal, that protect patient privacy. An example of a method that an ambulance service would use to safeguard patient confidentiality is:
   A. requiring employees to place completed PCRs in a locked box.
   B. using only patient last names during radio transmissions.
   C. allowing only PCRs with patient names to be distributed during QA meetings.
   D. none of these is an acceptable procedure.

D **40.** The policy an ambulance service develops concerning patient rights and confidentially must take into consideration:
   A. state regulations.
   B. local regulations.
   C. HIPAA.
   D. all of these.

COMPLETE THE FOLLOWING

1. List five examples of components of a communications system.

A. _____

B. _____

C. _____

D. _____

E. _____

2. List six interpersonal communications guidelines to use when dealing with patients, families, friends, and bystanders.

A. _____

B. _____

C. _____

D. _____

E. _____

F. _____

3. List ten examples of patient data on a prehospital care report (PCR).

A. _____

B. _____

C. _____

D. _____

E. _____

F. _____

G. _____

H. _____

I. _____

J. _____

STREET SCENES DISCUSSION

Review the Street Scene on page 421 of the textbook. Then answer the following questions.

1. Why was it difficult for the service a few years ago when the documentation was done in a different manner by another EMT?

2. If a patient refuses a treatment you feel is needed, what should you do?

3. What is the legal view of an incomplete PCR?

CASE STUDY

You are dispatched to a patient who was involved in a single-vehicle automobile crash. The patient may have fallen asleep at the wheel. There is significant damage to the front of the vehicle from stripping a tree.

On arrival, you conduct a scene size-up. You conclude that the scene is safe and you have plenty of help. Police officers are on the scene dealing with investigation, making notifications, and controlling traffic.

1. At this point in the call, what two types of radio communication have you most likely already used?

_____

_____

2. You conduct your primary assessment and there are no immediate life threats present. In the patient's own words, what would be the reason the ambulance was called to the scene?

_____

3. After determining there were no life threats, you proceed to interview the patient and conduct the secondary survey. As a precaution, based on the MOI, what should another EMS provider be doing while you examine the patient?

_____

Aside from a small cut on the head, which has already stopped bleeding, the 28-year-old patient is alert and denies any injuries. He states he just wants to get home and go to sleep. The police have already done a breathalizer and they tell you he has not been drinking. You obtain a set of baseline vital signs and they are all within normal limits. The patient states that he has no medical history, is not under a doctor's care, and takes no medications.

4. Should you just let the patient sign off as an RMA?

_____

5. Why or why not?

_____

6. If the patient simply wants to sign off and go home, what other strategies can you employ to attempt to convince him to be seen in the ED?

_____

After a lengthy discussion, you manage to convince the patient it is in his best interest to be seen in the local ED. You and your partner remove the patient from the vehicle using the KED and long backboard. En route to the hospital, you obtain another set of vital signs and prepare for the medical radio report.

7. What is an example of the medical radio report that you will be giving to the ED on this patient?

_____

_____

_____

On arrival at the ED, the triage nurse tells you to take the patient to room A-7. Once in the room, you begin to transfer the long backboard over to the hospital stretcher and at the same time give an oral report to the nurse who will be taking care of the patient.

8. What are some examples of the information passed along in the oral report to the nurse or physician in the ED?

_____

_____

EMT SKILLS PERFORMANCE CHECKLISTS

▶ RADIO REPORT (PP. 398–399)

Pick an ambulance call on which you were recently an observer, or pick a patient whom you examined during the hospital observation portion of the EMT course. Without releasing any confidential information about the call, such as the patient's name and address, take a moment and organize your thoughts so you can provide a mock radio report to another crew member or your instructor.

❑ Unit identification (ambulance number_____)

❑ Level of provider

❑ Estimated time of arrival (ETA)

❑ Patient's age and sex

❑ Chief complaint (why the patient called ambulance)

❑ Brief, pertinent history of the present illness or injury

❑ Major past illnesses

❑ Mental status (AVPU)

❑ Baseline vital signs

❑ Pertinent findings of the physical exam

❑ Emergency medical care given

❑ Response to emergency medical care

❑ Does medical direction have any questions or orders?

NOTE: There are a number of local formats for radio reports that may differ somewhat, yet they all adhere to the same principles. They should follow a logical order, be concise, and paint a picture of the patient's problem and the priorities for the hospital personnel.

▶ PATIENT REFUSAL PROCEDURE (PP. 412–415)

❑ Spend time communicating effectively with patient (includes reasoning, persistence, and strategies to convince the patient to go to the hospital).

❑ Clearly inform the patient of the consequences of not going to the hospital.

❑ Consult with medical direction.

❑ Contact family to help convince the patient.

❑ Call law enforcement, who may be able to order or "arrest" a serious patient in order to force the patient to go to the hospital.

❑ Try to determine why the patient is refusing care.

❑ Complete thorough documentation of the patient's refusal, have the patient sign the refusal release, and have a witness sign the release (e.g., bystander, police officer, family member).

NOTE: Procedures may differ by state and jurisdiction. Always follow your Medical Director's advice.

18

General Pharmacology

Standards: Pharmacology (Principles of Pharmacology, Medication Administration, Emergency Medications)

Competencies: Applies fundamental knowledge of the medications that the EMT may assist with/administer to a patient during an emergency.

OBJECTIVES

After reading this chapter you should be able to:

18.1 Define key terms introduced in this chapter.

18.2 List the drugs in your scope of practice.

18.3 For each medication you may administer or assist a patient in self-administering, describe the following:

   a. Generic and common trade names
   b. Indication(s)
   c. Contraindications
   d. Side effects and untoward effects
   e. Form(s)
   f. Route(s) of administration

18.4 Follow principles of medication administration safety, including the five rights of medication administration.

18.5 Discuss the importance of looking up medications and requesting information from medical direction when needed.

18.6 Identify the type of medical direction (on-line or off-line) required to administer each medication in the scope of practice.

18.7 Describe the characteristics of the oral, sublingual, inhaled, intravenous, intramuscular, subcutaneous, and endotracheal routes of administration.

©2012 Pearson Education, Inc.
Emergency Care, 12th Ed.

18.8 Identify special considerations in medication administration related to patients' ages and weights.

18.9 Explain the importance of accurate documentation of drug administration and patient reassessment following drug administration.

18.10 Discuss the importance of having readily available references to identify drugs commonly taken by patients.

18.11 Discuss the steps an EMT may take in assisting with IV therapy.

MATCH TERMINOLOGY/ DEFINITIONS

A. Specific signs or circumstances under which it is appropriate to administer a drug to a patient

B. A spray device with a mouthpiece that contains an aerosol form of a medication that a patient can spray directly into the airway

C. The study of drugs, their sources, characteristics, and effects

D. Medication given by mouth to treat an awake patient (who is able to swallow) with an altered mental status and a history of diabetes

E. A medication used to reduce the clotting ability of blood to prevent and treat clots associated with myocardial infarction

F. A drug that helps to constrict the blood vessels and relax passages of the airway. It may be used to counter a severe allergic reaction

G. A gas commonly found in the atmosphere; it is used as a drug to treat any patient whose medical or traumatic condition may cause him to be hypoxic

H. A powder, usually premixed with water, that will adsorb some poisons and help prevent them from being absorbed by the body

I. The study of the effects of medications on the body

J. An effect of a medication in addition to its desired effect that may be potentially harmful to the patient

K. Any action of a drug other than the desired action

L. Specific signs or circumstances under which it is not appropriate and may be harmful to administer a drug to a patient

M. A drug that helps to dilate the coronary vessels that supply the heart muscle with blood

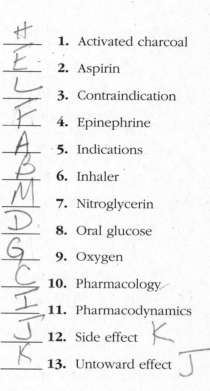

_H_ **1.** Activated charcoal

_E_ **2.** Aspirin

_L_ **3.** Contraindication

_F_ **4.** Epinephrine

_A_ **5.** Indications

_B_ **6.** Inhaler

_M_ **7.** Nitroglycerin

_D_ **8.** Oral glucose

_G_ **9.** Oxygen

_C_ **10.** Pharmacology

_I_ **11.** Pharmacodynamics

_J_ **12.** Side effect   K

_K_ **13.** Untoward effect   J

MULTIPLE-CHOICE REVIEW

_D_   **1.** The study of drugs, their sources, and their effects is called:
   A. anatomy.
   B. physiology.
   C. medicinology.
   D. pharmacology.

_D_   **2.** Medications that are routinely carried on the EMT-level EMS unit are:
   A. aspirin, oral glucose, and oxygen.
   B. oxygen and nitroglycerin.
   C. epinephrine and prescribed inhalers.
   D. all of these.

_C_   **3.** Aspirin is administered by the EMT in the field to:
   A. treat headaches.
   B. dilate the coronary arteries.
   C. help prevent clot formation.
   D. eliminate the pain from a serious injury.

_B_   **4.** When might administration of aspirin be contraindicated?
   A. When there is no water available
   B. If the patient has a history of GI bleeding
   C. If the patient may be having a heart attack
   D. All of these

_B_   **5.** Your patient is a teenager whose parent states, "She has not accepted her disease and is managing it poorly." Poorly managed diabetes can cause:
   A. hypoxia, or low oxygen.
   B. altered mental status.
   C. dilation of the coronary arteries.
   D. absorption of poisons.

_A_   **6.** You are treating a patient who is a diabetic with an altered mental status. He has a gag reflex, so oral glucose is your treatment. This is given between the patient's cheek and gum using a tongue depressor because:
   A. this method allows slow swallowing and absorption into the bloodstream.
   B. it will not be aspirated if the patient suddenly becomes unconscious.
   C. this area will cause the patient to regurgitate the stomach's contents.
   D. it will assist in dilating the coronary vessels as much as possible.

_C_   **7.** As an important part of your history taking, you will determine if the patient is taking any specific medications. Examples of medications a patient may have in his or her possession and that the EMT may assist the patient in taking under the appropriate circumstances are:
   A. glucose injections and anticonvulsants.
   B. home oxygen, antihypertensives, and anti-inflammatories.
   C. epinephrine auto-injector, a bronchodilator inhaler, nitroglycerin, and aspirin.
   D. insulin, antihypertensives, and anticonvulsants.

_C_   **8.** Your patient is a 52-year-old female who states that she has a long history of asthma and chronic bronchitis. It would not be unusual for her to carry _____ in her purse.
   A. nitroglycerin
   B. an epinephrine auto-injector
   C. a bronchodilator
   D. a bronchoconstrictor

©2012 Pearson Education, Inc.
Emergency Care, 12th Ed.

___C___ **9.** Your 62-year-old patient has a history of cardiac problems and takes nitro. The drug nitroglycerin is used to _____ vessels.
- **A.** dilate the peripheral
- **B.** constrict the peripheral
- **C.** dilate the coronary
- **D.** constrict the coronary

___A___ X ___C___ **10.** The comprehensive government publication listing all drugs in the United States is called the:
- **A.** *Physician's Desk Reference.*
- **B.** *Hazmat Guidebook.*
- **C.** *U.S. Pharmacopoeia (USP).*
- **D.** *National Medicine Guidebook.*

___B___ **11.** The name that the manufacturer uses in marketing a drug is called the _____ name.
- **A.** generic
- **B.** trade
- **C.** official
- **D.** original

___D___ **12.** Your patient tells you that he is not supposed to take a specific medication when his blood pressure is low or he feels dizzy. A circumstance in which a drug should not be used because it may cause harm to the patient or offer no effect in improving the patient's condition or illness is called a(n):
- **A.** indication.
- **B.** side effect.
- **C.** adverse reaction.
- **D.** contraindication.

___A___ **13.** You are administering a medication for a specific purpose according to your treatment protocols. An action of a drug that is other than the desired action is called a(n):
- **A.** side effect.
- **B.** overdose.
- **C.** contraindication.
- **D.** systemic effect.

___D___ **14.** Part of the treatment to a seriously ill patient will involve administration of a drug. Prior to administering the medication, you must know all of the following *except*:
- **A.** the route of administration.
- **B.** the proper dose to administer.
- **C.** the actions the medication will take.
- **D.** both the generic and chemical names.

___B___ **15.** You are treating a patient who is under a doctor's care for chronic pain and is taking medication for his condition. Drugs prescribed for pain relief are called:
- **A.** antidysrhythmics.
- **B.** analgesics.
- **C.** anticonvulsants.
- **D.** antihypertensives.

___D___ **16.** Your history reveals that the suspected cardiac patient is also taking a medication to control his hypertension. Drugs prescribed to reduce high blood pressure are called:
- **A.** antidysrhythmics.
- **B.** analgesics.
- **C.** anticonvulsants.
- **D.** antihypertensives.

C 17. Your patient tells you that she is taking a medication to control her irregular heartbeat. Drugs prescribed for heart rhythm disorders are called:
   A. antidiabetics.
   B. bronchodilators.
   C. antidysrhythmics.
   D. anticonvulsants.

B 18. Upon interviewing an asthmatic patient, you find that she is taking a medication for her disease. Drugs prescribed to relax the smooth muscles of the bronchial tubes are called:
   A. bronchospasms.
   B. bronchodilators.
   C. anticonvulsants.
   D. bronchoconstrictors.

C 19. Your patient has had a seizure. You find on interviewing her after she wakes up that she has not been taking her medicine this week. Drugs prescribed for prevention and control of seizures are called:
   A. antidiabetics.
   B. antihypertensives.
   C. anticonvulsants.
   D. antidepressants.

A 20. Your patient is taking a drug that was prescribed to help regulate his emotional activity and to minimize the psychological and emotional peaks and valleys. These kinds of drugs are called:
   A. antidepressants.
   B. analgesics.
   C. antidysrhythmics.
   D. anticonvulsants.

C 21. When a patient is administered tiny aerosol particles to treat a disease, such as asthma, this is considered the _____ route of administration.
   A. intravenous
   B. sublingual
   C. inhaled
   D. oral

B 22. EMTs who administer medications or assist patients in taking their prescribed meds according to protocols need to know about pharmacodynamics. An example of a result of understanding the pharmacodynamics of a specific medication is:
   A. pediatric patients would normally require larger doses.
   B. geriatric patients have difficulty eliminating medications.
   C. heavier patients require ten times the normal dose.
   D. all of these.

COMPLETE THE FOLLOWING

1. List six medications an EMT can administer or assist a patient in taking.

   A. _____

   B. _____

   C. _____

©2012 Pearson Education, Inc.
Emergency Care, 12th Ed.

D. _____

E. _____

F. _____

2. List the five "rights" to adhere to when administering a medication.

A. _____

B. _____

C. _____

D. _____

E. _____

STREET SCENES DISCUSSION

Review the Street Scene on page 442 of the textbook. Then answer the following questions.

1. Suppose the patient's wife had administered the nitroglycerin tablets before your arrival. What side effect should you be alert for?

2. What effect does a patient with chest pain expect from the nitroglycerin tablet? How does this effect occur?

3. Are there any "pertinent negatives" in the Sample Documentation? If so, what are they?

19
Respiratory Emergencies

Standards: Medicine (Respiratory)

Competency: Applies fundamental knowledge to provide basic emergency care and transportation based on assessment findings for an acutely ill patient.

OBJECTIVES

After reading this chapter you should be able to:

19.1 Define key terms introduced in this chapter.

19.2 Describe the anatomy and physiology of respiration.

19.3 Differentiate between adequate and inadequate breathing based on the rate, rhythm, and quality of breathing.

19.4 Discuss differences between the adult and pediatric airways and respiratory systems.

19.5 Recognize signs of inadequate breathing in pediatric patients.

19.6 Provide supplemental oxygen and assisted ventilation as needed for patients with inadequate breathing.

19.7 Assess the effectiveness of artificial ventilation.

19.8 Recognize the patient with difficulty breathing.

19.9 Given a scenario, perform an assessment and take the history of a variety of patients with difficulty breathing.

19.10 Recognize abnormal breath sounds, including wheezes, crackles, rhonchi, and stridor.

19.11 Assist a patient with administration of a prescribed bronchodilator by inhaler or small volume nebulizer, as permitted by medical direction.

19.12 Use CPAP to assist the patient with difficulty breathing, as permitted by medical direction.

19.13 Recognize the indications, contraindications, risks, and side effects of CPAP.

19.14 Describe the pathophysiology, signs, and symptoms of:

    a. COPD
    b. Asthma
    c. Pulmonary edema
    d. Pneumonia
    e. Spontaneous pneumothorax
    f. Pulmonary embolism
    g. Epiglottitis
    h. Pertussis
    i. Cystic fibrosis
    j. Viral respiratory infections

19.15 Given a scenario, provide treatment for a variety of patients with difficulty breathing.

MATCH TERMINOLOGY/ DEFINITIONS

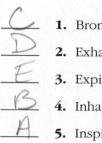
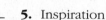

A. An active process in which the intercostal muscles and the diaphragm contract, expanding the size of the chest cavity and causing air to flow into the lungs

B. Another term for inspiration

C. Blockage of the bronchi that lead from the trachea to the lungs

D. Another term for expiration

E. A passive process in which the intercostal muscles and the diaphragm relax, causing the chest cavity to decrease in size and force air from the lungs

C **1.** Bronchoconstriction

D **2.** Exhalation

E **3.** Expiration

B **4.** Inhalation

A **5.** Inspiration

MULTIPLE-CHOICE REVIEW

C **1.** The structure that divides the chest cavity from the abdominal cavity is called the _____ muscle.
    A. intercostal
    B. sternocleidomastoid
    C. diaphragm
    D. inguinal

B **2.** Expiration is a(n):
    A. active process that involves the relaxation of the intercostal muscles and the diaphragm.
    B. passive process that involves the relaxation of the intercostal muscles and the diaphragm.
    C. active process that involves the contraction of the intercostal muscles and the diaphragm.
    D. passive process that involves the contraction of the intercostal muscles and the diaphragm.

C **3.** You are assessing a 32-year-old female who has breathing difficulty. To determine the *quality* of breathing, check for all of the following *except*:
    A. presence of breath sounds.
    B. chest expansion.
    C. breathing rhythm.
    D. depth of respirations.

_C_ **4.** You are evaluating an unresponsive male patient, in his fifties, who has only a few shallow, gasping breaths per minute. His treatment should involve:
   A. oxygen given via nasal cannula.
   B. immediate transport to a medical facility.
   C. immediate artificial ventilation with supplemental oxygen.
   D. oxygen given via nonrebreather mask.

_B_ **5.** Your patient is a 60-year-old male who is having difficulty breathing, and he is working very hard to breathe. He is using the muscles in his neck and abdomen to assist his breathing. These are referred to as the _____ muscles of breathing.
   A. extra
   B. accessory
   C. subdiaphragmatic
   D. smooth

_D_ **6.** Oxygenation of the body's tissue is reduced in a patient with inadequate breathing, so the skin may be _____ in color and feel _____.
   A. pale; dry and cool
   B. red; clammy and hot
   C. yellow; dry and warm
   D. blue; clammy and cool

_A_ **7.** You are treating an unresponsive adult male patient. If he is making _____ sounds, he may have a serious airway problem requiring immediate intervention.
   A. snoring or gurgling
   B. slight wheezing
   C. sniffling
   D. whistling or grunting

_C_ **8.** Statistically, a leading killer of infants and children is:
   A. motor vehicle collisions.
   B. heart attacks.
   C. respiratory conditions.
   D. infection.

_D_ **9.** Your patient is a child who is having difficulty breathing. You need to recall that the structure of an infant's or child's airway is different from an adult's in each of the following ways *except*:
   A. all airway structures are smaller and more easily obstructed.
   B. their tongues are proportionately larger than an adult's.
   C. the trachea is softer and more flexible.
   D. the cricoid cartilage is more rigid.

_B_ **10.** Because the chest wall is softer in infants and children, they:
   A. must inhale twice the amount of air to breathe.
   B. depend more heavily on the diaphragm for breathing.
   C. grunt and gurgle whenever they breathe.
   D. expend less energy than adults do when breathing.

_D_ **11.** The signs of inadequate breathing in infants and children include all of the following *except*:
   A. nasal flaring.
   B. grunting.
   C. seesaw breathing.
   D. lip quivering.

©2012 Pearson Education, Inc.
Emergency Care, 12th Ed.

_A_ ✗ _C_ **12.** When assessing your adult female patient, which one of the following would be *most* important to observe about her breathing?
   A. Presence of breathing and pulse rate
   B. Breathing pattern and adequacy of breathing
   C. Presence of breathing and adequacy of breathing
   D. Patient position and adequacy of breathing

_C_ ✗ _A_ **13.** Your 62-year-old female patient is going to need you to assist her ventilation. The best method for providing assisted ventilation is the:
   A. pocket face mask with supplemental oxygen.
   B. two-rescuer bag mask device with supplemental oxygen.
   C. flow-restricted, oxygen-powered ventilation device.
   D. one-rescuer bag mask device with supplemental oxygen.

_D_ **14.** If you are unsure whether the patient in multiple-choice question 13 requires artificial ventilation, you should:
   A. contact medical direction immediately.
   B. move to the ambulance and transport rapidly.
   C. increase the liter flow rate to the nonrebreather mask.
   D. provide artificial ventilation.

_B_ **15.** The adequate rate of artificial ventilations for a nonbreathing adult patient is _____ breaths per minute.
   A. 8
   B. 12
   C. 16
   D. 20

_C_ **16.** The adequate rate of artificial ventilations for a nonbreathing infant or child patient is _____ breaths per minute.
   A. 10
   B. 15
   C. 20
   D. 25

_C_ **17.** If an infant or a child has _____ in the setting of a respiratory emergency, this usually indicates trouble.
   A. a fever
   B. cold skin
   C. a low pulse
   D. a rapid pulse

_D_ ✗ _B_ **18.** You are artificially ventilating a 50-year-old male patient who is in respiratory arrest. His chest is not rising and falling with each ventilation. The *first* action you should take is to:
   A. increase the oxygen flow rate.
   B. increase the force of ventilations.
   C. change the ventilatory device.
   D. recheck the airway.

_C_ _B_ ✗ **19.** When assessing the breathing of an adult female patient, all of the following are important observations for the EMT to make *except*:
   A. the patient's positioning.
   B. the lung sounds.
   C. unusual anatomy such as a barrel chest.
   D. pale, cyanotic, flushed skin.

_D_ 20. The sign(s) of a lower airway problem include all of the following *except*:
  A. wheezing.
  B. increased breathing effort upon exhalation.
  C. rapid breathing without stridor.
  D. yellow skin color.

_C_ 21. Your 62-year-old female patient is only able to speak in short, choppy sentences. This may mean that she:
  A. has a language problem.
  B. is unable to hear you clearly.
  C. is experiencing breathing difficulty.
  D. is afraid of you.

_B_ 22. When you arrived on the scene, one of your first observations was the patient's position. When you note that she is in the tripod position due to her respiratory distress, this means that she is:
  A. holding herself up by two legs and one arm.
  B. leaning forward with hands resting on knees.
  C. in the recovery position.
  D. supine with knees flexed against the chest.

_D_ 23. Which pair of signs/symptoms is *not* commonly associated with breathing difficulty?
  A. Crowing/restlessness
  B. Retractions/shortness of breath
  C. Increased pulse/tightness in chest
  D. Vomiting/headache

_B_ 24. If the adult male patient you are treating is suffering from breathing difficulty but you decide he is breathing adequately, oxygen should be administered via:
  A. nasal cannula.
  B. nonrebreather mask.
  C. pocket face mask.
  D. bag mask device with supplemental oxygen.

_C_ 25. If a patient is experiencing breathing difficulty and is breathing adequately, it is usually best to place him in the _____ position.
  A. tripod
  B. supine
  C. sitting-up
  D. none of these

_C_ 26. A patient who has been diagnosed with obstructive sleep apnea may use a _____ to sleep.
  A. bronchoconstrictor
  B. metered dose aspirator
  C. CPAP device
  D. sedative medication

_C_ 27. Your patient is a 37-year-old male with a history of breathing distress. He has his prescribed inhaler with him. Once you receive permission from medical direction to assist a patient with an inhaler, make sure you have all of the following *except*:
  A. the right dose.
  B. an inhaler that is not expired.
  C. a large enough syringe.
  D. a patient who is alert enough to cooperate.

©2012 Pearson Education, Inc.
Emergency Care, 12th Ed.

_A___ **28.** Prior to coaching the patient from multiple-choice question 27 in the use of his inhaler, you should:
   A. shake the inhaler vigorously.
   B. test the unit by spraying into the air.
   C. ensure that the patient is no longer alert.
   D. call the patient's personal physician.

_B___ **29.** To ensure that the most medication is absorbed when using an inhaler, you should try to encourage the patient to:
   A. take short, shallow breaths.
   B. hold the breath as long as possible.
   C. take a short nap.
   D. hyperventilate.

_D___ **30.** Blowing oxygen or air continuously at a low pressure into the airway is a
_B_ x   means of:
   A. preventing the alveoli from collapsing at the end of inhalation.
   B. pushing fluid out of the alveoli and back into the capillaries.
   C. providing artificial ventilation to the apneic patient.
   D. all of these.

_C___ **31.** A physician realizes that his patient may become anxious and use his inhaler improperly. To help improve the volume of the medication that the patient is able to self-administer when in distress, the physician may prescribe a:
   A. tranquilizer.
   B. decongestant.
   C. spacer device.
   D. heat treatment.

_B___ **32.** Of the prescribed inhalers listed below, which is *not* considered a medication that would be used in an emergency to reverse airway constriction because its use is aimed at prevention of attacks by reducing inflammation?
   A. Ventolin
   B. Advair
   C. Proventil
   D. Albuterol

_D___ **33.** When assessing the lungs of a 55-year-old male who presented in respiratory distress, you hear a fine bubbling sound upon inspiration. This sound is caused by fluid in the alveoli and is called:
   A. wheezes.
   B. stridor.
   C. rhonchi.
   D. crackles.

_D___ **34.** Although CPAP is frequently effective in relieving a patient's difficulty with
x C   breathing, it can have a side effect of:
   A. producing hypotension.
   B. pneumothorax.
   C. gastric distention.
   D. any of these may occur.

_B___ **35.** If a patient who has been treated with CPAP for the past 10 minutes starts to experience a decrease in mental status, the EMT should:
   A. turn up the pressure.
   B. remove CPAP and ventilate with a BVM.
   C. lower the level of pressure in the CPAP device considerably.
   D. administer a bronchodilator treatment per medical control.

_B_ **36.** Your patient has a chronic respiratory disease that has episodic exacerbations
or flares. He most likely is suffering from:
   A. pulmonary edema.
   B. asthma.
   C. pneumonia.
   D. emphysema.

_B_ **37.** You are standing by at the finish line of a 5-kilometer road race when a runner
✗ _A_   crosses the line and is suddenly in distress. He is very thin and tall, and
complaining of a sudden sharp pain when he breathes. What is his most likely
respiratory condition?
   A. Spontaneous pneumothorax
   B. Pulmonary embolism
   C. Cystic fibrosis
   D. A viral respiratory infection

_D_ **38.** The use of CPAP may be indicated if the patient who you suspect has
✗ _C_   _____ also has stable vital signs.
   A. a viral respiratory infection
   B. epiglottitis
   C. acute pulmonary edema
   D. spontaneous pneumothorax

_C_ **39.** You are treating a patient who just came off an airplane arriving from an
✗ _D_   international destination. A respiratory condition that may be caused by a deep
vein thrombosis after sitting for a very long flight is called:
   A. epiglottitis.
   B. asthma.
   C. acute pulmonary edema.
   D. pulmonary embolism.

_B_ ✗ **40.** A respiratory condition that used to be prominent with children but has been
_A_   virtually eliminated due to vaccinations of infants is:
   A. epiglottitis.
   B. croup.
   C. asthma.
   D. emphysema.

COMPLETE THE FOLLOWING

1. List eight observations during your assessment of the patient with breathing
difficulty.

   A. _____

   B. _____

   C. _____

   D. _____

   E. _____

   F. _____

   G. _____

   H. _____

©2012 Pearson Education, Inc.
Emergency Care, 12th Ed.

2. List four of the six vital sign changes you should evaluate when assessing the patient with a chief complaint of breathing difficulty.

A. _____

B. _____

C. _____

D. _____

3. List four of the common abnormal lung sounds and describe each.

A. _____

B. _____

C. _____

D. _____

4. Oxygen should be administered to all patients with respiratory distress, regardless of their oxygen saturation readings. The oximeter reading in a normal, healthy person is typically (A) _____. An oximeter reading below (B) _____ indicates hypoxia.

A. _____

B. _____

LABEL THE DIAGRAMS

Fill in each phase of respiration on the line provided.

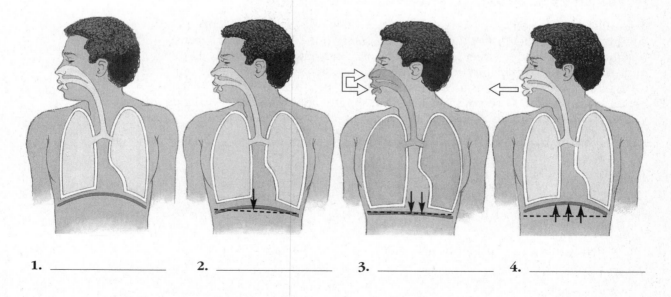

1. _____ 2. _____ 3. _____ 4. _____

STREET SCENES DISCUSSION

Review the Street Scene on page 468 of the textbook. Then answer the following questions.

1. You have already reported that the patient has emphysema. Imagine that you were also told the patient was coughing earlier in the day. Would it be worth documenting the cough on your PCR? Why or why not?

2. If advanced life support (ALS) had been available, would it have been appropriate to request its assistance?

3. Is it possible to assist the ventilations of a patient who is in a half-sitting position?

CASE STUDY

▶ THE THREE A.M. CALL: DAD SIMPLY CANNOT BREATHE

Your unit and the police are dispatched to the scene of a private residence in a suburban neighborhood. It is 3 A.M. and you can find the house easily because it is the only one with a street light on and police car out front. On arrival, you and your partner load up the stretcher with your assessment kit, the oxygen, and an extra blanket because it is a cold night. You are met at the front door by the patient's daughter, who nervously states, "Dad simply cannot breathe." She leads you to a bedroom, which is upstairs in the rear of the home.

1. As you approach the patient, what Standard Precautions should you take?

2. When would you consider using a HEPA mask or N-95 mask?

3. If the patient is awake and alert, what position would be best for him to be treated and transported in with a chief complaint of breathing difficulty?

You begin your assessment by introducing yourself, and you find out that the patient's name is Joe. He states he is 72 years old and cannot catch his breath. You notice that he is talking in short, choppy sentences. Your partner starts oxygen administration, and you ask a few more interview questions and obtain a set of baseline vital signs.

4. What is the significance of the short, choppy sentences?

5. What appliance is most appropriate for the initial oxygen administration to the patient?

6. If Joe was found with very rapid and very shallow breaths, would a different device be more appropriate to use?

The vital signs are: respirations of 24 and labored, pulse of 110 and irregular, BP of 140/82, and a pulse oximeter reading of 94 percent. Joe's mental status is alert and oriented times 3, and the oxygen has started to calm him down a bit. His daughter states that he usually takes his bronchodilator twice a day but has recently been feeling run down from "a touch of the flu." Joe denies any chest pain but is a little weak when he sits up at this point. His daughter also says that he is allergic to penicillin and sulfa drugs. Apparently he has not thought to try his bronchodilator early this morning.

7. If Joe has Albuterol prescribed to him and you have a standing order protocol to assist him, how is this administered and what is the usual dose?

8. If Joe's medication was not immediately available, but his daughter's medication was because she is an asthmatic, could you just administer her medication to Joe?

You are preparing to assist Joe in taking his medication by following your protocol. When you reassess him after a few minutes, he seems to be breathing better, he is talking in full sentences, and he is apologizing profusely for waking you and your partner up so early in the morning. You still insist that Joe take the ride to the hospital for follow-up care and possibly some additional tests. He is happy to go along with your plan.

9. If Joe's daughter handed you a spacer device, would you know what it is and know how to use it?

10. What side effects should you expect to see when administering Albuterol?

EMT SKILLS
PERFORMANCE CHECKLIST

▶ **PRESCRIBED (METERED-DOSE) INHALER (PP. 463–464)**

❑ Conduct a scene size-up.

❑ Take Standard Precautions.

❑ Perform a primary assessment.

❑ Obtain the patient's history and conduct a physical exam.

❑ Confirm indications for inhaler use.

❑ Obtain order from medical direction (either on-line or off-line).

❑ Ensure the right patient, right medication, right dose, and right route, and ensure that the patient is alert enough to use the inhaler.

❑ Check the expiration date of the inhaler.

❑ Check if the patient has already taken any doses.

❑ Ensure that the inhaler is at room temperature or warmer.

❑ Shake the inhaler vigorously several times.

❑ Have the patient exhale deeply.

©2012 Pearson Education, Inc.
Emergency Care, 12th Ed.

❑ Have the patient put his or her lips around the opening of the inhaler.

❑ Have the patient depress the handheld inhaler as he or she begins to inhale deeply.

❑ Instruct the patient to hold his or her breath for as long as comfortable so that the medication can be absorbed.

❑ Put oxygen back on the patient.

❑ Allow the patient to breathe a few times, and repeat the dose if so ordered by medical direction.

❑ If the patient has a spacer device for use with the inhaler, it should be used.

20
Cardiac Emergencies

Standards: Medicine (Cardiovascular)

Competencies: Applies fundamental knowledge to provide basic emergency care and transportation based on assessment findings for an acutely ill patient.

OBJECTIVES

After reading this chapter you should be able to:

20.1   Define key terms introduced in this chapter.

20.2   Describe the anatomy and physiology of the cardiovascular system.

20.3   Define acute coronary syndrome and discuss its most common signs and symptoms.

20.4   Discuss the management of a patient with acute coronary syndrome.

20.5   Discuss the indications, contraindications, dosage, and administration of nitroglycerin to a patient with chest pain.

20.6   Discuss the indications (including conditions that must be met), contraindications, and administration of aspirin to a patient with chest pain.

20.7   Discuss the following conditions and how each may lead to a cardiac emergency:
a. Coronary artery disease (CAD)
b. Aneurysm
c. Electrical malfunctions of the heart
d. Mechanical malfunctions of the heart
e. Angina pectoris
f. Acute myocardial infarction (AMI)
g. Congestive heart failure (CHF)

20.8   Discuss the following factors in the chain of survival and how each may contribute to patient survival of cardiac arrest:
a. Immediate recognition and activation
b. Early cardiopulmonary resuscitation (CPR)

c. Rapid defibrillation

d. Effective advanced life support

e. Integrated post-cardiac-arrest care

20.9 List the skills necessary for the EMT to manage a patient in cardiac arrest.

20.10 Discuss types of automated external defibrillators (AEDs) and how AEDs work.

20.11 Discuss the effective coordination of CPR and AED for a patient in cardiac arrest.

20.12 Discuss special considerations for AED use, including general principles, coordination with others, and post-resuscitation care.

20.13 Discuss the purpose and use of mechanical CPR devices.

MATCH TERMINOLOGY/ DEFINITIONS

▶ PART A

A. The failure of the heart to pump efficiently, leading to excessive blood or fluids in the lungs, the body, or both

B. Shortness of breath; labored or difficulty breathing

C. Diseases that affect the arteries of the heart

D. A blanket term used to represent any symptoms related to lack of oxygen (ischemia) in the heart muscle

E. The dilation, or ballooning, of a weakened section of the wall of an artery

F. Pain in the chest, which occurs when blood supply to the heart is reduced and a portion of the heart muscle is not receiving enough oxygen

G. The condition in which a portion of the myocardium dies as a result of oxygen starvation; often called a heart attack by laypersons

H. When the heart rate is slow, usually below 60 beats per minute

I. The heart and the blood vessels

J. A disturbance in heart rate and rhythm

D	1. Acute coronary syndrome (ACS)
G	2. Acute myocardial infarction (AMI)
F	3. Angina pectoris
E	4. Aneurysm
H	5. Bradycardia
I	6. Cardiovascular system
A	7. Congestive heart failure (CHF)
C	8. Coronary artery disease (CAD)
B	9. Dyspnea
J	10. Dysrhythmia

▶ PART B

A. A cardiac arrest that occurs within 2 hours of the onset of symptoms; the patient may have no prior symptoms of coronary artery disease

B. Swelling resulting from a build-up of fluid in the tissues

C. Accumulation of fluid in the lungs

D. A medication that dilates the blood vessels

E. Accumulation of fluid in the feet or ankles

F. A clot formed of blood and plaque attached to the inner wall of an artery or vein

B	1. Edema
J	2. Embolism
D	3. Nitroglycerin
H	4. Occlusion
E	5. Pedal edema
C	6. Pulmonary edema
I	7. Pulseless electrical activity (PEA)

G. A condition in which the heart's electrical impulses are disorganized, preventing the heart muscle from contracting normally

H. Blockage, as of an artery by fatty deposits

I. A condition in which the heart's electrical rhythm remains relatively normal, yet the mechanical pumping activity fails to follow the electrical activity, causing cardiac arrest

J. Blockage of a vessel by a clot or foreign material brought to the site by the blood current

K. A condition in which the heart has ceased generating electrical impulses

L. A condition in which the heartbeat is quite rapid; if rapid enough, it will not allow the heart's chambers to fill with enough blood between beats to produce blood flow sufficient to meet the body's needs

A **8.** Sudden death

F **9.** Thrombus

G **10.** Ventricular fibrillation (VF)

L **11.** Ventricular tachycardia (V-Tach)

K **12.** Asystole

MULTIPLE-CHOICE REVIEW

C **1.** Acute coronary syndrome (ACS) is a blanket term that refers to:
   A. a mild heart attack.
   B. sudden death of the cells in the heart muscle.
   C. any time the heart may not be getting enough oxygen.
   D. a period of time when the heart stops beating.

C **2.** Chest pain from the heart is typically described by the patient as a "crushing pain." It is also often described as any of the following *except*:
   A. dull.
   B. squeezing.
   C. tearing.
   D. heavy.

A **3.** Your 55-year-old male patient states that his pain seems to radiate from the chest. This sensation, when it is due to a heart problem, commonly radiates to the:
   A. arms and jaw.
   B. feet and head.
   C. stomach and lower abdomen.
   D. right arm and lower abdomen.

C **4.** In addition to chest pain or discomfort, the patient with cardiac compromise will also complain of:
   A. diarrhea.
   B. shivering.
   C. dyspnea.
   D. headache.

B **5.** Patients with heart problems may complain of any of the following *except*:
C   A. pain in the center of the chest.
     B. mild chest discomfort.
     C. sudden onset of sharp abdominal pain.
     D. difficulty breathing.

_D_ X B **6.** Early in your assessment of the 56-year-old male who presents with chest pain, you take his radial pulse. This is a very important vital sign because, if the heart is beating too fast or too slow, the patient with cardiac compromise may also:
  A. have stomach pain.
  B. lose consciousness.
  C. have a seizure or convulsion.
  D. have right-side weakness.

_A_ X C **7.** You are evaluating a 59-year-old female patient who you suspect may be exhibiting the signs and symptoms of an acute coronary syndrome. Her signs and symptoms may include any of the following *except*:
  A. difficulty breathing and abnormal pulse rate.
  B. sudden onset of sweating with nausea or vomiting.
  C. sharp lower abdominal pain and a fever.
  D. pain in the chest or upper abdomen.

_C_ **8.** You are treating a 62-year-old male patient who is complaining of crushing substernal chest pain and shortness of breath. His pulse is fast, BP is high, and pulse oxygen is in the low 90s. The EMT management of the patient with a suspected acute coronary syndrome should include all of the following *except*:
  A. placing the patient in the position of comfort.
  B. administering high-concentration oxygen by nonrebreather mask.
  C. administering high-flow oxygen by a nasal cannula.
  D. assisting the patient with nitroglycerin administration if medical direction authorizes.

_A_ **9.** What is the typical position of comfort that you should consider using for the patient in multiple-choice question 8?
  A. Fowler
  B. Supine
  C. Prone
  D. Lying down with knees bent

_C_ **10.** All of the following potential acute coronary syndrome patients are candidates for immediate transport *except* a patient with:
  A. no history of cardiac problems.
  B. a history of cardiac problems, who does not have nitroglycerin.
  C. prescribed nitroglycerin.
  D. a systolic blood pressure of less than 90–100.

_B_ **11.** You should consider using nitroglycerin when the 65-year-old female patient:
  A. is hypertensive and has a headache.
  B. has her own nitroglycerin and has crushing chest pain.
  C. loses consciousness after feeling dizzy.
  D. has chest pain for over 5 minutes and is hypotensive.

_C_ **12.** Which of the following is the best description of the role of medical direction in the treatment of a 55-year-old male who you suspect is having an acute coronary syndrome?
  A. Authorizing the EMT to administer oxygen via nonrebreather mask
  B. Prescribing nitroglycerin that the EMT can then assist the patient in taking
  C. Authorizing the EMT to assist the patient in taking his prescribed nitroglycerin
  D. Contacting the patient's physician to ensure that the patient's nitroglycerin prescription is not out of date

_C_ **13.** A patient is complaining of chest pain. In order for the EMT to administer nitroglycerin, all the following conditions must be met *except*:
   A. medical direction should authorize its administration.
   B. the patient's physician should have prescribed the medication.
   C. the patient's blood pressure is lower than 100 systolic.
   D. the patient's blood pressure is greater than 100 systolic.

_C_ **14.** The maximum number of doses of nitroglycerin routinely given by the EMT with medical control permission, or taken by the patient at the advice of his physician, is:
   A. one.
   B. two.
   C. three.
   D. four.

_C_ **15.** If the patient's blood pressure falls below 100 systolic after the EMT has administered nitroglycerin, the EMT should:
   A. administer another dose of nitroglycerin.
   B. reassess the patient's vital signs.
   C. treat for shock and transport promptly.
   D. do all of these.

_A_ **16.** Nitroglycerin is contraindicated for the patient who has:
   A. an obvious head injury and altered mental state.
   B. a systolic blood pressure of 110.
   C. not yet taken the maximum dose.
   D. been complaining of pain for at least 20 minutes.

_C_ **17.** You are treating a 62-year-old male patient who has a chief complaint of chest pain. You are considering administering aspirin to the patient. Of the following considerations, which would *not* be pertinent to administering this medicine?
   A. The patient has allergies.
   B. There is a history of asthma.
   C. The patient has taken Viagra.
   D. The patient is on anti-clotting meds.

_C_ **18.** You have administered aspirin to the patient with chest pain per your protocols. The patient has his own prescribed nitro and a stable BP, so you decide to assist him in administering one of his nitro pills. After administering the nitroglycerin, it is important for you to:
   A. immediately administer the next dose.
   B. discontinue the oxygen therapy.
   C. reassess the vital signs.
   D. lay the patient down.

_D_ **19.** The patient you are assessing who has been complaining of chest pain asks you what causes most cardiovascular emergencies. You explain that these conditions are caused, directly or indirectly, by all of the following *except*:
   A. changes in the inner walls of arteries.
   B. problems with the heart's electrical function.
   C. problems with the heart's mechanical function.
   D. complications resulting from cardiovascular surgery.

_A_ **20.** When the body is subjected to exertion or stress, the heart rate will normally:
   A. increase.
   B. decrease.
   C. become irregular.
   D. stop temporarily.

_B_ **21.** A condition that is often the result of the build-up of fatty deposits on the inner walls of the arteries is called:
  A. pulmonary embolism.
  B. coronary artery disease.
  C. obesity.
  D. congestive heart failure.

_D_ **22.** Factors that put a person at risk for developing acute coronary syndromes include:
  A. age.
  B. cigarette smoking.
  C. obesity.
  D. all of these.

_C_ **23.** Which of the following risk factors can be modified to reduce the risk of coronary artery disease?
  A. Age
  B. Heredity
  C. Hypertension
  D. None of these

_D_ **24.** The reason an emergency occurs in most cardiac-related medical emergencies is due to:
  A. reduced blood flow to the myocardium.
  B. cardiac arrest.
  C. loss of consciousness.
  D. breathing difficulty.

_B_ **25.** Angina pectoris means, literally:
  A. a small heart attack.
  B. a pain in the chest.
  C. paralyzed chest muscles.
  D. breathing difficulty.

_B_ **26.** Why is nitroglycerin administered to the patient with chest pain?
  A. It increases blood flow to the brain.
  B. It dilates the blood vessels and decreases the work of the heart.
  C. It constricts the blood vessels and raises the blood pressure.
  D. It is easy to administer in unconscious patients.

_B_ **27.** A condition in which a portion of the myocardium dies as a result of oxygen starvation is known as:
  A. coronary occlusion.
  B. acute myocardial infarction.
  C. myocardial starvation.
  D. acute angina attack.

_C_ **28.** A cardiac arrest that occurs within 2 hours of the onset of cardiac symptoms is referred to as:
  A. prehospital death.
  B. prehospital arrest.
  C. sudden death.
  D. ventricular tachycardia.

_B_ **29.** Unfortunately, nearly _____ of the patients who experience a cardiac arrest within 2 hours of the onset of symptoms have no previous history of cardiac problems.
  A. 10 percent
  B. 25 percent
  C. 60 percent
  D. 80 percent

A 30. Your 70-year-old female patient has a cardiovascular disorder that stems from
+ B weakened sections in the arterial walls. These weak spots begin to dilate to
      form a condition that is known as a(n):
   A. thrombosis.
   B. aneurysm.
   C. inflammation.
   D. infarction.

C 31. You are treating a 55-year-old male patient who has a history of three past MIs
*B^*   and angina. Due to his difficulty breathing and normally sedentary lifestyle, you
      suspect he may be experiencing congestive heart failure (CHF). CHF is a(n):
   A. clotting of the coronary artery.
   B. condition in which excessive fluids build up in the lungs and/or other
      organs.
   C. infection in the heart that makes it difficult to oxygenate the blood.
   D. chronic lung condition that requires a low concentration of oxygen
      administration.

B 32. Damage to the left ventricle and blood backing up into the lungs usually
      presents in the form of:
   A. pedal edema.   **C.** fibrinolyitics.
   B. pulmonary edema.   **D.** diaphoresis.

D 33. The five elements of the chain of survival include early access and each of the
      following links *except*:
   A. CPR.
   B. defibrillation.
   C. advanced care.
   D. prevention.

C 34. You are treating a 59-year-old male patient whose wife called EMS because he
      had difficulty breathing and was acting anxious and confused. He is diaphoretic
      and cyanotic, and his vitals are rapid respirations, tachycardia, and
      hypertension. He has swollen ankles and is coughing up pink sputum. What do
      you suspect is wrong with this patient?
   A. He is having an asthma attack.
   B. He is having an acute myocardial infarction.
   C. He has CHF as well as right heart failure.
   D. He is in the end stage of his emphysema.

B 35. Which of the following steps is *not* necessary to ensure that CPR can be
      delivered earlier to cardiac arrest victims?
   A. Send CPR-trained professionals to patients faster.
   B. Ensure that heart specialists are involved in CPR training.
   C. Train the public in CPR.
   D. Have EMDs instruct callers in how to perform hands-only CPR.

A 36. You just treated a 17-year-old male who was struck in the chest with a baseball
      and went into sudden cardiac arrest. Your Medical Director says that you did a
      good job on the call but this was not the typical cardiac arrest victim. Who is
      the typical cardiac arrest victim?
   A. A male in his sixties
   B. A female in her forties
   C. A male in his seventies
   D. There is no pattern to cardiac arrests.

D 37. The most common witness to a cardiac arrest is a:
   A. male in his forties.
   B. female in her forties.
   C. man in his sixties.
   D. female in her sixties.

©2012 Pearson Education, Inc.
Emergency Care, 12th Ed.

_D_ (handwritten, with _B_ crossed out) **38.** The single most important factor in determining survival from cardiac arrest is:
   A. nitroglycerin administration.
   B. training middle-aged and older people in CPR.
   C. early high-quality CPR.
   D. early defibrillation.

_B_ (handwritten) **39.** If the response time from the moment a call is received to arrival of the defibrillator is longer than _____ minutes, virtually no one survives a cardiac arrest.
   A. 6
   B. 8
   C. 10
   D. 12

_D_ (handwritten) **40.** When treating a cardiac arrest patient and there is no ALS unit in the community, the EMT should:
   A. discontinue resuscitative efforts and pronounce the patient dead.
   B. package quickly, provide high-quality CPR, and transport to the closest hospital.
   C. call for ACLS from another town and wait for its arrival.
   D. continue to provide CPR at the scene until the patient regains a pulse.

_D_ (handwritten) **41.** To manage a patient in cardiac arrest, the EMT should provide high-quality CPR as well as do all of the following *except*:
   A. use a bag-valve-mask device with oxygen.
   B. use an automated external defibrillator.
   C. request advanced life support backup (when available).
   D. administer epinephrine via IV.

_B_ (handwritten, with _D_) **42.** Which of the following steps is *not* necessary for the EMT to take when using a fully automated defibrillator?
   A. Assess the patient.
   B. Turn on the power.
   C. Put the pads on the patient's chest.
   D. Press the button to deliver the shock.

_B_ (handwritten) **43.** The primary electrical disturbance resulting in cardiac arrest is:
   A. asystole.
   B. ventricular fibrillation.
   C. ventricular tachycardia.
   D. pulseless electrical activity.

_A_ (handwritten) **44.** The shockable rhythms include all of the following *except*:
   A. asystole and PEA.
   B. ventricular fibrillation.
   C. pulseless ventricular tachycardia.
   D. ventricular tachycardia.

_A_ (handwritten) **45.** A nonshockable rhythm that can be the result of a terminally sick heart or severe blood loss is called:
   A. pulseless electrical activity.
   B. ventricular tachycardia.
   C. pulseless ventricular tachycardia.
   D. ventricular fibrillation.

_B_ (handwritten, with _C_) **46.** A nonshockable rhythm that is commonly called flatline is named:
   A. pulseless electrical activity.
   B. ventricular tachycardia.
   C. asystole.
   D. ventricular fibrillation.

_B_ **47.** When the AED is analyzing the patient's heart rhythm, the EMT must:
   A. continue the CPR compressions.
   B. avoid touching the patient.
   C. hyperventilate the patient.
   D. reassess for a carotid pulse.

_A_ **48.** The AED should routinely be used on:
   A. trauma victims.
   B. patients under 55 pounds.
   C. all patients under 8 years of age.
   D. adults, infants, and children in cardiac arrest.

_D_ **49.** The AED pads are first attached to the cables. Then the pad attached to the
   _____ cable goes on the _____ lower ribs.
   A. white; left
   B. white; right
   C. red; left
   D. red; right

_C_ **50.** After the first shock, the patient seems to move and you assess a strong carotid
   pulse. The patient is also breathing adequately. You should then
   _____ and transport.
   A. give high-concentration oxygen via bag-valve mask
   B. provide artificial ventilations with high-concentration oxygen
   C. give high-concentration oxygen via nonrebreather mask
   D. administer two more shocks

_B_ **51.** After three shocks, the EMT should _____ unless local protocol says
   otherwise.
   A. give two more shocks but this time, administer them in a row
   B. begin to transport the patient with high-quality CPR
   C. terminate the arrest because the patient will not survive
   D. increase the rate and volume of the ventilations

_A_ **52.** Which of the following is *not* a general principle of AED use?
   A. Hook up oxygen before beginning defibrillation.
   B. Avoid contact with the patient during rhythm analysis.
   C. Be sure everyone is "clear" before delivering each shock.
   D. Avoid defibrillation in a moving ambulance.

_B_ **53.** Of the cardiac arrest patients listed below, which one can be defibrillated
   immediately?
   A. Soaking-wet patient lying in the rain
   B. Trauma patient with severe blood loss
   C. Patient on a metal deck being cradled by another person
   D. Patient with an implanted defibrillator

_A_ **54.** If it is necessary to remove a nitroglycerin patch to defibrillate a patient,
   you should:
   A. wear gloves.
   B. wear goggles.
   C. ensure that you have a replacement patch.
   D. cleanse the patient's skin with alcohol.

_C_ **55.** If a 55-year-old patient who has a cardiac pacemaker needs to be defibrillated,
   the EMT should:
   A. perform the procedure as he or she would for other cardiac patients.
   B. remove the pacemaker before defibrillation.
   C. place the pad several inches away from the pacemaker battery.
   D. double the power setting on the AED.

©2012 Pearson Education, Inc.
Emergency Care, 12th Ed.

COMPLETE THE FOLLOWING

1. List the five elements (links) in the chain of survival.

A. _____

B. _____

C. _____

D. _____

E. _____

STREET SCENES DISCUSSION

Review the Street Scene on page 504 of the textbook. Then answer the following questions.

1. It was decided very quickly that ALS should be dispatched. This was an appropriate decision. Why is ALS needed in this type of call?

2. If the patient had prescribed nitroglycerin, would it have been appropriate to assist her in the administration of it? (Assume that you have a standing order to assist with nitroglycerin.)

3. If you had applied the AED and it did not shock the patient, what would that have meant?

4. How often should vital signs be taken on this patient? What is her priority?

EMT SKILLS
PERFORMANCE CHECKLISTS

▶ **MANAGING CHEST PAIN (PP. 473–474)**

❑ Take Standard Precautions.

❑ Perform focused assessment for cardiac patient.

❑ Take BP (systolic pressure must be above 90 mmHg).

❑ Contact medical direction for authorization to administer.

❑ Ensure that the patient is alert.

❑ Ensure right patient, right medication, right dose, and right route.

❑ Check expiration date.

❑ Assist the patient with nitroglycerin administration.

❑ Reassess vital signs and chest pain after each dose. Document findings.

NOTE: If the blood pressure falls below 90 systolic, treat the patient for shock (hypoperfusion). Transport promptly.

▶ **ASSESSING AND MANAGING A CARDIAC ARREST PATIENT (PP. 489–492)**

❑ Take Standard Precautions.

❑ Assess patient for responsiveness and normal breathing and a pulse (maximum 10 seconds).

❑ Assess pulse (maximum 10 seconds). If no pulse is present, begin CPR with chest compressions for 2 minutes (5 cycles) and attach AED cables to the patient.

❑ Direct the rescuer to stop CPR, stand clear, and analyze the patient's rhythm.

❑ If shockable rhythm is present, clear the patient and deliver a shock followed by immediate chest compressions.

❑ If nonshockable rhythm is present, immediately begin CPR with chest compressions.

❑ Provide CPR for 2 minutes (5 cycles of 30 compressions to 2 ventilations).

❑ Verify the presence or absence of a spontaneous pulse. If a spontaneous pulse is absent:

- Direct the resumption of CPR.
- Gather additional information on the arrest event.
    - Confirm the effectiveness of CPR (ventilation and compressions).
    - Direct the insertion of an airway adjunct (oropharyngeal/nasopharyngeal).
    - Direct the ventilation of the patient with high-concentration oxygen.
    - Ensure that CPR continues without unnecessary/prolonged interruption.

❑ After 2 minutes of CPR, reevaluate the patient.

❑ Repeat the defibrillator sequence.

❑ Check the carotid pulse.

❑ If there is a spontaneous pulse, check the patient's breathing.

©2012 Pearson Education, Inc.
Emergency Care, 12th Ed.

□ If breathing is adequate, provide high-concentration oxygen by nonre-breather mask. If breathing is inadequate, ventilate the patient with high-concentration oxygen.

□ Transport the patient without delay to a hospital prepared to provide post-resuscitative cardiac arrest care.

▶ CHECKING THE AED

□ Check the AED for the following:

- Unit, cables, connectors for cleanliness and condition.
- Supplies carried with AED.
- Power supply and its operation.
- Indicators on ECG display.
- ECG recorder operation.
- Charge display cycle with a simulator.
- Pacemaker feature, if applicable.

□ File a written report on status of AED.

NOTE: This list is derived from FDA Automated Defibrillator: Operator's Shift Checklist.

▶ USING THE THUMPER® (P. 500)

□ Take Standard Precautions.

□ Ensure that CPR is in progress and effective.

□ Attach the Thumper® base plate to a long backboard.

□ Stop CPR to slide the long backboard under the patient.*

□ Restart CPR and attach the shoulder straps to the patient.

□ Slide the Thumper® piston plate into position on the base plate (away from the chest).

□ Stop CPR and quickly pivot the piston arm into place, measuring anterior/posterior and middle sternum placement.*

□ Slowly adjust the depth of compression to the appropriate diagram.

□ Adjust ventilations.

□ Turn off compressions temporarily for pulse checks and defibrillation.*

□ Upon termination of arrest or return of spontaneous circulation, power down the unit.

▶ USING THE AUTO-PULSE® (P. 500)

□ Take Standard Precautions.

□ Ensure that CPR is in progress and effective.

□ Align the patient on the Auto-Pulse® platform.*

□ Close the Lifeband chest band over the patient's chest.

□ Press the start (Auto-Pulse® is designed to do the compressions automatically).

❏ Provide bag-mask ventilation at a rate of 2 ventilations for every 30 compressions. Each ventilation should be given over 1 second to provide visible chest rise.

❏ If an advanced airway (ETT, LMA, or Combitube) is in place, there are no longer cycles of compressions to ventilations. The compression rate is continuous at at least 100/min. and the ventilation rate is 8–10/min.

❏ After 2 minutes of CPR, reassess for pulse and/or shockable rhythm.*

*Always limit interruptions in chest compressions to 10 seconds or less.

©2012 Pearson Education, Inc.
Emergency Care, 12th Ed.

21
Diabetic Emergencies and Altered Mental Status

Standards: Medicine (Endocrine Disorders; Neurology)

Competency: Applies fundamental knowledge to provide basic emergency care and transportation based on assessment findings for an acutely ill patient.

OBJECTIVES

After reading this chapter you should be able to:

21.1 Define key terms introduced in this chapter.

21.2 Consider several possible causes of altered mental status when given scenarios involving patients with alterations in mental status.

21.3 Describe the basic physiological requirements for maintaining consciousness.

21.4 Perform primary and secondary assessments on patients with altered mental status.

21.5 Describe the pathophysiology of diabetes and diabetic emergencies.

21.6 Determine a patient's blood glucose level using a blood glucose meter, as allowed by local protocol.

21.7 Develop a plan to manage patients with diabetic emergencies involving hyperglycemia and hypoglycemia.

21.8 Recognize the signs, symptoms, and history consistent with other causes of altered mental status, including seizures, stroke, dizziness, and syncope.

21.9 Given a variety of scenarios involving patients with seizures, search for potential underlying causes.

21.10 Develop a plan to manage patients who are having or who have just had a seizure.

21.11 Explain the causes of strokes.

21.12 Develop a plan to manage patients who are exhibiting signs and symptoms of a stroke.

21.13 Given a scenario of a patient complaining of dizziness or syncope, search for potential underlying causes.

21.14 Develop a plan to manage patients with complaints of dizziness and syncope.

MATCH TERMINOLOGY/ DEFINITIONS

A. A form of sugar, the body's basic source of energy

B. Also called "sugar diabetes" or just "diabetes," the condition brought about by decreased insulin production or the inability of the body cells to use insulin properly

C. A hormone produced by the pancreas or taken as a medication by many diabetics

D. Fainting

E. A prolonged seizure or when a person suffers two or more convulsive seizures without regaining full consciousness

F. Low blood sugar

G. A medical condition that causes seizures; with proper medication, many of these patients no longer have seizures

H. High blood sugar

I. A sudden change in sensation, behavior, or movement; the most severe form produces violent muscle contractions called convulsions

J. A condition of altered function caused when an artery in the brain is blocked or ruptured, disrupting the supply of oxygenated blood or causing bleeding into the brain

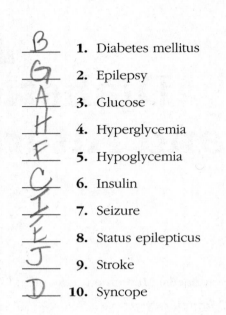

_B_ **1.** Diabetes mellitus

_G_ **2.** Epilepsy

_A_ **3.** Glucose

_H_ **4.** Hyperglycemia

_F_ **5.** Hypoglycemia

_C_ **6.** Insulin

_I_ **7.** Seizure

_E_ **8.** Status epilepticus

_J_ **9.** Stroke

_D_ **10.** Syncope

MULTIPLE-CHOICE REVIEW

_C_ **1.** The relationship of glucose to insulin is often described as:
   A. oppositional.
   B. synergistic.
   C. a lock-and-key mechanism.
   D. antagonistic.

x _C_ **2.** You are treating a 27-year-old female who has a condition that you suspect has been brought about by a decrease in insulin production. This condition is known as:
   A. diabetes mellitus.
   B. hypotension.
   C. hypoglycemia.
   D. stroke.

_C_ **3.** Your patient has a history of diabetes. You were called to her home because her family noticed her mental status was altered. The most common medical emergency for the diabetic patient is called:
   A. diabetes mellitus.
   B. hypotension.
   C. hypoglycemia.
   D. stroke.

_B_ X **4.** You are treating a diabetic patient who seems to have overdone his exercise routine today. He is a little confused about where he is and the day of the week. The most likely medical condition he has developed is called:

    A. hypoglycemia.
    B. hyperglycemia.
    C. diabetes mellitus.
    D. acute pulmonary edema.

_D_ X **5.** The hypoglycemia that EMTs see in the field has many causes. Which of the following is *not* a cause of hypoglycemia?

    A. The patient may have taken too much insulin by mistake.
    B. The patient ate a box of candy too fast.
    C. The patient has been vomiting.
    D. The patient has been fasting.

_A_ **6.** If sugar is not replenished quickly for the diabetic patient who has developed hypoglycemia, the patient:

    A. may have permanent brain damage.
    B. may go into pulmonary edema.
    C. will have chest pain.
    D. can live off his internal sugar supply for up to 2 weeks.

_C_ **7.** You are treating a patient who is unconscious for an unknown reason. The clues that a patient is a diabetic include all of the following *except*:

    A. a medical identification bracelet.
    B. the presence of insulin in the refrigerator.
    C. low-fat food in the freezer.
    D. information provided by family members.

_B_ **8.** In the patient with an altered mental status, the EMT should always consider _____ before proceeding with the secondary assessment and transport.

    A. hypothermia
    B. an airway or breathing problem
    C. that the patient may have had a seizure
    D. internal blood loss

_D_ **9.** An intoxicated appearance and uncharacteristic behavior are typical of:

    A. shock.
    B. dehydration.
    C. cardiac arrest.
    D. diabetic emergency.

_C_ X **10.** Your patient has a history of diabetes and takes medication by injection daily. Diabetics often present the EMT with all of the following signs and symptoms *except*:

    A. cold, clammy skin.
    B. decreased heart rate.
    C. anxiety.
    D. combativeness.

_A_ **11.** For the EMT to consider administering oral glucose, the patient must have an altered mental status, have a:

    A. history of diabetes, and be awake enough to swallow.
    B. prescribed medication, and have an absent gag reflex.
    C. history of seizures, and be awake.
    D. Medic Alert® tag that says "diabetic," and have a head injury.

_C_ **12.** You are treating a diabetic patient who has low blood sugar, as documented by a glucometer. When reassessing the patient after you administered oral glucose, you note the patient's condition has not improved. What action should you take?
  A. Call the patient's personal physician.
  B. Give glucose in orange juice.
  C. Consult medical direction about whether to administer more glucose.
  D. Administer oxygen by nasal cannula.

_C_ **13.** When it is time to transport the diabetic patient who does not respond to painful stimuli, which position is most appropriate?
  A. Supine
  B. Prone
  C. Recovery
  D. Fowler's

† _D_ **14.** Which statement about children with diabetes is *most* correct?
  A. Children are more likely than adults to eat correctly.
  B. Children are less likely than adults to exhaust blood sugar levels.
  — **C.** Children are more at risk than adults for developing hypoglycemia.
  D. Children have a greater risk for medical emergencies than do adults.

✗ _B_ **15.** Which of the following would *most* likely indicate an alteration in the patient's blood sugar level?
  A. Right lower abdominal pain
  B. Nausea and vomiting
  ◄ **C.** Change in mental status
  D. Rigid abdomen on palpation

_B_ **16.** Your patient is going to need oral glucose. Before and after administering the medication, you should make sure to:
  A. check for distal pulses in both arms.
  B. document the mental status of the patient.
  C. increase the oxygen flow rate by 5 liters per minute.
  D. have the patient drink a glass of water.

✗ _C_ **17.** A trade name for oral glucose is:
  A. D_5W.
  B. lactose.
  C. insulin.
  D. Insta-glucose.

✗ _B_ **18.** A patient is very confused and disoriented. Before deciding the patient has a behavioral problem, the EMT should consider all of the following *except*:
  A. a potential head injury.
  B. a brain tumor.
  C. hypoxia.
  — **D.** glucose allergy.

_B_ **19.** People with diabetes routinely test the level of sugar in their blood using a(n):
  A. capnograph.
  B. glucose meter.
  C. urinal.
  — **D.** oximeter.

_D_ **20.** Complications of diabetes include:
  A. kidney failure.
  B. heart disease.
  C. blindness.
  D. any of these.

©2012 Pearson Education, Inc.
Emergency Care, 12th Ed.

_C_ **21.** The reading on the device described in multiple-choice question 19 is reported in:
  A. grams of sugar per liter of blood.
  B. centimeters of blood per decimeter of sugar.
  C. milligrams of glucose per deciliter of blood.
  D. none of these.

_D_ **22.** If the diabetic is symptomatic and has a sugar level below _____, he is considered hypoglycemic.
  A. 140
  B. 120
  C. 100
  D. 80

_A_ **23.** If the diabetic is symptomatic and has a sugar level above _____, he is considered hyperglycemic.
  A. 120
  B. 100
  C. 80
  D. 60

_C_ **24.** You are assessing a patient who just had a seizure. The *most* common cause of seizures in adults is:
  A. taking a double dose of antiseizure medication.
  B. taking a small dose of antiseizure medication.
  C. not taking prescribed antiseizure medication.
  D. use of illicit street drugs.

_A_ **25.** Seizures are commonly caused by all of the following *except*:
  A. cold exposure.
  B. a high fever.
  C. a brain tumor.
  D. an infection.

_A_ **26.** Which of the following is *not* a characteristic of an idiopathic seizure?
  A. Lasts longer than 10 minutes
  B. Occurs spontaneously
  C. Cause is unknown
  D. Often starts in childhood

_A_ **27.** You are responding to a call for a 37-year-old male patient who has had a seizure. Convulsive seizures may be seen with:
  A. epilepsy or hypoglycemia.
  B. hyperventilation or AMI.
  C. anaphylaxis or pulmonary embolism.
  D. hyperglycemia or asthma.

_B_ **28.** You are interviewing the family member of a patient who just had a seizure. The best-known condition that results in seizures is:
  A. a stroke.
  B. epilepsy.
  C. measles.
  D. eclampsia.

_A_ **29.** Most members of the general public associate a _____ seizure with epilepsy.
  A. generalized tonic-clonic
  B. complex partial
  C. simple partial
  D. idiopathic

_D__ **30.** When obtaining the medical history of a seizure patient, interview the bystanders to find out all of the following *except*:
   A. how long the seizure lasted.
   B. what the patient did after the seizure.
   C. what the patient was doing prior to the seizure.
   D. what the family's reaction was to the seizure.

_C__ **31.** You are treating a patient who is actively seizing. He is rapidly becoming cyanotic. After convulsions end, what action should you take?
   A. Wait for the patient's color to return to normal.
   B. Place a nonrebreather mask with oxygen on the patient.
   C. Provide artificial ventilations with supplemental oxygen.
   D. Monitor the pulse closely for 2 minutes.

_B__ **32.** On your arrival at the scene, you notice that a bystander has placed a tongue blade in the corner of a seizure patient's mouth. What should you do?
   A. Begin oxygen therapy with a nonrebreather mask.
   B. Carefully remove the object from the patient's mouth.
   C. Immobilize the patient on a long spine board.
   D. Immediately transport the patient to the hospital.

_A__ **33.** A seizure will normally last about _____ minutes.
   A. 1 to 3   **C.** 7 to 10
   B. 4 to 6   **D.** 30

_B__ **34.** You are treating an elderly patient who has just had two back-to-back seizures without regaining consciousness. This is a serious condition called _____ and the treatment will include _____.
   A. repeating seizure; ventilation
   B. status epilepticus; ALS meds
   C. status asthmaticus; the recovery position
   D. convulsions; oxygen administration

X _A__ **35.** If you suspect a conscious 49-year-old female has had a stroke, you should transport her in the _____ position and pay close attention to her _____.
   A. recovery; heart rate
   B. supine; breathing rate
   C. prone; skin color
   D. semi-sitting; airway

_B__ **36.** When assessing your 53-year-old male patient, you determine he is having difficulty saying what he is thinking even though he clearly understands you. This condition found in stroke patients is called:
   A. receptive aphasia.
   B. expressive aphasia.
   C. miscommunication.
   D. confusion.

X _A__ **37.** When assessing your 42-year-old female patient, you determine that she can speak clearly but cannot understand what you are saying. This is called:
   A. expressive aphasia.
   B. hyperactivity.
   C. receptive aphasia.
   D. petit mal seizure.

_D__ **38.** Your patient is a suspected stroke patient. A common sign you would expect to find in this patient is:
   A. tingling in both legs.
   B. diminished urine flow.
   C. low blood pressure.
   D. headache.

©2012 Pearson Education, Inc.
Emergency Care, 12th Ed.

_____ **39.** You are treating a 58-year-old male patient who you suspect may be having a stroke. The signs and symptoms this patient presents with might include:
  A. vomiting.
  B. seizures.
  C. loss of bladder control.
  D. all of these.

_____ **40.** The 62-year-old male patient who presented with a number of the signs and symptoms of a stroke was taken to the ED yesterday. When talking with your Medical Director about the call, he tells you that the signs and symptoms were completely resolved within the past 24 hours. This patient was most likely suffering a(n):
  A. altered mental status (AMS).
  B. transient ischemic attack (TIA).
  C. acute myocardial infarction (AMI).
  D. hypoglycemic incident.

_____ **41.** You are treating a patient who passed out while waiting in a long line to get into a concert. When a patient faints, the medical term to describe this is usually a(n) _____ and the treatment would involve _____.
  A. hypoglycemic incident; oxygen administration
  B. stroke; Fowler position
  C. syncopal episode; oxygen administration
  D. hyperglycemic incident; Trendelenburg position

_____ **42.** When assessing your 45-year-old female patient, she says that she feels lightheaded. Lightheadedness, or dizziness, is a symptom that is often due to:
  A. too much blood being circulated to the brain.
  B. poor perfusion to the brain.
  C. too much fluid intake in too short a period of time.
  D. standing erect for too long a period of time.

INSIDE/OUTSIDE: HYPOGLYCEMIA

1. When the autonomic nervous system engages, what occurs?

_____

2. What signs or symptoms develop outside the body of the hypoglycemic patient?

_____

INSIDE/OUTSIDE: HYPERGLYCEMIA

1. As the blood sugar level creeps up, what does the patient complain of?

_____

2. What is the acetone or fruity smell on the diabetic's breath due to?

_____

INSIDE/OUTSIDE: TONIC-CLONIC SEIZURES

1. What happens in the tonic phase?

_____

2. What happens in the clonic phase?

_____

3. What is the postictal phase?

_____

COMPLETE THE FOLLOWING

1. List six signs and symptoms associated with a diabetic emergency.

A. _____

B. _____

C. _____

D. _____

E. _____

F. _____

2. Give four reasons a diabetic may develop *hyper*glycemia.

A. _____

B. _____

C. _____

D. _____

3. List the five categories of causes of dizziness and syncope.

A. _____

B. _____

C. _____

D. _____

E. _____

STREET SCENES DISCUSSION

Review the Street Scene on page 529 of the textbook. Then answer the following questions.

1. What advice should be given to this patient and his friend before they walk away?

2. Aside from the patient telling you he has not been eating all day, what are other possible causes of hypoglycemia?

3. If you did not have oral glucose with you, but you suspected his blood sugar was low, what else could you have used to help bring up this patient's sugar level?

CASE STUDY

▶ CALL FOR A MAN DOWN

You respond to an alleyway in the area of town where there are a number of factories. It is early evening, and this area is usually not well traveled on the weekends. The police are on the scene of an approximately 35-year-old male who was found unconscious by some kids who were riding by on their bikes. The scene is safe and you begin your primary assessment.

1. You do not see any apparent trauma. How would you open his airway?

_____

2. If the patient is breathing but very shallowly and very slowly, what should you do?

_____

In a couple of moments, the patient wakes up and is a bit nasty and combative. One of the police officers says that he remembers this guy. He has some medical problems and never takes his medicine.

3. You notice that the patient has urinated on himself. What may this be due to?

_____

4. With the assistance of the police, you carefully go through the patient's pockets and you come across an empty canister of dilantin. How does this contribute to the history?

_____

5. Is it safe to decide that this patient had a seizure and simply transport him?

_____

You decide to get a full set of baseline vital signs, administer some oxygen, and check the patient's blood sugar with the glucometer. Your partner goes back to the ambulance to return with the stretcher.

6. Why would you be doing all this when it may just be a seizure?

_____

7. The glucometer reads 70. What could this mean?

_____

At this point, the medics arrive and you share all the information you have with them. Because the patient is still "altered" and all of you are not confident in his gag reflex, the decision is made to start an IV and administer 25 grams of dextrose in 50 cc. Very soon thereafter, the patient becomes alert and tells you that he has developed type II diabetes in the last few years due to his poor eating habits and other factors.

8. What is type II diabetes, and do patients always have to take insulin?

_____

EMT SKILLS PERFORMANCE CHECKLISTS

▶ **MANAGEMENT OF A DIABETIC EMERGENCY (P. 512)**

❑ Conduct a scene size-up.

❑ Take Standard Precautions.

❑ Perform a primary assessment.

❑ Perform a focused history and physical exam, and take vital signs. Record the patient's mental status before glucose administration.

❑ Consult medical direction.

❑ Check for the signs and symptoms of altered mental status that result from a history of diabetes.

❑ Ensure that the patient is awake with a gag reflex.

❏ Place glucose on a tongue depressor and place between the cheek and gum.

❏ Perform ongoing assessment. Record the patient's mental status after glucose administration.

▶ USING A BLOOD GLUCOSE METER (PP. 512–513)

❏ Take Standard Precautions.

❏ Prepare the blood glucose meter and supplies (i.e., lancet, test strip, Band-aid, sharps container, alcohol preparation).

❏ Cleanse the skin with an alcohol prep. Allow the alcohol to dry before performing the stick.

❏ Use the lancet to perform a stick. Wipe away the first drop of blood that appears. Squeeze the puncture wound to get a second drop of blood.

❏ Apply the blood to the test strip. This may be done by holding the strip to the finger to draw the blood into the strip.

❏ Dispose of the lancet in a sharps container.

❏ Read the blood glucose level displayed on the glucose meter. It may take from 15 to 60 seconds for the device to provide a reading. (Newer devices take 5 seconds and less blood.)

❏ Assess the puncture site and apply direct pressure or a Band-aid to control the bleeding.

The reading is in mg/dl (milligrams of glucose per deciliter of blood.) Normal "fasting" blood sugar values are 70–110 mg/dl. If the patient has a value less than 60–80 mg/dl and is symptomatic, treatment should be provided following local medical control.

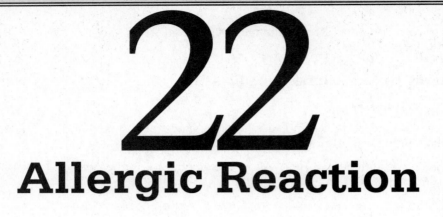

Allergic Reaction

Standards: Medicine (Immunology)

Competency: Applies fundamental knowledge to provide basic emergency care and transportation based on assessment findings for an acutely ill patient.

OBJECTIVES

After reading this chapter you should be able to:

22.1   Define key terms introduced in this chapter.

22.2   Differentiate between the signs and symptoms of an allergic reaction and an anaphylactic reaction.

22.3   Describe the relationship between allergens and antibodies necessary for an allergic reaction to occur.

22.4   Describe the effects of histamine and other chemicals in producing the signs and symptoms of anaphylaxis.

22.5   List common allergens.

22.6   Prioritize the steps in assessment and management of patients with allergic and anaphylactic reactions.

22.7   Recognize the indications for administering and assisting a patient in the use of an epinephrine auto-injector.

22.8   Describe the desired effects and side effects associated with the administration of epinephrine.

22.9   Demonstrate administration of epinephrine by auto-injector.

22.10 Describe the considerations in reassessment of patients with allergic and anaphylactic reactions.

MATCH TERMINOLOGY/ DEFINITIONS

A. Red, itchy, possibly raised blotches on the skin that often result from an allergic reaction

B. A severe or life-threatening allergic reaction in which the blood vessels dilate, causing a drop in blood pressure, and the tissues lining the respiratory system swell, interfering with the airway

C. Something that causes an allergic reaction

D. A hormone produced by the body; as a medication, it constricts blood vessels and dilates respiratory passages and is used to relieve severe allergic reactions

E. A syringe preloaded with medication that has a spring-loaded device and thus pushes the needle through the skin when the tip of the device is pressed firmly against the body

F. An exaggerated immune response

C 1. Allergen
F 2. Allergic reaction
B 3. Anaphylaxis
E 4. Auto-injector
D 5. Epinephrine
A 6. Hives

MULTIPLE-CHOICE REVIEW

C 1. A patient's exaggerated response of her body's immune system to any substance is called a(n) _____ reaction.
A. vasoconstricting
B. immune
C. allergic
D. syncopal

D 2. You are treating a 22-year-old female patient who you suspect is having an allergic reaction. Why would an allergic reaction sometimes be treated as a high-priority patient?
A. The patient can vomit.
B. The patient can become covered with hives.
C. An allergic reaction can speed up the heart rate.
D. An allergic reaction can cause airway obstruction.

C 3. The first time a person is exposed to an allergen, the person's immune system:
A. reacts violently.
B. shuts down.
C. forms antibodies.
D. ignores the allergen.

B X 4. The second time a person is exposed to an allergen, the body reactions may include all of the following *except*:
A. destruction of antibodies.
B. difficulty breathing.
C. massive swelling.
D. dilation of the blood vessels.

_D_ 5. When interviewing a patient, you should consider the common causes of allergic reactions; these causes include all of the following *except*:
A. hornet stings.
B. eggs and milk.
C. poison ivy and penicillin.
D. red fruits and vegetables.

_C_ 6. Why is it possible for a patient to be allergic to peanuts and not to walnuts or almonds?
A. Because walnuts have a protective quality to them
B. Because almonds cause vasoconstriction of the arteries
C. Because peanuts are legumes and not nuts
D. All of these

_B_ 7. You are treating a 35-year-old male patient who you suspect is having a life-threatening allergic reaction. He was stung by a few bees when mowing the lawn. The respiratory signs and symptoms of anaphylactic shock include all of the following *except*:
A. rapid breathing.
B. hives.
C. cough.
D. stridor.

_D_ 8. The effects on the cardiac system of an allergic reaction for the patient described in multiple-choice question 7 could include _____ heart rate and _____ blood pressure.
A. decreased; decreased
B. increased; increased
C. decreased; increased
D. increased; decreased

_C_ 9. For the situation in multiple-choice question 7 to be considered a severe allergic reaction, the patient must have signs and symptoms of shock or:
A. a history of allergies.
B. massive swelling.
C. respiratory distress.
D. increased blood pressure.

_B_ 10. Your patient who is experiencing a severe allergic reaction meets the protocol criteria and has his own self-injector. After you administer epinephrine by an auto-injector, you should:
A. prepare another dose.
B. reassess the patient after 2 minutes.
C. decrease the oxygen being administered.
D. allow the patient to remain at home.

_B_ 11. You are interviewing a 21-year-old female who states that she has no history of allergies. She is obviously having her first allergic reaction, so you should:
A. consult with medical direction.
B. treat for shock and transport immediately.
C. administer epinephrine via auto-injector.
D. attempt to determine the cause immediately.

_A_ 12. Your 22-year-old male patient has an epinephrine auto-injector in his backpack. Besides helping him take his medication, you should always:
A. ask if the patient has any spare auto-injectors for the trip to the hospital.
B. call the patient's physician and request another dosage of the medication.
C. determine if other family members have a history of allergic reactions.
D. take the insect or substance that caused the reaction to the hospital.

_B_ **13.** You are treating an adult patient who you suspect is having a severe allergic reaction. He has an Epi-pen® on him for situations like this. The recommended location for injection with the epinephrine auto-injector is the:
   A. center of the back.
   B. lateral mid-thigh.
   C. buttocks.
   D. biceps.

_B_ **14.** Your patient is a preschooler who has a history of peanut allergies. He has an epinephrine auto-injector that is held by the school nurse. These devices come in two different sizes. The child size (for children weighing fewer than 66 pounds) contains:
   A. 0.05 mg.
   B. 0.15 mg.
   C. 0.5 mg.
   D. 1.0 mg.

_B_ **15.** You are on a call involving a severe allergic reaction in a child patient. Which statement is *true* related to anaphylactic reactions in infants and children?
   A. Infants frequently experience anaphylactic reactions.
   B. Children outgrow allergies as they mature.
   C. Anaphylactic reactions are common in younger children.
   D. Parents seldom can provide useful information about the child's medical history.

_____ **16.** Which of the following is an example of a difference in the reaction of a patient experiencing an anaphylactic reaction compared to a patient experiencing a simple allergic reaction?
   A. The allergic reaction has generalized hives.
   B. The allergic reaction has localized swelling.
   C. The anaphylactic reaction includes bradycardia and mild anxiety.
   D. The anaphylactic reaction includes sneezing and coughing.

INSIDE/OUTSIDE: ALLERGIC REACTIONS

1. Histamine is a very important chemical that is released into the bloodstream in response to the release of antibodies to a particular antigen. During the release of histamine, when a patient is having a severe allergic reaction, what five things occur to the body?

   A. _____

   B. _____

   C. _____

   D. _____

   E. _____

2. What are four signs and symptoms that develop from histamine release and can be observed by the EMT when assessing the patient?

   A. _____

   B. _____

   C. _____

   D. _____

COMPLETE THE FOLLOWING

1. List ten signs and symptoms of allergic reaction or anaphylactic shock.

A. _____

B. _____

C. _____

D. _____

E. _____

F. _____

G. _____

H. _____

I. _____

J. _____

2. For a patient to be considered in anaphylaxis, list two signs, either of which must be evident.

A. _____

B. _____

LABEL THE DIAGRAMS

Fill in the name of each substance that may cause an allergic reaction on the line provided.

1. _____

2. _____

3. _____

4. _____

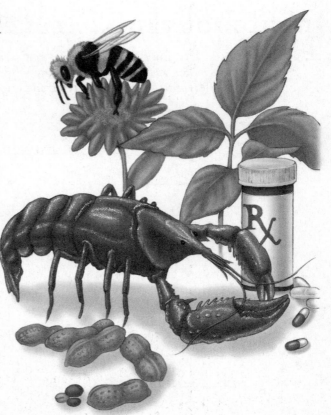

STREET SCENES DISCUSSION

Review the Street Scene on page 544 of the textbook. Then answer the following questions.

1. If the patient had an epinephrine auto-injector, would it be appropriate to use it in this situation? If so, where would you inject it?

2. Would it be appropriate to call for an estimated time of arrival (ETA) on the ALS unit? Why or why not?

3. If the patient went into cardiac arrest, what would be your patient-care priorities?

CASE STUDY

▶ THE LAKEFRONT EMERGENCY

You respond to a call from a woman having difficulty breathing while at a camp on a lake. Upon your arrival, you ensure that the scene is safe, and you find a woman in her forties who is clutching her chest and is having obvious breathing difficulty.

1. Is there a need for another ambulance?

2. Should you call for an ALS unit to respond?

After taking Standard Precautions, you begin your primary assessment. There is no reason to suspect trauma, and the patient has an open airway. She is responsive, although she talks in short, choppy sentences. She knows her name, where she is, and the day of the week.

©2012 Pearson Education, Inc.
Emergency Care, 12th Ed.

3. Why is she talking in short, choppy sentences?

4. What would be your assessment of her level of responsiveness?

A high-pitched musical tone is heard as she breathes. She shows other signs of respiratory distress.

5. What is the name of her breathing sound, and what are some of the potential causes of this sound?

6. What are some additional signs of breathing difficulty that you may observe in this patient?

You decide that beginning oxygen administration is an appropriate thing to do at this time.

7. How would you deliver the oxygen, and how many liters per minute would you administer?

You note the patient has a weak and rapid radial pulse. There is no reason to suspect any life-threatening external bleeding in this instance. The patient is very pale and is sweating profusely. She also complains of chest tightness and dizziness, which she denies she has ever had before.

8. Would you prioritize this patient as a low or high priority? Why?

©2012 Pearson Education, Inc.
Emergency Care, 12th Ed.

9. What would be the best position in which to transport the patient and why?

As you begin to prepare the patient for transport, you start the focused history and physical exam. The patient has chest tightness and breathing difficulty, which came on suddenly. The pain is across the upper chest, doesn't radiate, and is constant. Nothing the patient does makes the pain go away; she states it is a 7 on a scale of 1 to 10, with 10 being the worst pain she ever had. The pain has been present for approximately 15 minutes. You assign a crew member to obtain a complete set of vital signs as you quickly listen to her lungs. She has a weak and rapid pulse at 110, respirations are labored at 26 per minute, and her blood pressure is 88/50 mmHg.

10. As you load the patient into the ambulance, what additional history should you obtain?

Your patient states that she was cleaning out the gutter and may have been stung by a bee. She previously reacted severely to a bee sting and carries a bee-sting kit.

11. (A) What medicine is usually in these kits? **(B)** Should you help her take the medicine?

12. (A) Is it necessary to call a doctor? **(B)** What must be checked prior to administering the medicine?

As you leave the scene, the driver arranges for an ALS intercept on the way to the hospital. Other than reassessing the patient after administering the medication, you continue to monitor the patient. About 5 minutes en route, your driver pulls the ambulance to the side of the road momentarily as the ALS paramedic jumps in with his equipment. Then you proceed to the hospital.

13. What would be your quick report to the paramedic on **(A)** the patient's chief complaint, **(B)** your assessment of the situation, and **(C)** the treatment you have given?

14. What care would you expect to see the paramedic give en route to the hospital?

EMT SKILLS PERFORMANCE CHECKLIST

▶ **ASSESSING AND MANAGING AN ALLERGIC REACTION* (PP. 537–538)**

❏ Take Standard Precautions.

❏ Perform a primary assessment. Provide high-concentration oxygen by non-rebreather mask.

❏ Obtain the SAMPLE history.

❏ Take the patient's vital signs.†

❏ Obtain the patient's prescribed epinephrine auto-injector. Ensure that the:

  • Prescription is written for the patient who is experiencing the severe allergic reaction or your protocols permit carrying the auto-injector on the ambulance.
  • The medication is not discolored (if visible).

❏ Obtain an order from medical direction (either on-line or off-line).

❏ Remove the safety cap(s) from the auto-injector.

❏ Place the tip of the auto-injector against the patient's thigh (lateral portion, midway between the waist and knee).

❏ Push the injector firmly against the thigh until the injector activates.

❏ Hold the injector in place until the medication is injected (at least 10 seconds).

❏ Dispose of a single-dose injector, such as the EpiPen®, in biohazard container; save a two-dose injector, such as the Twinject®, and transport with the patient in case the second dose is later required.

❏ Record activity and time.

❏ Reassess the patient, paying special attention to the patient's ABCs and vital signs, while transporting.

*These patients change very quickly so move quickly!

†Initial reassessment 2 minutes post-epi administration.

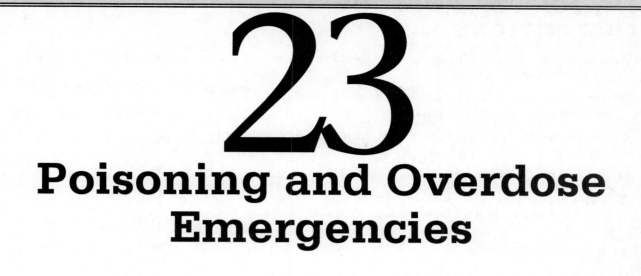

23

Poisoning and Overdose Emergencies

Standards: Medicine (Toxicology)

Competency: Applies fundamental knowledge to provide basic emergency care and transportation based on assessment findings for an acutely ill patient.

OBJECTIVES

After reading this chapter you should be able to:

23.1 Define key terms introduced in this chapter.

23.2 Describe the ways in which poisons can enter the body.

23.3 Identify potential dangers to EMS providers and others at scenes where poisoning, alcohol abuse, or substance abuse is involved.

23.4 Collect key elements in the history of a patient who has been poisoned.

23.5 Describe the use of activated charcoal in the management of ingested poisons.

23.6 Explain the management of patients who have ingested a poison.

23.7 Develop a plan for managing patients who have inhaled poisons.

23.8 Develop a plan for managing patients who have absorbed poisons through the skin.

23.9 Develop a plan for managing patients who have been poisoned through injection.

23.10 Describe the health risks associated with alcohol abuse.

23.11 Recognize the signs and symptoms of alcohol abuse and alcohol withdrawal.

23.12 Recognize signs, symptoms, and health risks associated with abuse of substances, including stimulants, depressants, narcotics, volatile chemicals, and hallucinogens.

23.13 Given a variety of scenarios, develop a treatment plan for patients with emergencies related to alcohol and substance abuse.

MATCH TERMINOLOGY/ DEFINITIONS

A. Any substance that can harm the body by altering cell structure or functions

B. Stimulants, such as amphetamines, that affect the central nervous system to excite the user

C. State in which a patient's body reacts severely when deprived of an abused substance

D. Poisons that are taken into the body through unbroken skin

E. Depressants, such as barbiturates, that depress the central nervous system, often used to bring on a more relaxed state of mind

F. Poisons that are swallowed

G. A class of drugs that affect the nervous system and change many normal body activities; their legal use is for relief of pain; illicit use is to produce an intense state of relaxation

H. A substance that adsorbs many poisons and prevents them from being absorbed by the body

I. Thinning down or weakening by mixing with something else

J. Poisons that are inserted through the skin, for example, by needle, snake fangs, or insect stinger

K. A severe reaction that can be part of alcohol withdrawal, characterized by sweating, trembling, anxiety, and hallucinations

L. Poisons that are breathed in

M. Mind-affecting or mind-altering drugs that act on the central nervous system to produce excitement and distortion of perceptions

N. A poisonous substance secreted by bacteria, plants, or animals

O. Vaporizing compounds, such as cleaning fluid, that are breathed in by an abuser to produce a "high"

P. A substance that neutralizes a poison or its effects

_D_ 1. Absorbed poisons

_P_ 2. Activated charcoal

____ 3. Antidote

_K_ 4. Delirium tremens

____ 5. Dilution

_E_ 6. Downers

_M_ 7. Hallucinogens

_F_ 8. Ingested poisons

_L_ 9. Inhaled poisons

_J_ 10. Injected poisons

_G_ 11. Narcotics

_A_ 12. Poison

_N_ 13. Toxin

_B_ 14. Uppers

_O_ 15. Volatile chemicals

____ 16. Withdrawal

MULTIPLE-CHOICE REVIEW

_B_ 1. You are on the scene of a 28-year-old female who you suspect may have been poisoned. Which of the following is an environmental clue at the scene that can be used to help you determine that your patient may have been poisoned?
A. The patient appears to have been vomiting.
B. There is an empty pill bottle on the night table.
C. The patient has an altered mental status.
D. The patient states that she has a headache.

_A_ 2. Which of the following is the most accurate definition of a poison?
   A. Any substance that can harm the body, sometimes seriously enough to create a medical emergency
   B. Any foreign substance swallowed by the patient
   C. Any substance that could kill the patient if it is injected into the body
   D. Any substance labeled with a hazardous material placard or label

_A_ 3. Most of the over 1 million poisonings yearly in the United States are due to:
   A. suicide attempts by adults.
   B. attempts to murder someone.
   C. accidents involving young children.
   D. teenagers using illicit drugs.

_B_ 4. A substance secreted by plants, animals, or bacteria that is poisonous to humans is called a:
   A. chemical.
   B. toxin.
   C. narcotic.
   D. drug.

_A_ 5. Due to the poisons they produce, plants such as _____ can be dangerous to humans or pets.
   A. mistletoe
   B. mushrooms
   C. rubber plants
   D. all of these

_B_ 6. Bacteria may produce toxins that cause deadly diseases such as:
   A. HIV.
   B. botulism.
   C. penicillin.
   D. steroids.

_B_ 7. For most poisonous substances, the reaction is more serious in:
   A. the evening hours.
   B. the elderly and the ill.
   C. smaller concentrations.
   D. the summer.

_C_ 8. Which one of the following is *not* a way that poisons damage the body?
   A. Destroying skin and other tissues
   B. Enhancing normal biochemical processes
   C. Overstimulating the central nervous system
   D. Displacing oxygen on the hemoglobin

_D_ 9. Poisons may enter the body through any of the following routes *except*:
   A. inhalation.
   B. ingestion.
   C. injection.
   D. excretion.

_A_ 10. Carbon monoxide, chlorine, and sulfur are examples of _____ poisons.
   A. ingested
   B. injected
   C. inhaled
   D. swallowed

_____ 11. You suspect that your 28-year-old male patient may have been exposed to a poison that was absorbed. Examples of absorbed poisons include:
   A. insecticides and agricultural chemicals.
   B. carbon monoxide and chlorine.
   C. insect stings and snake bites.
   D. aspirin and LSD.

_____ 12. The venom of a bite from a rattlesnake is an example of an _____ poison.
   A. ingested
   B. injected
   C. inhaled
   D. absorbed

_____ 13. You are treating a 32-year-old female who was found unconscious by her roommate when she got home late at night. Why is it important to determine when the ingestion of a poison occurred?
   A. Different poisons act on the body at different rates.
   B. Those who ingest poison in the evening tend to vomit more.
   C. Dilution of the poison is not effective after 10 minutes.
   D. The antidote works more effectively once the poison is in the intestines.

_____ 14. You suspect poisoning by ingestion in a child whom you have examined for a patent airway. You can now ask the parent for the child's:
   A. name.
   B. weight.
   C. last visit to a physician.
   D. favorite drink.

_____ 15. The most common results of poison ingestion are:
   A. altered mental status and diarrhea.
   B. nausea and vomiting.
   C. abdominal pain and diarrhea.
   D. chemical burns around the mouth and stomach pain.

_____ 16. You have a standing order to use activated charcoal if the patient meets the criteria. Activated charcoal is used to:
   A. act as an antidote.
   B. dilute the poisonous substance.
   C. reduce the amount of poison absorbed by the body.
   D. speed up the digestion of most chemicals in the body.

_____ 17. Why isn't the oral medication called syrup of ipecac routinely used for toxic ingestions when the patient is found still alert?
   A. Vomiting can occur after the mental status diminishes, increasing the chance of aspiration.
   B. It removes only about one-third of the stomach contents.
   C. It is slow to react compared with other substances or dilution.
   D. All of these are correct reasons.

_____ 18. The decision on when to use activated charcoal is best made:
   A. en route to the hospital.
   B. upon arrival at the emergency department.
   C. with medical direction or poison-control-center consultation.
   D. in consultation with the patient's family physician.

_____ 19. You are treating a 28-year-old male who accidentally ingested a poison. Activated charcoal is _not_ routinely used with ingestion of:
   A. caustic substances.
   B. strong acids.
   C. strong alkalis.
   D. all of these.

©2012 Pearson Education, Inc.
Emergency Care, 12th Ed.

_____ **20.** Your 8-year-old male child has ingested a caustic substance that he should not have been able to access. Examples of caustic substances include all of the following *except*:
  A. lye.
  B. venom.
  C. toilet bowl cleaner.
  D. oven cleaner.

_____ **21.** Your patient is a 22-year-old male who has been stealing fuel from his neighbor's cars at night. Tonight he may have sucked in too much gasoline, and his friend has called 911 because he continues to cough violently after the ingestion. The appropriate treatment for this patient should:
  A. not include activated charcoal.
  B. not include oxygen administration.
  C. include immediate transportation.
  D. be to treat him like a patient with an airway obstruction.

_____ **22.** When a physician orders dilution of an ingested substance, you can use either water or:
  A. a cola drink.
  B. coffee.
  C. milk.
  D. apple juice.

_____ **23.** Your patient is a 32-year-old male who is having signs and symptoms of an inhalation. The most common inhaled poison is:
  A. carbon dioxide.
  B. nitrogen.
  C. carbon monoxide.
  D. phosgene.

_____ **24.** As you approach a 35-year-old male patient who has passed out while cleaning a large tank, you smell an unusual odor. What should you do?
  A. Stand back and attempt to learn more about the chemical involved.
  B. Rapidly remove the patient from the area using a drag maneuver.
  C. Ignore the smell; it is probably a normal odor around industrial sites.
  D. Ask his coworkers to bring the patient to your ambulance.

_____ **25.** The principal prehospital treatment of a 40-year-old male patient who has inhaled poison is:
  A. administering activated charcoal to the patient.
  B. administering high-concentration oxygen.
  C. providing full spinal immobilization.
  D. administering an antidote.

_____ **26.** Besides motor vehicle exhaust, where else might you find carbon monoxide?
  A. In the patient compartment of your ambulance, there may be CO.
  B. Wherever you can smell its odor, there is a large quantity of CO.
  C. Around an improperly vented wood-burning stove, there is CO gas.
  D. Around the foundation of a house, there is often CO gas.

_____ **27.** Your patient is one of the five members of a family who may have been exposed to a leaky heating system and carbon monoxide. How does carbon monoxide affect the body?
  A. It causes severe respiratory burns.
  B. It prevents the normal carrying of oxygen by the red blood cells.
  C. It causes the tissues in the airway to swell, making breathing difficult.
  D. It stimulates the central nervous system to decrease oxygen consumption.

_____ 28. You are treating a family whose fireplace may not have been properly vented to the outside of their home. You might expect to see these patients exhibit any of the following *except*:
   A. cyanosis.
   B. altered mental status.
   C. dizziness.
   D. cherry-red lips.

_____ 29. You are treating a patient who has fertilizer all over his arms and legs. After ensuring your own safety with PPE, you should:
   A. brush off as much powder as possible, then irrigate.
   B. immediately start irrigation with very cold water.
   C. leave the powder in place and transport immediately.
   D. irrigate with water for 20 minutes.

_____ 30. You have responded to a call where a patient seems to have mixed a couple of cleaning agents and is now unconscious. There is a strong smell of rotten eggs in the air. What would you suspect?
   A. The mixture produced large quantities of chlorine.
   B. The mixture may have produced hydrogen sulfide, which can be deadly.
   C. The mixture contains cyanide because that chemical causes unconsciousness.
   D. One of the chemicals was eggs, and they are often deadly when mixed with salts.

_____ 31. Of the following signs and symptoms, which one is *not* seen with alcohol abuse but *is* seen with a diabetic emergency?
   A. Acetone breath
   B. Hallucinations
   C. Slurred speech
   D. Swaying and unsteadiness of movement

_____ 32. The sweating, trembling, anxiety, and hallucinations found in the alcohol withdrawal patient are called:
   A. withdrawal signs.
   B. seizures.
   C. delirium tremens.
   D. Parkinson tremors.

_____ 33. Your 40-year-old male patient has been mixing alcohol with drugs. He exhibits:
   A. uncontrolled shivering.
   B. depressed vital signs.
   C. extreme calmness.
   D. all of these.

_____ 34. When interviewing an intoxicated 32-year-old male patient, do not begin by asking if he has taken any drugs. The reason for this statement is that:
   A. the presence of drugs will negate the presence of the alcohol.
   B. the patient may feel you are accusing him of a crime.
   C. alcoholics generally do not take drugs.
   D. the patient will probably not tell the truth.

_____ 35. Your patient is a 35-year-old female who is very anxious and jittery. She has taken an overdose of a drug that stimulates the nervous system to cause extreme excitement. These drugs are called:
   A. uppers.
   B. downers.
   C. narcotics.
   D. antihypertensives.

©2012 Pearson Education, Inc.
Emergency Care, 12th Ed.

_____ **36.** The patient you are treating has difficulty sleeping, so she takes tranquilizers. These sleeping pills are examples of:

    A. uppers.   **C.** narcotics.

    B. downers.   **D.** hallucinogens.

_____ **37.** You are treating a 29-year-old male patient who has taken an overdose of a drug that has a depressant effect on the central nervous system. These types of drugs are called:

    A. uppers.

    B. downers.

    C. narcotics.

    D. hallucinogens.

_____ **38.** Your patient has taken an overdose of a drug that is capable of producing stupor or sleep; it is also normally used to relieve pain. These types of medications are called:

    A. uppers.

    B. downers.

    C. narcotics.

    D. hallucinogens.

_____ **39.** Your 25-year-old male patient has taken a mind-altering drug designed to act on the nervous system and produce intense excitement or distortion of the patient's perceptions. This drug was most likely a(n):

    A. upper.

    B. downer.

    C. narcotic.

    D. hallucinogen.

_____ **40.** Drugs that have few legal uses and are dissolved in the mouth are called:

    A. narcotics.

    B. uppers.

    C. hallucinogens.

    D. downers.

_____ **41.** Your patient is a 16-year-old male who was found huffing a rag drenched in chemicals. Cleaning fluid, glue, and model cement are examples of:

    A. hallucinogens.

    B. volatile chemicals.

    C. diuretics.

    D. narcotics.

_____ **42.** A 21-year-old female who has overdosed on an "upper" may have signs and symptoms such as:

    A. excitement, increased pulse and breathing rates, dilated pupils, and rapid speech.

    B. sluggishness, sleepiness, and lack of coordination of body and speech.

    C. fast pulse rate, dilated pupils, flushed face, and "seeing" or "hearing" things.

    D. reduced pulse rate and rate and depth of breathing, constricted pupils, and sweating.

_____ **43.** Your 22-year-old male patient has overdosed on a downer, according to his significant other. You can expect to see/observe signs and symptoms such as:

    A. excitement, increased pulse and breathing rates, dilated pupils, and rapid speech.

    B. sluggishness, sleepiness, and lack of coordination of body and speech.

    C. fast pulse rate, dilated pupils, flushed face, and "seeing" or "hearing" things.

    D. reduced pulse rate and rate and depth of breathing, constricted pupils, and sweating.

_____ **44.** A 32-year-old female patient who has overdosed on a hallucinogen may have signs and symptoms such as:

    A. excitement, increased pulse and breathing rates, dilated pupils, and rapid speech.

    B. sluggishness, sleepiness, and lack of coordination of body and speech.

    C. fast pulse rate, dilated pupils, flushed face, and "seeing" or "hearing" things.

    D. reduced pulse rate and rate and depth of breathing, constricted pupils, and sweating.

_____ **45.** Your 52-year-old male patient has been taking double to triple his pain relief medication, but that is not even touching the pain for him. If he was to overdose on the narcotic he takes, he may have signs and symptoms such as:

    A. excitement, increased pulse and breathing rates, dilated pupils, and rapid speech.

    B. sluggishness, sleepiness, and lack of coordination of body and speech.

    C. fast pulse rate, dilated pupils, flushed face, and "seeing" or "hearing" things.

    D. reduced pulse rate and rate and depth of breathing, constricted pupils, and sweating.

INSIDE/OUTSIDE: ACETAMINOPHEN OVERDOSE

1. The patient who overdoses on acetaminophen is likely to have what effects on the "inside"?

_____

2. The patient who overdoses on acetaminophen is likely to experience what symptoms during the first 4 to 12 hours on the "outside"?

_____

COMPLETE THE FOLLOWING

1. What information should the EMT document for medical direction when treating a patient the EMT suspects was poisoned?

    A. _____

    B. _____

    C. _____

    D. _____

    E. _____

    F. _____

    G. _____

    H. _____

2. List at least six signs and symptoms of alcohol abuse.

A. _____

B. _____

C. _____

D. _____

E. _____

F. _____

3. What is the phone number for the poison control center?

_____

LABEL THE DIAGRAMS

Fill in the way that each type of poison enters the body.

1. _____   1. _____

2. _____

3. _____

4. _____

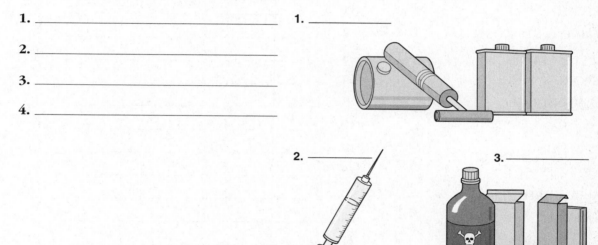

2. _____   3. _____

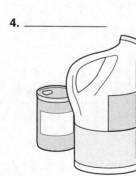 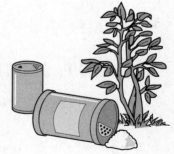

4. _____

COMPLETE THE CHART

Fill in the type of commonly abused drug on the line provided. Indicate on the chart whether each drug is an upper, downer, narcotic, mind-altering drug, or volatile chemical.

AMPHETAMINE   1. _____

CODEINE   2. _____

DMT   3. _____
LSD

PSILOCYBIN   4. _____

GASOLINE   5. _____

SECOBARBITAL   6. _____

METHAQUALONE   7. _____

COCAINE   8. _____

DEXTROAMPHETAMINE   9. _____

CHLORAL HYDRATE   10. _____

MESCALINE   11. _____

MORNING GLORY SEEDS   12. _____

STP   13. _____

HEROIN   14. _____

BUTYL NITRATE   15. _____

PCP   16. _____

FENTANYL   17. _____

METHADONE   18. _____

BARBITURATES   19. _____

DEMEROL   20. _____

PHENOBARBITAL   21. _____

MARIJUANA   22. _____

OPIUM   23. _____

AMYL NITRATE   24. _____

CARBON TETRACHLORIDE   25. _____

STREET SCENES DISCUSSION

Review the Street Scene on page 569 of the textbook. Then answer the following questions.

1. Imagine you were confronted with an infant who had an altered mental status and evidence of ingested poison. Would you quickly administer activated charcoal to the patient? Why or why not?

2. If the infant continues to vomit, what emergency care should be your highest priority?

3. Why is it necessary to take the oil to the hospital?

CASE STUDY

▶ NOT A FUN PARTY FOR EVERYONE!

Your ambulance responds to a private home in a suburban neighborhood. The police are on the scene, and they are trying to sort out the details of a party that seems to have taken place while the parents were away on a cruise.

On arrival it is clear that the scene is safe, although quite a few detectives are attempting to question the 10 teenagers who are left from the party. There are literally piles of beer cans all over the place and the house is obviously a mess. Apparently the reason the police were called was due to a fight breaking out.

1. Your patient is a16-year-old female who is unconscious and appears to have vomited all over herself. What is your first priority?

2. Her "friend" states that she downed about a six pack of beer and smoked some pot. That was the last she saw her friend until the police arrived a few hours later. The patient's name is Mary and she does not respond to her name or to painful stimuli. You notice that she has a raspy cough and there is still some gurgling when she breathes. What should you do?

3. Would an ALS unit be helpful for Mary?

Your partner gets a fast and faint radial pulse and very shallow respirations at about 8 to 10 per minute. You decide to begin ventilations with a BVM attached to high-concentration oxygen. You also decide to get Mary packaged and head for the hospital. You will be trying to meet with the ALS unit on the way to the ED.

4. What is this patient's priority?

5. What is the likely prehospital diagnosis for this patient?

About 5 minutes from the residence, your partner pulls into a gas station where the medic unit is waiting. The medic jumps into your unit along with some of his portable equipment and off you go to the ED.

6. Why is it important not to delay this patient's arrival at the ED?

7. Is this a patient where syrup of ipecac or activated charcoal would be indicated? Why or why not?

EMT SKILLS
PERFORMANCE CHECKLISTS

▶ **MANAGEMENT OF INGESTED POISONS (P. 551)**

❑ Take Standard Precautions.

❑ Conduct a primary assessment.

❑ Maintain an open airway.

❑ Obtain a SAMPLE history, vital signs, and the most appropriate physical exam.

❑ Quickly gather information about the substance.

❑ Call medical direction on the scene or en route.

❑ If directed, administer activated charcoal.

❑ Position patient for vomiting and save all vomitus. Have suction ready.

❑ Provide reassessment.

❑ Transport as soon as possible.

▶ MANAGEMENT OF INHALED POISONS (P. 555)

❑ Size up the situation, and take the necessary precautions to prevent injury to yourself and your crew.*

❑ Take Standard Precautions. Remove patient from the source. Avoid contaminating yourself with poison.

❑ Maintain open airway. Stay alert for vomiting. Properly position the patient and have suction equipment ready.

❑ Conduct a primary assessment.

❑ Administer high-concentration oxygen by nonrebreather mask.

❑ Obtain a SAMPLE history, vital signs, and the most appropriate physical exam.

❑ Remove contaminated clothing and other articles (e.g., shoes, jewelry).

❑ Quickly gather information about the product (containers, bottles, and labels).

❑ Call medical direction on the scene or en route.

❑ Transport as soon as possible.

❑ Provide reassessment en route.

▶ MANAGEMENT OF ABSORBED POISONS (P. 560)

❑ Size up the situation, and take the necessary precautions to prevent injury to yourself and your crew.

❑ Take Standard Precautions.

❑ Remove the patient from the source. Avoid contaminating yourself with the poison.

❑ Conduct a primary assessment.

❑ Maintain an open airway.

❑ Administer high-concentration oxygen.

❑ Obtain a SAMPLE history, vital signs, and the most appropriate physical exam.

❑ Brush powders from the patient. Be careful not to abrade the patient's skin.

❑ Remove contaminated clothing and other articles such as shoes and jewelry.

❑ Quickly gather information about the product.

❑ If appropriate, irrigate with a large amount of clear water for at least 20 minutes. Call medical direction.

❑ Provide reassessment.

❑ Be alert for shock, and transport as soon as possible.

*Safety Note: In the presence of hazardous fumes or gases, wear protective clothing and self-contained breathing apparatus or wait for those who are properly trained and equipped to enter the scene and bring the patient out to a safe area.

24
Abdominal Emergencies

Standard: Medicine (Toxicology)

Competency: Applies fundamental knowledge to provide basic emergency care and transportation based on assessment findings for an acutely ill patient.

OBJECTIVES

24.1   Define key terms introduced in this chapter.

24.2   Describe the location, structure, and function of the organs in the abdominal cavity.

24.3   Explain the origins and characteristics of visceral and parietal pain.

24.4   Associate areas of referred pain with the likely origins of the pain.

24.5   Explain the significance of pain described as tearing in nature.

24.6   Recognize the common signs and symptoms of abdominal conditions, including appendicitis, peritonitis, cholecystitis, pancreatitis, ulcers, abdominal aortic aneurysm, hernia, and renal colic.

24.7   Given various scenarios, demonstrate appropriate assessment and management of patients complaining of abdominal pain.

24.8   Elicit key information in the history of patients complaining of abdominal pain.

24.9   Incorporate special considerations into the assessment and management of female and geriatric patients, as well as patients of different cultures, who are complaining of abdominal pain.

MATCH TERMINOLOGY/ DEFINITIONS

A. Pain that is felt in a location other than where the pain originates

B. Sharp pain that feels as if body tissues are being torn apart

C. A poorly localized, dull, or diffuse pain that arises from the abdominal viscera

D. A localized, intense pain from the peritoneum, which lines the abdominal cavity

E. The abdominal cavity (parietal) and covering of the organs within it (visceral)

_____ 1. Parietal pain

_____ 2. Peritoneum

_____ 3. Referred pain

_____ 4. Tearing pain

_____ 5. Visceral pain

MULTIPLE-CHOICE REVIEW

_____ 1. The membrane that covers the abdominal organs is called the _____ peritoneum.
   A. pleural
   B. visceral
   C. parietal
   D. serius

_____ 2. The organs outside the peritoneum that are found between the abdomen and the back are in the _____ space.
   A. posterior pelvic
   B. subxiphoid
   C. retroperitoneal
   D. dorsal back

_____ 3. Pain originating from an organ in the abdomen is called:
   A. somatic.
   B. parietal.
   C. referred.
   D. visceral.

_____ 4. Pain from an organ is often described as intermittent and:
   A. dull.
   B. achy.
   C. diffuse.
   D. any of these.

_____ 5. You are assessing a 23-year-old female who has colicky pain, This pain is often _____ pain from a _____ organ in the abdomen.
   A. tearing; hollow
   B. referred; solid
   C. visceral; hollow
   D. parietal; solid

_____ 6. You are treating a patient who states that he is having another gall bladder attack. He says that he should not have eaten that fried food and that he has pain in his right shoulder blade. Why might the pain in his right shoulder blade be a symptom of gall bladder problems?
   A. The gallbladder is located under the right shoulder blade in most adult patients.
   B. Nerve pathways from the gallbladder return to the spinal cord by way of shared pathways with the shoulder.
   C. The muscle that holds the gallbladder in position is attached to the right scapula.
   D. It is not common for this to happen at all.

_____ 7. Why would last oral intake be an important part of your SAMPLE history to ask the patient if he has a chief complaint of abdominal discomfort?
   A. The food may have been spoiled.
   B. Food can lead to altered mental state in many instances.
   C. Visceral pain is more severe on an empty stomach.
   D. Referred pain is more severe on a full stomach.

_____ 8. You are treating a 22-year-old female with a chief complaint of abdominal discomfort. Why would it be appropriate to ask her where she is in her menstrual cycle?
   A. To file a complete PCR
   B. To begin to focus on the possibility of an ectopic pregnancy
   C. To definitively rule out an ectopic pregnancy
   D. To rule out the possibility that the patient could be pregnant

_____ 9. You are assessing a 25-year-old male who has abdominal pain. When you palpate his abdomen, be sure to palpate the area with the pain:
   A. last.
   B. first.
   C. second.
   D. third.

_____ 10. You are treating a male patient in his forties who has a chief complaint of abdominal discomfort. He denies any difficulty breathing yet has vital signs consistent with a patient in shock or hypoperfusion. You should:
   A. transport him in the semi-Fowler position.
   B. administer 10–15 lpm oxygen by nonrebreather mask.
   C. apply a cervical collar and long spine board.
   D. contact medical direction for permission to assist the patient with a nitro.

_____ 11. When a 61-year-old male patient tells you that he has a tearing sensation in the back and denies any recent injury, the EMT should suspect:
   A. an acute appendicitis.
   B. kidney stones.
   C. abdominal aortic aneurysm.
   D. a flare-up of pancreatitis.

_____ 12. Your 35-year-old female patient is experiencing a severe and sudden epigastric pain that seems to radiate to the shoulder. She says that it gets worse when she eats. Of the choices below, which is the most likely cause?
   A. Ectopic pregnancy
   B. Cholecystitis
   C. A hernia
   D. Renal colic

©2012 Pearson Education, Inc.
Emergency Care, 12th Ed.

_____ **13.** You are assessing a 25-year-old male who has no primary survey problems but is writhing in pain. He just cannot seem to find a comfortable position from his pain in the lower back and flank. What would you suspect is his most likely problem?
   A. Peritonitis
   B. A hernia
   C. AAA
   D. Renal colic

_____ **14.** You have responded to the local high school physical education center where a 17-year-old male is complaining of lower abdominal pain. On palpation, he has a lump he is concerned about. Because this came on suddenly during exercising, what do you suspect it could be?
   A. A tension pneumothorax
   B. A hernia
   C. A spontaneous embolism
   D. An AAA

_____ **15.** Your 55-year-old male patient called the ambulance because he has been feeling weak and dizzy most of the day. He states that he has no chest pain or difficulty breathing, but he is nauseated and has had very dark-colored diarrhea all day. What do you suspect is his most likely problem?
   A. An acute myocardial infarction
   B. An abdominal aneurism
   C. A bleeding ulcer
   D. Food poisoning

COMPLETE THE FOLLOWING

1. List four solid structures (organs) found in the abdomen.

   A. _____

   B. _____

   C. _____

   D. _____

2. List six hollow structures (organs) found in the abdomen.

   A. _____

   B. _____

   C. _____

   D. _____

   E. _____

   F. _____

3. When doing an assessment on a female patient with a chief complaint of abdominal pain, what are five important questions to ask?

A. _____

B. _____

C. _____

D. _____

E. _____

LABEL THE DIAGRAMS

Fill in the name of each structure on the line provided.

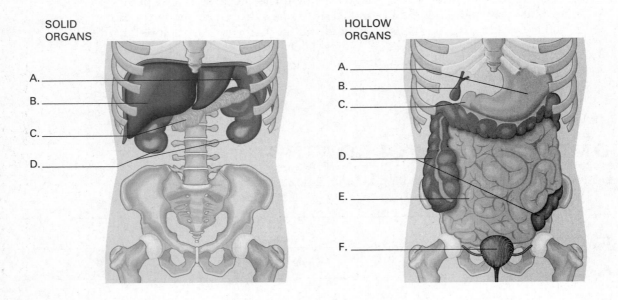

SOLID ORGANS

A. _____

B. _____

C. _____

D. _____

HOLLOW ORGANS

A. _____

B. _____

C. _____

©2012 Pearson Education, Inc.
Emergency Care, 12th Ed.

D. _____

E. _____

F. _____

STREET SCENES DISCUSSION

Review the Street Scene on page 586 of the textbook. Then answer the following questions.

1. Suppose this patient were 25 years old. Would you have more potential causes of her illness to consider and, if so, what would be the most serious ones?

2. When examining her abdomen, you notice that she has a mass that seems to have a pulse, and she has a tearing sensation in her abdomen radiating into her back. What could this be and is it a priority?

3. If the patient suddenly begins to complain of pain in the epigastric area and breaks out in a cold sweat, what should you consider?

25

Behavioral and Psychiatric Emergencies and Suicide

Standard: Medicine (Psychiatric)

Competency: Applies fundamental knowledge to provide basic emergency care and transportation based on assessment findings for an acutely ill patient.

OBJECTIVES

25.1 Define key terms introduced in this chapter.

25.2 Recognize behaviors that are abnormal in a given context.

25.3 Discuss medical and traumatic conditions that can cause unusual behavior.

25.4 Use a process of critical thinking to help differentiate between patients with possible physiological causes of behavioral emergencies and those with psychiatric causes.

25.5 Given a number of scenarios involving situational stressors or unusual patient behavior, demonstrate techniques to calm the patient and gain his cooperation.

25.6 Given a number of scenarios involving psychiatric conditions and behavioral emergencies, demonstrate effective assessment and history taking.

25.7 Prioritize the steps in managing patients presenting with behavioral emergencies.

25.8 Explain the special considerations for EMS provider, patient, and bystander safety on behavioral emergency calls.

25.9 Describe factors often associated with risk of suicide.

25.10 Recognize indications that a patient may become violent.

25.11 Explain considerations in using force and restraint when managing behavioral emergency calls.

25.12 Explain considerations when faced with a behavioral emergency patient who refuses treatment and transport.

MATCH TERMINOLOGY/ DEFINITIONS

A. Bizarre and/or aggressive behavior, shouting, paranoia, panic, violence toward others, insensitivity to pain, unexpected physical strength, and hyperthermia, usually associated with cocaine or amphetamine use

B. The manner in which a person acts

C. Inadequate breathing or respiratory arrest caused by a body position that restricts breathing

D. When a patient's behavior is not typical for the situation; when the patient's behavior is unacceptable or intolerable to the patient, his family, or the community; or when the patient may harm himself or others

B **1.** Behavior

D **2.** Behavioral emergency

A **3.** Excited delirium

C **4.** Positional asphyxia

MULTIPLE-CHOICE REVIEW

D **1.** Physical causes of altered behavior include all of the following *except*:
   A. inadequate blood flow to the brain.
   B. mind-altering substances.
   C. excessive heat or cold.
   D. differing lifestyles.

C **2.** Your 56-year-old male patient is exhibiting altered behavior ranging from irritability to altered mental status. This behavior can be due to any of the following *except*:
   A. lack of oxygen.
   B. head trauma.
   C. hypoactivity.
   D. hypoglycemia.

C **3.** You're assessing a 34-year-old male whom you suspect is experiencing a stress reaction. To calm this patient, you should:
   A. complete your assessment as quickly as possible.
   B. allow the patient to control the situation.
   C. explain things to the patient honestly.
   D. restrain the patient quickly.

B **4.** You are assessing a 25-year-old female whose family members called the ambulance because they felt she was having a behavioral emergency. Which one of the following is *not* usually a common presentation for a patient like this?
   A. Panic or anxiety
   B. Neat appearance
   C. Repetitive motions
   D. Pressured-sounding speech

B **5.** You are called to care for a 22-year-old male patient who has attempted suicide with a handgun or is threatening to attempt suicide. Your first concern should be:
   A. how you will restrain the patient.
   B. your personal safety.
   C. determining the patient's method for suicide.
   D. the patient's and family's safety.

_A_ 6. Of the following age groups, the highest suicide rates occur in the
_____ age group.
  A. 15–25
  B. 25–30
  C. 30–35
  D. 35–40

_C_ 7. As you arrive on the scene. the police officer tells you that the patient has been
exhibiting self-destructive activity. Which one of the following is *not* an
example of this type of activity?
  A. A defined lethal plan of action that has been verbalized
  B. Giving away personal possessions
  C. Denial of suicidal thoughts
  D. Previous suicide threats

_C_ 8. You are assessing a patient who has a long history of depression and suicidal
gestures or attempts. The family member who called the ambulance states that
she has actually been exhibiting a sudden improvement from depression over
the past few days. In this case, you should consider that the patient is:
  A. no longer suicidal.
  B. now ready to accept care.
  C. still at risk for suicide.
  D. none of these.

_D_ 9. When assessing an aggressive patient for a possible threat to you or your crew,
take all of the following actions *except*:
  A. try to determine the patient's history of aggressive behavior.
  B. pay attention to the patient's vocal activity.
  C. note the patient's posturing.
  D. assess the patient in the kitchen.

_A_ 10. If your 35-year-old male patient stands in a corner of the room with his fists
clenched, screaming obscenities, you should:
  A. request police backup and keep the doorway in sight.
  B. raise your voice to a higher level than the patient's.
  C. challenge the patient in an attempt to calm him.
  D. explain that you would respond in the same way.

_B_ 11. Use of reasonable force to restrain a patient should involve an evaluation of all
of the following *except* the:
  A. patient's size and strength.
  B. family's ability to pay for your services.
  C. patient's mental status.
  D. available methods of restraint.

_A_ 12. In some instances, the EMT may have to utilize force. The use of force by an
EMT is allowed:
  A. to defend against an attack by an emotionally disturbed patient.
  B. only when the police are present.
  C. whenever a patient refuses any of your treatments.
  D. whenever you suspect the patient has been drinking.

_A_ 13. Once the decision has been made to restrain your 22-year-old male patient,
which one of the following steps should be avoided?
  A. Use multiple straps to restrain the patient.
  B. Reassure the patient throughout the procedure.
  C. Reassess the patient's distal circulation frequently.
  _ D. Use two rescuers to secure the patient.

©2012 Pearson Education, Inc.
Emergency Care, 12th Ed.

_D_ **14.** Once restrained, the patient from multiple-choice question 13 begins spitting at you and your partner. This behavior can be managed best by:
A. placing the patient in a prone position on the stretcher.
B. wrapping the patient's mouth with roller gauze.
C. placing 3-inch tape across the patient's mouth.
D. placing a surgical mask on the patient's face.

_C_ **15.** You are treating a 28-year-old male patient who you feel is becoming a danger to himself or the others around him and will need to be transported against his will. You should:
A. restrain the patient immediately.
B. transport the patient with the family's assistance.
C. contact the police for assistance.
D. contact the patient's physician.

INSIDE/OUTSIDE: NEUROTRANSMITTERS

1. What is the purpose of a neurotransmitter?

_____

2. Medications such as Prozac®, Paxil®, and Zoloft® are in a class of medications called seratonin selective reuptake inhibitors. What are these medications used for and why?

_____

COMPLETE THE FOLLOWING

1. List nine factors associated with a risk for suicide.

A. _____

B. _____

C. _____

D. _____

E. _____

F. _____

G. _____

H. _____

I. _____

2. When a patient acts as if he may hurt himself or others, your first concern must be your own safety. List three precautions you should take.

A. _____

B. _____

C. _____

3. List behaviors you may expect to see in an aggressive or hostile patient.

A. _____

B. _____

C. _____

D. _____

E. _____

CASE STUDY

▶ TODAY IS NOT THE DAY TO DIE

You respond to a call for a 36-year-old male who is severely bleeding. It is late at night and the call is in a private residence, so the police are also responding. On arrival, a police officer meets your crew at the door and tells you that the patient had a razor and has slashed his wrists numerous times. They talked him into dropping the weapon, but he will need medical care.

As you approach the patient, you introduce yourself and see that there is blood all over the room.

1. Because you can have a conversation with the patient, what are the next steps of the primary assessment?

_____

2. If the patient still has considerable bleeding from his right wrist, what should you do?

_____

3. The bleeding is oozing from some wounds and flowing from others. What types of vessels did the patient likely cut?

_____

After beginning to control the bleeding wounds, you are able to get the patient to start talking. It seems he is very upset because his wife left him after months of being unemployed. He has no money and way too many bills, which has caused them to be near bankruptcy.

4. Would it be appropriate to ask the patient if he was trying to take his own life?

_____

5. The patient says that he does not want to go to the hospital because he does not want his wife to find out what happened here tonight. What should you do?

_____

After further questioning the patient starts to get very agitated and insists that he will not be going to the hospital. You feel strongly that he needs to go for wound care, stitches, and a mental health follow-up. The police officer calls you aside and states that he and his fellow officers will help you restrain the patient if you feel that he needs to go.

6. If it comes to having to restrain the patient, how should restraint be done?

_____

STREET SCENES DISCUSSION

Review the Street Scene on page 600 of the textbook. Then answer the following questions.

1. Suppose that the patient had suddenly become violent, flailing his arms and screaming obscenities. Should you help the police hold him down?

2. Once the patient is down, how should he be restrained?

3. Because the patient is having a behavioral emergency, is it acceptable to skip taking vital signs?

EMT SKILLS PERFORMANCE CHECKLIST

▶ **RESTRAINING A PATIENT* (P. 596)**

❑ Plan your approach to the patient in advance and remain outside the reach of arms and legs until you are ready to act.

❑ Assign one EMT to each limb and approach the patient at the same time.

❑ Place the patient on the stretcher, as his condition and local protocols indicate. Do not let go until he is properly secured.

❑ Use multiple straps or other soft restraints to secure the patient to the stretcher.

❑ When the patient is secure, assess his distal circulation and monitor his airway and breathing continually.

*Never perform this skill when the patient is prone.

26
Hematologic and Renal Emergencies

Standard: Medicine (Hematology; Abdominal and Gastrointestinal Disorders)

Competency: Applies fundamental knowledge to provide basic emergency care and transportation based on assessment findings for an acutely ill patient.

OBJECTIVES

After reading this chapter you should be able to:

26.1 Define key terms introduced in this chapter.

26.2 Describe the structure and function of the renal and hematologic systems.

26.3 Identify medications that can interfere with blood clotting.

26.4 Explain the pathophysiology and complications of sickle cell anemia.

26.5 Provide assessment and management for patients with emergencies related to sickle cell anemia.

26.6 Describe the causes and consequences of acute and chronic renal failure.

26.7 Explain the purpose of hemodialysis and peritoneal dialysis.

26.8 Recognize patients with complications of end-stage renal disease, dialysis, and missed dialysis.

26.9 Provide treatment for patients with complications of end-stage renal disease, dialysis, and missed dialysis.

26.10 Describe special considerations for patients who have received a kidney transplant.

MATCH TERMINOLOGY/DEFINITIONS

A. Irreversible renal failure to the extent that the kidneys can no longer provide adequate filtration and fluid balance to sustain life; survival usually requires dialysis

B. A mechanical process for peritoneal dialysis in which a machine fills and empties the abdominal cavity of dialysis solution

C. A gravity exchange process for peritoneal dialysis in which a bag of dialysis fluid is raised above the level of an abdominal catheter to fill the abdominal cavity and lowered below the level of the abdominal catheter to drain the fluid out

D. Lack of a normal number of red blood cells in the circulation

E. The process by which toxins and excess fluid are removed from the body by a medical system independent of the kidneys

F. An inherited disease in which a genetic defect in the hemoglobin results in abnormal structure of the red blood cells

G. Loss of the kidneys' ability to filter the blood and remove toxins and excess fluid from the body

H. A vibration felt on gentle palpation, such as that which typically occurs within an arterial-venous fistula

I. Bacterial infection within the peritoneal cavity

J. One cycle of filling and draining the peritoneal cavity in peritoneal dialysis

_____ **1.** Anemia

_____ **2.** Continuous ambulatory peritoneal dialysis (CAPD)

_____ **3.** Continuous cycle–assisted peritoneal dialysis (CCPD)

_____ **4.** Dialysis

_____ **5.** End-stage renal disease (ESRD)

_____ **6.** Exchange

_____ **7.** Peritonitis

_____ **8.** Renal failure

_____ **9.** Sickle cell anemia (SCA)

_____ **10.** Thrill

MULTIPLE-CHOICE REVIEW

_____ **1.** The medical specialty concerned with renal/kidney diseases is called:
   A. neurology.
   B. nephrology.
   C. histology.
   D. hematology.

_____ **2.** The functions of our blood include all of the following *except*:
   A. removal of oxygen from the cells.
   B. control of bleeding by clotting.
   C. delivery of waste products to the kidneys and the liver.
   D. removal of carbon dioxide from the cells.

_____ **3.** The medical specialty concerned with the blood disorders is called:
   A. nephrology.
   B. neurology.
   C. hematology.
   D. histology.

_____ **4.** A component of the blood that is critical to the body's response to infection is called:
   A. red blood cells.
   B. platelets.
   C. white blood cells.
   D. hemoglobin.

_____ **5.** A component of the blood that is designed to aggregate as a response to a bleeding injury is called the:
   A. red blood cells.
   B. platelets.
   C. white blood cells.
   D. hemoglobin.

_____ 6. The liquid in which the blood cells and platelets are suspended is called:
   A. interstitial fluid.   **C.** lymph.
   B. plasma.   **D.** coumadin.

_____ 7. The 45-year-old male patient you are assessing tells you that he has a history of chronic anemia. He is pale and complains of fatigue. This condition could be due to:
   A. recurrent heavy menstrual periods.
   B. a slow GI bleed.
   C. a disease that affects the white blood cells.
   D. all of these.

_____ 8. Your patient tells you he has a genetic disease but was not specific. He goes on to say that he had to have his spleen removed a few years ago. He called the ambulance today because he has severe pain in his arms, legs, and abdomen. What is a likely cause of this condition?
   A. A stroke   **C.** A sickle cell crisis
   B. A pulmonary embolism   **D.** A blood clot in the aorta

_____ 9. A complication that may be found in a 35-year-old male who has sickle cell anemia is:
   A. destruction of the spleen.   **C.** priapism.
   B. acute chest syndrome.   **D.** all of these.

_____ 10. If the patient in multiple-choice question 9 needs emergency treatment, the EMT should provide:
   A. high-flow supplemental oxygen.
   B. monitoring for a high fever.
   C. treatment for shock.
   D. all of these would be appropriate.

_____ 11. The patient has a long history of poorly controlled diabetes and hypertension. What life-ending disease is highly likely to occur in this patient?
   A. GI bleeding   **C.** Brain hemorrhage
   B. Renal failure   **D.** COPD

_____ 12. When a patient has been trapped in a building for several days, all of the following, including dehydration, are concerns of the EMT _except_:
   A. chronic renal failure.   **C.** acute renal failure.
   B. shock.   **D.** stroke.

_____ 13. The process by which an external medical system independent of the kidneys is used to remove toxins and excess fluid from the body is called:
   A. excretion.   **C.** dialysis.
   B. dehydration.   **D.** all of these.

_____ 14. Your 56-year-old male patient tells you that he has kidney problems and must go to the clinic three times a week. The reason he goes there is probably to:
   A. do blood tests.   **C.** receive hemodialysis.
   B. take blood transfusions.   **D.** undergo peritoneal dialysis.

_____ 15. A "vibration" that can be palpated at the fistula in the arm of the dialysis patient is called a(n):
   A. thrill.   **C.** hematoma.
   B. aneurism.   **D.** embolism.

_____ 16. A winter storm over the last few days has closed the schools and affected travel on the roads. You are called to the home of a 62-year-old male patient who states that he missed his dialysis twice this week because of the storm. What are the symptoms that he may exhibit?
   A. Shortness of breath   **C.** Swollen ankles, hands, and face
   B. Fluid in the lungs   **D.** All of these

©2012 Pearson Education, Inc.
Emergency Care, 12th Ed.

_____ **17.** The most commonly transported organ(s) is (are) the:
  A. kidneys.   **C.** heart.
  B. liver.   **D.** spleen.

_____ **18.** You are treating a 58-year-old female who states that she is not feeling well after returning home from her dialysis treatment. Each of the following is a complication of dialysis *except*:
  A. development of an aortic aneurism.
  B. bleeding from the site of the A-V fistula.
  C. clotting and loss of function of the A-V fistula.
  D. a bacterial infection of the blood.

COMPLETE THE FOLLOWING

1. List the two types of peritoneal dialysis.

  A. _____

  B. _____

2. What is the difference between the two types of peritoneal dialysis?

  A. _____

  B. _____

STREET SCENES DISCUSSION

Review the Street Scene on page 613 of the textbook. Then answer the following questions.

1. How would you handle the patient if the blood glucose was 68 mg/dl during your assessment?

2. Suppose the patient had a facial droop and weakness on the right side of the body. Would these symptoms change your destination? Why?

3. If the patient had obvious pulmonary edema and red frothy sputum, would these symptoms change the priority?

Interim Exam 2

Use the answer sheet on pages 254–256 to complete this exam. It is perforated, so it can be removed easily from this workbook.

1. During the primary assessment, all of the following are assessed *except*:
   A. airway.
   B. mental status.
   C. circulation.
   D. blood pressure.

2. Which is *not* a component of the primary assessment?
   A. Determining patient priority
   B. Evaluating extremity mobility
   C. Forming a general impression
   D. Assessing breathing

3. When forming your general impression of a child's condition, the environment can provide clues. An example would be a child:
   A. complaining of nausea or vomiting.
   B. holding pieces of a toy in his or her hand.
   C. with a blood pressure of 120/80.
   D. with a rapid heartbeat.

4. When forming a general impression, the EMT takes into consideration all of the following *except* the patient's:
   A. position.
   B. age and sex.
   C. blood pressure.
   D. sounds.

5. After forming a general impression, the next step of the primary assessment is:
   A. assessing breathing.
   B. assessing mental status.
   C. determining the priority of the patient.
   D. assessing the airway.

6. The "V" in AVPU stands for:
   A. virtual.
   B. visible.
   C. verbal.
   D. vertex.

7. The "P" in AVPU stands for:
   A. pulse.
   B. painful.
   C. paralysis.
   D. paresthesia.

8. The lowest and the most serious mental status is:
   A. A.
   B. V.
   C. P.
   D. U.

9. If a patient's level of responsiveness is lower than "Alert," you should:
   A. apply a cervical collar.
   B. administer high-concentration oxygen.
   C. place him or her in a recovery position.
   D. bandage all bleeding wounds.

10. If a patient is talking or crying, assume that the patient:
    A. is in little pain.
    B. has no life-threatening bleeding.
    C. has an open airway.
    D. has an "A" mental status.

11. If the patient is not alert and her breathing rate is slower than 8 breaths per minute, the EMT should:
    A. insert an oral airway.
    B. place the patient in a prone position.
    C. assist ventilations with a bag-valve mask.
    D. apply the PASG.

12. Pale and clammy skin indicates:
    A. nervous system damage.
    B. poor circulation.
    C. extremely high temperature.
    D. an airway problem.

13. A patient who gives a poor general impression should be considered a _____ priority.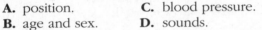
    A. high
    B. low
    C. delayed
    D. stable

14. Which one of the following is *not* an example of a high-priority condition?
    A. Difficulty breathing
    B. Nausea and vomiting
    C. A severed artery
    D. A mental status of "U"

15. The primary assessment takes different forms, which depend on the age of the patient and whether he or she:
    A. has a medical problem or a trauma problem.
    B. is alert or conscious.
    C. has a history of diabetes.
    D. has a history of head injury.

16. When evaluating circulation in infants, the EMT should use the:
    A. femoral pulse.
    B. distal pulse check.
    C. capillary refill test.
    D. radial pulse.

17. The mental status of an unconscious infant is typically checked by:
    A. splashing cold water on him.
    B. shouting and flicking his feet.
    C. performing a pin prick on the feet.
    D. applying a sternal rub.

©2012 Pearson Education, Inc.
Emergency Care, 12th Ed.

18. Which is *not* a high-priority condition?
    A. Shock
    B. A fever with a rash
    C. A complicated childbirth
    D. Severe pain anywhere

19. The difference between the general impression steps for a medical patient and those for a trauma patient is:
    A. manual stabilization of the head for a trauma patient.
    B. no SAMPLE is taken for a trauma patient.
    C. the medical patient is treated faster.
    D. the AVPU is not used for a medical patient.

20. The EMT documents that the chest pain patient denies shortness of breath. This is most appropriately termed:
    A. an informative objective.
    B. advisory information.
    C. a pertinent negative.
    D. run data information.

21. When writing the narrative section of a prehospital care report (PCR), the EMT should do all of the following *except*:
    A. use medical terminology correctly.
    B. avoid nonstandard abbreviations.
    C. write legibly and use correct spelling.
    D. state one's personal opinion of the patient's condition.

22. Which statement best describes an important concept of documentation?
    A. Always fill out a continuation sheet.
    B. If it is not written down, you didn't do it.
    C. It should include plenty of medical terms.
    D. Document everything you see.

23. If the patient does not wish to go to the hospital, the EMT should:
    A. document with a refusal-of-care form.
    B. take the patient to the hospital anyway.
    C. end the assessment immediately.
    D. call for another crew to subdue him.

24. An important part of the assessment or care was not performed. This is called:
    A. submission.   C. inhibition.
    B. omission.   D. commission.

25. An EMT makes up a set of vitals for inclusion on the prehospital care report (PCR). This is called:
    A. assault.
    B. libel.
    C. falsification.
    D. battery.

26. An objective statement is:
    A. one that is made from a particular point of view.
    B. one that is made by the patient or a family member.
    C. one that describes observable or measurable information.
    D. one's own assessment of what is wrong with the patient.

27. The EMT writes "The patient is alert and oriented" on the prehospital care report (PCR) This is an example of:
    A. objective information.
    B. a statement beyond his or her training.
    C. subjective information.
    D. nonfactual information.

28. When you are documenting exactly what a patient told you on the prehospital care report (PCR), you should:
    A. paraphrase for brevity.
    B. summarize the key points.
    C. use medical terminology.
    D. use quotes around the statement.

29. Writing a statement such as "The patient's daughter was rude to us" on a prehospital care report (PCR) is:
    A. not relevant.
    B. objective information.
    C. run data information.
    D. an example of what should be included in quotes.

30. The next step in the primary assessment after establishing unresponsiveness is to:
    A. ensure an open airway.
    B. check for adequate breathing.
    C. check for circulation.
    D. look for profuse bleeding.

31. The term *sixth sense* is used to describe:
    A. an EMT's clinical judgment.
    B. the six steps in a primary assessment.
    C. a patient's sensory functions.
    D. the ability to hear.

32. Which one of the following is a true vital sign?
    A. Nausea
    B. Skin temperature
    C. Level of responsiveness
    D. Age

33. The normal pulse rate for an adult at rest is between _____ beats per minute.
    A. 50 and 70   C. 65 and 95
    B. 60 and 100   D. 80 and 100

©2012 Pearson Education, Inc.
Emergency Care, 12th Ed.

34. During the determination of vital signs, the initial pulse rate for patients 1 year of age and older is normally taken at the _____ pulse.
    A. carotid
    B. femoral
    C. pedal
    D. radial

35. When the force of the pulse is weak and thin, it is described as:
    A. shallow.
    B. full.
    C. partial.
    D. thready.

36. Normal at-rest respiration rates for adults vary from _____ breaths per minute.
    A. 5 to 10
    B. 12 to 20
    C. 15 to 30
    D. 20 to 32

37. A noisy, harsh sound heard during inhalation that indicates a partial airway obstruction is:
    A. gurgling.
    B. snorting.
    C. stertorous respirations.
    D. crowing.

38. Systolic blood pressure indicates the arterial pressure created as the:
    A. artery contracts.
    B. artery relaxes.
    C. heart contracts.
    D. heart relaxes.

39. Diastolic blood pressure indicates the arterial pressure created as the:
    A. heart contracts.
    B. heart refills.
    C. artery contracts.
    D. artery relaxes.

40. The technique of measuring blood pressure with a sphygmomanometer and a stethoscope is called:
    A. palpation.
    B. auscultation.
    C. oscillation.
    D. priapism.

41. Determining blood pressure by palpation is:
    A. not as accurate as the auscultation method.
    B. used when there is no noise around a patient.
    C. documented as the "palp/diastolic."
    D. used whenever the patient is hypertensive.

42. Information that you can see, hear, feel, and smell is called:
    A. signs.
    B. sensations.
    C. symptoms.
    D. assessments.

43. When the EMT asks the patient "Have you recently had any surgery or injuries?" he is inquiring about the:
    A. patient's medications.
    B. patient's pertinent past history.
    C. events leading up to the illness.
    D. allergies that the patient may have.

44. When the EMT asks the patient "Are you on birth control pills?" she is inquiring about the:
    A. patient's medications.
    B. patient's pertinent past history.
    C. events leading up to the illness.
    D. allergies that the patient may have.

45. An acronym used to remember what questions to ask about the patient's present problem and past history is:
    A. AVPU.
    B. DCAP-BTLS.
    C. SAMPLE.
    D. PEARL.

46. When conducting a patient interview on an adult patient, the EMT should do all of the following *except*:
    A. position oneself close to the patient.
    B. identify oneself and reassure the patient.
    C. gently touch the patient's shoulder or rest a hand over the patient's hand.
    D. avoid asking the patient's age.

47. Normal diastolic pressures range from _____ mmHg.
    A. 50 to 80
    B. 50 to 90
    C. 60 to 80
    D. 60 to 90

48. Using the formula presented in the text, a 36-year-old man would have an estimated systolic blood pressure of _____ mmHg.
    A. 116
    B. 126
    C. 136
    D. 146

49. Using the formula presented in the text, a 26-year-old woman would have an estimated systolic blood pressure of _____ mmHg.
    A. 106
    B. 116
    C. 126
    D. 136

50. Why should the stethoscope *not* be placed under the cuff and then inflated when evaluating the blood pressure?
    A. It may give a false reading.
    B. It can dent the stethoscope.
    C. The patient will not like the feeling.
    D. It will prevent pumping the cuff to the proper pressure.

©2012 Pearson Education, Inc.
Emergency Care, 12th Ed.

51. When taking a patient's blood pressure, the stethoscope is placed over the _____ artery.
   A. carotid
   B. radial
   C. brachial
   D. femoral

52. The best indication of potential injury is the:
   A. type of accident.
   B. type of injury.
   C. mechanism of injury (MOI).
   D. position of the patient.

53. When there are no apparent hazards at the scene of a collision, the danger zone should extend _____ feet in all directions from the wreckage.
   A. 25
   B. 50
   C. 75
   D. 100

54. In the up-and-over injury pattern, the patient is most likely to sustain _____ injuries.
   A. knee
   B. hip
   C. head
   D. leg

55. A keen awareness that there may be injuries based on the mechanism of injury (MOI) is called a(n):
   A. sixth sense.
   B. general impression.
   C. index of suspicion.
   D. kinesthetic sense.

56. The purpose of the primary assessment is to:
   A. take the patient's vital signs.
   B. gather information about the collision.
   C. discover and treat life-threatening conditions.
   D. obtain the patient's history.

57. The first step in the focused history and physical exam for *any* trauma patient is to:
   A. make a status decision.
   B. check for an open airway.
   C. reconsider the mechanism of injury (MOI).
   D. treat life-threatening conditions.

58. The "A" in DCAP-BTLS stands for:
   A. allergies.
   B. alert.
   C. abrasions.
   D. arrhythmia.

59. All of the following are clues that help an EMT determine the need for cervical immobilization *except*:
   A. mechanism of injury (MOI).
   B. level of responsiveness.
   C. location of injuries.
   D. breathing rate.

60. Which of the following is *true* of the rapid trauma assessment?
   A. It begins with examination of the posterior body and ends with examination of the head.
   B. It evaluates areas of the body where the greatest threats to the patient may be.
   C. It is performed on a trauma patient who has no significant mechanism of injury.
   D. It includes careful examination of the face, eyes, ears, nose, and mouth.

61. On which type of patient is the secondary assessment most often performed?
   A. A trauma patient with a significant mechanism of injury
   B. A trauma patient with no significant mechanism of injury
   C. A responsive medical patient
   D. An unresponsive medical patient

62. To obtain a history of a patient's present illness:
   A. ask the OPQRST questions.
   B. conduct the subjective interview.
   C. ask the SAMPLE questions.
   D. use the look, listen, feel, and smell method.

63. The "P" in OPQRST stands for:
   A. punctures.
   B. penetrations.
   C. provokes.
   D. pulses.

64. The steps in the focused history and physical exam of the unresponsive medical patient include the following:
   1. Obtain baseline vital signs.
   2. Gather the history of the present illness from bystanders and family.
   3. Conduct a rapid physical exam.
   4. Gather a SAMPLE history from bystanders and family.

   Which is the correct order in which these steps should be performed?
   A. 3, 1, 2, 4
   B. 2, 3, 4, 1
   C. 3, 2, 4, 1
   D. 1, 2, 3, 4

65. For a stable patient, the EMT should perform the reassessment every _____ minutes.
   A. 5
   B. 10
   C. 15
   D. 20

66. During the reassessment, whenever you believe there may have been a change in the patient's condition, you should immediately:
   A. repeat the primary assessment.
   B. transport the patient immediately.
   C. document trends in vital signs.
   D. repeat the rapid trauma assessment.

67. Cool, clammy skin in a middle-aged male most likely indicates:
A. high fever.   C. mild fever.
B. exposure to cold.   D. shock.

68. As an EMT, your overriding concern at all times is:
A. the patient's safety.
B. the safety of patients and bystanders.
C. the patient's life.
D. your own safety.

69. During the secondary assessment of the head of a trauma patient, inspect the:
A. ears and nose for blood or clear fluids.
B. inner surface of the eyelids.
C. skin color of the cheeks.
D. mouth for blood and clear fluids.

70. Infants and young children under the age of _____ are abdominal breathers.
A. 2   C. 8
B. 4   D. 12

71. Repeaters are:
A. phones that transmit radio signals over airwaves instead of wires.
B. devices used to transmit radio signals over long distances.
C. patients who consistently call 911.
D. a type of cellular phone used in EMS.

72. Which of the following is an appropriate interpersonal communication technique?
A. Standing above a patient
B. Avoiding eye contact
C. Directly facing a patient
D. Standing with arms crossed

73. What is the *first* item given to the hospital in your medical radio report to the receiving facility?
A. The patient's age and sex
B. Unit identification and level of provider
C. Estimated time of arrival
D. Emergency medical care given

74. Which of the following is *not* considered an essential component of the verbal report to the receiving facility?
A. Patient's chief complaint
B. Additional treatment given en route
C. Additional vital signs taken en route
D. Patient's attitude

75. Which of the following is *true* of the medical radio report?
A. The EMT uses codes to communicate patient information.
B. The EMT makes sure to give his or her patient diagnosis.

C. The EMT paints a picture of the patient's problem in words.
D. The EMT speaks rapidly to limit transmission time.

76. To avoid misunderstanding and miscommunication when speaking with medical direction, you should do all of the following *except*:
A. give information clearly and accurately.
B. repeat back the order you are given word for word.
C. ask the physician to repeat the order if it is unclear.
D. avoid questioning the physician about the order.

77. Medications that are carried on the ambulance and that EMTs can administer include activated charcoal, oxygen, and:
A. oral glucose.   C. epinephrine.
B. nitroglycerin.   D. all of these.

78. Any action of a drug other than the desired action is called a(n):
A. contraindication. C. reflex.
B. indication.   D. side effect.

79. When a drug is administered subcutaneously, the drug is:
A. dissolved under the tongue.
B. injected into a vein.
C. rubbed into a muscle.
D. injected under the skin.

80. Which of the following is *true* of the structure of infants' and children's airways?
A. The trachea is more rigid and less flexible than an adult's.
B. The tongue is proportionately smaller than an adult's.
C. The cricoid cartilage is more rigid than an adult's.
D. They depend more on the diaphragm for respiration than adults do.

81. The means of providing artificial ventilation are:
1. Pocket face mask with supplemental oxygen
2. Two-person bag-valve mask with supplemental oxygen
3. Flow-restricted, oxygen-powered ventilator
4. One-person bag-valve mask with supplemental oxygen
Which of these is the best method to use?
A. 1   C. 3
B. 2   D. 4

©2012 Pearson Education, Inc.
Emergency Care, 12th Ed.

82. The adequate rate of artificial ventilations for a nonbreathing adult patient is _____ breaths per minute.
   A. 6–8
   B. 10–12
   C. 14–16
   D. 18–20

83. The adequate rate of artificial ventilations for a nonbreathing infant or child patient is _____ breaths per minute.
   A. 8–10
   B. 6–8
   C. 12–20
   D. 22–25

84. Which of the following respiratory sounds made by an unresponsive adult most likely indicates a serious airway problem requiring immediate intervention?
   A. Snoring or gurgling
   B. Slight wheezing
   C. Sniffling
   D. Whistling or grunting

85. The skin of a patient with inadequate breathing will most likely be:
   A. pale, cool, and dry.
   B. red, hot, and clammy.
   C. yellow, warm, and dry.
   D. blue, cool, and clammy.

86. If a patient is experiencing breathing difficulty but is breathing adequately, it is usually best to place him in the _____ position.
   A. tripod
   B. supine
   C. sitting-up
   D. recovery

87. Which one of the following is a name for adult chest pain due to a decreased blood supply to the heart muscle?
   A. Stroke
   B. Arrhythmia
   C. Congestive heart failure
   D. Angina pectoris

88. Most heart attacks are caused by the narrowing or occlusion of a _____ artery.
   A. cephalic
   B. brachial
   C. coronary
   D. carotid

89. Which of the following is the condition in which a portion of the myocardium dies because of oxygen starvation?
   A. Angina pectoris
   B. Mechanical pump failure
   C. Cardiogenic shock
   D. Acute myocardial infarction

90. An irregular heart rhythm is called:
   A. mechanical pump failure.
   B. arrhythmia.
   C. cardiogenic shock.
   D. congestive heart failure.

91. Which term applies to a pulse slower than 60 beats per minute?
   A. Bradycardia
   B. Ventricular fibrillation
   C. Tachycardia
   D. Atrial fibrillation

92. An at-rest heart beating faster than 100 beats per minute is referred to as:
   A. bradycardia.
   B. ventricular fibrillation.
   C. tachycardia.
   D. atrial fibrillation.

93. Which of the following is the name for a condition caused by excessive fluid build-up in the lungs because of the inadequate pumping of the heart?
   A. Congestive heart failure
   B. Acute heart failure
   C. Acute myocardial infarction
   D. Chronic myocardial infarction

94. The 52-year-old male conscious patient with a possible heart attack is best transported in the:
   A. recovery position.
   B. medical coma position.
   C. traumatic coma position.
   D. position of comfort.

95. A diabetic found with a weak, rapid pulse and cold, clammy skin who complains of hunger pangs suffers from:
   A. hypoglycemia.
   B. cardiogenic shock.
   C. hyperglycemia.
   D. ulcers.

96. Which of the following conditions frequently results in an acetone smell on the patient's breath?
   A. Stroke
   B. Hyperglycemia
   C. Ulcers
   D. Hypoglycemia

97. A conscious hypoglycemic patient who is able to swallow is frequently administered:
   A. oral glucose.
   B. insulin.
   C. nitroglycerin.
   D. epinephrine.

98. You are treating a 25-year-old female diabetic patient. If you cannot administer glucose gel because she is not alert enough to swallow, you should:
   A. wait until her mental status improves.
   B. contact medical direction immediately.
   C. treat her like any other patient with altered mental status.
   D. place her in a position of comfort.

99. The first time a person is exposed to an allergen, the immune system:
   A. reacts violently.
   B. shuts down.
   C. forms antibodies.
   D. ignores the allergen.

100. To be considered a severe allergic reaction, a patient must have signs and symptoms of shock and/or:
   A. a history of allergies.
   B. massive swelling.
   C. respiratory distress.
   D. increased blood pressure.

101. A 21-year-old male patient has no history of allergies and is having his first allergic reaction. What action should you take?
   A. Consult with medical direction.
   B. Treat for shock and transport immediately.
   C. Administer epinephrine via auto-injector.
   D. Attempt to determine the cause immediately.

102. Carbon monoxide, chlorine, and ammonia are examples of _____ poisons.
   A. ingested
   B. injected
   C. inhaled
   D. absorbed

103. It is important for the EMT to determine when the ingestion of a poison occurred because:
   A. different poisons act on the body at different rates.
   B. those who ingest poison in the evening tend to vomit frequently.
   C. dilution of the poison is never effective after 10 minutes.
   D. the antidote is more effective once the poison reaches the stomach.

104. The principal prehospital treatment of a patient who has inhaled poisonous gas is:
   A. administering activated charcoal.
   B. administering high-concentration oxygen.
   C. rapidly administering an antidote.
   D. irrigating the respiratory tract with water.

105. Drinking alcohol along with taking other drugs frequently results in:
   A. uncontrolled shivering.
   B. depressed vital signs.
   C. extreme agitation.
   D. all of these.

106. Activated charcoal is contraindicated for patients who have ingested:
   A. alkalis.
   B. gasoline.
   C. acids.
   D. all of these.

107. Most cases of poisoning:
   A. are intentional in nature.
   B. involve elderly patients.
   C. involve young children.
   D. lead to disability or death.

108. Poisons that are swallowed are _____ poisons.
   A. absorbed
   B. inhaled
   C. ingested
   D. injected

109. What is the name for a gravity exchange process for peritoneal dialysis in which a bag of dialysis fluid is raised above the level of an abdominal catheter to fill the abdominal cavity and lowered below the level of the abdominal catheter to drain the fluid out?
   A. Continuous cycler–assisted peritoneal dialysis
   B. Continuous ambulatory peritoneal dialysis
   C. Abdominal dialysis
   D. Primary fluid exchange process

110. You are called to the home of a dialysis patient who has extreme abdominal pain and a fever. She said that she spent the whole day at the clinic and was not feeling well since she got home. What could be her most likely problem today?
   A. Diabetes
   B. An ulcer
   C. Peritonitis
   D. Appendicitis

111. Your patient in multiple-choice question 110 tells you that she was told she has a thrill in the arm used for the dialysis. What does that mean?
   A. There is a hairline fracture in the bone in that extremity.
   B. She is missing a number of vessels in the extremity.
   C. It is a very tight bandage applied after the procedure to minimize blood clots.
   D. It is a vibration felt on palpation, which typically occurs within an arterial-venous fistula.

112. Common presentations of patients experiencing psychiatric emergencies include each of the following except:
   A. panic or anxiety.
   B. severe pain after falling and striking the head.
   C. suicidal or self-destructive behavior.
   D. unusual speech patterns (i.e., too rapid or pressured-sounding speech).

113. Emergency care of a patient having a behavioral or psychiatric emergency includes each of the following *except*:
    A. plenty of physical contact.
    B. encouraging the patient to discuss what is troubling him.
    C. not lying to the patient.
    D. being prepared to spend time talking to the patient.

114. In a limited number of situations, you may have to utilize force. The use of force by an EMT is allowed:
    A. to defend against an attack by an emotionally disturbed patient.
    B. whenever the patient refuses to be transported.
    C. if the patient refuses to follow your care plan.
    D. if the patient has taken any drugs.

115. The organs found outside the peritoneum and between the abdomen and the back are in the:
    A. posterior pelvic compartment.
    B. retroperitoneal space.
    C. periumbilical region.
    D. posterior buttocks.

116. The spleen is located in the _____ quadrant.
    A. upper right
    B. lower right
    C. upper left
    D. lower left

117. Your 60-year-old male patient tells you that he has a tearing sensation going into the middle of his back. He states that he has no back problems and has a history of hypertension. What is possibly wrong with him?
    A. A kidney stone
    B. Acute pulmonary edema
    C. Acute appendicitis
    D. An abdominal aortic aneurysm

118. Your patient has a history of alcoholism and is complaining of stomach pains and feeling weak and dizzy. He states that he vomited twice and has had very dark, foul-smelling diarrhea all day. What is the likely cause of today's problem?
    A. He also has diabetes and needs insulin.
    B. He has a bleeding ulcer.
    C. He is having a stroke.
    D. His spleen is malfunctioning.

119. Your first step when called to care for any attempted suicide victim is to:
    A. gain access to the patient.
    B. wait for police assistance.
    C. survey for behavioral changes.
    D. ensure your own safety.

120. You are on the scene of a patient whom the police have been talking with for quite some time. They were originally called to the private residence because a neighbor thought she had heard shots fired. Apparently no one was injured, but there are weapons in the home. You are unable to perform normal assessment and care procedures because the patient is aggressive and hostile. What action should you take?
    A. Restrain the patient immediately.
    B. Ask a family member to assist you.
    C. Seek advice from medical direction.
    D. Call the patient's physician.

121. When is the EMT allowed to use reasonable force?
    A. Only when the police are on the scene
    B. To defend against attack by an emotionally disturbed patient
    C. Whenever a patient refuses treatment
    D. Whenever alcohol abuse is suspected

122. The limited number of interventions an EMT can provide include all of the following *except*:
    A. administration of intravenous fluids.
    B. application of an AED.
    C. application of oxygen.
    D. insertion of oral or nasal airways.

123. When a 42-year-old patient presents with more than one condition or with a familiar condition but under unusual circumstances, the EMT should:
    A. call medical direction right away.
    B. call for an ALS unit right away.
    C. assess the patient as usual.
    D. assign a higher priority to the patient.

124. When a 45-year-old male patient tells you that he has a disease with which you are not familiar, it is best to respond by saying:
    A. "I'm not familiar with that disease. Could you tell me about it?"
    B. "That doesn't concern me. My job is to treat emergencies."
    C. "Interesting disease. I studied it during EMS training."
    D. "I'm not a physician. Just tell me what's wrong today."

125. When a patient has two or more medical conditions that are presenting symptoms at the same time, it is good to:
    A. treat them all at once.
    B. treat them one at a time.
    C. consult with medical direction for advice.
    D. just manage the ABCs and forget the rest.

126. The 59-year-old female patient with slurred speech may have had:
   A. a stroke.
   B. an overdose.
   C. a seizure.
   D. any combination of these.

127. The 46-year-old male with chest pain may have any of the following conditions, *except:*
   A. angina.
   B. acute myocardial infarction.
   C. seizure.
   D. rib fracture.

128. A 45-year-old female patient who is vomiting coffee-ground-like material and complaining of abdominal pain probably has:
   A. internal bleeding.
   B. a seizure history.
   C. gallbladder problems.
   D. ingested a strong acid.

129. A wheeze is a common breathing sound found in a patient having:
   A. an asthma attack.
   B. an allergic reaction.
   C. bronchospasm.
   D. any one of these.

130. There is no specific EMT intervention for the patient with:
   A. chest pain.
   B. abdominal pain.
   C. a fractured leg.
   D. a serious laceration.

131. Each one of the following is an example of patient problems that have no specific EMT intervention *except*:
   A. headache.
   B. sickle-cell crisis.
   C. hyperthermia.
   D. post-surgical complications.

132. The term used to describe the conclusion that an EMT makes about a patient's condition, after assessing that patient, is called the:
   A. presumptive diagnosis.
   B. EMT diagnosis.
   C. EMS diagnosis.
   D. all of these are correct.

133. The analytical process that assists the EMT in reaching a field diagnosis is referred to as:
   A. active assessment.
   B. passive assessment.
   C. critical thinking.
   D. detailed assessment.

134. The basic approach that clinicians use to arrive at a diagnosis includes each of the following *except*:
   A. gather information.
   B. administer many lab tests.
   C. consider the possibilities.
   D. reach a conclusion.

135. You are on the scene of a 60-year-old female complaining of difficulty breathing and a fever. You draw up a list of conditions that may be the cause of her problems today. This is referred to as the:
   A. admission diagnosis.
   B. presenting problem.
   C. differential diagnosis.
   D. assessment finding.

136. The signs or symptoms that suggest the possibility of a particular problem that is very serious are referred to as a(n):
   A. red flag.   C. unstable situation.
   B. black triage tag. D. none of these.

137. When a highly experienced physician comes to a diagnosis, he or she most likely used:
   A. heuristics.
   B. pattern recognition.
   C. shortcuts.
   D. all of these.

138. The traditional approach to diagnosis involves:
   A. narrowing down a long list.
   B. jumping to conclusions.
   C. taking lots of shortcuts.
   D. eliminating similar conditions.

139. Each of the following are considered common heuristics or biases *except*:
   A. illusory correlation.
   B. availability.
   C. respresentativeness.
   D. underconfidence.

140. When an EMT is specifically looking for evidence that supports the diagnosis he or she already has in mind, he or she is committing a(n) _____ bias.
   A. anchoring   C. satisfying
   B. confirmation   D. illusionary

141. When a patient does not fit the "classic pattern," such as a cardiac patient without crushing substernal chest pain radiating down the left arm, you have to be careful not to make a(n) _____ error or bias.
   A. confirmation   C. overconfidence
   B. representativeness   D. availability

©2012 Pearson Education, Inc.
Emergency Care, 12th Ed.

142. You once treated a 50-year-old female with heat stroke. The next time you have a female patient and you are in a warm environment, you may be more likely to think of this as the diagnosis as opposed to more common problems, such as dehydration. This bias is referred to as:

A. overconfidence.   **C.** confirmation.
B. illusory correlation. **D.** availability.

143. You should be skeptical about one condition being the actual cause of another condition that a patient presents with. Drawing conclusions about the cause of a diagnosis can lead to a(n):

A. anchoring adjustment.
B. illusory correlation.
C. search-satisfying bias.
D. availability bias.

144. You are treating a patient who was found on the floor in the basement of his son's house. It seems evident that he has a fractured hip as he lies on the floor in pain. If you stop the search for a diagnosis as soon as you come up with the cause of today's problem, this can lead to:

A. missing out on the secondary diagnosis.
B. overconfidence and misdiagnosis.
C. overestimating the frequency of the problem.
D. all of these.

145. You are treating a respiratory patient who is conscious, alert, and in severe distress. He took an Albuterol treatment prior to your arrival on the scene. At this point, you have been administering CPAP for about 10 minutes. You notice that his mental status is rapidly diminishing. What should you do next?

A. Administer another bronchodilator treatment per medical control.
B. Remove the CPAP and ventilate the patient with a BVM device.
C. Lower the level of pressure in the CPAP device considerably.
D. Turn up the pressure of the oxygen going into the CPAP device.

146. You receive a high-priority call to meet an incoming airplane on the tarmac at the regional airport. A 60-year-old female patient with a history of deep vein thrombosis and 35 years of smoking a pack a day of cigarettes is acutely short of breath. This shortness of breath began about 20 minutes ago, and the EMTs are administering oxygen by nonrebreather mask at this time. The duration of the flight was approximately 6 hours.

What do you suspect is the patient's prehospital diagnosis?

A. An acute exacerbation of her COPD
B. The development of epiglottitis
C. A pulmonary embolism
D. Acute pulmonary edema

*147. You arrive on the scene of a family who is very anxious because the father, a 45-year-old male, and the 17-year-old daughter were piling wood when they found a beehive. They both have numerous stings, but the daughter is experiencing the signs of an anaphylactic reaction while the father is experiencing a simple allergic reaction. You will most likely find that:

A. the daughter has hypotension.
B. the father has hypertension.
C. the daughter has hives.
D. the father has swelling of the airway structures.

*148. You respond to a call for a woman who was described as sleeping in her car. The police have arrived, and a car window needed to be broken to gain access to the 35-year-old female because the doors were locked and she is unconscious. As you enter the vehicle, there is a strong smell of rotten eggs. What should you suspect happened?

A. The exhaust fumes were not well vented on the vehicle, causing a CO_2 leak.
B. She may have attempted suicide by mixing chemicals to produce hydrogen sulfide.
C. There was a cyanide leak into the vehicle.
D. She may have taken double dose of a strong sleeping pill.

149. Each of the components of the blood has specialized functions. The _____ are the cells that are critical in response to infection and the mediators of the body's immune response.

A. red blood cells
B. white blood cells
C. platelets
D. plasma

150. The complications of sickle cell disease can include each of the following *except*:

A. destruction of the pancreas.
B. acute chest syndrome.
C. priapism.
D. stroke.

Interim Exam 2 Answer Sheet

Fill in the correct answer for each item. When scoring, note that there are 150 questions valued at 0.67 points each.

1. [ ] A	[ ] B	[ ] C	[ ] D
2. [ ] A	[ ] B	[ ] C	[ ] D
3. [ ] A	[ ] B	[ ] C	[ ] D
4. [ ] A	[ ] B	[ ] C	[ ] D
5. [ ] A	[ ] B	[ ] C	[ ] D
6. [ ] A	[ ] B	[ ] C	[ ] D
7. [ ] A	[ ] B	[ ] C	[ ] D
8. [ ] A	[ ] B	[ ] C	[ ] D
9. [ ] A	[ ] B	[ ] C	[ ] D
10. [ ] A	[ ] B	[ ] C	[ ] D
11. [ ] A	[ ] B	[ ] C	[ ] D
12. [ ] A	[ ] B	[ ] C	[ ] D
13. [ ] A	[ ] B	[ ] C	[ ] D
14. [ ] A	[ ] B	[ ] C	[ ] D
15. [ ] A	[ ] B	[ ] C	[ ] D
16. [ ] A	[ ] B	[ ] C	[ ] D
17. [ ] A	[ ] B	[ ] C	[ ] D
18. [ ] A	[ ] B	[ ] C	[ ] D
19. [ ] A	[ ] B	[ ] C	[ ] D
20. [ ] A	[ ] B	[ ] C	[ ] D
21. [ ] A	[ ] B	[ ] C	[ ] D
22. [ ] A	[ ] B	[ ] C	[ ] D
23. [ ] A	[ ] B	[ ] C	[ ] D
24. [ ] A	[ ] B	[ ] C	[ ] D
25. [ ] A	[ ] B	[ ] C	[ ] D
26. [ ] A	[ ] B	[ ] C	[ ] D
27. [ ] A	[ ] B	[ ] C	[ ] D
28. [ ] A	[ ] B	[ ] C	[ ] D
29. [ ] A	[ ] B	[ ] C	[ ] D
30. [ ] A	[ ] B	[ ] C	[ ] D
31. [ ] A	[ ] B	[ ] C	[ ] D
32. [ ] A	[ ] B	[ ] C	[ ] D
33. [ ] A	[ ] B	[ ] C	[ ] D

34. [ ] A	[ ] B	[ ] C	[ ] D
35. [ ] A	[ ] B	[ ] C	[ ] D
36. [ ] A	[ ] B	[ ] C	[ ] D
37. [ ] A	[ ] B	[ ] C	[ ] D
38. [ ] A	[ ] B	[ ] C	[ ] D
39. [ ] A	[ ] B	[ ] C	[ ] D
40. [ ] A	[ ] B	[ ] C	[ ] D
41. [ ] A	[ ] B	[ ] C	[ ] D
42. [ ] A	[ ] B	[ ] C	[ ] D
43. [ ] A	[ ] B	[ ] C	[ ] D
44. [ ] A	[ ] B	[ ] C	[ ] D
45. [ ] A	[ ] B	[ ] C	[ ] D
46. [ ] A	[ ] B	[ ] C	[ ] D
47. [ ] A	[ ] B	[ ] C	[ ] D
48. [ ] A	[ ] B	[ ] C	[ ] D
49. [ ] A	[ ] B	[ ] C	[ ] D
50. [ ] A	[ ] B	[ ] C	[ ] D
51. [ ] A	[ ] B	[ ] C	[ ] D
52. [ ] A	[ ] B	[ ] C	[ ] D
53. [ ] A	[ ] B	[ ] C	[ ] D
54. [ ] A	[ ] B	[ ] C	[ ] D
55. [ ] A	[ ] B	[ ] C	[ ] D
56. [ ] A	[ ] B	[ ] C	[ ] D
57. [ ] A	[ ] B	[ ] C	[ ] D
58. [ ] A	[ ] B	[ ] C	[ ] D
59. [ ] A	[ ] B	[ ] C	[ ] D
60. [ ] A	[ ] B	[ ] C	[ ] D
61. [ ] A	[ ] B	[ ] C	[ ] D
62. [ ] A	[ ] B	[ ] C	[ ] D
63. [ ] A	[ ] B	[ ] C	[ ] D
64. [ ] A	[ ] B	[ ] C	[ ] D
65. [ ] A	[ ] B	[ ] C	[ ] D
66. [ ] A	[ ] B	[ ] C	[ ] D

67.	[ ] A	[ ] B	[ ] C	[ ] D		104.	[ ] A	[ ] B	[ ] C	[ ] D
68.	[ ] A	[ ] B	[ ] C	[ ] D		105.	[ ] A	[ ] B	[ ] C	[ ] D
69.	[ ] A	[ ] B	[ ] C	[ ] D		106.	[ ] A	[ ] B	[ ] C	[ ] D
70.	[ ] A	[ ] B	[ ] C	[ ] D		107.	[ ] A	[ ] B	[ ] C	[ ] D
71.	[ ] A	[ ] B	[ ] C	[ ] D		108.	[ ] A	[ ] B	[ ] C	[ ] D
72.	[ ] A	[ ] B	[ ] C	[ ] D		109.	[ ] A	[ ] B	[ ] C	[ ] D
73.	[ ] A	[ ] B	[ ] C	[ ] D		110.	[ ] A	[ ] B	[ ] C	[ ] D
74.	[ ] A	[ ] B	[ ] C	[ ] D		111.	[ ] A	[ ] B	[ ] C	[ ] D
75.	[ ] A	[ ] B	[ ] C	[ ] D		112.	[ ] A	[ ] B	[ ] C	[ ] D
76.	[ ] A	[ ] B	[ ] C	[ ] D		113.	[ ] A	[ ] B	[ ] C	[ ] D
77.	[ ] A	[ ] B	[ ] C	[ ] D		114.	[ ] A	[ ] B	[ ] C	[ ] D
78.	[ ] A	[ ] B	[ ] C	[ ] D		115.	[ ] A	[ ] B	[ ] C	[ ] D
79.	[ ] A	[ ] B	[ ] C	[ ] D		116.	[ ] A	[ ] B	[ ] C	[ ] D
80.	[ ] A	[ ] B	[ ] C	[ ] D		117.	[ ] A	[ ] B	[ ] C	[ ] D
81.	[ ] A	[ ] B	[ ] C	[ ] D		118.	[ ] A	[ ] B	[ ] C	[ ] D
82.	[ ] A	[ ] B	[ ] C	[ ] D		119.	[ ] A	[ ] B	[ ] C	[ ] D
83.	[ ] A	[ ] B	[ ] C	[ ] D		120.	[ ] A	[ ] B	[ ] C	[ ] D
84.	[ ] A	[ ] B	[ ] C	[ ] D		121.	[ ] A	[ ] B	[ ] C	[ ] D
85.	[ ] A	[ ] B	[ ] C	[ ] D		122.	[ ] A	[ ] B	[ ] C	[ ] D
86.	[ ] A	[ ] B	[ ] C	[ ] D		123.	[ ] A	[ ] B	[ ] C	[ ] D
87.	[ ] A	[ ] B	[ ] C	[ ] D		124.	[ ] A	[ ] B	[ ] C	[ ] D
88.	[ ] A	[ ] B	[ ] C	[ ] D		125.	[ ] A	[ ] B	[ ] C	[ ] D
89.	[ ] A	[ ] B	[ ] C	[ ] D		126.	[ ] A	[ ] B	[ ] C	[ ] D
90.	[ ] A	[ ] B	[ ] C	[ ] D		127.	[ ] A	[ ] B	[ ] C	[ ] D
91.	[ ] A	[ ] B	[ ] C	[ ] D		128.	[ ] A	[ ] B	[ ] C	[ ] D
92.	[ ] A	[ ] B	[ ] C	[ ] D		129.	[ ] A	[ ] B	[ ] C	[ ] D
93.	[ ] A	[ ] B	[ ] C	[ ] D		130.	[ ] A	[ ] B	[ ] C	[ ] D
94.	[ ] A	[ ] B	[ ] C	[ ] D		131.	[ ] A	[ ] B	[ ] C	[ ] D
95.	[ ] A	[ ] B	[ ] C	[ ] D		132.	[ ] A	[ ] B	[ ] C	[ ] D
96.	[ ] A	[ ] B	[ ] C	[ ] D		133.	[ ] A	[ ] B	[ ] C	[ ] D
97.	[ ] A	[ ] B	[ ] C	[ ] D		134.	[ ] A	[ ] B	[ ] C	[ ] D
98.	[ ] A	[ ] B	[ ] C	[ ] D		135.	[ ] A	[ ] B	[ ] C	[ ] D
99.	[ ] A	[ ] B	[ ] C	[ ] D		136.	[ ] A	[ ] B	[ ] C	[ ] D
100.	[ ] A	[ ] B	[ ] C	[ ] D		137.	[ ] A	[ ] B	[ ] C	[ ] D
101.	[ ] A	[ ] B	[ ] C	[ ] D		138.	[ ] A	[ ] B	[ ] C	[ ] D
102.	[ ] A	[ ] B	[ ] C	[ ] D		139.	[ ] A	[ ] B	[ ] C	[ ] D
103.	[ ] A	[ ] B	[ ] C	[ ] D		140.	[ ] A	[ ] B	[ ] C	[ ] D

141.	[ ] A	[ ] B	[ ] C	[ ] D		146.	[ ] A	[ ] B	[ ] C	[ ] D
142.	[ ] A	[ ] B	[ ] C	[ ] D		147.	[ ] A	[ ] B	[ ] C	[ ] D
143.	[ ] A	[ ] B	[ ] C	[ ] D		148.	[ ] A	[ ] B	[ ] C	[ ] D
144.	[ ] A	[ ] B	[ ] C	[ ] D		149.	[ ] A	[ ] B	[ ] C	[ ] D
145.	[ ] A	[ ] B	[ ] C	[ ] D		150.	[ ] A	[ ] B	[ ] C	[ ] D

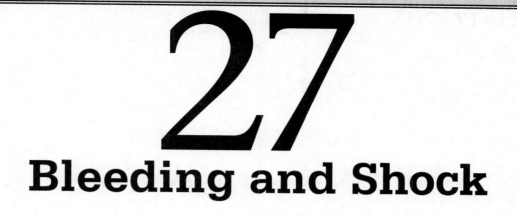

27
Bleeding and Shock

Standards: Shock and Resuscitation; Trauma (Bleeding)

Competency: Applies fundamental knowledge of the causes, pathophysiology, and management of shock, respiratory failure or arrest, cardiac failure or arrest, and postresuscitation management.

Applies fundamental knowledge to provide basic emergency care and transportation based on assessment findings for an acutely injured patient.

▌OBJECTIVES

After reading this chapter you should be able to:

27.1   Define key terms introduced in this chapter.

27.2   Describe the structure and function of the circulatory system, including the functions of the blood.

27.3   Explain the concept of perfusion.

27.4   Compare and contrast arterial, venous, and capillary bleeding.

27.5   Discuss causes and effects of severe external bleeding.

27.6   Discuss assessment and management of external bleeding, including methods of controlling external bleeding.

27.7   Identify patients at risk for internal bleeding.

27.8   Recognize signs of internal bleeding and discuss patient care for internal bleeding.

27.9   Discuss the causes of shock and its effects on the body.

27.10 Explain the concepts of compensated, decompensated, and irreversible shock.

27.11 Discuss the types of shock.

27.12 Relate the signs and symptoms of shock to the body's attempts to compensate for blood loss.

27.13 Discuss the management of patients in shock.

MATCH TERMINOLOGY/ DEFINITIONS

▶ **PART A**

A. The major artery of the upper arm

B. When the patient is developing shock but the body is still able to maintain perfusion

C. Bleeding that is characterized by a slow, oozing flow of blood

D. Shock resulting from blood loss

E. Occurs when the body can no longer compensate for low blood volume or lack of perfusion; a late sign such as decreasing shock but the body is still able to maintain perfusion

F. Inability of the body to adequately circulate blood to the body's cells to supply them with oxygen and nutrients

G. Bleeding, especially severe bleeding

H. Shock, or lack of perfusion, brought on not by blood loss but by inadequate pumping action of the heart

I. The major artery supplying the thigh

J. Bleeding from an artery, which is characterized by bright red blood and is rapid, profuse, and difficult to control

_____ 1. Arterial bleeding

_____ 2. Brachial artery

_____ 3. Capillary bleeding

_____ 4. Cardiogenic shock

_____ 5. Compensated shock

_____ 6. Decompensated shock

_____ 7. Femoral artery

_____ 8. Hemorrhage

_____ 9. Hemorrhagic shock

_____ 10. Hypoperfusion

▶ **PART B**

A. A device used for bleeding control that constricts all blood flow to and from an extremity

B. Bleeding from a vein, which is characterized by dark red or maroon blood and is a steady flow that is easy to control

C. Hypoperfusion due to nerve paralysis resulting in the dilation of blood vessels that increases the volume of the circulatory system beyond the point where it can be filled

D. A site where a main artery lies near the surface of the body and directly over a bone; pressure on such a point can stop distal bleeding

E. When the body has lost the battle to maintain perfusion to vital organs; even if adequate vital signs return, the patient may die days later due to organ failure

F. Shock resulting from blood or fluid loss

G. A bulky dressing held in position with a tightly wrapped bandage to apply pressure that helps control bleeding

H. The inability of the body to adequately circulate blood to the body's cells and thus supply them with oxygen and nutrients

I. The supply of oxygen to and removal of wastes from the cells and tissues of the body as a result of the flow of blood through the capillaries

_____ 1. Hypovolemic shock

_____ 2. Irreversible shock

_____ 3. Neurogenic shock

_____ 4. Perfusion

_____ 5. Pressure dressing

_____ 6. Pressure point

_____ 7. Shock

_____ 8. Tourniquet

_____ 9. Venous bleeding

MULTIPLE-CHOICE REVIEW

_____ 1. Blood that has been depleted of oxygen and loaded with carbon dioxide empties into the _____, which carry it back to the heart.
- A. arteries
- B. veins
- C. capillaries
- D. tissues

_____ 2. Cells and tissues of the brain, spinal cord, and _____ are the *most* sensitive to inadequate perfusion.
- A. kidneys
- B. lungs
- C. stomach
- D. heart

_____ 3. Your 22-year-old male patient was stabbed multiple times in a bar fight. Police are on the scene and it is safe to begin your assessment and treatment. The use of _____ is essential whenever bleeding is discovered or simply anticipated.
- A. full protective gear
- B. Standard Precautions
- C. universal isolation precautions
- D. Tyvek overalls

_____ 4. You will be doing a complete body scan search of the patient from multiple-choice question 3 to look for bleeding. Bleeding is classified as all of the following *except*:
- A. arterial.
- B. venous.
- C. cellular.
- D. capillary.

_____ 5. Finding arterial bleeding quickly is very important when assessing the patient in multiple-choice question 3. Which statement about arterial bleeding is correct?
- A. Clot formation takes place rapidly.
- B. It is often rapid and profuse.
- C. It is the least difficult to control.
- D. It causes the blood pressure to rise.

_____ 6. A steady flow of dark red or maroon blood is a result of _____ bleeding.
- A. arterial
- B. venous
- C. capillary
- D. pulmonary

_____ 7. Your patient has sustained a large road rash from sliding along the highway when he laid down his motorcycle. Bleeding described as oozing usually is a result of _____ bleeding.
- A. arterial
- B. venous
- C. capillary
- D. bronchiole

_____ 8. You are treating a 52-year-old male whose throat was slashed in a robbery. When a large bleeding vein in the neck sucks in debris or an air bubble, this can cause:
- A. an evisceration.
- B. heart stoppage.
- C. infection.
- D. severe bleeding.

_____ 9. Sudden blood loss of _____ in an adult is considered serious.
- A. 250 cc
- B. 500 cc
- C. 600 cc
- D. 1,000 cc

_____ 10. Sudden blood loss of _____ in a child is considered serious.
- A. 200 cc
- B. 300 cc
- C. 400 cc
- D. 500 cc

_____ 11. Sudden blood loss of _____ in a 1-year-old infant is considered serious.
- A. 25 cc
- B. 50 cc
- C. 100 cc
- D. 150 cc

©2012 Pearson Education, Inc.
Emergency Care, 12th Ed.

Chapter 27 • *Bleeding and Shock* **259**

_____ 12. When a patient cuts a blood vessel, the body attempts to protect the patient even prior to the first bandage being applied by an EMT. The body's natural responses to bleeding are constriction of the injured blood vessel and:
   A. perfusion.
   B. hypoperfusion.
   C. compensation.
   D. clotting.

_____ 13. You are treating a 19-year-old who experienced a series of lacerations. Your assessment of external bleeding includes all of the following items *except*:
   A. estimating the amount of blood lost in order to predict potential shock.
   B. waiting for signs and symptoms of shock to appear before beginning treatment.
   C. triaging, or prioritizing, bleeding patients properly.
   D. identifying bleeding that must be treated during the primary assessment.

_____ 14. The major methods used to control external extremity bleeding include all of the following *except*:
   A. direct pressure.
   B. elevation.
   C. tourniquet.
   D. vessel clamps.

_____ 15. Why is administration of supplemental oxygen an important treatment for any trauma patient?
   A. It enhances blood clotting.
   B. It improves oxygenation of the tissues.
   C. It constricts the blood vessels.
   D. It is important for all of these reasons.

_____ 16. You are treating a 28-year-old female who sustained several deep lacerations when she fell off her bike and then fell onto a guardrail. The most common and effective way to control severe external extremity bleeding is by:
   A. cold application.
   B. elevation.
   C. tourniquet.
   D. direct pressure.

_____ 17. The patient has already bled through a small pile of gauze pads. You will be applying some additional sterile pads to the injury. The initial layer of dressing should not be removed from a bleeding wound because it:
   A. can become a biohazard.
   B. takes too long to remove.
   C. is a necessary part of clot formation.
   D. may increase the chance of infection.

_____ 18. After controlling bleeding from an extremity using a pressure dressing, be sure to:
   A. loosen the tourniquet.
   B. check the distal pulse.
   C. apply a PASG.
   D. administer oxygen by nasal cannula.

_____ 19. Elevation is used to assist in bleeding control for all of the following reasons *except*:
   A. it slows bleeding.
   B. it raises the limb above the heart.
   C. it helps to reduce blood pressure in the limb.
   D. it speeds up the pulse rate.

_____ 20. When is it *inappropriate* to use elevation to assist in bleeding control?
   A. As you apply direct pressure
   B. While trying to bandage an extremity
   C. If you suspect musculoskeletal injuries
   D. When a patient is found lying down

©2012 Pearson Education, Inc.
Emergency Care, 12th Ed.

_____ **21.** A patient fell through a store window and has sustained a large cut, which is flowing blood from his forehead. What is the method of bleeding control that should be utilized?

   A. A tourniquet will need to be applied to control the bleeding.

   B. Direct pressure with a dressing and bandage should work.

   C. Apply cold directly to the wound right away.

   D. Lower the head below the heart and the bleeding will stop.

_____ **22.** You are treating a 22-year-old male who has a deep laceration that is continuing to bleed. Use of direct pressure may *not* be effective if the wound:

   A. was caused by an impaled object.

   B. was accompanied by spinal injury.

   C. is at the distal end of a limb.

   D. is a profusely bleeding artery.

_____ **23.** You are going to use an air splint to manage the bleeding on the lower leg of a 22-year-old male patient. Which of the following is *true* about the use of an air splint?

   A. It is effective for controlling venous and capillary bleeding.

   B. It should be used only if there is no suspected bone injury.

   C. It is most effective for controlling arterial bleeding.

   D. It should be used before other manual methods of bleeding control.

_____ **24.** Which of the following is *not* a guideline for supplementing bleeding control with cold application?

   A. Wrap the ice pack in a cloth or towel.

   B. Do not apply the cold application directly onto the skin.

   C. Do not leave the cold pack in place for more than 20 minutes.

   D. Insert the ice directly into the wound.

_____ **25.** Use of the pneumatic antishock garment (PASG) is controversial, and its use should be defined by your service's Medical Director. Some "experts" agree that the PASG is useful for:

   A. controlling bleeding from head trauma.

   B. controlling bleeding from the areas the garment covers.

   C. penetrating chest trauma.

   D. the patient in cardiogenic shock.

_____ **26.** You are treating a 29-year-old female factory worker who was involved in an accident where a machine has amputated her right forearm. Bleeding from a clean-edged amputation is usually cared for initially with:

   A. a pressure dressing.   **C.** a tourniquet.

   B. cold application.   **D.** a pneumatic antishock garment.

_____ **27.** Rough-edged amputations, usually produced by crushing or tearing injuries:

   A. are easily controlled by a pressure bandage.

   B. tend to stop bleeding on their own.

   C. often bleed very heavily.

   D. constrict quickly to control bleeding.

_____ **28.** You have decided that the most appropriate method of bleeding control for your patient is to apply a tourniquet. Once a tourniquet is in place, it must:

   A. not be removed or loosened unless ordered by medical direction.

   B. be covered immediately to prevent accidental removal.

   C. be loosened every 15 minutes to dislodge clots.

   D. be used under the pneumatic antishock garment.

_____ 29. Your 35-year-old male patient has severe bleeding from a large laceration on his right forearm. You tried direct pressure and it obviously did not work. A blood pressure cuff:
A. can be used as a tourniquet if it is inflated to 70 mmHg.
B. should never be used for bleeding control.
C. can be used as a temporary tourniquet if it is inflated to 150 mmHg.
D. should always be used to control arterial bleeding.

_____ 30. If your 20-year-old female patient, who fell off her bike, has a head injury, and you note bleeding or loss of cerebrospinal fluid (CSF) from the patient's ears or nose, you should:
A. apply direct pressure to the skull.
B. apply direct pressure to the ears and nose.
C. apply cold packs to the ears and nose.
D. allow the drainage to flow freely.

_____ 31. You are treating a 58-year-old woman who has had a nosebleed for the last hour. The medical term for a nosebleed is:
A. hemorrhage.
B. epistaxis.
C. epihemorrhage.
D. nostrium.

_____ 32. You are treating a 50-year-old female patient who called the ambulance because her nose has been bleeding for quite a while. To stop a nosebleed, try each of the following _except_:
A. place the patient in a sitting position, leaning forward.
B. apply direct pressure by pinching the nostrils.
C. keep the patient calm.
D. apply cold packs to the bridge of the nose.

_____ 33. The leading cause of internal injuries and bleeding is:
A. blunt trauma.
B. penetrating trauma.
C. auto collisions.
D. large lacerations.

_____ 34. Which is _not_ an example of a penetrating trauma?
A. Blast injury
B. Gunshot wound
C. Knife wound
D. Ice-pick wound

_____ 35. You suspect that your 52-year-old male patient may have internal bleeding. Signs of internal bleeding include all of the following _except_:
A. vomiting a coffee-ground-like substance.
B. bradycardia and a flushed face.
C. dark, tarry stools.
D. tender, rigid, or distended abdomen.

_____ 36. A 28-year-old male patient fell and you suspect he has sustained internal bleeding. He may have all of the following _except_:
A. painful, swollen, or deformed extremities.
B. signs and symptoms of shock.
C. bright red blood in the stool.
D. a laceration to the forearm.

_____ 37. Because of internal bleeding, the patient is developing inadequate tissue perfusion. This condition is referred to as:
A. hyperperfusion.
B. hypoxia.
C. hypoperfusion.
D. hypotension.

_____ 38. You suspect that your patient may be going into shock. Shock may develop as a result of all of the following _except_:
A. pump failure.
B. lost blood volume.
C. dilated blood vessels.
D. injury to the head.

_____ **39.** The type of shock most commonly seen by EMTs is _____ shock.
  A. cardiogenic   **C.** neurogenic
  B. irreversible   **D.** hypovolemic

_____ **40.** The most common mechanism of shock for a heart attack patient is:
  A. vasoconstriction.   **C.** pump failure.
  B. fluid loss.   **D.** vasodilation.

_____ **41.** Your patient was involved in a car crash and it took all night to find his car. He is unable to move his lower extremities and you suspect he is in shock. Shock caused by the failure of the nervous system to control the diameter of blood vessels is called _____ shock.
  A. hypovolemic   **C.** neurogenic
  B. cardiogenic   **D.** reversible

_____ **42.** Your 46-year-old male patient is in shock, yet his body is still able to maintain perfusion to his vital organs. This is often referred to as _____ shock.
  A. compensated   **C.** delayed
  B. decompensated   **D.** irreversible

_____ **43.** Early signs of shock that are actually the body's compensating mechanisms include all of the following _except_:
  A. increased heart rate.
  B. increased respirations.
  C. pale, cool skin.
  D. decreased capillary refill time.

_____ **44.** Your patient with severe internal bleeding is struggling to deal with the blood loss. When the body has lost the battle to maintain perfusion to the organ systems, the patient is experiencing _____ shock.
  A. delayed   **C.** decompensated
  B. compensated   **D.** irreversible

_____ **45.** You are treating a 45-year-old female patient who has sustained considerable blood loss after slicing her hand while preparing food. She states that she feels nauseated. What is causing this symptom of feeling nauseated?
  A. Blood is diverted from the digestive system.
  B. Blood rushes rapidly to the digestive system.
  C. Shock increases the production of digestive juices.
  D. The patient has swallowed a great amount of blood.

_____ **46.** The pulse of the patient in multiple-choice question 45 will likely:
  A. decrease.   **C.** increase.
  B. be absent.   **D.** be irregular.

_____ **47.** The patient from multiple-choice question 45 has a drop in her blood pressure, and this is:
  A. an early sign of shock.
  B. an early sign of shock in a child.
  C. always present in shock.
  D. a late sign of shock.

_____ **48.** When observing the patient who you suspect may be in shock, additional signs may include any of the following _except_:
  A. thirst.
  B. dilated pupils.
  C. cyanosis around the lips and nail beds.
  D. flushed, warm skin.

_____ **49.** Your patient is a 6-year-old male who fell off his skateboard and has numerous injuries to both of his legs. You should be especially careful when evaluating pediatric patients for shock because they:

    A. cannot be administered oxygen at low flow rates.

    B. may display few signs and/or symptoms until a large percentage of blood volume is lost.

    C. can decompensate for blood loss very quickly.

    D. may exhibit erratic capillary refill times.

_____ **50.** Which of the following is the best description of the concept of a "platinum 10 minutes"?

    A. The maximum on-scene time when caring for a trauma or shock patient

    B. The optimum time limit from the time of injury until surgery

    C. The maximum time limit for controlling arterial bleeding before shock occurs

    D. The optimum time limit for applying PASG to the shock patient

INSIDE/OUTSIDE: FIGHT-OR-FLIGHT

1. What happens to the patient when the blood vessels constrict?

_____

2. What happens when the blood vessels in the kidneys constrict?

_____

3. What happens when the blood vessels in the GI tract constrict?

_____

COMPLETE THE FOLLOWING

1. List three major types of shock.

    A. _____

    B. _____

    C. _____

2. List six signs and symptoms of shock.

    A. _____

    B. _____

    C. _____

    D. _____

    E. _____

    F. _____

STREET SCENES DISCUSSION

Review the Street Scene on page 640 of the textbook. Then answer the following questions.

1. This patient may have broken a rib or two. What abdominal organs are protected by the rib cage?

2. Would an ALS unit be appropriate for this patient?

3. You observe that the patient's mental status is changing. What might this indicate to you?

CASE STUDY

▶ CONVENIENCE STORE SHOOTING

You respond to a local convenience store where there has been an armed robbery. The call was dispatched as a shooting, and the police have already secured the scene. A bystander who pulled up to the store just as the shooter was running out the front door states, "The injured clerk is sitting on the floor, clutching his stomach."

1. What is the importance of a secure scene?

2. As you enter the store, what other scene size-up procedures are important?

You find the 18-year-old male clerk holding the right upper quadrant of his abdomen with a piece of cloth soaked in blood. He is conscious and alert, and he knows his name, where he is, and the day of the week. His name is Tom. He complains of pain and says that he is very thirsty. You reach down and feel for his radial pulse. You can barely feel it because it is so fast and weak.

3. What important information have you just found out about this patient?

4. What phase and what type of shock is your patient in based on the information you know?

5. What is the relevance of his being thirsty?

When you check Tom's carotid pulse, it is about 120 per minute and thready. His respirations are 24 per minute, shallow, and regular. You quickly assess his chest; you find no entry into the chest and equal breath sounds on both lungs. You immediately search for other injuries, and you ask him about other complaints and find he has none. You do a very quick search from head to toe for additional external hemorrhage and an exit bullet wound. Your partner begins to control the bleeding and administer oxygen to the patient. Together, you and your partner carefully lay Tom down on a long spine board.

6. Because Tom was shot in the abdomen, what is the importance of listening to his lungs?

7. What device should be used and at what liter flow rate should the regulator be set for this patient?

8. Should an ALS unit be called for if one was not dispatched with you? If so, should you wait on the scene for ALS or arrange an intercept?

The patient is very pale and sweating profusely. He is beginning to get anxious about dying. You and your partner rapidly move him to the ambulance.

9. On a call like this, what is the maximum time you should spend on the scene? What is this time frame commonly called?

10. To give the surgeons a fighting chance to save Tom's life, what is the maximum time you should spend in assessment and transportation of the patient to the trauma center? What is this time frame commonly called?

The patient is loaded in the ambulance. His level of responsiveness is reassessed, and he is responding to painful stimuli only. ALS will intercept you en route.

11. Aside from reassessing the vitals, what airway care should be considered at this time?

©2012 Pearson Education, Inc.
Emergency Care, 12th Ed.

12. Would the PASG be indicated in this case?

13. Is this patient critical?

You meet the ALS unit. They jump aboard your ambulance with their portable equipment. The driver quickly continues to the hospital.

14. What procedures would you suspect an ALS unit might do en route to the hospital?

15. Briefly write down the radio report that you would give to the hospital en route. The patient initially told you he has no allergies, takes no medications, and has been healthy; his last meal was lunch a few hours ago. The paramedics establish two large-bore IVs and prepare to intubate the patient endotracheally. His pulse oximeter reading is 85 percent, and his ECG is sinus tachycardia at a rate of 136.

Radio Report:

_____

_____

_____

_____

_____

EMT SKILLS PERFORMANCE CHECKLISTS

▶ **CONTROLLING EXTERNAL BLEEDING/MANAGING SHOCK (PP. 624–625; P. 637)**

❑ Take Standard Precautions.

❑ Apply direct pressure to the wound.

❑ Elevate the extremity.

❑ Apply a dressing to the wound.

❑ If the wound continues to bleed, apply an additional dressing to it.

❑ If the wound appears on an extremity and continues to bleed profusely, consider application of an arterial tourniquet.

❑ Administer high-concentration oxygen by nonrebreather mask.

❑ Properly position the patient.

❑ Initiate steps to prevent heat loss from the patient.

❑ Determine the need for immediate transportation.

▶ APPLICATION OF PASG (P. 638)

❑ Take Standard Precautions.

❑ Ensure that patient meets local protocol for PASG.

❑ Check for contraindications (e.g., pulmonary edema, penetrating chest injury).

❑ Remove clothing and check for sharp objects.

❑ Quickly assess the areas that will be under the PASG.

❑ Position the PASG with the top of the abdominal section at or below the last set of ribs.

❑ Secure the PASG around the patient.

❑ Attach the hoses.

❑ Check the patient's blood pressure.

❑ Begin the inflation sequence.

❑ Stop the inflation sequence (106 mmHg or pop-off valves release).

❑ Operate the PASG to maintain air pressure in the device.

❑ Reassess the patient's vital signs.

WARNINGS: Do not actually inflate a PASG on a mock victim in a classroom setting. Do not inflate the abdominal section if the patient is pregnant.

▶ APPLICATION OF A TOURNIQUET (PP. 627–629)

❑ Take Standard Precautions.

❑ Assign another rescuer to apply direct pressure and use a pressure point.

❑ Select a site no farther than 2 inches from the wound (if the wound is on a joint or just distal to the joint, apply the tourniquet above the joint).

❑ If using a commercial tourniquet, place the strap around the limb, pull the free end through the buckle or catch, and tighten this end over the pad. Tighten to the point where bleeding is controlled. Do not tighten beyond that point.

❑ If you are using cravats, or triangular bandages, wrap the material around the injured limb and tie a knot over the pad. Slip a pen, stick, or similar device into the knot and rotate to tighten the tourniquet. Tighten to the point that bleeding is controlled and no more. Secure the device in place with tape or by tying the ends of the cravat.

❑ Keep the tourniquet in place. Do not loosen or remove.

❑ Advise the hospital staff of the application of a tourniquet during your radio report and in person on your arrival at the emergency department.

❑ Do not cover the extremity; visually monitor the wound site and the effectiveness of the tourniquet.

❑ Document on the PCR.

28

Soft-Tissue Trauma

Standard: Trauma (Soft-Tissue Trauma)

Competency: Applies fundamental knowledge to provide basic emergency care and transportation based on assessment findings for an acutely injured patient.

▌OBJECTIVES

After reading this chapter you should be able to:

28.1 Define key terms introduced in this chapter.

28.2 Describe the structure and function of the skin.

28.3 Describe types of closed soft-tissue wounds and the assessment and management of closed soft-tissue wounds.

28.4 Predict internal injuries that may be indicated by various contusion (bruise) types and locations.

28.5 Describe types of open soft-tissue wounds and general assessment and care for open soft-tissue wounds.

28.6 Describe specific treatment for abrasions and lacerations, puncture wounds, impaled objects, avulsions, amputations, and genital injuries.

28.7 Discuss complications associated with burns.

28.8 Classify burns by agent, source, depth, and severity.

28.9 Describe specific treatment for thermal burns and chemical burns.

28.10 Describe assessment and management for electrical burns.

28.11 Describe considerations in the dressing and bandaging of open wounds.

MATCH TERMINOLOGY/ DEFINITIONS

▶ **PART A**

A. Swelling caused by the collection of blood under the skin or in damaged tissues as a result of an injured or broken blood vessel

B. The outer layer of the skin

C. Any material used to hold a dressing in place

D. A cut

E. An injury in which the skin is interrupted, exposing the tissue beneath

F. An internal injury with no open pathway from the outside to the injured site

G. A burn in which all the layers of the skin are damaged; also called a third-degree burn. There are usually areas of the skin that are charred black or areas that are dry and white.

H. The tearing away or tearing off of a piece or flap or other soft tissue; this term may also be used for an eye pulled from its socket or a tooth dislodged from the gum

I. Any material used to cover a wound that will help control bleeding and prevent additional contamination

J. An injury caused when force is transmitted from the body's exterior to its internal structures: Bones can be broken; muscles, nerves, and tissues can be damaged; and internal organs can rupture, causing internal bleeding

K. Any dressing that forms an airtight seal

L. The inner layer of the skin found below the epidermis; this inner layer is rich in blood vessels and nerves

M. A bruise

N. A scratch or scrape

O. The surgical removal or traumatic severing of a body part, usually an extremity

_____ **1.** Abrasion

_____ **2.** Amputation

_____ **3.** Avulsion

_____ **4.** Bandage

_____ **5.** Closed wound

_____ **6.** Contusion

_____ **7.** Crush injury

_____ **8.** Dermis

_____ **9.** Dressing

_____ **10.** Epidermis

_____ **11.** Full thickness burn

_____ **12.** Hematoma

_____ **13.** Laceration

_____ **14.** Occlusive dressing

_____ **15.** Open wound

▶ **PART B**

A. A bulky dressing

B. A method for estimating the extent of a burn. For an adult, each of the following areas represents 9 percent of the body surface: the head and neck, each upper extremity, the chest, the abdomen, the upper back, the lower back and buttocks, the front of each lower extremity, and the back of each lower extremity. The remaining 1 percent is assigned to the genital region.

C. A method for estimating the extent of a burn. The palm of the patient's hand, which equals about 1 percent of the body's surface area, is compared with the patient's burn to estimate its size.

_____ **1.** Partial thickness burn

_____ **2.** Pressure dressing

_____ **3.** Puncture wound

_____ **4.** Rule of nines

_____ **5.** Rule of palm

_____ **6.** Subcutaneous layers

_____ **7.** Superficial burn

_____ **8.** Universal dressing

D. A burn that involves only the epidermis, the outer layer of the skin; also called a first-degree burn. It is characterized by reddening of the skin and perhaps some swelling.

E. A burn in which the epidermis is burned through and the dermis is damaged; also called a second-degree burn. Burns of this type cause reddening, blistering, and a mottled appearance.

F. An open wound that tears through the skin and destroys underlying tissues. A penetrating puncture wound can be shallow or deep. A perforating puncture wound has both an entrance and an exit wound.

G. The layers of fat and soft tissues found below the dermis

H. A dressing applied tightly to assist in bleeding control

MULTIPLE-CHOICE REVIEW

_____ **1.** The soft tissues of the body include all of the following *except*:
  A. skin, fatty tissue, and muscles.
  B. blood vessels and fibrous tissues.
  C. teeth, bones, and cartilage.
  D. nerves, membranes, and glands.

_____ **2.** Which of the following is *not* a function of the skin?
  A. Protection
  B. Shock absorption
  C. Temperature regulation
  D. Blood insulation

_____ **3.** The layers of the skin include all of the following *except*:
  A. epidermis.   **C.** subcutaneous.
  B. dermis.   **D.** epithelial.

_____ **4.** The skin has multiple layers. The layer called the _____ is composed of dead cells, which are rubbed or sloughed off and are replaced continuously.
  A. epidermis   **C.** subcutaneous
  B. dermis   **D.** epithelial

_____ **5.** Specialized nerve endings in the skin layer called the _____ are involved with the senses of touch, cold, heat, and pain.
  A. epidermis   **C.** subcutaneous layers
  B. dermis   **D.** epithelial cells

_____ **6.** Shock absorption and insulation are major functions of which layer of the skin?
  A. Epidermis   **C.** Subcutaneous
  B. Dermis   **D.** Epithelial

_____ **7.** You are treating a 35-year-old male who sustained an injury from an impact with a blunt object. There is no external bleeding. This wound is called a _____ injury.
  A. stabbing   **C.** closed
  B. laceration   **D.** perforation

_____ **8.** A closed wound that involves tissue damage and a collection of blood at the injury site is called a:
  A. crush injury.   **C.** contusion.
  B. hematoma.   **D.** penetration.

_____ 9. A soft-tissue injury caused by a force that can cause rupture or bleeding of internal organs is called a _____ injury.
    A. contusion   **C.** crush
    B. hematoma   **D.** high-force

_____ 10. A(n) _____ is an injury in which the skin is interrupted, exposing the tissues underneath.
    A. hematoma   **C.** open wound
    B. closed wound   **D.** crush injury

_____ 11. A 19-year-old male patient crashed his bike and slid along the road on the rainy pavement. The oozing of blood from his capillary beds is from an injury called a(n):
    A. amputation.   **C.** laceration.
    B. abrasion.   **D.** puncture.

_____ 12. A 21-year-old female sustained a cut on her hand while slicing carrots for a stew. This wound is called a(n):
    A. abrasion.   **C.** laceration.
    B. puncture.   **D.** avulsion.

_____ 13. When a sharp or pointed object, such as an ice pick or a bullet, passes through the skin or other tissue, a(n) _____ wound has occurred.
    A. abrasion   **C.** amputation
    B. puncture   **D.** crush injury

_____ 14. You are treating a 35-year-old male patient whose tip of the nose was cut or torn off. This is a(n) _____ injury.
    A. avulsion   **C.** crush
    B. penetration   **D.** amputation

_____ 15. You are treating a 27-year-old female patient who has sustained a severe open wound. Your first priority, as it relates to this type of wound, is to:
    A. control bleeding.
    B. clean the wound.
    C. prevent contamination.
    D. bandage the wound.

_____ 16. Your 40-year-old female patient has sustained a 3-inch laceration on her right forearm. Care for this injury includes:
    A. applying a tourniquet above the elbow.
    B. applying a butterfly bandage, then releasing the patient.
    C. pulling apart the edges to inspect the wound.
    D. checking the pulse distal to the injury.

_____ 17. You are on the scene of a local bar where there was just a shooting. The police are there, and the scene is now considered "safe at this point." Various types of guns, when fired at close range, can cause all of the following _except_:
    A. burns around the entry wound.
    B. injection of air into the tissues.
    C. large contusion to the tissue.
    D. significant cold injuries.

_____ 18. You are treating a 38-year-old female who has a large shard of glass impaled in her right leg. Care in the field for this patient includes:
    A. stabilizing the object in place.
    B. using direct pressure on the site.
    C. leaving the object alone and rapidly transporting.
    D. carefully removing the object.

©2012 Pearson Education, Inc.
Emergency Care, 12th Ed.

_____ 19. Which of the following is *not* correct about an injury caused by an impaled object?
   A. The object may plug bleeding from a major artery.
   B. Removal may cause further injury to the nerves, muscles, and soft tissue.
   C. Pressure should be applied to the object to stabilize it.
   D. All of these are incorrect.

_____ 20. To control profuse bleeding resulting from an injury caused by an impaled object:
   A. position your gloved hands on either side of the object and exert downward pressure.
   B. use a pressure point distal to the injury to control the bleeding.
   C. let the blood flow freely from the wound left by removal of the object.
   D. stabilize the object with gloved hands and then immediately apply a tourniquet.

_____ 21. The 18-year-old male you are assessing was running with a sharp tool and tripped, impaling the tool in his right cheek. Which of the following is *false* about this impaled object?
   A. It should never be removed.
   B. It can create an airway obstruction.
   C. It can cause nausea and vomiting.
   D. It is pulled out in the direction it entered.

_____ 22. If a 22-year-old male patient has an impaled object in his right eye, the care you provide should include use of a:
   A. pressure bandage placed over the eye.
   B. loose bandage placed over the eye.
   C. combination of 4 × 4s and a paper cup.
   D. combination of 3-inch gauze and a Styrofoam cup.

_____ 23. Your 33-year-old male patient has sustained an injury that tore open his left leg. There is no break in the bone, but there is a large avulsed flap of tissue that has been torn loose but not off. You should do all of the following *except*:
   A. fold the skin back to its normal position.
   B. control bleeding and dress the wound.
   C. clean the wound surface.
   D. tear off the remainder of the flap and put it on ice.

_____ 24. You are treating a 37-year-old male patient who managed to stick his hand into the chute of an operating snow blower. He was severely injured and all of his fingers are severed. The amputated parts torn from his body should be wrapped and placed in a:
   A. cup of dry ice placed in an airtight container.
   B. plastic bag filled with ice.
   C. plastic bag on top of a sealed bag of ice.
   D. saline and ice solution.

_____ 25. You are treating a 35-year-old male whose lower leg has been amputated by a train. The most effective treatment for an amputation is to:
   A. apply a tourniquet.
   B. place the amputated part in ice.
   C. place a snug pressure dressing over the stump.
   D. apply ice over the stump.

_____ 26. For the patient in multiple-choice question 25, who sustained an amputation, whenever possible you should:
   A. place the amputated body part in ice and transport before the patient.
   B. transport the patient and the amputated body part in the same ambulance.
   C. apply a tourniquet after completing a partial amputation.
   D. immerse the amputated part in saline and transport before the patient.

_____ **27.** Your patient has a suspected air bubble that may have been sucked into a large vein in his neck. This is called a(n):

A. air embolus.
B. blood clot.
C. occlusion.
D. case of the "bends."

_____ **28.** The treatment of neck vein injury includes all of the following *except*:

A. compressing the region of injury.
B. preventing an embolus.
C. preventing shock.
D. stopping bleeding.

_____ **29.** Your 32-year-old male patient was taking money out of an ATM when suddenly someone slashed his throat from behind and stole his money. To treat a neck laceration like this, you should use a(n):

A. pressure bandage.
B. thin dressing.
C. ACE bandage.
D. occlusive dressing.

_____ **30.** When applying pressure to the neck wound of the patient in multiple-choice question 29, be sure you do *not*:

A. apply pressure over the laceration.
B. compress both carotids at the same time.
C. administer oxygen to the patient.
D. treat the patient for shock.

_____ **31.** You are dispatched to the scene of an explosion. On arrival, you find a 35-year-old male who bystanders say was in an area of the explosion. In terms of injuries, you expect to find a(n):

A. mixture of open and closed injuries.
B. series of penetrating objects.
C. impaled object.
D. amputation.

_____ **32.** You are evaluating a 52-year-old male patient who was the driver of a vehicle involved in a head-on collision. He was not wearing his seat belt. When he pitched forward, he smashed his chest into the steering column. This type of injury is called:

A. closed lung injury.
B. penetrating trauma.
C. compression injury.
D. puncture trauma.

_____ **33.** Blast injuries often include each of the following *except*:

A. potentially infectious disease.
B. tertiary injuries from air injection into the skin.
C. primary lacerations and abrasions.
D. secondary projectile injuries.

_____ **34.** You are assessing the chest of a 25-year-old male who was shot. An injury that has both an entrance and an exit is called a _____ wound.

A. puncture
B. penetrating
C. perforating puncture
D. compression injury

_____ **35.** Burn injuries often involve structures below the skin, including muscles and:

A. nerves.
B. bones.
C. blood vessels.
D. all of these.

_____ **36.** Your patient has serious thermal burns to his face and forearm. In addition to the physical damage caused by burns, patients often suffer:

A. heart attacks.
B. emotional and psychological problems.
C. diabetic emergencies.
D. delayed reactions such as developing skin cancer.

©2012 Pearson Education, Inc.
Emergency Care, 12th Ed.

_____ **37.** When caring for a 22-year-old male burn patient:
   A. think beyond the burn to possible medical causes and results.
   B. always begin transport before treatment.
   C. obtain the name of the product that caused the burn.
   D. determine the duration of the exposure.

_____ **38.** When caring for a 22-year-old male who was burned:
   A. do not neglect assessment to begin burn care.
   B. transport immediately.
   C. take the patient to the closest hospital.
   D. run cold water on the patient for at least 20 minutes.

_____ **39.** Examples of agents causing burns include all of the following *except*:
   A. AC current.   **C.** dry lime.
   B. hydrochloric acid.   **D.** distilled water.

_____ **40.** A burn that involves only the epidermis is called a _____ burn.
   A. superficial   **C.** full thickness
   B. partial thickness   **D.** epi thickness

_____ **41.** Which of the following burns will result in deep, intense pain; blisters; and mottled skin?
   A. Superficial   **C.** Full thickness
   B. Partial thickness   **D.** Medium layer

_____ **42.** To distinguish between a partial thickness burn and a full thickness burn, look for _____, which indicate(s) a full thickness burn.
   A. blisters   **C.** dry and white areas
   B. mottled skin   **D.** swelling

_____ **43.** Your patient is a 22-year-old male who sustained an electrical burn when improperly installing an outlet. Electrical burns are of special concern because they:
   A. cause respiratory burns if superheated gas is inhaled.
   B. pose a great risk of severe internal injuries.
   C. may remain on the skin and continue to burn for hours.
   D. cause the patient to lose hair over time.

_____ **44.** A patient who was working in a chemistry lab sustained a burn when a beaker of a strong acid spilled all over him. Chemical burns are of special concern because they:
   A. cause respiratory burns if superheated gas is inhaled.
   B. pose a great risk of internal injury.
   C. may remain on the skin and continue to burn for hours.
   D. jump from one extremity to another.

_____ **45.** Burns to the face are of special concern because they:
   A. continue to burn for hours.
   B. can cause heart irregularities.
   C. increase the potential for shock.
   D. may involve airway injury.

_____ **46.** One type of burn that can interrupt circulation to distal tissues is called a _____ burn.
   A. circulation   **C.** circumferential
   B. radiation   **D.** distal

_____ **47.** You are treating a 35-year-old male patient who has partial thickness burns to the entire left arm, chest, face, and neck. Using the rule of nines, approximate the size of the burn area.
   A. 18 percent   **C.** 27 percent
   B. 22 percent   **D.** 32 percent

_____ 48. You are treating a 45-year-old female patient who has partial thickness burns totally covering the legs, chest, and abdomen. Using the rule of nines, approximate the size of the burn area.
   A. 18 percent   C. 45 percent
   B. 36 percent   D. 54 percent

_____ 49. Your patient has sustained a burn injury that is about the size of five of his palms. This burn would cover approximately _____ percent of the patient's total body surface area.
   A. 5   C. 15
   B. 10   D. 20

_____ 50. The age of the patient is an important factor in burns. Patients under _____ and over _____ years of age have the most severe body responses to burns.
   A. 3; 50   C. 10; 65
   B. 5; 55   D. 15; 70

_____ 51. A partial thickness burn that involves less than 15 percent of the body surface is classified as:
   A. minor.   C. critical.
   B. moderate.   D. unnecessary to treat.

_____ 52. A partial thickness burn that involves between 15 and 30 percent of the body surface area is classified as a _____ burn.
   A. minor   C. critical
   B. moderate   D. life-threatening

_____ 53. A partial thickness burn that involves more than 30 percent of the body surface area is classified as a _____ burn.
   A. minor   C. critical
   B. moderate   D. fatal

_____ 54. Critical burns include all of the following _except_:
   A. circumferential burns.
   B. moderate burns in an infant or elderly patient.
   C. burns complicated by musculoskeletal injuries.
   D. partial thickness burns on the wrist.

_____ 55. A partial thickness burn that involves between 10 and 20 percent of the body surface area of a child under 5 years of age is considered a _____ burn.
   A. minor   C. critical
   B. moderate   D. fatal

_____ 56. You are treating a 35-year-old female who was scalded by a pot full of boiling water. Which of the following is _not_ considered a critical burn in this case?
   A. Entire genital area
   B. Full thickness burn to the entire chest and abdomen
   C. Full thickness burn to the front of the right forearm
   D. Partial thickness burn to both lower extremities

_____ 57. If a 22-year-old male patient has a partial thickness burn to the entire back, he should be:
   A. wrapped in a dry, sterile burn sheet.
   B. cooled down with ice for 15 minutes.
   C. wrapped in moist sterile dressings.
   D. dried and wrapped in an airtight dressing.

©2012 Pearson Education, Inc.
Emergency Care, 12th Ed.

_____ **58.** The primary care for a patient with a chemical burn is to:
  A. wrap the patient in a dry, sterile burn sheet.
  B. wash away the chemical with flowing water.
  C. dry the patient and wrap in an airtight dressing.
  D. wrap the patient with moist sterile dressings.

_____ **59.** You are treating a 22-year-old female patient who was burned. She is having visual difficulties, is restless and irritable, and has an irregular pulse rate and muscle tenderness. This patient probably suffered a(n) _____ burn.
  A. chemical   **C.** electrical
  B. thermal   **D.** radiation

_____ **60.** If _____ is the burn agent, brush it from the patient's skin and then flush the patient with water.
  A. dry lime   **C.** radiation
  B. electricity   **D.** acid

_____ **61.** Your 19-year-old male patient has sustained a very serious injury, and it will be necessary to apply an occlusive dressing to the wound. An occlusive dressing is used to:
  A. form an airtight seal.
  B. stabilize an impaled object.
  C. control severe bleeding.
  D. secure sprain injuries.

INSIDE/OUTSIDE: ACIDS AND ALKALIS

1. Why should an alkali burn be irrigated for a longer time than an acid burn?_____

_____

2. Which acid is the "exception to the rule" addressed in Inside/Outside question 1? Why?

_____

COMPLETE THE FOLLOWING

1. List three types of burns.

  A. _____

  B. _____

  C. _____

2. List the parts of the adult body that account for 9 percent each, using the rule of nines.

  A. _____

  B. _____

  C. _____

  D. _____

E. _____

F. _____

G. _____

H. _____

3. List five signs and symptoms of an electrical injury.

A. _____

B. _____

C. _____

D. _____

E. _____

LABEL THE DIAGRAM

Fill in the name of each type of burn and how the skin is damaged.

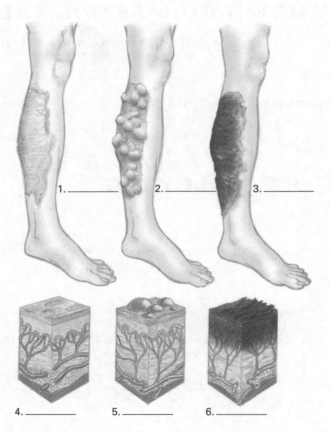

1. _____ 2. _____ 3. _____

4. _____ 5. _____ 6. _____

STREET SCENES DISCUSSION

Review the Street Scene on page 678 of the textbook. Then answer the following questions.

1. Your patient had a serious laceration, but the bleeding had stopped by the time you arrived. Suppose it was a different situation, and when you uncovered the wound, blood spurted across the room. How should the bleeding be controlled?

2. Suppose that the patient's wound, when uncovered, was only bleeding slowly but there was a large piece of glass impaled in her arm. How would you manage this injury?

3. On assessment of the patient's vital signs, it is apparent that she already has low blood pressure. How should the patient be managed?

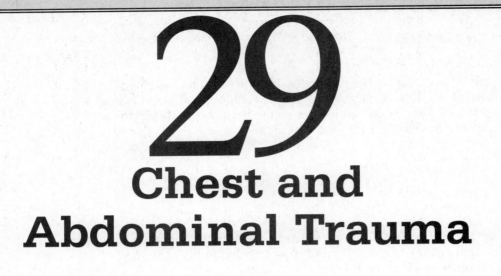

Chest and Abdominal Trauma

Standard: Trauma (Chest Trauma; Abdominal and Genitourinary Trauma)

Competency: Applies fundamental knowledge to provide basic emergency care and transportation based on assessment findings for an acutely injured patient.

OBJECTIVES

After reading this chapter you should be able to:

29.1   Define key terms introduced in this chapter.

29.2   Describe mechanisms of injury commonly associated with chest injuries.

29.3   Describe specific chest injuries, including flail chest, open chest wounds, pneumothorax, tension pneumothorax, hemothorax, traumatic asphyxia, cardiac tamponade, aortic injury, and *commotio cordis*, and the assessment and management for each of these specific injuries.

29.4   Discuss mechanisms and types of abdominal injury.

29.5   Demonstrate the assessment and management of patients with blunt and penetrating abdominal injuries, including management of evisceration.

MATCH TERMINOLOGY/ DEFINITIONS

A. Movement of ribs in a flail segment that is opposite to the direction of movement of the chest cavity

B. Air in the chest cavity

C. An injury in which the skin is interrupted, exposing the tissue beneath

D. Any dressing that forms an airtight seal

_____ **1.** Closed wound

_____ **2.** Dressing

_____ **3.** Evisceration

_____ **4.** Flail chest

E. An open chest wound in which air is sucked into the chest cavity

F. A bulky dressing

G. Fracture of two or more adjacent ribs in two or more places that allows for free movement of the fractured segment

H. An intestine or other internal organ protruding through a wound in the abdomen

I. A type of pneumothorax in which air that enters the chest cavity is prevented from escaping

J. Any material (preferably sterile) used to cover a wound that will help control bleeding and help prevent additional contamination

K. An internal injury with no open pathway from the outside

_____ **5.** Occlusive dressing

_____ **6.** Open wound

_____ **7.** Paradoxical motion

_____ **8.** Pneumothorax

_____ **9.** Sucking chest wound

_____ **10.** Tension pneumothorax

_____ **11.** Universal dressing

MULTIPLE-CHOICE REVIEW

_____ **1.** The chest can be injured due to:
- **A.** compression.
- **B.** penetrating trauma.
- **C.** blunt trauma.
- **D.** all of these.

_____ **2.** A 25-year-old male patient sustains an injury to his chest wall in which he has two or more consecutive ribs that are fractured in two or more places. This patient most likely has a(n):
- **A.** sternal contusion.
- **B.** tension pneumothorax.
- **C.** flail chest.
- **D.** abdominal evisceration.

_____ **3.** When the patient described in multiple-choice question 2 breathes, he may exhibit
- **A.** hyperventilation.
- **B.** paradoxical motion.
- **C.** apnea.
- **D.** an injury to his kidneys.

_____ **4.** When the delicate pressure balance within the chest cavity is compromised, initially the:
- **A.** diaphragm stops working.
- **B.** lung on the injured side may collapse.
- **C.** lung on the uninjured side may collapse.
- **D.** patient will stop breathing.

_____ **5.** The chest cavity that is open to the atmosphere is referred to as a:
- **A.** flail chest.
- **B.** hemothorax.
- **C.** sucking chest wound.
- **D.** rib fracture.

_____ **6.** The treatment for a 22-year-old male who has sustained an open wound to the chest includes all of the following *except*:
- **A.** maintaining an open airway.
- **B.** binding the chest tightly.
- **C.** administering high-concentration oxygen.
- **D.** sealing the open wound.

_____ **7.** When air becomes trapped in the chest cavity, it can affect the body in all of the following ways *except* by
- **A.** putting pressure on the unaffected lung and heart.
- **B.** reducing cardiac output.
- **C.** affecting oxygenation of the blood.
- **D.** increasing the ventilatory volume of the chest.

_____ 8. The signs of pneumothorax or tension pneumothorax include all of the following *except*:
A. tracheal deviation to the uninjured side.
B. distended neck veins.
C. uneven chest wall movement.
D. increased depth of respiration.

_____ 9. Which of the following is *not* a sign of traumatic asphyxia?
A. Distended neck veins
B. Coughed-up, frothy blood
C. Head, neck, and shoulders that appear dark blue
D. Bloodshot and bulging eyes

_____ 10. When taping an occlusive dressing in place:
A. have the patient inhale as you tape.
B. have the patient exhale as you tape.
C. tape the dressing in place quickly because this is a life-threatening situation.
D. have the patient hold his or her breath.

_____ 11. An open wound to the abdomen that is so large and deep that organs protrude through the opening is called an:
A. impaled object.
B. evisceration.
C. avulsion.
D. amputated intestine.

_____ 12. The signs of an abdominal injury include all of the following *except*:
A. lacerations and puncture wounds to the lower back.
B. large bruises on the abdomen.
C. indications of developing shock.
D. contusions over the upper ribs.

_____ 13. Your 56-year-old male patient may have a GI bleed. Partially digested blood that is vomited looks like:
A. black and tarry material.
B. coffee grounds.
C. stained mucus.
D. meconium staining.

_____ 14. You are treating a 35-year-old female who fell and may have injured her abdomen. Which of the following is *not* a symptom of an abdominal injury?
A. Cramps
B. Nausea
C. Headache
D. Thirst

_____ 15. How would you consider positioning the patient described in multiple-choice question 14?
A. Prone, with her arms outstretched
B. Supine, with her legs flexed at the knees
C. In the left lateral recumbent position
D. Supine, with her legs straight

_____ 16. When covering an exposed abdominal organ, the EMT should apply a(n) _____ directly over the wound site.
A. plastic wrap from a sterile roll of Saran wrap
B. occlusive dressing that is warm and dry
C. sterile saline-moistened dressing and then an occlusive dressing
D. aluminum foil wrapping

_____ 17. Your patient is a 17-year-old lacrosse player who suddenly collapsed after being hit in the chest with the lacrosse ball. What is his likely condition?
A. Pneumothorax
B. Tension pneumothorax
C. Traumatic asphyxia
D. *Commotio cordis*

©2012 Pearson Education, Inc.
Emergency Care, 12th Ed.

_____ **18.** You are evaluating a 25-year-old male patient whose abdomen was slashed open. The treatment of an evisceration should *never* include:

    A. using an occlusive dressing.

    B. cutting away the clothing.

    C. replacing or touching the exposed organ.

    D. applying a sterile, saline-soaked dressing.

INSIDE/OUTSIDE: THE PATH OF THE BULLET

1. A patient has a gunshot wound in the lower rib with an exit at the same level in the back. Is it possible for this to be both a chest injury and an abdominal injury? If so, how?

2. Refer to the patient in Inside/Outside question 1. Is there a way in which the spleen or liver, which are abdominal organs, may have been injured?

COMPLETE THE FOLLOWING

1. Explain what the following injuries are:

    A. *Commotio cordis:* _____

    B. Cardiac tamponade: _____

    C. Traumatic asphyxia: _____

    D. Hemothorax: _____

    E. Pneumothorax: _____

STREET SCENES DISCUSSION

Review the Street Scene on page 694 of the textbook. Then answer the following questions.

1. In this case, the patient had a bleeding injury. If the patient had slashed her abdomen, how would you manage her?

2. Imagine that, after you controlled the bleeding, the patient became dizzy, weak, and very pale. What might you consider doing to help her?

3. If the patient had a penetrating chest injury, how would you manage her?

4. What should be your primary concern with the patient who has sustained an open injury to the chest wall?

30

Musculoskeletal Trauma

Standard: Trauma (Orthopedic Trauma)

Competency: Applies fundamental knowledge to provide basic emergency care and transportation based on assessment findings for an acutely injured patient.

▌OBJECTIVES

After reading this chapter you should be able to:

30.1 Define key terms introduced in this chapter.

30.2 Describe the anatomy of elements of the musculoskeletal system.

30.3 Associate mechanisms of injury with the potential for musculoskeletal injuries.

30.4 Describe the four types of musculoskeletal injury (fracture, dislocation, sprain, and strain) and define open and closed extremity injuries.

30.5 Discuss the assessment of musculoskeletal injuries, including compartment syndrome.

30.6 Discuss the general care of musculoskeletal injuries.

30.7 Discuss specific considerations for splinting.

30.8 Discuss considerations in the assessment and management of specific types of injuries, including:

   a. Shoulder girdle injuries
   b. Pelvic injuries
   c. Hip dislocation
   d. Hip fracture
   e. Femur shaft fracture
   f. Knee injury
   g. Tibia or fibula injury
   h. Ankle or foot injury

MATCH TERMINOLOGY/ DEFINITIONS

A. Tissues or fibers that cause movement of body parts and organs

B. The disruption or "coming apart" of a joint

C. An extremity injury in which the skin has been broken or torn through from the inside by an injured bone, or from the outside by something that has caused a penetrating wound with associated injury to the bone

D. A splint that applies constant pull along the length of the lower extremity to help stabilize the fractured bone and to reduce muscle spasms in the limb; this type of splint is used primarily on femoral shaft fractures

E. A grating sensation or sound made when fracture bone ends rub together

F. Tissue that binds muscles to bones

G. Any break in a bone

H. The portions of the skeleton that include the clavicles, scapulae, arms, wrists, and hands (upper extremities) and the pelvis, thighs, legs, ankles, and feet (lower extremities)

I. Tough tissue that covers the joint ends and bones and helps to form certain body parts such as the outer ear

J. Muscle injury caused by overstretching or overexertion of the muscle

K. The process of applying tension to straighten and realign a fractured limb before splinting; also called tension

L. Places where bones articulate, or meet

M. The stretching and tearing of ligaments

N. Connective tissues that connect bone to bone

O. An incomplete fracture

P. Fracture in which the broken bone segments are at an angle to each other

Q. An injury to an extremity with no associated opening in the skin

R. Hard but flexible living structures that provide support for the body and protection to vital organs

S. A fracture in which the bone is broken in several places

T. Injury caused when tissue such as blood vessels and nerves are constricted within a space from swelling or from a tight dressing or cast

_____ 1. Angulated fracture

_____ 2. Bones

_____ 3. Cartilage

_____ 4. Closed extremity injury

_____ 5. Comminuted fracture

_____ 6. Compartment syndrome

_____ 7. Crepitus

_____ 8. Dislocation

_____ 9. Extremities

_____ 10. Fracture

_____ 11. Greenstick fracture

_____ 12. Joints

_____ 13. Ligaments

_____ 14. Manual traction

_____ 15. Muscles

_____ 16. Open extremity injury

_____ 17. Sprain

_____ 18. Strain

_____ 19. Tendons

_____ 20. Traction splint

©2012 Pearson Education, Inc.
Emergency Care, 12th Ed.

MULTIPLE-CHOICE REVIEW

_____ 1. As we age, our bones become _____, resulting in bones that are more brittle and easy to break.
   A. deficient in magnesium
   B. deficient in calcium
   C. high in iron
   D. high in potassium

_____ 2. The strong white fibrous material covering the bones is called the:
   A. perineum.
   B. marrow.
   C. periosteum.
   D. shell.

_____ 3. Your patient is a 6-year-old who has a leg fracture. In children, the majority of the long bone growth occurs in the:
   A. bone marrow.
   B. growth plate.
   C. periosteum.
   D. growth shaft.

_____ 4. Musculoskeletal injuries are caused by direct, indirect, and _____ force.
   A. positive
   B. penetrating
   C. negative
   D. twisting

_____ 5. Fractures of the femur typically cause a _____-pint blood loss over the first 2 hours.
   A. 1
   B. 2
   C. 3
   D. 4

_____ 6. The death rate from closed fracture of the femur dropped from 80 percent to under 20 percent in the post–World War I period due to the invention of the:
   A. PASG.
   B. IV bag.
   C. traction splint.
   D. tourniquet.

_____ 7. Bone marrow is the site of production for which of the following?
   A. Calcium
   B. Protein
   C. Red blood cells
   D. Fat

_____ 8. The stretching or tearing of ligaments is called a:
   A. dislocation.
   B. fracture.
   C. sprain.
   D. strain.

_____ 9. A break in the continuity of the skin of a fractured extremity is considered a(n) _____ bone or joint injury.
   A. simple
   B. open
   C. closed
   D. grating

_____ 10. Your 19-year-old male patient fell while playing basketball. You suspect that he broke his right tibia. Proper splinting of a closed fracture is:
   A. done with an air splint and gentle traction.
   B. done with the pneumatic antishock garment.
   C. designed to prevent closed injuries from becoming open ones.
   D. completed in the hospital by a surgeon.

_____ 11. The signs and symptoms of a bone or joint injury include all of the following *except*:
   A. grating.
   B. swelling.
   C. vomiting.
   D. bruising.

_____ 12. Your 19-year-old female patient was snowboarding when she injured her right shoulder. It appears to be out of the socket and in an unusual position. When a joint is locked into a position like this, the EMT should:
   A. splint the joint in the position found.
   B. pull traction and straighten the joint.
   C. use a long backboard as a full body splint.
   D. disregard splinting and transport immediately.

_____ 13. Which procedure is done at least twice whenever a splint is applied?
   A. Elevation of the injured extremity
   B. Manual stabilization of the injured extremity
   C. Assessment for circulation, sensation, and motor function distal to the injury
   D. Application of gentle manual traction

_____ 14. You are treating a 22-year-old male who you suspect has sustained a fracture to his right forearm. The treatment of a possible fracture includes the steps below:
   1. Take Standard Precautions.
   2. Elevate the extremity.
   3. Splint the injury.
   4. Apply a cold pack.

   What is the correct order of the steps?
   A. 2, 3, 4, 1   **C.** 3, 2, 4, 1
   B. 1, 3, 2, 4   **D.** 1, 4, 2, 3

_____ 15. Your 52-year-old male patient stepped off the curb into the street when a large truck cut the corner too close and ran him over. He has numerous fractures and is in a lot of pain. Multiple fractures, especially of the _____, can cause life-threatening external and internal bleeding.
   A. radius   **C.** femur
   B. ulna   **D.** tibia

_____ 16. After splinting and treating the patient in multiple-choice question 15 for shock, you decide en route to the ED to apply cold, too. Applying cold packs to fractures:
   A. helps to reduce the swelling.
   B. stops bleeding from the bone.
   C. eliminates the need for a pressure bandage.
   D. stops all the pain and discomfort.

_____ 17. You are treating a 22-year-old female who fell off the roof of her house. Your primary assessment of this patient with multiple musculoskeletal injuries reveals that the patient is unstable; care should include all of the following *except*:
   A. manage the ABCs.
   B. immobilize the patient on a long spine board.
   C. transport the patient immediately.
   D. splint each injury individually.

_____ 18. You have a 22-year-old female who fell on an outstretched arm. A splint properly applied to a closed bone injury, such as a colles fracture, should help prevent all of the following *except*:
   A. damage to muscles, nerves, or blood vessels.
   B. an open bone injury.
   C. motion of bone fragments.
   D. circulation to the extremity.

_____ 19. Fracture management is not generally the highest priority compared to other problems identified during the primary survey of the patient. Fractures can introduce complications, however, which may include all of the following *except*:
   A. excessive bleeding.
   B. increased pain from movement.
   C. paralysis of the extremity.
   D. increased distal sensation.

_____ 20. Your 45-year-old female patient has a grossly deformed ulnar and radius fracture that will need to be properly splinted. The objective of realignment is to:
   A. minimize blood loss and reduce pain.
   B. immobilize the bone ends and adjacent joints.
   C. assist in restoring circulation and to fit the extremity into a splint.
   D. prevent incorrect healing and avoid surgery.

©2012 Pearson Education, Inc.
Emergency Care, 12th Ed.

_____ **21.** You are treating a 62-year-old female patient who fell down the basement stairs. She did not strike her head, but she is in a lot of pain from lower extremity fractures. There is a severe deformity of the right distal extremity, and it is cyanotic or pulseless. You should:
   A. align with gentle traction before splinting.
   B. apply a pillow splint to the extremity.
   C. delay splinting until you are en route to the hospital.
   D. contact medical direction immediately.

_____ **22.** What are the three basic types of splints?
   A. Rigid, formable, and traction
   B. PASG, board, and ladder
   C. Padded, soft, and anatomical
   D. Air, cardboard, and vacuum

_____ **23.** Which of the following is *not* true about rigid splints?
   A. They require that the limb be moved into anatomical position.
   B. They tend to provide the greatest support.
   C. They are ideally used to splint long bones.
   D. They can immobilize joint injuries in the position found.

_____ **24.** Your patient has a serious fracture to which you will be applying a traction splint. What is the bone that is most likely fractured?
   A. Pelvis   **C.** Femur
   B. Humerus   **D.** Clavicle

_____ **25.** When splinting the patient in multiple-choice question 24, the EMT should:
   A. first move the patient to a stretcher.
   B. leave any open leg wounds exposed so bleeding can be monitored.
   C. replace protruding bones as soon as priorities are arranged.
   D. secure the injury site and the joints above and below.

_____ **26.** Your 50-year-old female patient has sustained a fracture to her right tibia. To ensure proper stabilization and increase comfort when applying a rigid splint:
   A. place the patient on a stretcher before splinting.
   B. place the patient on a long spine board before splinting.
   C. pad the spaces between the body part and the splint.
   D. ensure that the splint conforms to the body curves.

_____ **27.** The method of splinting should be dictated by the:
   A. time when the injury occurred.
   B. severity of the patient's condition and the priority decision.
   C. distance to the destination hospital.
   D. presence or absence of pain.

_____ **28.** If you decide that the 35-year-old male patient you are treating for musculoskeletal injuries is unstable, you should do all of the following *except*:
   A. care for life-threatening problems first.
   B. align the injuries in an anatomical position.
   C. immobilize the entire body to a long spine board.
   D. apply two traction splints prior to securing the patient on a long spine board.

_____ **29.** Hazards of improper splinting include:
   A. aggravation of a bone or joint injury.
   B. reduced distal circulation.
   C. delay in transport of the patient with a life-threatening injury.
   D. all of these.

_____ **30.** You are treating a 35-year-old female who was the front-seat, unrestrained passenger in a rear-end collision. Her right tibia struck the lower dashboard of the car. If the lower leg is cyanotic or lacks a pulse when a knee joint injury is assessed, the EMT should:
   A. splint it in the position in which it was found.
   B. transport the patient to the hospital immediately.
   C. realign with gentle traction if no resistance is met.
   D. call for assistance from a paramedic unit.

_____ **31.** Examples of a bipolar traction splint include all of the following *except*:
   A. Hare®.   C. Fernotrac®.
   B. Sager®.   D. half-ring.

_____ **32.** The amount of traction that the EMT should pull when applying a Sager® traction splint is:
   A. enough until the patient verbalizes relief.
   B. about 10 percent of the patient's body weight up to 15 pounds.
   C. minimal because it doesn't require traction.
   D. about 15 percent of the patient's body weight up to 30 pounds.

_____ **33.** The indications for a traction splint are a possible mid-shaft femur fracture with:
   A. either knee or ankle involvement.   C. extensive blood loss.
   B. no joint or lower leg injury.   D. an open fracture.

_____ **34.** Whenever possible, _____ rescuers should be used to apply a traction splint.
   A. two   C. four
   B. three   D. five

_____ **35.** The 52-year-old male patient you are treating has multiple leg fractures and exhibits the signs of shock. You should:
   A. apply two traction splints and pull tension to 30 pounds.
   B. align in a normal position and transport on a backboard.
   C. apply PASG as a splint and treat for shock.
   D. apply a vacuum splint to each leg and transport quickly.

_____ **36.** You are treating a 19-year-old who twisted his left knee playing racquet ball. The signs and symptoms of a knee injury may include any of the following *except*:
   A. pain and tenderness.   C. deformity.
   B. swelling.   D. discoloration to the thigh.

_____ **37.** Elderly patients are more susceptible to _____ fractures because of brittle bones or bones weakened by disease.
   A. hip   C. heel
   B. tibia   D. spine

_____ **38.** You are treating a 68-year-old male who was found on the floor in the hallway at the county nursing home. You suspect that he may have had a syncopal episode and also sustained a fractured hip. This decision is based on the injured limb appearing:
   A. slightly swollen.   C. longer than the other extremity.
   B. shorter than the other extremity. D. mottled and cold.

_____ **39.** Your 36-year-old female patient had a serious fall. She is complaining of an unexplained sensation of having to empty her bladder. She may have experienced a _____ fracture.
   A. femur
   B. hip
   C. pelvic
   D. none of these

_____ **40.** Your 55-year-old female patient was crushed by a vehicle. You suspect that she may have a pelvic injury. When stabilizing her, you should do all of the following *except*:

    A. assume there is a spinal injury.

    B. determine distal function.

    C. apply PASG if the patient is hypotensive.

    D. raise the lower legs.

COMPLETE THE FOLLOWING

1. List eight signs and symptoms of musculoskeletal injury.

    A. _____

    B. _____

    C. _____

    D. _____

    E. _____

    F. _____

    G. _____

    H. _____

2. List eight signs and symptoms of a hip fracture.

    A. _____

    B. _____

    C. _____

    D. _____

    E. _____

    F. _____

    G. _____

    H. _____

LABEL THE DIAGRAM

Fill in the name of each bone on the line provided.

Skeletal System

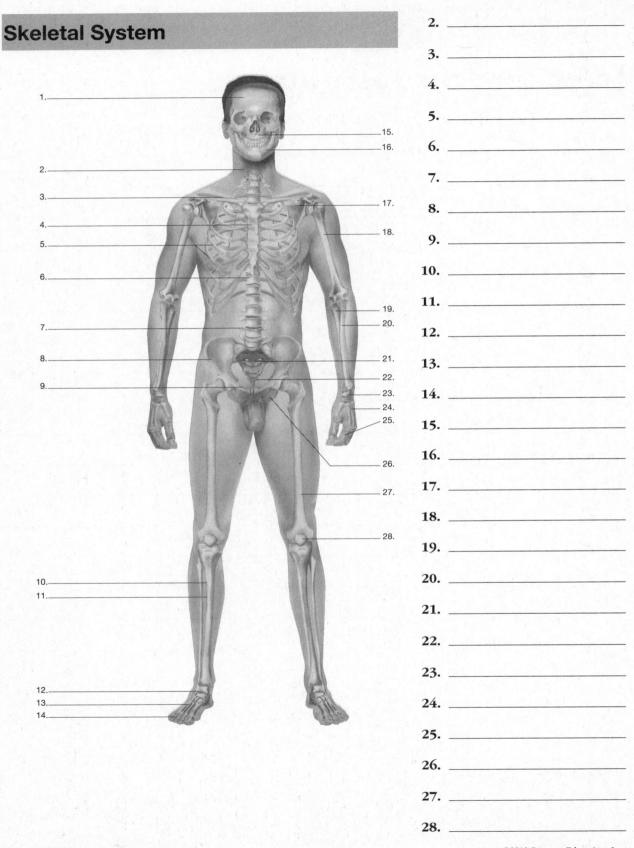

1. _____

2. _____

3. _____

4. _____

5. _____

6. _____

7. _____

8. _____

9. _____

10. _____

11. _____

12. _____

13. _____

14. _____

15. _____

16. _____

17. _____

18. _____

19. _____

20. _____

21. _____

22. _____

23. _____

24. _____

25. _____

26. _____

27. _____

28. _____

INSIDE/OUTSIDE: FRACTURE . . . OR NO FRACTURE?

1. Why do patients who experience a long bone fracture often experience shock?

   _____

2. Why should the EMT splint based on the suspicion of a fracture rather than actually confirming the presence of a fracture?

   _____

3. What is the significance of the swelling when a patient has a suspected fracture?

   _____

STREET SCENES DISCUSSION

Review the Street Scene on page 745 of the textbook. Then answer the following questions.

1. When the injured leg was examined, it was found to be swollen. If it had been an open fracture, what would you have observed?

2. Imagine that the patient is found lying on the ground with the injured leg grossly deformed in the mid-shaft area. Should you attempt to straighten it? Explain.

3. Suppose the patient does not have a distal pulse in the injured leg. What can you do?

4. Should you have called for ALS in this case?

EMT SKILLS
PERFORMANCE CHECKLISTS

▶ **REALIGNING AN EXTREMITY (PP. 709–710)**

❑ Take Standard Precautions.

❑ Assess distal circulation, sensation, and motor function.

❑ One EMT grasps the distal extremity while a partner places one hand above and one hand below the injury site.

❑ The partner supports the injury site while the first EMT pulls gentle manual traction in the direction of the long axis of the body. If resistance is felt or if it appears that bone ends will come through the skin, stop realignment and splint the extremity in the position found.

❑ If no resistance is felt, maintain gentle traction until the extremity is properly splinted.

❑ Reassess distal circulation, sensation, and motor function.

▶ **IMMOBILIZATION: LONG BONE (PP. 713–714)**

❑ Take Standard Precautions.

❑ Direct application of manual stabilization.

❑ Assess distal circulation, sensation, and motor function.

❑ Measure a splint.

❑ Apply the splint.

❑ Immobilize the joints above and below the injury.

❑ Secure the entire injured extremity from the distal to the proximal direction.

❑ Immobilize the hand or foot in a functional position.

❑ Reassess distal circulation, sensation, and motor function.

▶ **IMMOBILIZATION: JOINT (P. 715)**

❑ Take Standard Precautions.

❑ Direct application of manual stabilization of the injured extremity.

❑ Assess distal circulation, sensation, and motor function.

❑ Select the proper splinting device.

❑ Immobilize the site of injury and the bones above and below.

❑ Reassess distal circulation, sensation, and motor function.

▶ **IMMOBILIZATION: PELVIC FRACTURE SPLINTING (P. 720, 722)**

❑ Take Standard Precautions.

❑ Move the patient as little as possible. Never lift an unsupported patient. If you must log roll, gently roll onto the uninjured side when possible.

❑ Assess distal circulation, sensation, and motor function.

❑ Straighten the lower limbs into the anatomical position if there are no injuries to the hip joints and lower limbs and if it can be done without meeting resistance or causing excessive pain.

- Prevent additional injury by stabilizing the lower limbs. Place a folded blanket between the patient's legs, from the groin to the feet, and bind them together with wide cravats. The cravats can be adjusted for proper placement at the upper thigh, above the knee, and above the ankle.

- If permitted by local protocol, apply PASG to stabilize the pelvis in a patient with hypotension (BP below 90 mmHg).

- Assume that there are spinal injuries. Immobilize the patient on a long spine board. When securing the patient, avoid placing the straps over the pelvic area.

- Reassess distal circulation, sensation, and motor function.

- Care for shock, providing high-concentration oxygen.

- Transport the patient as soon as possible.

- Monitor vital signs.

► IMMOBILIZATION: TRACTION SPLINTING (PP. 710–714)

- Take Standard Precautions.

- Direct manual stabilization of the injured leg.

- Assess distal circulation, sensation, and motor function.

- Direct application of manual traction.

- Adjust and position the splint on the injured leg.

- Apply a proximal securing device (e.g., ischial strap).

- Apply a distal securing device (e.g., ankle hitch).

- Apply mechanical traction.

- Position and secure the support straps.

- Reassess distal circulation, sensation, and motor function.

- Secure the patient's torso and traction the splint to a long backboard for transport.

31

Trauma to the Head, Neck, and Spine

Standards: Trauma (Head, Facial, Neck, and Spine Trauma)

Competency: Applies fundamental knowledge to provide basic emergency care and transportation based on assessment findings for an acutely injured patient.

OBJECTIVES

After reading this chapter you should be able to:

31.1   Define key terms introduced in this chapter.

31.2   Describe the components and function of the nervous system and the anatomy of the head and spine.

31.3   Describe types of injuries to the skull and brain.

31.4   Describe the general assessment and management of skull fractures and brain injuries.

31.5   Describe specific concerns in management of cranial injuries with impaled objects.

31.6   Describe specific concerns in management of injuries to the face and jaw.

31.7   Define nontraumatic brain injuries.

31.8   Explain the purpose and elements of the Glasgow Coma Scale.

31.9   Discuss the assessment and management of open wounds to the neck.

31.10 List types and mechanisms of spine injury.

31.11 Discuss the assessment and management of spine and spinal cord injury.

31.12 Discuss issues in the immobilization of the head, neck, and spine, specifically for the following:

   a. Applying a cervical collar
   b. Immobilizing a seated patient, including rapid extrication for high-priority patients
   c. Applying a long backboard

©2012 Pearson Education, Inc.
Emergency Care, 12th Ed.

d. Rapid extrication from a child safety seat

e. Immobilizing a standing patient

f. Immobilizing a patient wearing a helmet

31.13 Discuss issues in selective spine immobilization.

MATCH TERMINOLOGY/ DEFINITIONS

A. The nerves that enter and exit the spinal cord between the vertebrae, 12 pairs of cranial nerves that travel between the brain and organs without passing through the spinal cord, and all of the body's other motor and sensory nerves

B. Mild closed head injury without detectable damage to the brain; complete recovery is usually expected

C. Provides overall control of thought, sensation, and the voluntary and involuntary motor functions of the body; the major components of the nervous system are the brain and the spinal cord

D. The cheek bone; also called the zygomatic bone

E. The bony bump on a vertebra

F. The bones of the spinal column (singular vertebrae)

G. The movable joint formed between the mandible and the temporal bones; also called the TMJ

H. The bony structure making up the forehead and the top, back, and upper sides of the skull

I. The fluid that surrounds the brain and spinal cord

J. In brain injuries, a bruised brain caused when the force of a blow to the head is great enough to rupture blood vessels

K. The brain and the spinal cord

L. Bone that forms part of the sides of the skull and floor of the cranial cavity

M. The bones that form the upper third, or bridge, of the nose

N. The bony structures around the eyes; the eye sockets

O. A state of shock caused by nerve paralysis that is sometimes caused by spinal injuries

P. Controls involuntary functions

Q. The lower jaw bone

R. In brain injuries, a cut to the brain

S. The opening at the base of the skull through which the spinal cord passes from the brain

T. Pressure inside the skull

U. The two fused bones forming the upper jaw

V. Pushing of a portion of the brain through the foramen magnum as a result of increased intracranial pressure

_____ **1.** Autonomic nervous system

_____ **2.** Central nervous system

_____ **3.** Cerebrospinal fluid (CSF)

_____ **4.** Concussion

_____ **5.** Contusion

_____ **6.** Cranium

_____ **7.** Dermatome

_____ **8.** Foramen magnum

_____ **9.** Hematoma

_____ **10.** Herniation

_____ **11.** Intracranial pressure (ICP)

_____ **12.** Laceration

_____ **13.** Malar

_____ **14.** Mandible

_____ **15.** Maxillae

_____ **16.** Nasal bones

_____ **17.** Nervous system

_____ **18.** Neurogenic shock

_____ **19.** Orbits

_____ **20.** Peripheral nervous system

_____ **21.** Spinous process

_____ **22.** Temporal bone

_____ **23.** Temporomandibular joint

_____ **24.** Vertebrae

W. In a head injury, a collection of blood within the skull or brain

X. An area of the skin that is innervated by a single spinal nerve

MULTIPLE-CHOICE REVIEW

_____ **1.** The function of the spinal column is to:
  A. produce cerebrospinal fluid.
  B. protect the spinal cord.
  C. allow for back movement in all directions.
  D. manufacture platelets.

_____ **2.** The spine is made up of _____ vertebrae.
  A. 35   C. 33
  B. 23   D. 38

_____ **3.** When a patient has a scalp injury:
  A. expect minimal bleeding.
  B. determine the wound depth.
  C. expect profuse bleeding.
  D. palpate the site with the fingertips.

_____ **4.** You are assessing a 22-year-old male who was involved in a bar fight earlier this evening. It is now 4 a.m. and the family called the ambulance because he has been vomiting. You notice he has a bruise behind the ear. This is called:
  A. Cushing's syndrome.
  B. raccoon eyes.
  C. Battle's sign.
  D. posturing syndrome.

_____ **5.** Further assessment of the patient in multiple-choice question 4 reveals that he also has discoloration of the soft tissues under both eyes. This finding is called:
  A. Cushing syndrome.
  B. raccoon eyes.
  C. Battle's sign.
  D. posturing syndrome.

_____ **6.** You suspect that your patient may have a traumatic brain injury. His signs and symptoms may include:
  A. blood or fluid flowing from the ears and/or nose.
  B. yellow discoloration in the eyes.
  C. bruising around the base of the nose.
  D. pain at the base of the neck.

_____ **7.** Skull or traumatic brain injury may result in:
  A. airway swelling and dizziness.
  B. altered mental status and unequal pupils.
  C. difficulty moving below the waist.
  D. headache and hypoperfusion.

_____ **8.** Which of the following is a late sign of skull or traumatic brain injury?
  A. Temperature increase
  B. Raccoon eyes
  C. Irregular breathing patterns
  D. Battle's sign

_____ 9. Which of the following is generally *not* a sign of traumatic brain injury, except in infants?
  A. Bleeding from the nose and ears
  B. Unequal pupils
  C. Hypoperfusion
  D. Seizures

_____ 10. What is the significance of an increase in carbon dioxide in the injured brain?
  A. It decreases the blood pressure.
  B. It causes brain tissue swelling.
  C. It raises the heart rate.
  D. It causes brain tissue shrinkage.

_____ 11. You are treating a 35-year-old female who failed to wear a helmet and struck her head when she fell off her bike. In most EMS systems, she would be taken to a trauma center if her Glasgow Coma Scale (GCS) score was less than:
  A. 8   C. 12
  B. 10   D. 15

_____ 12. You are treating a patient who has a steel rod penetrating the skull. You should:
  A. shorten lengthy objects, using any available tools.
  B. elevate the patient's legs immediately.
  C. remove the object and quickly control the bleeding.
  D. stabilize the object with bulky dressings.

_____ 13. You are treating a 19-year-old male who was in a fight. His face has multiple fractures, his nose is broken, and his jaw may be fractured. The primary concern for emergency care of a facial fracture or jaw injury is the:
  A. external bleeding.   C. loss of teeth.
  B. patient's airway.   D. basilar skull fracture.

_____ 14. You are treating a 35-year-old female who has an injury to one of her spinal vertebrae. Based on the frequency of injury, it is most likely one of the:
  A. lumbar and sacral.
  B. thoracic and cervical.
  C. coccygeal and thoracic.
  D. cervical and lumbar.

_____ 15. When the spine is excessively pulled, which commonly occurs during a hanging, this is called a(n) _____ injury.
  A. excessive rotation
  B. lateral bending
  C. distraction
  D. compression

_____ 16. On your size-up of an automobile collision, you notice that both sides of the windshield have a spider-web crack. It is wise to call for a backup ambulance because:
  A. every collision should have a two-ambulance response.
  B. patients hitting their heads on the windshield will be critical.
  C. both the driver and the passenger require spinal injury treatment.
  D. it takes four EMS personnel to properly immobilize one patient.

_____ 17. Which of the following would *not* create a high index of suspicion of a spine injury?
  A. Motor vehicle or motorcycle collisions
  B. Falls that cause open fractures to the ankles
  C. Trauma patients who are found unconscious
  D. A fall from two times the patient's height

_____ **18.** All of the following are examples of cervical-spine injuries that can result from a diving accident *except*:
   A. excessive extension.
   B. compression.
   C. excessive flexion.
   D. lateral bending.

_____ **19.** You are treating an approximately 20-year-old male trauma patient who was found unconscious at the bottom of a stairway. The unconscious trauma patient should be:
   A. treated as if he has a spine injury.
   B. rolled immediately to check for back injuries.
   C. placed in the recovery position.
   D. placed in a prone position for fluid to drain.

_____ **20.** Within moments of your arrival at the side of the patient described in multiple-choice question 19, he regains consciousness. The most reliable sign of spinal-cord injury in the conscious patient is:
   A. pain with movement.
   B. impaired breathing.
   C. tenderness on the spine.
   D. paralysis of the extremities.

_____ **21.** The patient does not complain of any spinal pain. It is important to remember that a lack of spinal pain does not rule out the possibility of spinal-cord injury because:
   A. spinal injuries seldom cause pain.
   B. other painful injuries may mask it.
   C. spinal injuries are not painful until shock sets in.
   D. a patient may feel the pain but cannot verbalize it.

_____ **22.** When assessing a suspected spine-injured patient, you note a reversal of the normal breathing pattern. This is likely a result of damage to the nerves that control the:
   A. rib cage.
   B. diaphragm.
   C. abdomen.
   D. lungs.

_____ **23.** If a patient is found on her back with arms extended above the head, this may indicate a _____ spine injury.
   A. thoracic
   B. lumbar
   C. sacral
   D. cervical

_____ **24.** You are treating a 52-year-old man who was involved in a serious high-speed collision. If the patient is up and walking around at the scene, you should:
   A. assess for a potential spinal injury.
   B. check with medical direction for orders.
   C. check with bystanders about the patient's mental status.
   D. assume that the patient is uninjured.

_____ **25.** If a responsive patient has the mechanism of injury for a spinal injury, the EMT should do all of the following *except*:
   A. assess for spinal pain by asking the patient to move.
   B. keep the patient still while asking him or her questions.
   C. assess for equality of strength in the extremities.
   D. assess for tingling in the extremities.

_____ **26.** After performing the primary assessment and rapid trauma exam on a spine-injured patient, your next step is to:
   A. determine the patient's priority.
   B. administer high-concentration oxygen.
   C. immobilize the patient on a long spine board.
   D. determine the mechanism of injury.

©2012 Pearson Education, Inc.
Emergency Care, 12th Ed.

_____ **27.** You are assessing a 27-year-old male who you suspect has a spine injury. If he complains of pain when you attempt to place his head in a neutral in-line position, you should:
  A. pad the neck before immobilizing.
  B. steady the head in the position found.
  C. continue with the stabilization procedure.
  D. contact medical direction immediately.

_____ **28.** When treating the patient in multiple-choice question 27, who you suspect has a spine injury, one EMT on your crew should:
  A. strap the patient's head, then the torso, to the long spine board.
  B. maintain constant manual in-line immobilization until the patient is secured to a backboard.
  C. assess for range of cervical spine motion.
  D. pad the neck before stabilizing.

_____ **29.** Which of the following statements about the rigid cervical collar is _false?_
  A. A collar of an incorrect size can hyperextend the neck.
  B. Maintain manual stabilization when applying a rigid cervical collar.
  C. The collar completely eliminates neck movement.
  D. The collar should never obstruct the airway.

_____ **30.** If a stable 22-year-old male patient is found in a sitting position on the ground and is complaining about back pain, the EMT should:
  A. apply a cervical collar and rapidly transport the patient.
  B. ask the patient to lie down, then immobilize.
  C. immobilize with a short spine board or extrication vest.
  D. perform a rapid take-down procedure with a long spine board.

_____ **31.** You are treating a 45-year-old male who was involved in a high-speed car crash. You have decided to use the rapid extrication technique, which is typically used in all of the following situations _except_ when
  A. moving a patient rapidly from an unsafe scene.
  B. a stable, low-priority patient must be immobilized.
  C. more seriously injured patients must be accessed.
  D. moving a high-priority patient.

_____ **32.** When immobilizing a 6-year-old or younger child on a long backboard:
  A. provide padding beneath the shoulder blades.
  B. it is unnecessary to apply a cervical collar.
  C. place a chin cup or chin strap on the patient.
  D. secure the head first and then secure the torso.

_____ **33.** Your patient is a 19-year-old male who was involved in a motorcycle crash. You should consider keeping the helmet on the patient:
  A. if it interferes with breathing management.
  B. if it has a snug fit that allows no head movement.
  C. by using a two-rescuer procedure.
  D. if it hinders immobilization.

_____ **34.** Which is the correct order of steps for applying a short spine immobilization device?
  1) Secure the device to the patient's torso.
  2) Secure the patient's head to the device.
  3) Position the device behind the patient.
  4) Evaluate torso fixation and pad behind the neck as necessary.
  A. 3, 2, 1, 4
  B. 3, 1, 4, 2
  C. 4, 3, 1, 2
  D. 3, 4, 1, 2

_____ **35.** Prior to and after immobilization, the EMT should assess:
   A. pulses in all extremities.
   B. motor function in all extremities.
   C. sensation in all extremities.
   D. all of these.

_____ **36.** You are treating a patient who fell backward and struck his head. You suspect that he is developing increased ICP. The time it takes to develop the symptoms from an increased ICP depend on:
   A. the rate of bleeding into the head.
   B. the location of the bleed.
   C. the age of the patient
   D. all of these are important factors.

_____ **37.** You are treating a 22-year-old male who was assaulted with a knife. The attacker slashed the patient's throat. Initially there was considerable blood, but you were able to control it and bandage the wound. The patient went into sudden cardiac arrest. What is the most likely cause?
   A. A stroke
   B. A heart attack
   C. An air embolism
   D. Infection from the wound

_____ **38.** Your patient fell down the stairs and may have injured his spine. Examples of findings that may lead you to consider a spine injury include all of the following *except*:
   A. the presence of priapism.
   B. the loss of bladder control.
   C. an increased pulse rate.
   D. nerve impairment to the extremities.

INSIDE/OUTSIDE: THREE EXAMPLES OF DYSFUNCTION FROM SPINAL INJURY

1. Your 35-year-old male patient was involved in a car crash and sustained an injury to the third, fourth, or fifth cervical vertebrae. He may have an injury to which nerve? What would be the effect on the patient?

_____

2. At a point in the development of the patient's injury in Inside/Outside question 1, the patient begins to exhibit hypotension. Why does this develop?

_____

3. Why doesn't the patient's pulse increase like that of most other patients who are in shock?

_____

COMPLETE THE FOLLOWING

1. List ten signs of a skull fracture or brain injury.

   A. _____

   B. _____

   C. _____

D. _____

E. _____

F. _____

G. _____

H. _____

I. _____

J. _____

2. List four types of traumatic brain injury (TBI).

A. _____

B. _____

C. _____

D. _____

LABEL THE DIAGRAM

Fill in the name of each division of the spine on the line provided.

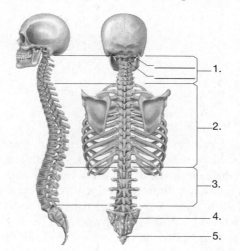

1. _____

2. _____

3. _____

4. _____

5. _____

STREET SCENES DISCUSSION

Review the Street Scene on page 790 of the textbook. Then answer the following questions.

1. Suppose that this patient had a lucid interval followed by decreasing mental status. What would be your highest priority in the treatment of this patient?

2. If the patient tells you he has no neck pain, why is it necessary to continue to immobilize him?

3. If the patient has a serious head injury, what would you expect to happen with his vital signs (provided he had no other injury)?

CASE STUDY

▶ **DEEP DIVE IN A SHALLOW POOL**

You respond to a call for an injury in a pool at a private residence in your district. The EMS dispatcher tells you they have received numerous 911 calls on this incident and they are trying to calm someone down to obtain better information. Fortunately, your EMS station is only about a mile from the location. As you pull up in front, you see lots of cars parked outside. A bystander runs up to the ambulance and says, "Please come quickly. He is still in the swimming pool. Can I help you carry anything?" Hearing this, you notify the dispatcher to continue the ALS unit and have the police respond also.

Both you and your partner are experienced swimmers. As you enter the backyard with your equipment, you ask her quickly, "Wet or dry?" She says, "Go. I'll take care of coordinating the poolside activities."

When you first see the patient, he is face up and being assisted in floating on his back by one other person in the pool, who states that his name is Bill. He says that he was a lifeguard 20 years ago. The patient is an adult male about 40 years old, and he is in about 5 feet of water. There is some blood in the pool from a large laceration to the patient's forehead.

You quickly empty your pockets, remove your shoes, hand the radio to your partner, and carefully enter the shallow end of the pool without making any waves. You also happen to notice that everyone has a soccer team shirt on.

1. What would you want to know about the patient from Bill right away?

2. How would you move the patient from the deep water to the shallow end of the pool?

Seeing that most of the adults are a bit intoxicated and most of the children at poolside are a bit small, you ask your partner to get an ETA on the backup unit. Just then, the members of the backup unit come walking into the backyard. There are two paramedics and an EMT who is a student in the paramedic course. You ask them to assist with the patient removal (if they are good swimmers).

3. What equipment will be needed?

In talking with Bill, you find that the party is a celebration for the children winning the soccer tournament. The patient, whose name is Tom, is the coach and apparently is not a drinker, so after two beers he did something he never would have done normally. Apparently, they were horsing around near the edge of the pool and he flipped head-first into the shallow end. The laceration was from striking his head. He was initially unconscious. Bill had entered the pool and carefully turned him over, as he was trained years ago to do, and Tom regained consciousness after a moment or two. Bill said that he did not believe Tom swallowed any water.

4. What other information should you obtain?

As one of the medics and the student enter the water with a long backboard and a rigid collar, you instruct Bill to continue to stabilize the patient's head and neck in a neutral position. You assist the patient in floating. The patient is very scared because he is unable to feel his arms or legs.

5. When the patient asks you what are you going to do, what should you tell him?

You carefully float the patient to the shallow end of the pool and do the immobilization there. The voids are padded, and the patient is strapped to the board. By this time, the police have arrived and have asked the soccer team members and their parents to move to the deck area and watch from there. Your partner has found two more helpers who are not intoxicated to assist in the lifting at poolside. Your in-water team lifts the immobilized patient onto the edge of the pool, and the out-of-water team carefully lifts the patient and backboard onto a stretcher.

6. What are some of the initial management steps your partner should take while you get out of the pool?

Once it is clear that your patient does not have any movement of his arms and legs, your partner and the paramedic call for a helicopter and ask the police to set up a landing zone. Fortunately, there is an elementary school with a large field about two blocks away. The patient will be going directly to the Regional Trauma Center, and a paramedic will be going along.

When the patient is loaded into your ambulance, the paramedic inserts an IV, the patient's clothing is cut off and he is covered with a blanket, the pulse oximeter is attached, and ECG electrodes are placed on him. His vital signs are still within normal range at this time.

After the patient and paramedic fly off in the helicopter, you look at your partner and say, "Can you imagine? Forty years old. Life can change so fast!" You talk about the call as you clean up back at the station. Although the situation is very sad, and life will change dramatically for the patient and his family, you are satisfied that the response, assessment, management, and teamwork went well. You and your partner agree that you will both stop at the hospital tomorrow to visit the patient. The report that was relayed back to you from the helicopter team was that the patient sustained a fracture of C-4, which severed his spinal cord.

7. Before handing in your PCR, is there anything that you should make sure is clearly documented? If so, what?

EMT SKILLS PERFORMANCE CHECKLISTS

▶ SPINAL IMMOBILIZATION: SEATED PATIENT (PP. 770–771)

❑ Take Standard Precautions.

❑ Direct assistant to manually stabilize the head in a neutral, in-line position.

❑ Assess distal circulation, sensory response, and motor function.

❑ Apply a rigid extrication collar of the correct size.

❑ Position the immobilization device behind the patient.

❑ Secure the device to the patient's torso.

❑ Evaluate and pad behind the patient's head as needed.

❑ Secure the patient's head to the device.

❑ Evaluate and adjust the straps.

❑ Secure the patient's wrists and legs and transfer to a long spine board.

❑ Reassess distal circulation, sensory response, and motor function.

▶ **SPINAL IMMOBILIZATION: SUPINE PATIENT (P. 777)**

❑ Take Standard Precautions.

❑ Direct assistant to place/maintain head in a neutral, in-line position and maintain manual stabilization until the patient is completely immobilized.

❑ Assess distal circulation, sensory response, and motor function.

❑ Apply a rigid extrication collar of the proper size.

❑ Position the immobilization device appropriately.

❑ Move the patient onto the device without compromising the integrity of the spine. Apply padding to the voids between the torso and the board as necessary.

❑ Immobilize the patient's torso to the device.

❑ Evaluate and pad behind the patient's head as necessary, or behind the shoulders with patients age 6 and under.

❑ Pad and immobilize the patient's head.

❑ Secure the patient's arms and legs to the board.

❑ Reassesses distal circulation, sensory response, and motor function.

▶ **RAPID TAKEDOWN OF STANDING PATIENT (PP. 781–783)**

STEP 1: RESCUERS GET IN POSITION

❑ Rescuer A: Get in position behind the patient and hold manual in-line stabilization of the head and neck. Maintain manual stabilization until the patient is completely immobilized on a long backboard.

❑ Rescuer B: Get in position in front of the patient. Explain the procedure so patient does not move.

STEP 2: ASSESS CSM AND APPLY A CERVICAL COLLAR

❑ Rescuer B: Quickly assess distal circulation, sensory response, and motor function in all four extremities.

❑ Rescuer B: Apply a rigid extrication collar of the correct size.

STEP 3: POSITION THE LONG BACKBOARD

❑ Rescuer B or C: Position the long backboard behind the patient, being careful not to disturb manual stabilization in any way.

❑ Rescuers B and C: Standing in front of patient and to each side, reach under the patient's armpit and grasp the backboard handhold at the level of the armpit or higher. Both rescuers must hold the same level.

❑ Rescuers B and C: Then place your other hand on the patient's upper arm, securing the patient to the backboard by holding his upper arm on the board.

STEP 4: SLOWLY LOWER THE PATIENT

❑ Rescuers B and C: Slowly lower the patient backward, communicating with Rescuer A behind the board so it is clear when the scapulae are beginning to rest on the board. Remember to lift with your legs, bending at the knees and not at the waist. Rescuer A gently allows the head to come back to the board as the shoulders come back.

❑ Once the patient's head is on the board, it is never lifted off the board again as Rescuer A kneels down at the patient's head.

❑ Reassess CSM when the patient is finally down.

STEP 5: SECURE THE PATIENT TO THE BACKBOARD

▶ RAPID EXTRICATION PROCEDURE FOR HIGH-PRIORITY PATIENTS (PP. 772–773)

STEP 1: PERFORM A PRIMARY ASSESSMENT

❑ Rescuer A: Maintain manual stabilization of the patient's head and neck.

❑ Rescuer B: Conduct a primary assessment of the patient and determine the need for rapid extrication based on patient status. Assess distal circulation, sensory response, and motor function in four extremities.

STEP 2: APPLY A CERVICAL COLLAR

❑ Rescuer B: Apply a cervical rigid collar of the correct size.

❑ Rescuer A: Continue to maintain manual stabilization before, during, and after application of the collar.

STEP 3: LIFT THE PATIENT AND POSITION THE LONG BACKBOARD

❑ Rescuer B: Hold the patient's armpit, and join hands with Rescuer C under the patient's thighs.

❑ Rescuer A: Call for a lift, while maintaining manual stabilization.

❑ Rescuer B: Lift patient approximately 1.5 to 2 inches (just enough) off the seat with Rescuer C.

❑ Bystander (or Fourth Rescuer): Insert a long backboard under the patient on the seat (and support the end of the board).

STEP 4: BEGIN TO POSITION THE PATIENT FOR EXTRICATION

❑ Rescuer B: Reach across the patient's chest and support by both armpits.

❑ Rescuer A: While maintaining manual stabilization, call for one-fourth turn, so the patient is moved perpendicular to the steering wheel, ready to exit the car head first.

❑ Rescuer C: Free the patient's lower legs from any obstructions.

❑ Rescuer B: Begin to turn the patient's back toward the door until Rescuer A says, "Stop turn."

❑ Rescuer A: Turn the patient. Call for "stop turn" just before being unable to hold the patient's head anymore.

❑ Rescuer C: Begin to turn the patient's back toward the door, freeing the legs, then sliding up to the thighs until Rescuer A says, "Stop."

STEP 5: COMPLETE ANOTHER ONE-QUARTER TURN

❑ Rescuer B: Stop move and wait for Rescuer C. Then take over manual stabilization of the head and neck from Rescuer A.

❑ Rescuer A: Maintain head/neck stabilization until Rescuer B takes over, allowing him or her to either exit the car and work from outside or reach over the seat from inside if there is room or if the roof has been removed.

❑ Rescuer C: Move hands from the thighs to the patient's armpits. Then replace Rescuer B.

❑ Rescuers A, B, and C: Complete another one-quarter turn.

STEP 6: LOWER THE PATIENT ONTO THE LONG BACKBOARD

❑ Rescuer B: Lower the patient onto the long backboard.

❑ Rescuer A: Call for the move to lower the patient's torso into a supine position onto the long backboard.

❑ Rescuer C: Lower the patient onto the long backboard.

❑ Bystander (or Fourth Rescuer): Stabilize the board.

STEP 7: POSITION THE PATIENT ON THE BACKBOARD

❑ Rescuer B: Slide the patient as a unit.

❑ Rescuer A: Call for the move to slide the patient toward the head end of the backboard. Once in position, tell partners to stop. Slide the chest as a unit.

❑ Rescuer C: Slide the pelvis as a unit until Rescuer A says, "Stop."

❑ Bystander (or Fourth Rescuer): Stabilize the head end of the long backboard.

STEP 8: SECURE THE PATIENT TO THE BACKBOARD

❑ Crew carefully strap the patient's torso first, head last, and then move the backboard to the stretcher.

❑ Reassess CSM.

▶ CHILD SAFETY SEAT IMMOBILIZATION: ASSESSMENT (PP. 779–780)

❑ Take Standard Precautions.

❑ EMT #1 gets in position or positions him- or herself behind the patient and holds manual in-line stabilization of the head/neck. This remains his or her job throughout the procedure.

❑ Based on the primary assessment and the patient's status, determine if the infant/toddler should be immobilized in the child safety seat or rapidly extricated from the seat.

❑ EMT #2 assesses distal circulation, sensation, and motor function in all four extremities before and after the immobilization.

▶ IMMOBILIZING THE PATIENT IN A CHILD SAFETY SEAT* (PP. 779–780)

❑ Take Standard Precautions.

❑ EMT #1: Stabilize the child safety seat in an upright position. Maintain manual head/neck stabilization of the head and neck throughout procedure until the patient is completely immobile.

❑ EMT #2: Prepare equipment. Apply a rigid extrication collar or improvise with a rolled hand towel for the newborn/infant.

❏ EMT #2: Place a small blanket or bath towel on the child's lap. Either strap or use wide tape to secure the pelvis and chest area to the seat.

❏ EMT #2: Place a towel roll on either side of the head to fill the voids. Tape the forehead in place. Then place tape across collar or maxilla. Avoid taping the chin, which would place pressure on the child's neck.

❏ EMT #1: Carry the child and seat to the ambulance and strap onto the stretcher with the stretcher head raised.

❏ Reassess distal circulation, sensation, and motor function.

▶ RAPID EXTRICATION FROM A CHILD SAFETY SEAT (PP. 779–780)

❏ Take Standard Precautions.

❏ EMT #1: Stabilize the child safety seat in the upright position. Maintain manual stabilization of the head and neck throughout the procedure until the patient is completely immobilized.

❏ EMT #2: Prepare the equipment. Loosen or cut the seat straps and raise the front guard.

❏ Apply the rigid extrication collar or improvise with a rolled hand towel in the newborn/infant.

❏ EMT #2: Place the child safety seat on the center of the long backboard and slowly tilt it back into a supine position, being careful not to allow the child to slide out of the chair. If the child has a large head, it is helpful to place a towel under the area where his or her shoulders will end up on the board.

❏ EMT #1: Call for a coordinated long-axis move onto the board.

❏ EMT #2: Grasp the chest and armpits with each hand and do a coordinated long-axis move onto the board. Make sure the child is positioned at the end of the board and not in the middle.

❏ EMT #2: Place a rolled blanket on each side of the patient.

❏ EMT #2: Strap the pelvis and upper chest to the board. Do not strap the abdomen down. Tape the lower legs to the board with wide tape.

❏ EMT #2: Place a towel roll on each side of the head to fill the voids. Tape the forehead in place. Then place the tape across the collar or the maxilla. Do not tape across the chin to avoid pressure on the child's neck.

*As long as the seat is not damaged.

32
Multisystem Trauma

Standard: Trauma (Multisystem Trauma)

Competency: Applies fundamental knowledge to provide basic emergency care and transportation based on assessment findings for an acutely injured patient.

OBJECTIVES

After reading this chapter you should be able to:

32.1   Define key terms introduced in this chapter.

32.2   Describe the considerations for teamwork, timing, and transport decisions in assessing and managing patients with multisystem trauma or multiple trauma.

32.3   Discuss the physiologic, anatomic, and mechanism of injury criteria for determining patient severity with regard to trauma triage and transport decisions.

32.4   Recognize special patient considerations that increase the patient's priority for transport, such as age, anti-coagulation bleeding disorders, burns, time-sensitive extremity injuries, end-stage renal disorders requiring dialysis, and pregnancy.

32.5   Discuss general principles of multisystem trauma management.

32.6   Describe the purposes of trauma scoring systems.

MATCH TERMINOLOGY/ DEFINITIONS

A. One or more injuries that affect more than one body system

B. A way of evaluating trauma patients according to a numerical rating system to determine the severity of the patient's trauma

C. More than one serious injury

_____ **1.** Multiple trauma

_____ **2.** Multisystem trauma

_____ **3.** Trauma score

MULTIPLE-CHOICE REVIEW

_____ 1. You were called to the scene of a motor vehicle collision where two cars collided in an intersection and one vehicle pinned a pedestrian, a 22-year-old male, against a telephone pole. The 22-year-old male patient has a fractured right leg and a suspected crushed pelvis. This would be called a _____patient.
  - **A.** lower extremity
  - **B.** multiple-trauma
  - **C.** shock
  - **D.** stable

_____ 2. The driver of one of the vehicles in multiple-choice question 1 is a 55-year-old female who has an obvious angulated forearm, and is unresponsive and lying across the front seat of her vehicle. What is the highest priority for her?
  - **A.** Splinting the arm
  - **B.** Immobilizing her neck
  - **C.** Managing her airway
  - **D.** Assessing distal pulses

_____ 3. At what point will the male patient described in multiple-choice question 1 most likely be considered stabilized?
  - **A.** At the emergency department
  - **B.** Once splints have been provided
  - **C.** In the surgical suite
  - **D.** Once the ALS has been called

_____ 4. To save the life of the critical patient in multiple-choice question 1, it will be important for the EMT to remember the three "Ts" in the management of a multiple-trauma patient. The three "Ts" are timing, transport, and:
  - **A.** teamwork.
  - **B.** trauma.
  - **C.** treatment.
  - **D.** thorax.

_____ 5. The guidelines for trauma triage and transport, as released by the Centers for Disease Control and Prevention, take into consideration each of the following factors _except_:
  - **A.** physiological determinants.
  - **B.** patient's sex.
  - **C.** MOI.
  - **D.** anatomic criteria.

_____ 6. A 25-year-old male trauma patient begins to make gurgling sounds as he breathes. What should you do?
  - **A.** Ventilate him.
  - **B.** Suction the airway.
  - **C.** Hyperextend the neck.
  - **D.** Apply oxygen with a nonrebreather mask.

_____ 7. Your 35-year-old female patient has numerous fractures in her legs from being run over by a pickup truck that cut the street corner too tight. Sometimes a_____can act as a full-body splint when the critical patient must be immobilized quickly.
  - **A.** wheeled stretcher
  - **B.** short KED
  - **C.** warm blanket
  - **D.** long backboard

_____ 8. Your 35-year-old female patient was changing her tire on a major highway when another vehicle ran into her and her vehicle. She has two fractured femurs, a crushed pelvis, and a possible abdominal injury. You should:
  - **A.** not apply a traction splint.
  - **B.** consider the PASG if your protocols allow.
  - **C.** set up an ALS intercept en route to the hospital.
  - **D.** do all of these.

_____ 9. You are treating the patient described in multiple-choice question 8 and have decided it is appropriate to minimize your scene care in accordance with your established protocols. You will most likely perform any or all of the following skills *except*:

A. suction the airway.

B. ventilate with a BVM.

C. bandage all of the lacerations.

A. immobilize the cervical spine.

_____ 10. Even when you are trying to limit on-scene time for a multiple-trauma patient, the one thing you do *not* leave out is:

A. applying traction splints if needed.

B. the secondary assessment.

C. ensuring scene safety.

D. immobilization to a long backboard.

_____ 11. An example of a patient who requires triage to a higher level of care would be the:

A. child with a headache after being struck by a golf ball.

B. geriatric patient who fell and is on anticoagulant medications.

C. adolescent with a femur fracture from playing basketball.

D. middle-aged man who may have fractured his forearm.

_____ 12. In some EMS systems, the EMTs are asked to assign a number to the severity of the trauma patient utilizing the trauma score. The scoring system for trauma patients also helps to:

A. allow the trauma centers to evaluate themselves.

B. determine which steps in the primary survey come first.

C. determine if a patient should go to a trauma center.

D. all of these.

INSIDE/OUTSID: INTERNAL INJURIES

1. A patient is exhibiting an elevated pulse, respiratory distress, and diminished or absent lung sounds on the left side of his chest after being stabbed with an ice pick in the left chest. You should suspect that he has sustained what type of injury on the "inside"?

2. A patient has audible lung sounds on both sides of the chest but has distended neck veins, a narrowing pulse pressure, and increased pulse and respiration. You should suspect that he has what type of injury on the "inside"?

COMPLETE THE FOLLOWING

1. List five examples of treatments that would be appropriate on the scene of a critical trauma patient.

A. _____

B. _____

C. _____

D. _____

E. _____

STREET SCENES DISCUSSION

Review the Street Scene on page 803 of the textbook. Then answer the following questions.

1. In this case, the use of rapid extrication seems appropriate, considering the mechanism of injury and the patient findings. But suppose the patient is alert, obviously pregnant, lying supine on the seat, and complaining of dizziness. Would rapid extrication still be appropriate? Explain.

2. Imagine that, after immobilizing the patient on a long backboard, she developed breathing difficulty due to blood in the airway. What might you consider doing to help her?

3. If the patient has a fractured femur, would a traction splint be appropriate?

4. What should be your concern for the other patients on the scene?

33
Environmental Emergencies

Standard: Trauma (Environmental Emergencies)

Competency: Applies fundamental knowledge to provide basic emergency care and transportation based on assessment findings for an acutely injured patient.

OBJECTIVES

33.1 Describe processes of heat loss and heat production by the body.

33.2 Recognize predisposing factors and exposure factors in relation to hypothermia.

33.3 Recognize signs and symptoms of hypothermia.

33.4 Describe the indications, contraindications, benefits, and risks of passive and active rewarming techniques.

33.5 Prioritize steps in assessment and management of patients with varying degrees of hypothermia.

33.6 Discuss assessment and management for early or superficial local cold injury and for late or deep local cold injury.

33.7 Discuss the effects of heat on the human body.

33.8 Differentiate between assessment and management priorities for heat emergency patients with moist, pale, normal-to-cool skin, and those with hot skin that is either dry or moist.

33.9 Anticipate the types of injuries and medical conditions that may be associated with water-related accidents. Discuss the assessment and management of the following water-related emergencies:

   a. Drowning (including rescue breathing and care for possible spinal injuries)
   b. Diving accidents
   c. Scuba diving accidents

33.10 Discuss the assessment and management of the following types of bites and stings:

    a. Insect bites and stings
    b. Snake bites
    c. Poisoning from marine life

MATCH TERMINOLOGY/ DEFINITIONS

▶ PART A

A. The change from liquid to gas; when the body perspires or gets wet, evaporation of the perspiration or other liquid into the air has a cooling effect on the body

B. An increase in the body temperature above normal; life-threatening in its extreme

C. Application of an external heat source to rewarm the body of a hypothermic patient

D. Carrying away of heat by currents of air or water or other gases or liquids

E. Generalized cooling that reduces body temperature below normal; life-threatening in its extreme

F. The transfer of heat from one material to another through direct contact

G. A condition resulting from nitrogen trapped in the body's tissues caused by coming up too quickly from a deep, prolonged dive; a symptom of this condition is "the bends," or deep pain in the muscles and joints

H. Application of heat to the lateral chest, neck, armpits, and groin of a hypothermic patient

I. The process of experiencing respiratory impairment from submersion/immersion in liquid, which may result in death, morbidity (illness or other adverse effects), or no morbidity

J. Gas bubble in the bloodstream; the more accurate term is arterial gas embolism (AGE)

    _____ **1.** Active rewarming

    _____ **2.** Air embolism

    _____ **3.** Central rewarming

    _____ **4.** Conduction

    _____ **5.** Convection

    _____ **6.** Decompression sickness

    _____ **7.** Drowning

    _____ **8.** Evaporation

    _____ **9.** Hyperthermia

    _____ **10.** Hypothermia

▶ PART B

A. Chilling caused by convection of heat from the body in the presence of air currents

B. Covering a hypothermic patient and taking other steps to prevent further heat loss and help the body rewarm itself

C. Sending out energy, such as heat, in waves into space

D. Breathing; during breathing, body heat is lost as warm air is exhaled from the body

E. Cooling or freezing of particular (local) parts of the body

F. A toxin (poison) produced by certain animals such as snakes, spiders, and some marine life forms

    _____ **1.** Local cooling

    _____ **2.** Passive rewarming

    _____ **3.** Radiation

    _____ **4.** Respiration

    _____ **5.** Toxins

    _____ **6.** Venom

    _____ **7.** Water chill

    _____ **8.** Wind chill

G. Substances produced by animals or plants that are poisonous to humans

H. Chilling caused by conduction of heat from the body when the body or clothing is wet

MULTIPLE-CHOICE REVIEW

_____ **1.** Heat will flow from a warmer material to a cooler one. Water conducts heat away from the body_____than still air.
  A. 25 times faster
  B. 25 times slower
  C. 50 times faster
  D. 50 times slower

_____ **2.** The body loses heat from respiration, radiation, conduction, convection, and:
  A. excretion.
  B. induction.
  C. evaporation.
  D. condensation.

_____ **3.** When there is_____wind, there is _____ heat loss.
  A. more; less
  B. less; greater
  C. more; greater
  D. no; maximum

_____ **4.** Most radiant heat loss occurs from a person's:
  A. arms and legs.
  B. chest and back.
  C. head and neck.
  D. feet and hands.

_____ **5.** You are treating a patient who you suspect may have been predisposed to hypothermia. The factors that could predispose your patient include all of the following _except_:
  A. burns.
  B. diabetes.
  C. spinal-cord injuries.
  D. headache.

_____ **6.** Which one of the following is _not_ a reason that infants and children are more prone to hypothermia?
  A. They have small muscle mass.
  B. They have large skin surface in relation to their total body mass.
  C. They are unable to shiver effectively.
  D. They have more body fat than adults do.

_____ **7.** You are treating a 58-year-old male patient with an open right tibia fracture. He was found lying on his cold garage floor by his son, who states, "He must have been lying there all night." You should also consider:
  A. stroke.
  B. hypothermia.
  C. pulmonary edema.
  D. hyperperfusion.

_____ **8.** You are treating a 68-year-old female who was found wandering around intoxicated on a cold evening. She did not have a coat on, and you determine her body temperature is below 90°F. With a core body temperature in this range, she:
  A. may be shivering uncontrollably.
  B. may no longer be shivering.
  C. will be pulseless.
  D. will suddenly become alert.

_____ **9.** All of the following are signs and symptoms of hypothermia _except_:
  A. high blood pressure and low pulse.
  B. stiff or rigid posture.
  C. cool abdominal skin temperature.
  D. loss of motor coordination.

_____ **10.** You are treating a 65-year-old male who stepped out of his house in his pajamas on a winter morning to grab the newspaper but ended up locking himself out of the house. He wandered around the neighborhood for 20 minutes, until he found a neighbor who would let him in and call 911 for help. Your protocol calls for passive rewarming of this patient. This procedure involves:
  A. applying heat packs to the patient.
  B. covering the patient.
  C. administering heated oxygen to the patient.
  D. massaging the patient's limbs.

_____ **11.** You are assessing a 22-year-old male patient who did not plan well and got caught outdoors in a cold rain for hours. He is alert and responding, but he is very cold and you suspect he may be hypothermic. His treatment may include all of the following *except*:
  A. removal of all the patient's wet clothing.
  B. actively rewarming the patient during transport.
  C. rapidly giving the patient plenty of hot liquids.
  D. providing care for shock and providing oxygen.

_____ **12.** You are actively rewarming a patient. If your Medical Director has authorized this treatment, you should:
  A. apply heat to the chest, neck, armpits, and groin.
  B. quickly rewarm the patient.
  C. give the patient stimulants to drink.
  D. immerse the arms and feet in hot water.

_____ **13.** Once the decision is made to rewarm a hypothermic patient, central rewarming should be used. The reason why you should rewarm the body's core first is to:
  A. prevent blood from collecting in the extremities due to vasodilation.
  B. quickly circulate cold blood throughout the body.
  C. speed up the blood flow to the extremities.
  D. increase blood flow to the brain to prevent unconsciousness.

_____ **14.** After checking the core body temperature for the patient in multiple-choice question 11, you determine he is in mild hypothermia. When transporting this alert patient, it is recommended that you:
  A. transport in Fowler position.
  B. massage his legs so he can walk to the ambulance.
  C. keep him at rest and avoid unnecessary exercise.
  D. leave his wet clothes in place to expedite transport.

_____ **15.** In a heat emergency, EMT care of a patient with moist, pale, normal-to-cool skin includes all of the following *except*:
  A. place the patient in an air-conditioned ambulance.
  B. fan the patient so he begins to shiver.
  C. elevate the patient's legs.
  D. administer oxygen.

_____ **16.** In a heat emergency, if a patient with moist, pale, normal-to-cool skin is responsive and not nauseated, the EMT should:
  A. skip the oxygen.
  B. place cold packs in the patient's armpits.
  C. have the patient drink water.
  D. do all of these.

©2012 Pearson Education, Inc.
Emergency Care, 12th Ed.

_____ 17. When treating the unresponsive hypothermia patient who is not responding appropriately:
A. keep the patient's head raised above the feet for transport to the hospital.
B. place the patient in a bath of warm for at least 20 minutes.
C. provide high-concentration oxygen that has been passed through a warm humidifier.
D. massage the extremities for 35 to 45 seconds.

_____ 18. You are treating a patient who was found by her mailbox in the snow. She may have slipped, fell on the ice, and struck her head because she is unconscious and very cold to the touch. Once in the ambulance, you check her core body temperature and it is below 80°F. Because patients with extreme hypothermia may not reach biological death for over 30 minutes, the medical philosophy is:
A. if there is a pulse, start CPR.
B. they are not dead until they're warm and dead.
C. resuscitate for no longer than 30 minutes.
D. always resuscitate very aggressively.

_____ 19. A cold injury usually occurring to exposed areas of the body that is brought about by direct contact with a cold object or exposure to cold air is called:
A. an early local cold injury.
B. a superficial late cold injury.
C. frostbite.
D. a deep local cold injury.

_____ 20. The skin color of a patient with a superficial local cold injury will change from _____ to _____.
A. red; white   C. red; blue
B. white; red   D. white; blue

_____ 21. Your 45-year-old female patient fell on an outstretched arm and sustained a fractured right radius and ulna. While waiting for help to arrive, the extremity was exposed and you suspect there is also a local superficial cold injury. You should:
A. splint and leave uncovered.
B. rub the extremity briskly.
C. not re-expose the injury to cold.
D. immerse the extremity in hot water.

_____ 22. If the muscles, bones, deep blood vessels, and organ membranes became frozen in the patient from multiple-choice question 21, this type of injury would be referred to as:
A. a superficial local cold injury.
B. frostnip.
C. a deep local cold injury.
D. local cooling.

_____ 23. In frostbite, the affected area first appears:
A. black and stiff.   C. red and blotchy.
B. white and waxy.   D. blue and abraded.

_____ 24. Do not allow the frostbite patient to smoke or drink alcohol because:
A. the patient may suffer altered mental status or fall asleep.
B. these substances stimulate the patient to move, which could cause further injury.
C. constriction of blood vessels and decreased circulation to the injured tissues may result.
D. either could contaminate the frostbitten area.

_____ 25. You are treating a patient who has local deep frostbite injuries to his fingers. You have contacted medical control and received permission to provide active rewarming of the frozen part(s). This procedure:
  A. is seldom recommended in the field.
  B. includes using very hot water.
  C. is performed without removing the patient's clothing.
  D. includes covering the patient's face.

_____ 26. When assessing an unconscious patient who you suspect is in extreme hypothermia, check the carotid pulse for _____ seconds.
  A. 5–10
  B. 15–25
  C. 30–45
  D. 50–60

_____ 27. The environment associated with hyperthermia includes heat and:
  A. high winds.
  B. light rain.
  C. high humidity.
  D. low humidity.

_____ 28. You hear on the news that today will be both a very hot and a very humid day. The higher the humidity is, the:
  A. less you perspire.
  B. less your perspiration evaporates.
  C. less you radiate heat.
  D. more you lose heat from your body.

_____ 29. The medical problems resulting from dry heat are often worse than those from moist heat because:
  A. dry heat is more common.
  B. moist heat tires people quickly.
  C. dry heat causes more sunburn.
  D. dry heat affects the respiratory system more quickly.

_____ 30. When salts are lost by the body through sweating, the patient may have all of the following _except_:
  A. muscle cramps.
  B. weakness or exhaustion.
  C. dizziness or periods of faintness.
  D. fluid buildup in the lungs.

_____ 31. You are treating a patient who was outside installing a new roof on a hot day. You suspect that he may have heat exhaustion and he is likely to have:
  A. dry, hot skin.
  B. moist, pale, normal-to-cool skin.
  C. a lack of sweating.
  D. a rapid, strong pulse.

_____ 32. The signs and symptoms of a heat emergency in patients who have hot, dry, or moist skin include:
  A. slow and shallow breathing.
  B. seizures.
  C. constricted pupils.
  D. muscle cramps.

_____ 32. When you are responding to a water-related emergency, the EMT should suspect each of the following situations in addition to a drowning _except_:
  A. substance abuse may have contributed to the incident.
  B. the patient may have sustained an internal injury.
  C. profuse perspiration is the likely cause.
  D. the patient may have struck his or her head or neck.

©2012 Pearson Education, Inc.
Emergency Care, 12th Ed.

_____ **34.** Which of the following is a large contributor to adolescent and adult drownings?
  A. Inexperience with equipment
  B. Substance abuse
  C. Stomach cramps
  D. Car crash immersions

_____ **35.** During a drowning submersion incident, water flowing past the epiglottis causes:
  A. a reflex to close the mouth.
  B. the patient to gasp for more air.
  C. a reflex spasm of the larynx.
  D. the patient to begin hyperventilating.

_____ **36.** About 10 percent of drowning submersion victims die from:
  A. too much fluid in their lungs.
  B. the lack of air.
  C. cervical spine injuries.
  D. crushing chest injury.

_____ **37.** You have been called to the river's edge, where a 19-year-old female has been pinned against a rock and some debris. If you are not an experienced swimmer, you should:
  A. never attempt to go into the water to do a rescue.
  B. don a flotation device prior to going into the water.
  C. use a boat as your first approach to conduct the rescue.
  D. coach the patient in floating techniques.

_____ **38.** You were called to a backyard swimming pool for a patient who was seen diving into the shallow end of the pool. There is a cut on his forehead and blood in the pool, and he is floating face up in the pool. If you suspect that this patient has a possible spine injury, you should:
  A. spineboard the patient as you pull him from the water.
  B. immobilize and spineboard the patient while he is still in the water.
  C. quickly remove the patient from the water to prevent hypothermia.
  D. encourage the patient to swim to the side of the pool.

_____ **39.** Two special medical problems seen in scuba diving accidents are decompression sickness and:
  A. carbon monoxide poisoning.
  B. oxygen toxicity.
  C. air embolism.
  D. arthritis.

_____ **40.** The risk of decompression sickness is increased by:
  A. air travel within 12 hours of a dive.
  B. breathing 100 percent oxygen immediately after the dive.
  C. drinking fluids before and after the dive.
  D. none of these.

_____ **41.** A toxin produced by some animals that is harmful to humans is called:
  A. poison.   C. venom.
  B. lymph.   D. allergen.

_____ **42.** Typical sources of injected poisons include _____ bites or stings.
  A. spider   C. snake
  B. scorpion   D. all of these

_____ **43.** While cleaning out the crawl space below the house, a 50-year-old female experienced blotchy skin, redness in her arm, weakness, and nausea. Her daughter has called the ambulance. After getting the history and doing an assessment, you believe it is possible that she:
  A. is developing heat stroke.
  B. was bitten by a poisonous spider.
  C. is having a diabetic reaction.
  D. is allergic to something in the air.

_____ **44.** You suspect that the patient from multiple-choice question 43 may have sustained an injected poisoning. The signs and symptoms include all of the following *except*:
  A. lack of sensation in one side of the body.
  B. puncture marks.
  C. muscle cramps, chest tightening, and joint pain.
  D. excessive saliva formation and profuse sweating.

_____ **45.** Just as you load the patient from multiple-choice question 43 into the ambulance, her daughter calls you back to the porch. Apparently a snake has crawled out into the sunshine, and you suspect that the patient has been bitten by that snake. You should do all of the following *except*:
  A. call for medical direction.
  B. clean the injection site with soap and water.
  C. remove rings, bracelets, or other constricting items on the bitten limb.
  D. capture the live snake and bring it in the ambulance to the emergency department.

_____ **46.** You have been called to the river's edge where a small craft will be meeting you with a patient on board. Apparently, a 28-year-old male was taking lessons in scuba diving and today was his checkout dive. The instructor tells you that his student was very nervous because all of his diving instruction has been in a swimming pool or shallow water. They were diving at an old shipwreck that is about 80 to 100 feet down. The patient got nervous and ascended way too fast. Which of the following signs and symptoms would *not* be likely in this patient?
  A. Frothy blood in the mouth or nose
  B. Inability to move both legs
  C. Blurred vision or convulsions
  D. Chest pain

_____ **47.** If the patient in multiple-choice question 46 has convulsions or lapses rapidly into unconsciousness leading to respiratory or cardiac arrest, you should suspect:
  A. decompression sickness.
  B. internal bleeding.
  C. that he was bitten by a large fish.
  D. that he may have an air embolism.

_____ **48.** The patient in multiple-choice question 46 is conscious and confused. He is experiencing personality changes and fatigue, and he is acting like he is intoxicated, although there is no way he could have taken anything. You should suspect:
  A. decompression sickness.
  B. a TIA.
  C. anaphylactic shock.
  D. hypoglycemia.

©2012 Pearson Education, Inc.
Emergency Care, 12th Ed.

INSIDE/OUTSIDES: HYPOTHERMIA AND HYPERTHERMIA

1. When the patient's skin is hot and the patient has a body temperature over 103°F, you should suspect that he has what problem on the "outside"?

2. The patient who is cold, has hypothermia, and exhibits an altered mental status on the "outside" most likely has what body temperature on the "inside"?

COMPLETE THE FOLLOWING

1. List six signs and symptoms of a heat emergency patient with moist, pale, and normal-to-cool skin.

   A. _____

   B. _____

   C. _____

   D. _____

   E. _____

   F. _____

2. List six signs and symptoms of a heat emergency patient with hot and dry or hot and moist skin.

   A. _____

   B. _____

   C. _____

   D. _____

   E. _____

   F. _____

3. List twelve signs and symptoms of an insect-, spider-, or scorpion-injected poisoning.

A. _____

B. _____

C. _____

D. _____

E. _____

F. _____

G. _____

H. _____

I. _____

J. _____

K. _____

L. _____

4. List five signs and/or symptoms of a snake bite.

A. _____

B. _____

C. _____

D. _____

E. _____

STREET SCENES DISCUSSION

Review the Street Scene on page 883 of the textbook. Then answer the following questions.

1. If the condition of the patient requires that you actively rewarm him, what should you do?

2. If the patient goes into cardiac arrest at the scene, should CPR be performed?

©2012 Pearson Education, Inc.
Emergency Care, 12th Ed.

3. Patients in hypothermia usually have a slow pulse. In this case, the vital signs showed tachycardia. What might this indicate in a patient?

CASE STUDY

▶ Too Cold for Comfort

You respond to a call for a child with an altered mental status in the backyard of a private residence. It is late in the afternoon on a windy day, so you grab your uniform jacket as you jump into the ambulance. On arrival, you are met by three children, ages approximately 9 to 12, who state that their little sister has been acting "funny." Their parent is at the store, and they called her on the cell phone. She was the one who called 911 and should be home momentarily.

Apparently the children have been practicing diving in the pool for the past 4 hours. The youngest child, Robin—a very thin, small 7-year-old—is sitting by the edge of the pool shivering.

1. What are your primary assessment concerns with the patient?

2. Is it necessary for you to wait until the parent arrives to question the children?

3. Besides obtaining a set of baseline vital signs, what additional history may be helpful to obtain?

Upon questioning, you find that Robin has not been playing as part of the group for at least the last hour. When you ask the children if they were cold, they say that they did not notice the temperature, just the wind, until a few minutes ago when the sun went down. They are also able to confirm that Robin has no medical history, takes no meds, has no allergies, and has not eaten since lunchtime. When you question Robin, it is clear that she is confused and shivering, cool to the touch, and breathing rapidly.

4. After ruling out trauma, you place the child on your stretcher. What would be the best position?

5. When the mother arrives, you advise her of your findings. She is in agreement that the child should be checked in the hospital. What do you suspect may be wrong with this child?

6. Would it be appropriate to administer oxygen to Robin?

7. If you took her temperature, what do you suspect you would find?

8. Why might this child be prone to hypothermia?

The parent tells you that the children are all very good swimmers and they are practicing for a diving competition. She ran out for only a half hour to go to the store. The children are quick to call her on the cell phone whenever there is a problem. She also says that she told them to get out of the pool before she left for the store.

9. When she asks you how a similar incident could be prevented in the future, what should you say?

EMT SKILLS PERFORMANCE CHECKLISTS

▶ **ACTIVE, RAPID REWARMING OF FROZEN PARTS (P. 809)**

❏ Take Standard Precautions.

❏ Conduct a primary assessment.

❏ Conduct secondary assessment and baseline vital signs.

❏ Consider administering oxygen by nonrebreather mask.

❏ Heat water to a temperature between 100°F and 105°F.

©2012 Pearson Education, Inc.
Emergency Care, 12th Ed.

- ❑ Fill a container with the heated water and prepare the injured part by removing clothing, jewelry, bands, and straps.

- ❑ Fully immerse the injured part. Do not allow the injured area to touch the sides or bottom of the container. Do not place any pressure on the affected part. Continuously stir the water. When the water cools below 100°F, remove the affected part and add more warm water. The patient may complain of moderate pain as the affected area rewarms or may experience some period of intense pain.

- ❑ If you complete rewarming of the part, gently dry the affected area and apply a dry sterile dressing.

- ❑ Place dry sterile dressings between the fingers and toes before dressing the hands and feet.

- ❑ Cover the site with blankets or whatever is available to keep the affected area warm. Do not allow these coverings to come in contact with the injured area or to put pressure on the site.

- ❑ Keep the patient at rest. Do not allow the patient to walk if a lower extremity has been frostbitten or frozen.

- ❑ Keep the entire patient warm.

- ❑ Continue to monitor the patient.

- ❑ Assist circulation according to local protocol. (Some systems recommend rhythmically and carefully raising and lowering the affected limb.)

- ❑ Do not allow the limb to refreeze.

- ❑ Transport the patient as soon as possible with the affected limb slightly elevated.

▶ WATER RESCUE—POSSIBLE SPINAL INJURY (PP. 824–826)

- ❑ Take Standard Precautions.

- ❑ Conduct a primary assessment.

- ❑ Splint the patient's head and neck with arms.*

- ❑ Roll the patient over into the supine position.

- ❑ Ensure airway and breathing. (*Note:* If the patient is not breathing, remove him or her from the water on a backboard as soon as possible.)

- ❑ Provide manual stabilization of the head and neck.

- ❑ Assess distal circulation, sensation, and motor function in all four extremities.

- ❑ Slide the backboard under the patient.

- ❑ Apply a rigid extrication collar of the correct size.

- ❑ Tie down the torso, then the head and neck with the straps.

- ❑ Float the board to the edge of the water.

- ❑ Remove the patient from the water with as much assistance as needed.

- ❑ Obtain baseline vital signs.

- ❑ Conduct a secondary assessment.

❑ Reassess distal circulation, sensation, and motor function in all four extremities.

❑ Administer oxygen, and prepare to transport the patient.

Safety Note: Unless you are a very good swimmer and trained in water rescue, do not go into the water to save someone.

▶ ASSESSMENT AND MANAGEMENT OF SUSPECTED AIR EMBOLISM OR DECOMPRESSION SICKNESS (P. 822)

❑ Take Standard Precautions.

❑ Conduct a primary assessment.

❑ Maintain an open and clear airway.

❑ Administer the highest possible flow and concentration of oxygen by non-rebreather mask.

❑ Conduct a secondary assessment and baseline vital signs.

❑ Rapidly transport all patients with possible air emboli or decompression sickness.

❑ Contact medical direction for specific instructions concerning where to take the patient. You may be sent directly to a hyperbaric trauma care center.

❑ Keep the patient warm.

❑ Position the patient either supine or on either side. Continue to monitor the patient. You may have to reposition the patient to ensure an open airway.

❑ Consider the need for consult with Diver's Alert Network (DAN) emergency number (919) 684-8111 or non-emergency number (919) 684-2948.

34

Obstetrics and Gynecologic Emergencies

Standards: Medicine; Special Patient Populations (Gynecology; Obstetrics)

Competency: Applies fundamental knowledge to provide basic emergency care and transportation based on assessment findings for an acutely ill patient.

Applies fundamental knowledge of growth, development, and aging and assessment findings to provide basic emergency care and transportation for a patient with special needs.

OBJECTIVES

After reading this chapter you should be able to:

34.1 Define key terms introduced in this chapter.

34.2 Identify the anatomy of the female reproductive system and fetal development.

34.3 Explain the physiology of pregnancy and childbirth.

34.4 Discuss anatomical and physiological differences between pregnant and nonpregnant women.

34.5 Explain supine hypotensive syndrome.

34.6 Take measures to prevent and correct supine hypotensive syndrome.

34.7 Given a scenario involving a pregnant patient, select the proper questions to ask in the history and the proper techniques of physical examination.

34.8 Given a scenario, identify the stage of labor associated with the patient's history, signs, and symptoms.

34.9 Incorporate therapeutic communication and awareness of the mother's emotional needs and cultural considerations into your assessment and management of a pregnant patient.

34.10 Identify complications of pregnancy requiring emergency care.

34.11 Provide emergency care for patients with pregnancy complications.

34.12 Demonstrate assessment and management of the pregnant trauma patient.

34.13 Anticipate complications in the pregnant trauma patient.

34.14 Identify indications of impending delivery.

34.15 Differentiate between patients who should be transported prior to delivery and those who should be prepared for field delivery.

34.16 Anticipate the potential need for neonatal resuscitation.

34.17 Demonstrate preparation for a field delivery.

34.18 Demonstrate techniques for assisting with uncomplicated field delivery.

34.19 Demonstrate techniques for managing complications of field delivery.

34.20 Recognize complications of delivery that require additional EMS resources or immediate transport to the hospital.

34.21 Discuss the dos and don'ts of assisting with both uncomplicated and complicated field delivery.

34.22 Demonstrate assessment of the newborn, including determining 1-minute and 5-minute APGAR scores.

34.23 Differentiate between newborns requiring routine care and those needing resuscitation.

34.24 Demonstrate routine care of a newborn.

34.25 Demonstrate techniques of neonatal resuscitation.

34.26 Determine priorities for caring for both the mother and newborn, recognizing indications of the need for additional resources and immediate transportation.

34.27 Assess and manage a patient with a gynecological emergency.

34.28 Identify the medical, legal, and psychosocial considerations in managing the patient who has been sexually assaulted.

MATCH TERMINOLOGY/ DEFINITIONS

▶ **PART A**

A. The baby appears head first during birth; the normal presentation for birth

B. The neck of the uterus at the entrance to the birth canal

C. Implantation of the fertilized egg is not in the body of the uterus, occurring instead in the oviduct (fallopian tube), cervix, or abdominopelvic cavity

D. The placenta, membranes of the amniotic sac, part of the umbilical cord, and some tissues from the lining of the uterus that are delivered after the birth of the baby

E. The baby as he or she develops in the womb

F. Spontaneous abortion

G. Expulsion of a fetus as a result of deliberate actions taken to stop the pregnancy

H. The sensation of the fetus moving from high in the abdomen to low in the birth canal

_____ **1.** Abortion

_____ **2.** Abruptio placentae

_____ **3.** Afterbirth

_____ **4.** Amniotic sac

_____ **5.** Breech presentation

_____ **6.** Cephalic presentation

_____ **7.** Cervix

_____ **8.** Crowning

_____ **9.** Eclampsia

_____ **10.** Ectopic pregnancy

I. Spontaneous (miscarriage) or induced termination of pregnancy

J. Three stages of the delivery of a baby that begin with the contractions of the uterus and end with the expulsion of the placenta

K. The "bag of waters" that surrounds the developing fetus

L. Amniotic fluid that is greenish or brownish-yellow rather than clear; an indication of possible maternal or fetal distress during labor

M. The buttocks or both legs of a baby deliver first during birth

N. An infant's limb protrudes from the vagina before the appearance of any other body part

O. Part of the baby is visible through the vaginal opening

P. More than one baby is born during a single delivery

Q. A severe complication of pregnancy that produces seizures and coma

R. A condition in which the placenta separates from the uterine wall; a cause of prebirth bleeding

_____ **11.** Fetus

_____ **12.** Induced abortion

_____ **13.** Labor

_____ **14.** Lightening

_____ **15.** Limb presentation

_____ **16.** Meconium staining

_____ **17.** Miscarriage

_____ **18.** Multiple birth

▶ **PART B**

A. When the umbilical cord presents first and is squeezed between the vaginal wall and the baby's head

B. Dizziness and a drop in blood pressure caused when the mother is in a supine position and the weight of the uterus, infant, placenta, and amniotic fluid compresses the inferior vena cava, reducing return of blood to the heart and cardiac output

C. Any newborn weighing less than 5½ pounds or born before the thirty-seventh week of pregnancy

D. Fallopian tube; tube that carries eggs from an ovary to the uterus

E. Born dead

F. The phase of the female reproductive cycle where an ovum is released from the ovary

G. Fetal structure containing the blood vessels that carry blood to and from the placenta

H. The birth canal

I. Condition in which the placenta is formed in an abnormal location (usually low in the uterus and close to or over the cervical opening) that will not allow for a normal delivery of the fetus

J. The female reproductive organ that produces ova

K. The muscular abdominal organ where the fetus develops; the womb

_____ **1.** Ovary

_____ **2.** Ovulation

_____ **3.** Oviduct

_____ **4.** Perineum

_____ **5.** Placenta

_____ **6.** Placenta previa

_____ **7.** Preeclampsia

_____ **8.** Premature infant

_____ **9.** Prolapsed umbilical cord

_____ **10.** Spontaneous abortion

_____ **11.** Stillborn

_____ **12.** Supine hypotensive syndrome

_____ **13.** Umbilical cord

_____ **14.** Uterus

_____ **15.** Vagina

L. When the fetus and placenta deliver before the twentieth-eighth week of pregnancy; commonly called a miscarriage

M. A complication of pregnancy where the woman retains large amounts of fluid and has hypertension; she may also experience seizures and/or coma during birth, which is very dangerous to both mother and infant

N. The surface area between the vagina and the anus

O. The organ of pregnancy where exchange of oxygen, foods, and wastes occurs between a mother and her fetus

MULTIPLE-CHOICE REVIEW

_____ **1.** The 9 months of pregnancy are divided into 3-month trimesters. During the second trimester, the:
  A. fetus is being formed and there is little uterine growth during this period.
  B. uterus grows very rapidly while the woman's blood volume, cardiac output, and heart rate increase.
  C. uterus is often seen reaching up to the epigastrium by this time.
  D. uterus develops to full size.

_____ **2.** The normal birth position is _____ and is called a _____ birth.
  A. head first; breech   **C.** feet first; breech
  B. head first; cephalic   **D.** feet first; cephalic

_____ **3.** The first stage of labor starts:
  A. with conception.
  B. at the 9-month point.
  C. with regular contractions of the uterus.
  D. when the cervix is dilated.

_____ **4.** The second stage of labor starts with the:
  A. birth of the baby.   **C.** delivery of the afterbirth.
  B. regular contractions of the uterus. **D.** entry of the baby into the birth canal.

_____ **5.** The third stage of labor begins:
  A. after the birth of the baby.   **C.** with dilation of the cervix.
  B. with delivery of the afterbirth. **D.** with full growth of the uterus.

_____ **6.** The third stage of labor is complete when:
  A. the baby is born.
  B. the afterbirth is expelled.
  C. 20 minutes have passed since the delivery.
  D. the uterus is firm again.

_____ **7.** The process by which the cervix gradually widens and thins out is called:
  A. delivery.   **C.** staining.
  B. dilation.   **D.** contraction.

_____ **8.** As the fetus moves downward and the cervix dilates, normally the amniotic sac breaks and fluid leaks out. If this fluid is greenish or brownish-yellow in color, this may indicate:
  A. fetal or maternal distress.
  B. the fetus is dead.
  C. the mother is pushing too hard.
  D. the amniotic sac broke too early.

©2012 Pearson Education, Inc.
Emergency Care, 12th Ed.

_____ 9. You are assisting in the delivery for a 22-year-old female who is about to have her third child. She states that she has had prenatal care and is not aware of any complications. The baby is due next week. There is greenish or brownish-yellow fluid being expelled from the amniotic sac. This is called _____ and could indicate_____.
   A. a bloody show; a normal delivery
   B. vena cava syndrome; that the mother is being stressed
   C. meconium staining; potential fetal distress
   D. amniotic bile; that the infant will be a diabetic

_____ 10. When the mother, who is in labor and whom you are assessing, suddenly states, "I need to go to the bathroom right now!" this most likely means that the:
   A. birth will be delayed.   C. birth moment is nearing.
   B. uterus is almost dilated.   D. baby is in distress.

_____ 11. You are treating an 18-year-old woman who is full-term and has labor pains. When timing the contraction duration, it should be timed from the:
   A. start of the pain until the delivery of the infant.
   B. beginning of the contraction to when the uterus relaxes.
   C. end of a contraction to the beginning of the next one.
   D. peak of the contraction to the end of the contraction.

_____ 12. You will also need to determine the contraction interval for the patient in multiple-choice question 11. The contraction interval, or frequency, is timed from the:
   A. start of one contraction to the start of the next.
   B. beginning of the contraction to when the uterus relaxes.
   C. peak of the contraction to the end of the contraction.
   D. start of the pain until the delivery of the infant.

_____ 13. Delivery is imminent when the contractions last _____ seconds and are _____ minutes apart.
   A. 15; 5 to 8   C. 45; 8 to 10
   B. 30; 2 to 3   D. 90; 5 to 8

_____ 14. The EMT's primary roles at a normal childbirth scene are to determine whether the delivery will occur at the scene and, if so, to:
   A. determine if the delivery can be delayed.
   B. assist the mother as she delivers the infant.
   C. carefully deliver the infant.
   D. immobilize the patient.

_____ 15. The sterile obstetrical kit does _not_ contain:
   A. a rubber bulb syringe for suctioning.
   B. several individually wrapped sanitary napkins.
   C. heavy flat twine to tie the cord.
   D. cord clamps or hemostats.

_____ 16. When you are evaluating the mother for a possible home delivery, you should ask:
   A. if pregnancy problems run in the family.
   B. the frequency and duration of contractions.
   C. if the mother feels she needs to urinate.
   D. the father's blood type and medical history.

_____ 17. An important part of your assessment of the woman who you suspect is going to deliver soon is to examine for crowning. It is important to ask the mother if you can examine for crowning if the mother:
   A. is straining during contractions.
   B. is in her ninth month of pregnancy.
   C. is pregnant for the first time.
   D. It is not important to ask permission to examine the mother.

_____ 18. You are treating a 25-year-old female who is 8 months pregnant. She states she has contractions every 15 minutes or so, which last for about 20 seconds. She is not exactly sure what labor pain is like because this is her first pregnancy. Her vital signs are pulse of 96, blood pressure of 130/70, and respirations of 22. What should you do next?
   A. Administer oxygen and transport immediately.
   B. Prepare for a home delivery immediately.
   C. Ask if her water broke and prepare for a quiet ride to the hospital.
   D. Tell her to call you back when the contractions are more frequent.

_____ 19. If you determine that the delivery is imminent based on the presence of crowning and other signs, you should:
   A. contact medical direction.
   B. transport as quickly as possible.
   C. ask the mother to go to the bathroom first.
   D. ask the mother to hold her legs closed.

_____ 20. When a full-term pregnant woman in a supine position complains of dizziness and you note a drop in her blood pressure, this could be due to a condition called _____ syndrome.
   A. diabetes mellitus   C. Cushing reflex
   B. supine hypotension   D. fluid retention

_____ 21. To counteract the pressure of the uterus on the inferior vena cava, you should:
   A. raise the patient's legs.   C. raise the patient's head.
   B. transport the patient on her left side. D. apply the PASG.

_____ 22. You are preparing for a home delivery for a 30-year-old woman who is full-term with her third child. During the delivery, the EMT will need all of the following infection control gear _except_:
   A. surgical gloves.   C. eye protection.
   B. a mask.   D. a Tyvek suit.

_____ 23. During the delivery, you should encourage the mother to:
   A. breathe rapidly and deeply.
   B. hold her breath every 2 minutes.
   C. close her mouth and breathe through her nose.
   D. breathe deeply through her mouth.

_____ 24. When supporting the baby's head during a delivery, the EMT should do all of the following _except_:
   A. pull on the baby's shoulders when they appear.
   B. apply gentle pressure to control the delivery.
   C. place one hand below the baby's head.
   D. spread fingers evenly around the baby's head.

_____ 25. You are assisting a 23-year-old female who is about to deliver. She states that her water did not break. If the amniotic sac has not broken by the time the baby's head is delivered, you should:
   A. stop the delivery and transport immediately.
   B. use your finger to puncture the membrane.
   C. contact medical direction immediately.
   D. delay the delivery until it breaks.

_____ 26. If you cannot loosen or unwrap the umbilical cord from around the infant's neck, you should:
   A. stop the delivery and transport immediately.
   B. tell the mother to push more forcefully.
   C. clamp the cord in two places and cut between the clamps.
   D. contact medical direction for advice.

©2012 Pearson Education, Inc.
Emergency Care, 12th Ed.

_____ **27.** Most babies are born:
  A. face down and then rotate to either side.
  B. face up and then rotate to either side.
  C. feet and buttocks first and do not rotate.
  D. face up and do not rotate.

_____ **28.** When suctioning a newborn:
  A. compress the bulb syringe while it is inside the baby's mouth.
  B. compress the bulb syringe before placing it in the baby's mouth.
  C. suction the nose and then the mouth.
  D. insert the syringe about 22 inches into the baby's mouth.

_____ **29.** Once the baby's feet are delivered:
  A. pick the baby up by the feet using a firm grasp.
  B. lay the baby on her side with her head slightly lower than her torso.
  C. lay the baby on her side and massage her back.
  D. pick the baby up by the feet and massage her back.

_____ **30.** To assess the newborn, the EMT should do all of the following _except_:
  A. note ease of breathing.
  B. check movement in the extremities.
  C. note skin coloration.
  D. check the response to a sternal rub.

_____ **31.** Why is it necessary to suction the baby's mouth before the nose?
  A. So the baby can gasp and begin breathing
  B. So the baby is stimulated to cry
  C. To prevent aspiration of materials from his mouth
  D. Because this will open the nasopharynx passageway

_____ **32.** If assessment of the infant's breathing reveals shallow, slow, or absent respirations, the EMT should:
  A. provide oxygen by nonrebreather mask.
  B. use a gentle but vigorous rubbing of the infant's back.
  C. provide artificial ventilations at 40 to 60 per minute.
  D. provide artificial ventilations at 20 to 30 per minute.

_____ **33.** In a normal birth, the infant must be breathing on her own:
  A. before you clamp and cut the cord.
  B. prior to transportation to the hospital.
  C. prior to considering ventilation.
  D. in order to use an oral airway.

_____ **34.** The first umbilical cord clamp should be placed about _____ inches from the baby.
  A. 4   **C.** 8
  B. 6   **D.** 10

_____ **35.** The second umbilical cord clamp should be placed about _____ inches from the baby.
  A. 3   **C.** 7
  B. 5   **D.** 9

_____ **36.** If the placenta does not deliver within _____ minutes of the baby's birth, transport the mother and baby to a medical facility without delay.
  A. 5   **C.** 15
  B. 10   **D.** 20

_____ **37.** During the delivery of a full-term newborn, the mother sustains a tear in her perineum. The EMT should:
  A. massage the uterus for at least 15 minutes.
  B. apply a sanitary napkin and gentle pressure.
  C. transport the patient on her left side immediately.
  D. contact medical direction immediately.

_____ **38.** You will be assisting in the delivery for a 22-year-old female who was told by her doctor that the child is in the breech position. Which of the following is an appropriate action to take for a breech presentation?
  A. Place the mother on her left side.
  B. Provide low-concentration oxygen.
  C. Pull on the baby's legs to deliver.
  D. Initiate rapid transport upon recognition.

_____ **39.** During the examination of a 26-year-old woman with labor pains, you see the umbilical cord presenting first. You should:
  A. gently push up on the baby's head or buttocks to take pressure off of the cord.
  B. use two gloved fingers to check the cord for a pulse and keep the cord cool.
  C. raise the mother's head and lower the buttocks to lessen pressure on the birth canal.
  D. attempt to push the cord back if it is not wrapped around the baby's neck.

_____ **40.** You are about to assist in the delivery for a full-term 22-year-old female. When you check for crowning, you do not see the head but you do see one foot. When a baby's limb presents first, the EMT should:
  A. push gently on the extremity to prevent it from advancing.
  B. pull gently on the limb to encourage delivery.
  C. administer low-concentration oxygen to the mother.
  D. begin rapid transport of the patient immediately.

_____ **41.** You are assisting in the delivery for a 28-year-old female who is full-term; this is her third child. She said that she had frequent prenatal visits and they told her that she may be having twins. When assisting with the delivery of twins:
  A. the afterbirth will be delivered after each individual infant.
  B. clamp the cord of the first baby before the second baby is born.
  C. labor contractions will stop after the first delivery.
  D. transport the mother immediately.

_____ **42.** Newly born infants lose heat rapidly. Heat loss not only affects their comfort but also can:
  A. increase their glucose level.
  B. affect their ability to carry oxygen in their blood.
  C. cause them to develop a fever.
  D. decrease their ability to shiver.

_____ **43.** When oxygen is administered to an infant, it should be given by:
  A. a nonrebreather mask.
  B. flowing it past the baby's face.
  C. a pediatric nasal cannula.
  D. a transport ventilator.

_____ **44.** If you suspect meconium staining when the infant is born:
  A. contact medical direction for advice.
  B. avoid stimulating the infant before suctioning the oropharynx.
  C. suction the nose, then the mouth.
  D. provide oxygen to the mother.

©2012 Pearson Education, Inc.
Emergency Care, 12th Ed.

_____ **45.** A condition in which the placenta is formed low in the uterus and close to the cervical opening, preventing the normal delivery of the fetus, is called:
A. abruptio placentae.   **C.** placenta toxemia.
B. stillborn birth.   **D.** placenta previa.

_____ **46.** You are treating a 22-year-old female who is 8 months pregnant and just had a seizure. Which one of the following is true of seizures in pregnancy?
A. They are usually associated with low blood pressure.
B. They tend to occur early in pregnancy.
C. They pose a threat to the mother but not the unborn baby.
D. They are usually associated with extreme swelling of the extremities.

_____ **47.** The greatest danger associated with blunt trauma to the pregnant woman's abdomen and pelvis is:
A. cramping abdominal pains.   **C.** massive bleeding and shock.
B. spontaneous abortion.   **D.** elevated blood pressure.

_____ **48.** Which one of the following is *true* about the physiology of a pregnant woman?
A. Vital signs may be interpreted as suggestive of shock when they are actually normal.
B. The pregnant woman has a pulse rate that is 10–15 beats per minute slower than the nonpregnant female.
C. A woman in later pregnancy may have a blood volume that is up to 48 percent lower than her nonpregnant state.
D. Assessing for shock is easier in the pregnant patient than it is in a nonpregnant patient.

_____ **49.** Unless a back or neck injury is suspected, all pregnant women who have suffered blunt trauma injury should be transported in the _____ position.
A. supine   **C.** Trendelenburg
B. left lateral recumbent   **D.** Fowler

_____ **50.** You are called to the scene of a 35-year-old woman who has a complaint of abdominal pain. She tells you that she also has unexpected vaginal bleeding. Which of the following is *true* of the treatment necessary for this patient?
A. Massage the abdomen vigorously.
B. Assume the woman is pregnant and transport.
C. Treat as if she has a potentially life-threatening condition.
D. Determine the cause before treatment is begun.

COMPLETE THE FOLLOWING

1. List seven things you should do when evaluating the woman in labor.

A. _____

B. _____

C. _____

D. _____

E. _____

F. _____

G. _____

2. List the six steps you should take when providing care for a woman who presents with a prolapsed cord.

A. _____

B. _____

C. _____

D. _____

E. _____

F. _____

3. Complete the following chart:

APGAR SCORE

	0	1	2
Appearance	Blue (or pale) all over	**(A)**	Pink all over
Pulse	0	<100	**(B)**
Grimace (reaction to suctioning or flicking of the feet)	**(C)**	Facial grimace	Sneeze, cough, or cry
Activity	No movement	**(D)**	Moving around normally
Respiratory effort	None	Slow or irregular breathing; weak cry	**(E)**

LABEL THE DIAGRAMS

Fill in the name of each structure of pregnancy on the line provided.

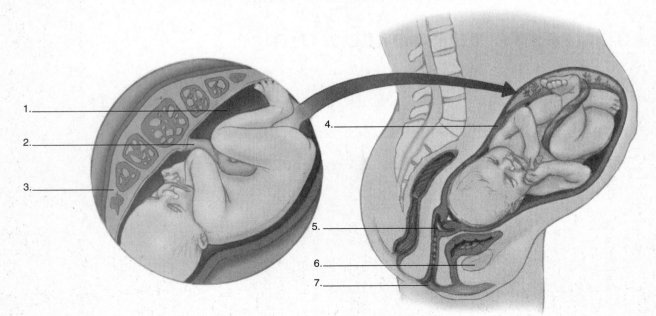

1. _____

2. _____

3. _____

4. _____

5. _____

6. _____

7. _____

©2012 Pearson Education, Inc.
Emergency Care, 12th Ed.

1. _____

2. _____

3. _____

4. _____

5. _____

6. _____

7. _____

INSIDE/OUTSIDE: PHYSIOLOGIC CHANGES OF PREGNANCY

1. For the pregnant woman who has a pink coloration to her skin, what is going on "inside" that this color relates to?

   _____

2. For the pregnant woman who has nausea, vomiting, and heartburn, what is going on "inside" that these conditions relate to?

   _____

3. In the woman who is in active labor when she has uterus contractions on the "inside," what would be observed on the "outside"?

   _____

4. If the woman who is in labor has a fetus that is not presenting its head first into the birth canal, what would the EMT observe on the "outside" of the patient?

   _____

STREET SCENES DISCUSSION

Review the Street Scene on page 875 of the textbook. Then answer the following questions.

1. Imagine that, when you observe crowning, you also observe that the amniotic sac is intact. What should you do?

2. When the amniotic fluid is expelled from the bag, you notice that it is dark green. What is this called? What does it indicate? What should you do about it?

3. Suppose that, after delivery of the placenta, you observe that the mother is continuing to bleed excessively. Is there anything you can do to help her?

EMT SKILLS PERFORMANCE CHECKLIST

▶ **EVALUATING THE MOTHER FOR IMMINENT DELIVERY (PP. 845–847)**

❑ Take Standard Precautions.

❑ Conduct a primary assessment.

❑ Obtain the mother's history to determine active labor. History includes:

- Length of pregnancy
- Number of previous pregnancies and births
- If the "bag of waters" has broken
- Frequency and duration of uterine contractions
- Recent vaginal discharge or hemorrhage
- If she is straining or feels the urge to move her bowels

❑ With the mother's permission, examine her for crowning.

❑ Feel for uterine contractions when she says that she is having a contraction.

❑ Take another set of vitals and make the decision to prepare for a delivery or to begin transport.

35

Pediatric Emergencies

Standard: Special Patient Populations (Pediatrics)

Competency: Applies fundamental knowledge of growth, development, and aging and assessment findings to provide basic emergency care and transportation for a patient with special needs.

▌ OBJECTIVES

After reading this chapter you should be able to:

35.1 Define key terms introduced in this chapter.

35.2 Describe the anatomic and physiologic characteristics of infants and children compared to adults and the implications of each for assessment and care of the pediatric patient.

35.3 Discuss the normal vital signs ranges for infants and children.

35.4 Adapt history-taking and assessment techniques to patients in each pediatric age group.

35.5 Discuss special considerations in dealing with adolescent patients.

35.6 Discuss the importance of involving caretakers in the assessment and emergency care of pediatric patients and anticipate reactions of parents and caregivers in response to an ill or injured child.

35.7 Discuss the use of the pediatric assessment triangle in assessing pediatric patients.

35.8 Explain special aspects of the steps of assessment for pediatric patients, including the scene size-up, primary assessment, secondary assessment with physical exam, and reassessment.

35.9 Demonstrate adaptations to techniques and equipment to properly manage the airway, ventilation, and oxygenation of pediatric patients.

35.10 Compare and contrast the causes, presentation, and management of shock in pediatric and adult patients.

©2012 Pearson Education, Inc.
Emergency Care, 12th Ed.

341

35.11 Recognize the particular concern for preventing heat loss in pediatric patients.

35.12 Recognize the signs, symptoms, and history associated with common pediatric medical emergencies, including:

    a. Difficulty breathing
    b. Croup
    c. Epiglottitis
    d. Fever
    e. Meningitis
    f. Diarrhea and vomiting
    g. Seizures
    h. Altered mental status
    i. Poisoning
    j. Drowning
    k. Sudden infant death syndrome (SIDS)

35.13 Discuss injury patterns common in pediatric trauma patients.

35.14 Discuss care for burns in pediatric patients.

35.15 Recognize indications of child abuse and neglect, and explain your ethical and legal responsibilities when you suspect child abuse or neglect.

35.16 Manage pediatric special needs patients, including those dependent on tracheostomy tubes, home artificial ventilators, central intravenous lines, gastrostomy tubes, and shunts.

MATCH TERMINOLOGY/ DEFINITIONS

A. Child from 3 to 6 years of age

B. Pulling in of the skin and soft tissue between the ribs when breathing; typically a sign of respiratory distress in children

C. Child from 12 to 18 years of age

D. Child from 6 to 12 years of age

E. Child from 1 to 3 years of age

F. Of or pertaining to a patient who has yet to reach puberty

G. Child between birth and 1 year of age

H. A soft spot on the infant's anterior scalp formed by the joining of not-yet-fused bones of the skull

_____ **1.** Adolescent

_____ **2.** Fontanelle

_____ **3.** Newborn or infant

_____ **4.** Pediatric

_____ **5.** Preschooler

_____ **6.** Retractions

_____ **7.** School-aged child

_____ **8.** Toddler

MULTIPLE-CHOICE REVIEW

_____ **1.** When a child is considered a toddler, his age group is between _____ year(s).

    A. birth and 1
    B. 1 and 3
    C. 3 and 6
    D. 6 and 12

_____ **2.** When a child is considered school age, her age group is between _____ years.

    A. 1 and 3
    B. 3 and 6
    C. 6 and 12
    D. 12 and 18

©2012 Pearson Education, Inc.
Emergency Care, 12th Ed.

_____ **3.** Which of the following is *not* appropriate when assessing a toddler?
   A. Have the child sit on the parent's lap.
   B. Avoid lying to the patient.
   C. Explain what you are doing.
   D. Perform the head exam first.

_____ **4.** Until about age 4, a child's head is proportionately _____ than the adult's.
   A. smaller and lighter
   B. smaller and heavier
   C. larger and heavier
   D. larger and lighter

_____ **5.** The soft spot on an infant's skull is called a:
   A. croup.
   B. fontanelle.
   C. depression.
   D. shunt.

_____ **6.** You are assessing an infant who has an altered level of consciousness. You notice that she has a sunken fontanelle, which may be an indication of:
   A. dehydration.
   B. rising intracranial pressure.
   C. external hemorrhage.
   D. hypertension.

_____ **7.** You are assessing an infant who was found by a caregiver lying on the floor. You notice that there is a bulging fontanelle, which may be an indication of:
   A. dehydration.
   B. elevated intracranial pressure.
   C. external hemorrhage.
   D. hypertension.

_____ **8.** You are treating a newborn baby who may have had a seizure. When evaluating the respirations, it is important to remember that newborns usually breathe:
   A. over 60 times a minute.
   B. less than 8 times a minute.
   C. through their mouths.
   D. through their noses.

_____ **9.** You find that it is necessary to do a manual maneuver to help keep the airway open in the infant you are treating. As opposed to treating an adult patient, in an infant, hyperextension of the neck:
   A. is necessary to open the airway.
   B. may result in obstructing the airway.
   C. is necessary if trauma is suspected.
   D. is a procedure reserved for respiratory distress.

_____ **10.** If the EMT suctions the unresponsive child's airway for longer than a few seconds at a time, this will most likely lead to:
   A. gag reflex activation.
   B. vagus nerve stimulation.
   C. airway blockage.
   D. cardiac arrest.

_____ **11.** The tongues of infants and children are more likely than an adult's to fall back into and block the airway because their tongues are:
   A. proportionately larger than an adult's.
   B. larger than an adult's.
   C. proportionately smaller than an adult's.
   D. smaller than an adult's.

_____ **12.** You are treating a 5-year-old child who fell off a small bike and struck his head. He is unconscious, and you will need to open his airway and insert an oropharyngeal airway (OPA). The insertion procedure for an OPA in a child this age is performed:
   A. much more quickly than in an adult.
   B. with the tip pointing toward the tongue and throat.
   C. the same way it is done for adults.
   D. without inserting a tongue depressor.

_____ **13.** When assessing the capillary refill of the child in multiple-choice question 12, peripheral perfusion is considered satisfactory if the color returns in less than _____ seconds.

A. 2   **C.** 4
B. 3   **D.** 5

_____ **14.** You suspect that your 3-year-old patient may be developing a partial airway obstruction. You carefully open the airway and assess the ventilations. Which of the following is *not* a sign of a partial airway obstruction in an infant or a child?

A. Normal skin color
B. Adequate peripheral perfusion
C. Noisy breathing (stridor and crowing)
D. Loss of consciousness

_____ **15.** Your patient was playing in the sandbox with other children when suddenly he seemed to be in distress. There is a good possibility he may have swallowed part of a small toy. Signs of a severe partial airway obstruction or complete airway obstruction in an infant or a child include all of the following *except*:

A. cyanosis.   **C.** crying or coughing.
B. altered mental status.   **D.** inability to speak.

_____ **16.** The effects of hypoxia on an infant or a child are:

A. slowed heart rate and improved mental status.
B. increased heart rate and decreased mental status.
C. slowed heart rate and altered mental status.
D. increased heart rate and coma.

_____ **17.** You decide it will be necessary to begin ventilations on the 5-year-old you are treating. All of the following are appropriate guidelines to follow when ventilating the infant or child *except*:

A. avoid breathing too hard through the pocket face mask.
B. avoid using excessive bag pressure and volume.
C. use a properly sized mask to ensure a good mask seal.
D. omit the use of infection control barriers.

_____ **18.** To ventilate the child in multiple-choice question 17, you decide to use a manual bag mask device with supplementary oxygen rather than the flow-restricted, oxygen-powered ventilation device (FROPVD). The FROPVD is:

A. used with caution in an infant.
B. contraindicated in infants and children.
C. preferred during the resuscitation of a child.
D. used only with the pop-off valve engaged in children.

_____ **19.** Common causes of shock in infants and children include:

A. allergic reactions.
B. diarrhea and/or vomiting that results in dehydration.
C. poisoning.
D. cardiac events.

_____ **20.** Less common causes of shock in a child include all of the following *except*:

A. allergic reactions.   **C.** poisoning.
B. cardiac events.   **D.** croup.

_____ **21.** The blood volume of infants and children is approximately _____ percent of the total body weight.

A. 6   **C.** 10
B. 8   **D.** 12

©2012 Pearson Education, Inc.
Emergency Care, 12th Ed.

_____ **22.** When children are in shock, they do all of the following *except*:
   A. compensate for a long time.
   B. appear better than they actually are.
   C. decompensate very rapidly.
   D. decompensate very slowly.

_____ **23.** You are managing a 7-year-old child who fell onto his abdomen, and you suspect he may be bleeding internally. You should avoid:
   A. administering too much oxygen.
   B. transporting too quickly.
   C. waiting for signs of decompensated shock before treating for shock.
   D. placing the child in the Trendelenburg position if respiratory distress is not evident.

_____ **24.** Decreased urine output and absence of tears are signs of _____ in infants and children.
   A. epiglottitis   **C.** hypothermia
   B. shock   **D.** croup

_____ **25.** When treating a child in shock, unless there are injuries that would contraindicate it, the EMT should:
   A. lower the patient's legs.   **C.** have the patient sit up.
   B. elevate the patient's legs.   **D.** have the patient lie supine.

_____ **26.** Because children have a large skin surface area in proportion to their body mass, they can easily become victims of:
   A. hypothermia.   **C.** airway obstruction.
   B. high fever.   **D.** hypovolemia.

_____ **27.** If a child has an airway respiratory disease, it is very important that the EMT avoid:
   A. opening the airway.
   B. inserting a tongue blade into the mouth.
   C. positioning the child in the parent's lap.
   D. administering blow-by oxygen.

_____ **28.** The signs of an airway disease in a child include all of the following *except*:
   A. stridor on inspiration.   **C.** rapid breathing.
   B. breathing effort on exhalation. **D.** wheezing.

_____ **29.** A viral illness that causes inflammation of the upper airway and bronchi, which is often accompanied by a "seal bark" cough, is called:
   A. bronchitis.   **C.** croup.
   B. asthma.   **D.** epiglottitis.

_____ **30.** You are assessing a pediatric patient who you suspect is exhibiting the early signs of respiratory distress. Of the following signs you observe, which would you *not* expect to see in the early phase of respiratory distress?
   A. Nasal flaring   **C.** Grunting
   B. Slow or irregular respiratory rate   **D.** Use of abdominal muscles

_____ **31.** You are treating a toddler who has been irritable all morning. His mother believes he has been running a fever but does not have a thermometer in the house. Causes of fever in children include all of the following *except*:
   A. upper respiratory infection.   **C.** pneumonia.
   B. hypothermia.   **D.** infection.

_____ **32.** In the out-of-hospital setting, which of the following is the most appropriate manner to determine an infant's skin temperature?
   A. Ungloved hand
   B. Rectal thermometer
   C. Oral thermometer
   D. Pulse oximeter

_____ **33.** When treating an infant or a child who you suspect has a high fever, you should:
   A. submerge the patient in cold water.
   B. use rubbing alcohol to cool the patient.
   C. monitor for shivering while cooling with tepid water.
   D. cover the patient with a towel soaked in ice water.

_____ **34.** Infants are more susceptible to _____ because, compared to adults, a greater percentage of their body is water.
   A. shock   **C.** high fever
   B. dehydration   **D.** all of these

_____ **35.** Which of the following is _false_ regarding seizures in the pediatric patient?
   A. Seizures require medical evaluation.
   B. Seizures should be considered life-threatening.
   C. Seizures are rarely caused by fever.
   D. Seizures may be a sign of an underlying condition.

_____ **36.** Severe aspirin poisoning in children can cause all of the following _except_:
   A. seizures.   **C.** coma.
   B. dehydration.   **D.** shock.

_____ **37.** A common cause of lead poisoning in children is:
   A. ingesting or licking chips of lead-based paint.
   B. chewing on pencils.
   C. drinking water from a well.
   D. eating fish from freshwater lakes.

_____ **38.** You are treating a 5-year-old child who accidentally ingested a handful of her mother's vitamin tablets, thinking they were candy. Should you be concerned?
   A. No. The body eliminates excess vitamins.
   B. No. The child will just have diarrhea for a few days.
   C. Yes. Many vitamin pills contain iron, which can be fatal to a child.
   D. Yes. Adult vitamins are too concentrated for children.

_____ **39.** The majority of meningitis cases occur between the ages of 1 month and:
   A. 6 months.   **C.** 3 years.
   B. 1 year.   **D.** 5 years.

_____ **40.** You respond to a private residence early in the morning. The parents are very upset because they went to wake up their infant and she was not breathing. In cases of sudden infant death syndrome, the EMT should:
   A. not deliver care and transport immediately.
   B. pronounce the infant's death.
   C. look for evidence of child neglect.
   D. provide resuscitation and transport.

_____ **41.** The number one cause of death in infants and children is:
   A. respiratory arrest.   **C.** cardiac arrest.
   B. trauma.   **D.** child abuse.

_____ **42.** The child who has been struck by a vehicle may present with a triad of injuries that include head injury, lower extremity injury, and _____ injury.
   A. chest   **C.** abdominal
   B. neck   **D.** upper extremity

_____ **43.** You are treating a 7-year-old child who was not wearing a helmet and skied off the trail into a tree. He struck his head. Which of the following is _true_ of a head-injured child?
   A. The most frequent sign is altered mental status.
   B. Respiratory arrest is a common secondary effect.
   C. Suspect internal injuries whenever the patient presents with shock.
   D. All of these are true.

©2012 Pearson Education, Inc.
Emergency Care, 12th Ed.

_____ **44.** Because the musculoskeletal structures of the chest are less developed in infants and children:
  A. they are able to maintain rapid respiratory rates for a long time.
  B. they are more likely than adults to fracture their ribs.
  C. the chest is less easily deformed.
  D. they are more likely to incur injury to structures beneath the ribs.

_____ **45.** Because the abdominal muscles of infants and small children are immature, they:
  A. have less visible signs of breathing difficulty.
  B. use their chest muscles for breathing.
  C. have less protection for underlying organs.
  D. rarely have distention of the abdomen.

_____ **46.** You are treating a school-age child who was critically burned when experimenting with a chemistry set in his basement. The guidelines for managing pediatric burn patients include all of the following *except*:
  A. use the rule of nines to estimate the extent of burns.
  B. identify candidates for transportation to burn centers.
  C. cover the burn with sterile dressing.
  D. keep the patient cool to reduce pain.

_____ **47.** You are treating a 6-year-old female who shows indications that child abuse may be a contributing factor in the "accident" that occurred today. Evidence of child abuse can include all of the following *except*:
  A. repeated responses to provide care for the same child or family.
  B. poorly healing wounds or improperly healed fractures.
  C. indications of past injuries.
  D. a parent who seems concerned about the child's injuries.

_____ **48.** When you respond to the home of a person whom you think may be a child abuser, look for all of the following *except*:
  A. a family member who has trouble controlling anger.
  B. indications of alcohol and drug abuse.
  C. torn clothing on the child.
  D. any adult who appears in a state of depression.

_____ **49.** Aside from assessment and management of the injuries sustained in the patient in multiple-choice question 47, which of the following is *not* part of your role when child abuse is suspected?
  A. Control your emotions and hold back accusations.
  B. Gather information from parents/caregivers away from the child.
  C. Talk to the child separately and ask her if she has been abused.
  D. Report your suspicions of abuse to the emergency department.

_____ **50.** When treating a child who you suspect is suffering from epiglottitis, it is important to:
  A. immediately transport the child.
  B. not place anything in the child's mouth.
  C. constantly monitor the respiratory status.
  D. do all of these.

_____ **51.** The primary cause of cardiac arrest in children is:
  A. electrocution.   **C.** respiratory disorders.
  B. drowning.   **D.** meningitis.

_____ **52.** You are assessing a 6-year-old patient who fell off his bike. He was not wearing his helmet and has a bruise on the forehead. His mother is now at the scene and is helping to hold him still. In assessing breathing, you should observe all of the following *except*:
  A. the emotional state.   **C.** the effort of breathing.
  B. chest expansion.   **D.** sounds of breathing.

_____ 53. You determine that the child in multiple-choice question 52 is verbally responsive but confused, and his lips are cyanotic. His capillary refill takes 3 seconds, and his respiratory rate is slightly over 30 per minute. What care should this child receive?
   A. Bag-valve-mask device ventilations and an OPA
   B. Spinal immobilization
   C. Assistance with an epinephrine self-injector
   D. An albuterol treatment

_____ 54. Why would it be appropriate to identify the patient in multiple-choice question 52 as a priority patient?
   A. He is unconscious.
   B. He did not wear a helmet.
   C. He may be suffering from shock and altered level of consciousness.
   D. He was riding a bike.

INSIDE/OUTSIDE: AIRWAY POSITION

1. How can the EMT compensate for the 4-year-old child's proportionately larger head when immobilizing the neck?

_____

2. How can the EMT compensate for the 4-year-old child's flexible trachea when opening the airway?

_____

INSIDE/OUTSIDE: PEDIATRIC HYPOVOLEMIC SHOCK

1. When the body of a child who is losing blood starts to compensate, what happens on the "inside"?

_____

2. What happens on the "outside" of the child's body when compensating for blood loss?

_____

INSIDE/OUTSIDE: RESPIRATORY DISTRESS VS. RESPIRATORY FAILURE

When a child has an airway or breathing problem, he or she will begin to compensate for the problem.

1. What happens on the "inside" during respiratory distress?

_____

2. What happens on the "outside" during respiratory distress?

_____

3. What happens on the "inside" during respiratory failure?

_____

4. What happens on the "outside" during respiratory failure?

_____

COMPLETE THE FOLLOWING

List ten signs of respiratory distress in a child.

A. _____

B. _____

C. _____

D. _____

E. _____

F. _____

G. _____

H. _____

I. _____

J. _____

COMPLETE THE CHART

Fill in each numbered box to complete the chart.

Artificial Ventilation (Rescue Breathing)

	Puberty and Older	Over Age 1 to Puberty	Birth to 1 Year
Ventilation Duration	1.	2.	3.
Ventilation Rate	4.	5.	6.

STREET SCENES DISCUSSION

Review the Street Scene on page 929 in the textbook. Then answer the following questions.

1. The mother reported seeing her child "shake." What do you suppose happened to this child?

2. This child's mental status improved. Suppose it had not improved, and the child was warm to the touch and had a rash. What Standard Precautions would be appropriate?

3. Why would it be important for you to follow up on the hospital admission of this child?

CASE STUDY

▶ THE CASE OF THE POISONED JUICE

You are dispatched to a community childcare center that called 911 because a number of the children suddenly became ill after lunch. On arrival, you determine that the scene is safe to enter and size up the situation. There are at least six children of different ages, ranging from infant to 6 years old, who have become nauseated after drinking apple juice that was left over from a few days ago. They are vomiting and complaining of stomach cramps. You have decided to call for an ALS unit and another BLS unit for backup at this time.

1. What Standard Precautions should you take?

2. How could you prepare for additional patients with the assistance of the childcare workers?

As your crew begins to evaluate each of the children, the childcare supervisor notifies you that all the parents of the sick children have been called. It appears that all of the children are in various stages of vomiting and most also have diarrhea. Initial assessment doesn't reveal any patients who are high priority except one infant who normally requires special care.

3. What can be a complication of children who are vomiting and suffering from diarrhea?

4. The infant who receives special care is normally healthy except that she is closely watched because she has had a shunt installed since birth. What is a shunt? Why are shunts used frequently in infants?

The other ambulances arrive. The decision is made to immediately transport the infant with the shunt as a high priority and call for an additional ambulance to respond to the scene. Each of the EMTs begins obtaining complete sets of vital signs on the remaining children. Most of the 60 children in the childcare center are being evaluated for complaints and a full set of vitals; a prehospital care report has been completed on each child. Most of the children are not sick; however, you notice a trend of "sympathy" pains from children who could not possibly have had a drink from the contaminated can of juice.

5. What would be the normal vital signs to expect from the infants?

6. What would be the normal vital signs to expect from the toddlers?

7. What would be the normal vital signs to expect from the preschoolers?

8. As you examine the infants, are there any assessment strategies that would be helpful?

9. As you examine the toddlers, are there any assessment strategies that would be helpful?

10. As you examine the preschoolers, are there any assessment strategies that would be helpful?

When the parents arrive, some of them decide to sign the appropriate documentation and to take their children to their pediatricians. Eight other parents have agreed to be transported with their children to the local hospital so the children can be examined further in the emergency department.

11. For the infants and toddlers who are being transported by ambulance, what is the safest way to transport them provided they are stable and their parents are nearby to assist?

12. For the infants being transported by ambulance, what is the best way to determine their level of responsiveness with the assistance of their parents?

13. One of the paramedics suggests taking a sample of the juice that all the children drank. Why might this be helpful?

▶ ABUSER OR LOVING PARENT?

You respond to a call for a motor vehicle collision at an intersection. A police officer explains that two cars were involved and that car 1 did not stop at the stop sign and broadsided car 2. The driver of car 1, a middle-aged man, is limping outside his vehicle. He says that he has no injury but appears to be very anxious about the damage to the side of his new car. The driver of car 2 is sitting in the front seat of her car and consoling her toddler, who is still crying. Both the mother, who appears to be approximately 20 years old, and her young son have lacerations to the front of their heads and blood stains on the front of their clothing. As you approach the vehicle, you note that there are two spider-web cracks in the windshield, one in front of the driver's seat and the other in front of the passenger seat.

1. At the scene of an automobile collision in an intersection, what is your greatest scene-safety hazard?

2. Is there a need for another ambulance at the scene? Why or why not?

After taking Standard Precautions, you approach car 2 and begin your assessment of the mother and child. You notice there is no car seat in the vehicle. After introducing yourself, you explain to the mother that she should keep her head and neck still and that your partner would like to do the same for her child. She cooperates because she is concerned that her son has become a little confused since he smashed his head on the windshield.

3. Aside from manual stabilization of the head and neck, what are your initial concerns for the assessment of the child?

4. You note that the child is no longer crying and does not seem to care that you are evaluating him. Is this a significant finding? Explain.

5. Aside from AVPU, how else can you determine if the toddler's mental status is "normal"?

6. What is the significance of the cracks in the car's windshield to the patient assessment process?

7. When you ask the mother if the child was restrained, she says, "He does not like the belt and there is no way I can keep him still enough to sit in a special seat." What is the significance of this statement in relation to the child's current mental status?

During your assessment, you note that the inside of the vehicle smells like "cheap wine" and the mother is acting as if she is intoxicated. When you assess the mother, you ask if she has eaten this afternoon or had anything to drink. She says that she was upset today and had a few glasses of wine, but begs you not to tell the police officers. By this time, her child has been immobilized and is being placed into the ambulance by your partner and the First Responders. You proceed to immobilize the mother in the seated position with a vest-style immobilization device because her baseline vital signs are all normal and her other injuries are minor. The child, on the other hand, is being closely monitored because he has already vomited twice. You and your partner decide to go to the hospital as soon as the mother is loaded.

8. Should oxygen be administered to the child?

9. Would it be appropriate to set up an ALS intercept en route to the hospital?

After arrival at the hospital, while you are cleaning up your equipment, the emergency department physician comes out to talk to you. He says that the child did not have a spine injury but the head trauma was serious.

10. What should you say if he asks you how this incident and the child's injuries could have been prevented?

EMT SKILLS
PERFORMANCE CHECKLIST

▶ THE PEDIATRIC PHYSICAL EXAMINATION* (PP. 892–896)

❑ Examine the head for D-CAP-BTLS. Look for blood or clear fluid draining from the nose and ears. Palpate gently for soft or spongy areas, skull irregularities, or crepitus. Check the fontanelle in infants.

❑ Check the eyes. The pupils should be equal in size and react to light.

❑ Examine the neck. Check for D-CAP-BTLS, equal chest rise and fall, and crepitus.

❑ Examine the chest. Check for D-CAP-BTLS, equal chest rise and fall, and crepitus. Watch for signs of difficulty breathing.

❑ Auscultate for breath sounds over all lung fields. While examining the chest, be aware of the contents of the thorax.

❑ Examine the abdomen. Check for D-CAP-BTLS and guarding. Look for swelling that may indicate swallowed air. Divide the abdomen into quadrants and examine each one, while remembering which organs are located in each quadrant.

❑ Examine the pelvis for D-CAP-BTLS and crepitus. If the patient complains of pain, injury, or other problems in the genital area, assess that area for bruising, swelling, or tenderness.

❑ Examine the extremities for D-CAP-BTLS and crepitus. Evaluate for distal circulation, sensory function, motor function, and warmth. Look for unequal movement.

❑ If you have immobilized an extremity, check capillary refill and peripheral pulses, comparing them with the opposite arm or leg.

❑ Examine the back and buttocks for D-CAP-BTLS and crepitus. If the child requires immobilization, the back can be checked while the child is being log-rolled onto the long backboard.

*Conduct toe-to-head on toddlers.

©2012 Pearson Education, Inc.
Emergency Care, 12th Ed.

36
Geriatric Emergencies

Standard: Special Patient Populations (Geriatrics)

Competency: Applies fundamental knowledge of growth, development, and aging and assessment findings to provide basic emergency care and transportation for a patient with special needs.

OBJECTIVES

After reading this chapter you should be able to:

36.1 Describe common changes in body systems that occur in older age.

36.2 Discuss adaptations that may be required in communicating with and assessing older patients.

36.3 Discuss the need for awareness of and the special considerations regarding medical conditions and injuries to which older patients are prone, including effects of medications, shortness of breath, chest pain, altered mental status, gastrointestinal complaints, dizziness/weakness/malaise, depression/suicide, rash, pain, flulike symptoms, and falls, and the possible significance of general or nonspecific complaints in older adults.

36.4 Recommend changes to improve safety in the home of an elderly person.

36.5 Discuss possible indications of elder abuse.

36.6 Discuss psychosocial concerns of older patients, including the fear of loss of independence.

MATCH TERMINOLOGY/ DEFINITIONS

A. Elderly person, generally considered 65 years of age or older

B. Chronic disorder resulting in dementia

C. An inflammation in the tissue of the lung

D. An abnormal heart rhythm

E. A separation of the layers of the artery described as a tearing sensation

_____ 1. Alzheimer's disease

_____ 2. Aortic dissection

_____ 3. Pneumonia

_____ 4. Dysrhythmia

_____ 5. Geriatric

MULTIPLE-CHOICE REVIEW

_____ 1. Starting at age _____, our organ systems lose about _____ percent of their function each year.
   A. 20; 1   C. 30; 1
   B. 20; 2   D. 40; 2

_____ 2. Older patients are twice as likely to use EMS as younger patients. Older patients' traumatic complaints are often due to:
   A. a medical problem.   C. a car crash or fall.
   B. sporting events.   D. none of these.

_____ 3. Assessing the airway of an older patient is often difficult because of dentures and:
   A. large, poorly chewed pieces of food are often found.
   B. dysrhythmias occur frequently.
   C. an older person's trachea is usually narrower.
   D. of arthritic changes in the bones of the neck.

_____ 4. Because older patients are less likely to show severe symptoms in certain conditions, it can be difficult to:
   A. find a radial pulse.
   B. determine a patient's priority.
   C. assess for foreign body obstruction.
   D. note sudden onset of weakness.

_____ 5. After interviewing an elderly patient, the family members, who were listening in, tell you that some of the patient's responses were incorrect. This is sometimes the result of neurological problems as well as:
   A. paranoia.   C. medications.
   B. depression.   D. all of these.

_____ 6. When a patient replaces lost circumstances with imaginary ones, this is known as:
   A. depression.   C. flustering.
   B. confabulation.   D. dysrhythmia.

_____ 7. Many older people have a _____ pain.
   A. high threshold for   C. decreased sensitivity to
   B. low threshold for   D. all of these

_____ 8. As a person ages, the systolic blood pressure has a tendency to:
   A. decrease.   C. become erratic.
   B. increase.   D. stay constant.

9. You were called to the senior citizen center to treat a 69-year-old woman who was found on the floor in the hallway. She was coming back from the bathroom when she must have slipped on the waxed floor. You suspect she may have fractured her left hip. These injuries are especially common in elderly women because of:

  A. women's shorter legs.
  B. motor vehicle collisions.
  C. abnormal curvature of the hip.
  D. loss of calcium.

10. You are assessing an 80-year-old woman who has an injury. You should consider that any injury to an elderly patient could be a sign of:

  A. a severe fall.   **C.** abuse or neglect.
  B. Alzheimer's disease.   **D.** depression.

11. Your patient is a 67-year-old female who has very painful arthritis. She says that she has good days and bad ones, but today she had to take double the usual dose of ibuprofen and naproxen. She states that, in addition to the pain, her stomach is hurting, she is very lightheaded, and she vomited a coffee-brown substance just before calling the ambulance. What could be the problem with this woman?

  A. She is allergic to NSAIDs.
  B. She may have aggravated her ulcers.
  C. She is having an acute myocardial infarction.
  D. The combined effect of the two medicines lowered her blood pressure.

12. It seems that the patient in multiple-choice question 11 is on many other medications, too. She tells you that she does not always have enough money to fill her prescriptions on time. What problems can this lead to?

  A. Insufficient anticonvulsant medication can lead to seizures occurring.
  B. Less medication than usual can be difficult for the elderly patient to excrete.
  C. The medication can be too strong for the patient to take if it is taken in an underdose.
  D. The patient is likely to have excessive pain and miss sleep.

INSIDE/OUTSIDE: WHAT APPEARANCES REVEAL

When you are assessing and managing the care of a sick or injured elderly patient, it is important to remember what is going on inside the patient when you observe various things on the outside of the patient.

1. The patient has thinner, wrinkled skin. What is happening on the "inside"?

_____

2. The patient has graying hair. What is happening on the "inside"?

_____

3. The patient has a stooped posture and arthritic joint deformities. What is happening on the "inside"?

_____

4. The patient has a loss of central nervous system neurons on the "inside." What will he or she likely exhibit on the "outside"?

_____

COMPLETE THE FOLLOWING

The Physiological Effects of Aging and Implications for Assessment

Change	Result	Implications for Assessment
Depositing of cholesterol on arterial walls that have become thicker	(1)	Heart attack and stroke more likely
Degeneration of valves and muscles	(2)	More prone to falls
Decreased elasticity of lungs and decreased activity of cilia	(3)	Higher risk of pneumonia and other respiratory infections
Fewer taste buds, less saliva; less acid production and slower movement in digestive system	(4)	Maintain high index of suspicion for bowel obstruction
Diminished liver and kidney function	(5)	Need for reduced doses of medication; bleeding tendencies
Diminished function of thyroid	(6)	Increased risk of hypothermia and hyperthermia
Diminished muscle mass, loss of minerals from bones	(7)	Falls more likely; minor falls more likely to cause fractures
Increased risk of dementia	(8)	Assess degree of orientation and be aware of signs of neglect
Increased risk of depression and sleep disorders	(9)	Increased risk of suicide
Loss of skin elasticity; shrinking of sweat glands	(10)	Increased risk of injury (The EMT must handle the patient gently to avoid injuring skin and subcutaneous tissues.)

1. _____

2. _____

3. _____

4. _____

5. _____

6. _____

7. _____

8. _____

9. _____

10. _____

©2012 Pearson Education, Inc.
Emergency Care, 12th Ed.

STREET SCENES DISCUSSION

Review the Street Scene on page 948 of the textbook. Then answer the following questions.

1. Should an ALS unit be called for an intercept en route to the hospital?

2. Imagine that you found the apartment to be very cold and the patient wearing many layers of clothing. Why is it common for elderly people to keep their living quarters cold and wear more layers? What might you expect as a consequence?

3. Unlike the patient in the Street Scenes, some elderly patients become very anxious about going to the hospital in an ambulance. Why do you think that is true? What can you do about it?

37

Emergencies for Patients with Special Challenges

Standard: Special Patient Populations (Patients with Special Challenges)

Competency: Applies fundamental knowledge of growth, development, and aging and assessment findings to provide basic emergency care and transportation for a patient with special needs.

OBJECTIVES

After reading this chapter you should be able to:

37.1 Define key terms introduced in this chapter.

37.2 Describe special challenges patients may have, including various disabilities, terminal illness, obesity, homelessness/poverty, and autism.

37.3 Describe general considerations in responding to patients with special challenges.

37.4 Recognize physical impairments and common medical devices used in the home care of patients with special challenges, including respiratory devices, cardiac devices, gastrourinary devices, and central IV catheters, and discuss EMT assessment and transport considerations for each.

37.5 Explain why patients with special challenges are often especially vulnerable to abuse and neglect and what the EMT's obligations are in such situations.

MATCH TERMINOLOGY/ DEFINITIONS

A. A physical, emotional, behavioral, or cognitive condition that interferes with a person's ability to carry out everyday tasks, such as working or caring for oneself

B. A device that breathes for a patient

_____ **1.** Autism spectrum disorders (ASD)

_____ **2.** Automatic implanted cardiac defibrillator (AICD)

©2012 Pearson Education, Inc.
Emergency Care, 12th Ed.

C. A battery-powered mechanical pump implanted in the body to assist a failing left ventricle in pumping blood to the body

D. A device implanted under the skin that can detect life-threatening cardiac dysrhythmias and respond by delivering one or more high-energy shocks to correct the rhythm

E. A tube used to provide delivery of nutrients to the stomach; a nasogastric type is inserted through the nose and into the stomach, and a gastric type is surgically implanted through the abdominal wall and into the stomach

F. A surgical opening in the neck into the trachea

G. A surgically created opening into the body, as with a tracheostomy, colonostomy, or ileostomy

H. A tube inserted into the bladder through the urethra to drain urine from the bladder

I. The process of filtering the blood to remove toxic or unwanted wastes and fluids

J. A catheter surgically inserted for long-term delivery of medications or fluids into the central circulation

K. An external pouch that collects fecal matter diverted from the colon or ileum

L. A device worn by a patient that blows oxygen or air under constant low pressure through a tube and mask to keep airway passages from collapsing at the end of a breath

M. A condition of having too much body fat, defined as a body mass index of 30 or greater

N. A device implanted under the skin with wires implanted into the heart to modify the heart rate as needed to maintain an adequate heart rate

O. Developmental disorders that affect, among other things, the ability to communicate, report medical conditions, self-regulate behaviors, and interact with others

P. The branch of medicine that deals with the causes, prevention, and treatment of obesity

_____ **3.** Bariatrics

_____ **4.** Central IV catheter

_____ **5.** Continuous positive airway pressure (CPAP)

_____ **6.** Dialysis

_____ **7.** Disability

_____ **8.** Feeding tube

_____ **9.** Left ventricular assist device (LVAD)

_____ **10.** Obesity

_____ **11.** Ostomy bag

_____ **12.** Pacemaker

_____ **13.** Stoma

_____ **14.** Tracheostomy

_____ **15.** Urinary catheter

_____ **16.** Ventilator

MULTIPLE-CHOICE REVIEW

_____ **1.** To ensure proper care for the patient with special needs, the EMT must be able to _____ the patient's specific special health care needs in addition to the chief complaint.
   A. recognize
   B. understand
   C. evaluate
   D. do all of these

_____ **2.** The EMT may find patients with special care needs when responding to calls in any of the following locations *except*:
   A. the emergency department.
   B. nursing homes.
   C. specialty rehabilitation centers.
   D. specialized care facilities.

_____ **3.** One of the best resources to help you when confronted with a special needs patient who is on a specific device would be to use the:
   A. instruction manual for the device.
   B. web site for the product.
   C. family member who is with the patient.
   D. medical direction physician over the radio.

_____ **4.** You are interviewing your patient and she tells you that she has had a heart murmur since birth. A condition that is present at the birth of the special needs patient is considered:
   A. acquired.   **C.** congenital.
   B. adopted.   **D.** inflamed.

_____ **5.** This device is used by patients at home to help them sleep as well as by EMS providers in certain medical emergencies. It is designed to keep the air passages from collapsing at the end of a breath and is called a(n):
   A. positive-pressure ventilator.   **C.** bag-mask device.
   B. CPAP.   **D.** endotracheal tube.

_____ **6.** You have responded to the home of a 50-year-old female patient who has a tracheostomy tube and needs to be suctioned occasionally. Her husband tells you that this is especially common:
   A. during times of distress.
   B. within the first few weeks after the tube insertion.
   C. if the patient has an infection.
   D. if any of these conditions exists.

_____ **7.** You are called to the home of an elderly woman who sustained a cervical spine injury a number of years ago. Her caregiver tells you that she is on a device that is programmed to take over the timing and rate of her breathing. This device is called a(n):
   A. inhalator.   **C.** ventilator.
   B. exhalator.   **D.** CPAP device.

_____ **8.** There was a severe electrical storm and the power is out in a number of neighborhoods in your district. The patient on the device in multiple-choice question 7 has an electrical or battery failure, so you need to begin:
   A. CPAP.   **C.** bag-mask ventilation.
   B. using a nonrebreather mask.   **D.** attaching the AED.

_____ **9.** You are treating a 65-year-old male patient who has a long history of heart problems. He has had multiple heart attacks, and a cardiac device was implanted in his left upper abdominal quadrant. This device is most likely called a(n):
   A. pacemaker.   **C.** heart valve.
   B. AED.   **D.** AICD.

_____ **10.** Your patient is a special needs heart patient. The family member tells you that he has a cardiac chamber that pumps blood through the aorta to the body. This is called a(n):
   A. pacemaker.   **C.** left ventricular assist device.
   B. bypass machine.   **D.** AICD.

_____ **11.** A tube that is inserted into a patient who has lost the ability to regulate his urine is called a(n):
   A. colostomy.   **C.** ileostomy.
   B. urinary catheter.   **D.** stoma.

_____ 12. You are interviewing a 55-year-old female who has a history of hypertension and diabetes. She tells you that she needs to go for dialysis every other day in a local clinic. This procedure is done to:
   A. detoxify her blood.
   B. increase her blood sugar.
   C. remove fecal material from her bowel.
   D. do all of these.

_____ 13. Examples of devices commercially available as a Groshong®, Hickman®, and a Broviac® are called:
   A. peripherally inserted central catheters.
   B. angiocaths.
   C. central venous lines.
   D. implanted port devices.

_____ 14. A special needle is required to access a device called a(n):
   A. implanted port.   C. Mediport®.
   B. Port-a-Cath®.   D. all of these.

_____ 15. A major health risk that is on the rise in the United States is _____, which will ultimately increase the occurrence of _____.
   A. stroke; liver disease   C. obesity; type 2 diabetes
   B. heart disease; sleep apnea   D. cancer; heart failure

_____ 16. Hearing loss is more common in elderly people than in younger persons, but it is not restricted to older patients. One of the easiest ways to communicate with a patient with hearing loss is to:
   A. write questions on a pad of paper.
   B. expect him or her to read your lips.
   C. find a TDD/TTY phone.
   D. scream at the patient.

_____ 17. If a cardiac patient who has an AICD is suddenly shocked by the device, he or she is usually instructed to call EMS for any of the following reasons *except* if:
   A. he or she continues to have chest pain.
   B. he or she becomes dizzy and does not feel well.
   C. the shock was momentarily painful.
   D. this was the second shock in a 24-hour period.

_____ 18. When dealing with a patient who has a history of autism and who is having a "melt-down," the best advice for the EMT is to:
   A. loudly command the patient to calm down.
   B. do not allow the patient to express frustration.
   C. provide a show of force.
   D. remember that "calm creates calm."

_____ 19. The patient in multiple-choice question 18 is very upset. Your interaction during this crisis should be as basic as possible. This includes each of the following *except*:
   A. keep your instructions basic.
   B. ask basic questions.
   C. provide all treatments as quickly as possible.
   D. use less equipment (i.e., radios, pagers, cell phones) because they are distractions.

STREET SCENES DISCUSSION

Review the Street Scene on page 971 in the textbook. Then answer the following questions.

1. The ambulance was called because Amber was experiencing a fever and beginning to look gray. What is most likely wrong with the patient?

2. Why is it necessary to suction Amber's trach tube?

3. What do you suppose was causing the gurgling sounds when Amber was breathing?

©2012 Pearson Education, Inc.
Emergency Care, 12th Ed.

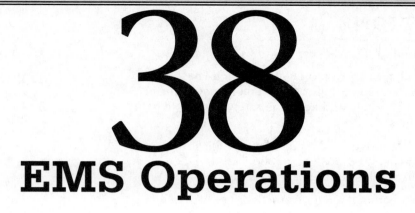

EMS Operations

Standard: EMS Operations (Principles of Safety Operating a Ground Ambulance; Air Medical)

Competency: Applies fundamental knowledge of operational roles and responsibilities to ensure patient, public, and personnel safety.

▌OBJECTIVES

After reading this chapter you should be able to:

38.1 Recognize the four types of ambulances currently specified by the U.S. Department of Transportation.

38.2 Describe the types of equipment required to be carried by EMS response units.

38.3 Describe the components of the vehicle and equipment checks done at the start of every shift.

38.4 Describe the roles and responsibilities of the Emergency Medical Dispatcher.

38.5 Discuss the principles of safe ambulance operation while responding to the scene.

38.6 Explain laws that typically apply to ambulance operations.

38.7 Discuss how to maintain safety at highway incidents.

38.8 Describe the steps necessary for transferring the patient to the ambulance.

38.9 Describe the EMT's responsibilities while transporting a patient to the hospital.

38.10 Describe the EMT's responsibilities when transferring care of patients to the emergency department staff.

38.11 Describe the EMT's responsibilities in terminating the call and readying the vehicle for the next response after the call and returning to quarters.

38.12 Identify when and how to call for air rescue, how to set up a landing zone, and how to approach a helicopter when assisting with an air rescue.

MATCH TERMINOLOGY/ DEFINITIONS

A. Emergency Medical Dispatcher

B. Legal term that appears in most states' driving laws and refers to the responsibility of the emergency vehicle operator to drive safely and keep the safety of all others in mind at all times

C. Call in which the driver of the emergency vehicle responds with lights and siren because he or she is of the understanding that loss of life or limb is possible

D. Large, flat area without aerial obstruction in which a helicopter can land to pick up a patient

_____ 1. Due regard

_____ 2. EMD

_____ 3. Landing zone (LZ)

_____ 4. True emergency

MULTIPLE-CHOICE REVIEW

_____ 1. The federal agency that develops specifications for ambulance vehicle designs is the:
A. U.S. Department of Motor Vehicles.
B. Food and Drug Administration.
C. U.S. Department of Transportation.
D. U.S. Department of Health, Education, and Welfare.

_____ 2. The purpose(s) for carrying an EPA-registered, intermediate-level disinfectant on the ambulance is to:
A. clean up blood spills.
B. destroy mycobacterium tuberculosis.
C. disinfect patient wounds.
D. do all of these.

_____ 3. Which of the following is *not* a piece of equipment that should be in the portable first-in kit, which is taken directly to a patient's side?
A. Suction unit   C. Blood pressure cuff
B. Rigid cervical collar   D. Telemetry repeater

_____ 4. Supplies used for the "C" step of the primary assessment of a trauma victim include all of the following *except*:
A. disposable gloves.   C. the AED.
B. occlusive dressings.   D. a suction unit.

_____ 5. On each call, you will need to take in the kit that has the equipment you need to take the patient's baseline vital signs. Each of the following is a piece of equipment used to obtain vital signs *except*:
A. rubber bulb syringe.   C. sphygmomanometer.
B. adult and pediatric stethoscope. D. penlight.

_____ 6. A device used to carry patients over long distances is called a:
A. Stokes basket.   C. Reeves stretcher.
B. scoop stretcher.   D. wheeled ambulance stretcher.

_____ 7. Which one of the following pieces of patient transfer equipment is *incorrectly* matched with its function?
A. Wheeled ambulance stretcher: transporting patients in sitting, supine, or Trendelenburg position
B. Folding stair chair: moving patients down stairs in a sitting position
C. Reeves stretcher: carrying patients from a high-angle rescue
D. Scoop stretcher: picking up patients found in tight spaces

©2012 Pearson Education, Inc.
Emergency Care, 12th Ed.

_____ 8. Components of a typical fixed oxygen delivery system include:
    A. 3,000-liter reservoir.
    B. a two-stage regulator.
    C. the necessary reducing valve and yokes.
    D. all of these.

_____ 9. Of the following devices carried on the ambulance or EMS vehicle for prehospital respiratory care, which is an optional item?
    A. Six adult and four pediatric nasal cannula
    B. Flow-restricted, oxygen-powered ventilation device (FROPVD)
    C. Automatic transport ventilator (ATV)
    D. Plastic cup for blow-by oxygen

_____ 10. The fixed suction unit in the ambulance or EMS vehicle should:
    A. provide an airflow of over 15 liters per minute.
    B. be usable by a person seated beside the patient.
    C. have a current hydrostat test date.
    D. reach a vacuum of at least 300 mmHg within 4 seconds.

_____ 11. Which of the following pieces of equipment carried on an ambulance or EMS vehicle for defibrillation or assisting with cardiopulmonary resuscitation is optional?
    A. Short or long spine board   **C.** Automated external defibrillator
    B. Mechanical CPR compressor   **D.** Kit with oral and nasal airways

_____ 12. Equipment that is carried on an ambulance or EMS vehicle for immobilization includes all of the following _except_:
    A. a Hare traction splint.   **C.** padded aluminum splints.
    B. triangular bandages.   **D.** a burn sheet.

_____ 13. Chemical cold packs are carried on an ambulance or EMS vehicle primarily for use with _____ injuries.
    A. musculoskeletal   **C.** respiratory
    B. abdominal   **D.** cardiac

_____ 14. Supplies used for wound care should include all of the following _except_:
    A. sterile burn sheets.   **C.** self-adhering roller bandages.
    B. 5 × 9-inch combine dressings.   **D.** Hare or Sager traction device.

_____ 15. What is the purpose of carrying sterilized aluminum foil on the ambulance or EMS vehicle?
    A. To wrap body parts in
    B. To maintain body heat
    C. To make a shield over an avulsed eye
    D. For warming minor abrasions

_____ 16. The supplies for childbirth include all the following _except_:
    A. a rubber bulb syringe.   **C.** large safety pins.
    B. sanitary napkins.   **D.** sterile surgical gloves.

_____ 17. Every shift, both you and your partner should:
    A. wash and wax the ambulance.
    B. change the oil in the ambulance.
    C. complete the equipment checklist.
    D. do preventive maintenance on the ambulance.

_____ 18. Of the following items checked on the ambulance or EMS vehicle, which is checked with the engine off?
    A. Dash-mounted gauges   **C.** Windshield wiper operation
    B. Battery   **D.** Vehicle's warning lights

_____ 19. The responsibilities of the Emergency Medical Dispatcher (EMD) include all of the following *except*:
A. dispatching and coordinating EMS resources.
B. interrogating the caller and prioritizing the call.
C. coordinating with other public safety agencies.
D. advising the caller that an ambulance is not needed.

_____ 20. When an Emergency Medical Dispatcher (EMD) questions a patient or caller, which of the following is *not* routinely asked?
A. What is the exact location of the patient?
B. What's the problem?
C. Has the patient been in the hospital recently?
D. How old is the patient?

_____ 21. When speaking with a caller who is at the scene of a traffic collision, the Emergency Medical Dispatcher (EMD) should ask all the following *except*:
A. Is traffic moving?
B. What brand vehicle was involved in the collision?
C. How many lanes of traffic are open?
D. Are any of the vehicles on fire?

_____ 22. To be a safe ambulance operator, the EMT should:
A. be tolerant of other drivers.
B. always wear glasses or contact lenses if required.
C. have a positive attitude about his or her ability as a driver.
D. do all of these.

_____ 23. Every state has statutes that regulate the operation of emergency vehicles. Under certain circumstances, vehicle operators can do all of the following *except*:
A. park the vehicle anywhere as long as it does not damage personal property.
B. proceed past red stop signals, flashing red stop signals, and stop signs.
C. exceed the posted speed limit as long as life and property are not endangered.
D. pass a school bus that has its red lights blinking.

_____ 24. You were dispatched to a priority assignment involving a motor vehicle collision. Once at the scene, you find one patient and determine that she is stable. This situation is no longer a:
A. true emergency.   C. cold response.
B. due regard.   D. priority-one response.

_____ 25. Which guideline for the use of the ambulance siren is *inappropriate*?
A. Use the siren sparingly.
B. Never assume that all motorists will hear your signal.
C. Be prepared for erratic movements of motorists.
D. Keep it on until the call is completed.

_____ 26. Which of the following is *true* about the use of lights and sirens?
A. Motorists are more inclined to give way to ambulances when sirens are continually sounded.
B. The decision about their use should be based on the patient's medical condition.
C. The use of the siren has little effect on the ambulance operator.
D. Four-way flashers should be used in addition to emergency lights.

_____ 27. Use of escorts or multivehicle responses is a:
A. very quick and successful means of response.
B. very dangerous means of response.
C. means of decreasing the chance of collision.
D. standard operating procedure in most communities.

_____ **28.** Factors that can affect ambulance response include all of the following *except*:
    A. the time of day.
    B. the weather.
    C. road maintenance and construction.
    D. the type of emergency.

_____ **29.** You are the first vehicle on the scene of an auto collision in which one of the automobiles is on fire. You should park your vehicle _____ the wreckage until the fire apparatus arrives.
    A. 50 feet from
    B. in front (upstream) of
    C. beyond (downstream)
    D. downwind from

_____ **30.** A sequence of operations to ready a patient for transfer is called:
    A. stabilization.
    B. packaging.
    C. transport.
    D. removal.

_____ **31.** You are loading a 52-year-old male patient on your stretcher into the ambulance. He is an unconscious patient with no potential spine injury and no signs of impending shock. You should position him in the ambulance:
    A. in the recovery position.
    B. with legs raised 8 to 12 inches.
    C. in the supine position.
    D. in a sitting-up position.

_____ **32.** Which of the following is an action you would *not* perform en route to the hospital?
    A. Recheck the patient's bandages and splints.
    B. Form a general impression of the patient.
    C. Perform ongoing assessment and continue to monitor vital signs.
    D. Notify the receiving facility of your estimated time of arrival.

_____ **33.** You are transporting a critically ill patient in severe respiratory failure to the nearest ED. If a patient develops cardiac arrest en route to the hospital, the EMT's *first* action should be to:
    A. apply and operate the AED.
    B. begin cardiopulmonary resuscitation.
    C. notify the emergency department.
    D. tell the operator to stop the ambulance.

_____ **34.** When delivering the patient to the hospital, the EMT should *never*:
    A. complete the prehospital care report (PCR) at the hospital.
    B. move a patient onto the hospital stretcher and just leave.
    C. transfer the patient's personal effects.
    D. obtain a release from the hospital.

_____ **35.** When approaching a helicopter, first wait for the pilot or medic to wave you in. Then approach from the _____ of the craft.
    A. rear
    B. uphill slope side
    C. front or side
    D. downhill slope rear

_____ **36.** Of the following patients, which is the *least* likely to be transported in a helicopter?
    A. Carbon monoxide poisoning victim
    B. Patient with a suspected stroke
    C. Cardiac arrest patient
    D. Patient with a critical burn

_____ **37.** The first-arriving EMS unit on the scene of a collision on a highway should park the vehicle in the _____ location. The ideal location for an ambulance would be in the _____ location.
    A. downstream; upstream
    B. traveling lane; second lane
    C. upstream; downstream
    D. slow lane; shoulder

_____ **38.** Some ambulance services have purchased GPS units for the dash of the ambulance to assist the vehicle operator in finding the location of the call. The EMT should remember that the GPS is all of the following *except*:

    A. an excellent substitute for knowledge of the response area.

    B. another type of distraction for the vehicle operator.

    C. occasionally inaccurate due to recent road construction.

    D. a device for the crew chief or other front seat passenger to deal with.

COMPLETE THE FOLLOWING

1. List the seven questions an EMD should ask a caller who is reporting a medical emergency.

    A. _____

    B. _____

    C. _____

    D. _____

    E. _____

    F. _____

    G. _____

2. List seven factors that can affect an ambulance response.

    A. _____

    B. _____

    C. _____

    D. _____

    E. _____

    F. _____

    G. _____

3. List the four major ways the EMT on the scene of a collision should describe the landing zone (LZ) to the air rescue service.

    A. _____

    B. _____

    C. _____

    D. _____

LABEL THE PHOTOGRAPHS

Fill in the name of each level of disinfecting shown in the photo on the line provided.

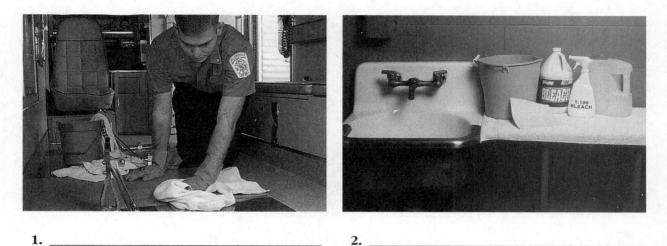

1. _____

2. _____

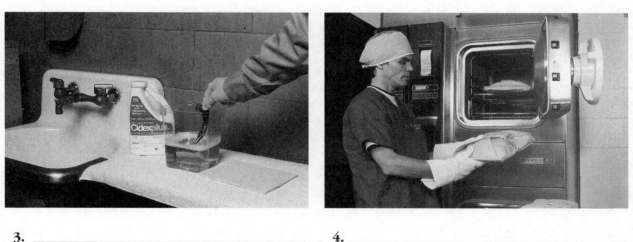

3. _____

4. _____

STREET SCENES DISCUSSION

Review the Street Scene on page 1005 of the textbook. Then answer the following questions.

1. Imagine that the ambulance had gone through a red light and had a collision en route to the call. What should you do right away?

2. If the collision involved another motorist, whose fault would it be?

3. Why is it an unsafe practice to drive an ambulance through a red light?

CASE STUDY

▶ **THE AMBULANCE COLLISION**

You are notified by dispatch to respond to the neighboring district for a mutual aid call—an ambulance has collided with a passenger vehicle at an intersection. Responding with emergency lights and siren, the ambulance had approached the red light and had attempted to pass through it without stopping. The other vehicle's occupants are an elderly couple who were on their way to the store.

As you arrive on the scene, it is obvious that there are a number of very seriously injured patients due to the speed and size of the ambulance that broadsided the car. You are assigned to look after the ambulance operator, who has minor cuts and scrapes. Fortunately for him, he was wearing his seat belt. His EMT-B partner was not as fortunate; another ambulance had already removed her from the scene with serious head and neck injuries from being ejected through the windshield of the ambulance. She had not been wearing her shoulder harness. Two other ambulance crews are in the process of removing the elderly man, who is in critical condition, and his wife, who has sustained leg fractures and is having a heart attack from the stress of the incident.

1. Was this a preventable collision?

2. Could the serious injuries to the female EMT-B have been prevented?

3. What happened to the patient to whom the ambulance was responding?

4. What is the first rule of medicine?

The next day, the headlines in the local newspaper are: "Ambulance Kills Two En Route to Third." The story goes on to say how the initial patient had basically minor medical problems and was taken by an ambulance to the local hospital for the flu and released within 3 hours. The newspaper concludes: "The driver was suspended. The district attorney requests that a grand jury inquiry be conducted."

©2012 Pearson Education, Inc.
Emergency Care, 12th Ed.

5. Aside from the reputation of the EMT-B who was driving, what might this "negative publicity" cost the service and other EMT-Bs who work there?

6. Why can the district attorney request a grand jury for this incident?

7. Is the operator of an emergency vehicle held to a higher standard than other motorists?

8. Who pays for the court defense of the EMT who was driving?

9. Could the EMT be personally sued for the injuries (deaths) that occurred?

10. How can an ambulance service prevent a collision like this from happening in its community?

EMT SKILLS PERFORMANCE CHECKLISTS

▶ TRANSFERRING THE PATIENT (PP. 989–991, 994)

❑ Take Standard Precautions.

❑ Transfer the patient as soon as possible. In a routine admission or when an illness or injury is not life threatening, first check to see what is to be done with the patient.

❑ An EMT should remain with the patient until transfer is complete.

❑ Assist the emergency department staff as required.

❑ Give a complete verbal report of the patient's condition and treatment administered.

❑ Complete your prehospital care report (PCR) and turn a copy over to the hospital staff.

❑ Transfer the patient's personal effects.

❑ Obtain your release from the hospital if required in your region.

▶ ACTIVITIES AT THE HOSPITAL (PP. 995–996; 998–1000)

❑ Take Standard Precautions.

❑ Clean the ambulance interior as required by your service exposure control plan.

❑ Replace respiratory equipment as required.

❑ Replace disposable items according to local policies.

❑ Exchange equipment according to local policies.

❑ Make up the ambulance stretcher.

▶ CHECKING THE AED

❑ Check the AED for the following:

- Unit, cables, and connectors for cleanliness
- Supplies carried with the AED
- Power supply and its operation
- Indicators on the ECG display
- ECG recorder operation
- Charge display cycle with a simulator
- Pacemaker feature, if applicable

❑ File a written report on the status of the AED.

NOTE: The specifics can be found in the FDA Automated Defibrillator: Operator's Shift Checklist.

©2012 Pearson Education, Inc.
Emergency Care, 12th Ed.

39

Hazardous Materials, Multiple-Casualty Incidents, and Incident Management

Standard: EMS Operations (Incident Management; Multiple-Casualty Incidents; Hazardous Materials)

Competency: Applies fundamental knowledge of operational roles and responsibilities to ensure patient, public, and personnel safety.

OBJECTIVES

After reading this chapter you should be able to:

39.1 Define key terms introduced in this chapter.

39.2 Anticipate situations in which hazardous materials may be involved.

39.3 Describe the roles in hazardous materials response of providers trained at each of the four levels of hazardous materials training specified by OSHA.

39.4 Describe the responsibilities of the EMT at a hazardous materials incident.

39.5 Given a description of a hazardous materials incident, identify the safe and danger zones, and then the hot, warm, and cold zones.

39.6 Explain how to identify specific hazardous materials using the NFPA 704 and Department of Transportation placard systems, packaging labels, invoices, bills of lading, shipping manifests, and Material Safety Data Sheets.

39.7 Identify sources of information on initial actions to take once the hazardous material has been identified, including the *Emergency Response Guidebook*, hotlines, and poison control centers.

39.8 Discuss how to establish a treatment area and decontamination and care for patients at a hazardous materials incident.

39.9 Describe multiple-casualty-incident operations.

39.10 Describe the principles and features of the Incident Command System.

39.11 Describe the principles of primary triage, secondary triage, and the START triage system.

39.12 Discuss transportation and staging logistics at a multiple-casualty incident.

39.13 Recognize the psychological aspects of multiple-casualty incidents for patients and responders.

MATCH TERMINOLOGY/ DEFINITIONS

A. Color-coded tag indicating the priority group to which a patient has been assigned

B. The area in which secondary triage takes place at a multiple-casualty incident (MCI)

C. Process of quickly assessing patients at a multiple-casualty incident (MCI) and assigning each a priority for receiving treatment; from a French word meaning "to sort"

D. Person responsible for overseeing triage at a multiple-casualty incident (MCI)

E. The area in which patients are treated at a multiple-casualty incident (MCI)

F. Person responsible for overseeing treatment of patients who have been triaged at a multiple-casualty incident (MCI)

G. Person responsible for communicating with sector officers and hospitals to manage transportation of patients to hospitals from a multiple-casualty incident (MCI)

H. Area in which ambulances are parked and other resources are held until needed

I. Person responsible for overseeing ambulances and ambulance personnel at a multiple-casualty incident (MCI)

J. Any medical or trauma event incident involving multiple patients

K. The management system used by federal, state, and local governments to manage emergencies in the United States

L. The first on the scene to establish order and initiate the Incident Command System

M. Any substance or material in a form that poses an unreasonable risk to health, safety, and property when transported in commerce

N. Area immediately surrounding a hazmat incident; extends far enough to prevent adverse effects outside the zone

O. Area in which the Incident Command post and support functions are located

P. Command organization in which a single agency controls all resources and operations

Q. The person who assumes overall direction of an incident

R. A subset of the National Incident Management System (NIMS)

_____ **1.** Cold zone

_____ **2.** Command

_____ **3.** Decontamination

_____ **4.** Disaster plan

_____ **5.** Hazardous material

_____ **6.** Hot zone

_____ **7.** Incident Command

_____ **8.** Incident Command System (ICS)

_____ **9.** Multiple-casualty incident (MCI)

_____ **10.** National Incident Management System (NIMS)

_____ **11.** Single incident command

_____ **12.** Staging area

_____ **13.** Staging supervisor

_____ **14.** Transportation supervisor

_____ **15.** Treatment area

_____ **16.** Treatment supervisor

_____ **17.** Triage

_____ **18.** Triage area

_____ **19.** Triage supervisor

_____ **20.** Triage tag

_____ **21.** Unified command

_____ **22.** Warm zone

©2012 Pearson Education, Inc.
Emergency Care, 12th Ed.

S. Area where personnel and equipment decontamination and hot zone support take place; it includes control points for the access corridor and thus assists in reducing the spread of contamination

T. Command organization in which several agencies work independently but cooperatively

U. A predefined set of instructions for a community's emergency responders

V. A chemical and/or physical process that reduces or prevents the spread of contamination from persons or equipment; the removal of hazardous substances from employees and their equipment to the extent necessary to preclude foreseeable health effects

MULTIPLE-CHOICE REVIEW

_____ **1.** On arrival at the scene of collision, you observe a large truck with placards on each of its sides. Using the *Emergency Response Guidebook*, you would find that ethyl acetate is a chemical that:
   A. irritates the eyes and respiratory tract.
   B. destroys the bone marrow.
   C. damages internal organs.
   D. is extremely explosive.

_____ **2.** On arrival at the scene of a vehicle fire involving a large truck, you observe that the large truck has placards on each of its sides. Using the *Emergency Response Guidebook*, you would find that Benzene (benzol) is a chemical that:
   A. damages the eyes by eliminating moisture.
   B. has toxic vapors that can be absorbed through the skin.
   C. is used as an industrial blasting agent.
   D. is used in surgical techniques to control pain.

_____ **3.** The regulations that are meant to enhance the knowledge, skills, and safety of emergency response personnel, as well as bring about a more effective response to hazmat emergencies, are found in:
   A. the Ryan White CARE Act.   **C.** NFPA 1200.
   B. FEMA 1910.1030.   **D.** OSHA 29 CFR 1910.120.

_____ **4.** "Those who initially respond to releases or potential releases of hazardous materials in order to protect people, property, and the environment. They stay at a safe distance, keep the incident from spreading, and protect others from any exposures." What level of training does this regulation statement describe?
   A. First Responder Awareness   **C.** Hazardous Materials Technician
   B. First Responder Operations   **D.** Hazardous Materials Specialist

_____ **5.** "Rescuers who are likely to witness or discover a hazardous substance release. They are trained only to recognize the problem and initiate a response from the proper organizations." What level of training does this regulation statement describe?
   A. First Responder Awareness   **C.** Hazardous Materials Technician
   B. First Responder Operations   **D.** Hazardous Materials Specialist

_____ **6.** The standard that deals with competencies for EMS personnel at a hazardous materials incident is called:
   A. OSHA 1910.1030.   **C.** NFPA 473.
   B. NFPA 472.   **D.** OSHA 1910.1200.

_____ 7. You are responding to a location in your district. The dispatcher informs you that the caller states, "There may be hazardous materials stored at the location." Which of the following is *not* likely to be a potential hazardous material location?
   A. Garden center
   B. Chemical plant
   C. Trucking terminal
   D. Pet store

_____ 8. Unless EMS personnel are trained to the level of_____, they must remain in the cold zone.
   A. First Responder Awareness
   B. First Responder Operations
   C. Hazardous Materials Technician
   D. Hazardous Materials Specialist

_____ 9. All victims leaving the _____ zone should be considered contaminated until proven otherwise.
   A. cold
   B. warm
   C. hot
   D. decontamination

_____ 10. What is the primary concern at the scene of a hazardous materials incident?
   A. The safety of the EMT and crew, patients, and the public
   B. Stabilizing the incident as fast as possible
   C. Quickly removing all exposed patients from the scene
   D. Determining the extent and cost of the damage

_____ 11. Upon arrival at a tanker truck crash where the vehicle has overturned and is rapidly leaking its contents onto the street, the EMT should:
   A. quickly apply a short spine board to the truck driver in the tanker.
   B. isolate the area and call for the appropriate backup assistance.
   C. try to stop or seal the leak as quickly as possible.
   D. send the least-senior EMT in to assess the patient.

_____ 12. The safe zone of a hazardous materials incident should be established in a _____ location.
   A. downwind/downhill
   B. upwind/same level
   C. downwind/same level
   D. upwind/downhill

_____ 13. The role of Command at a hazardous materials incident is to delegate responsibility for all the following *except*:
   A. directing bystanders to a safe area.
   B. establishing a perimeter.
   C. immediately initiating rescue attempts.
   D. evacuating people if necessary.

_____ 14. You are on the scene of a hazmat incident. One of your roles is to limit the spread of the materials. When a contaminated victim of a hazardous materials incident comes in contact with other people who are not contaminated, this is referred to as _____ contamination.
   A. secondary
   B. chemical
   C. contact
   D. clone

_____ 15. The designations on the sides of tanker trucks are called hazardous material:
   A. license plates.
   B. waybills.
   C. placards.
   D. shipping papers.

_____ 16. The commonly used placard system for fixed facilities is called the:
   A. MSDS.
   B. NFPA 704.
   C. CHEM 369 System.
   D. UN Classification System.

_____ 17. All employers are required to post in an obvious spot the information about all the chemicals in the workplace on a form called a(n):
   A. NFPA 704.
   B. MSDS.
   C. OSHA Chemical listing.
   D. fair trade posting.

_____ **18.** Resources that the EMT should use at a hazardous materials incident include all of the following *except*:
  A. copies of NFPA rules.
  B. the local hazmat team.
  C. the *Emergency Response Guidebook.*
  D. CHEM-TEL.

_____ **19.** The Incident Commander at the hazmat incident is collecting needed information so that he can contact CHEMTREC. What is CHEMTREC?
  A. Twenty-four-hour service for identifying hazardous materials
  B. Oil refinery and manufacturer
  C. National hazmat response team
  D. Round-the-clock special rescue teams

_____ **20.** EMS personnel at the scene of a hazardous materials incident are responsible for taking care of the injured and:
  A. identifying and controlling the substance involved.
  B. monitoring and rehabilitating hazmat team members.
  C. decontaminating patients exiting the hot zone.
  D. moving patients from the hot zone to the warm zone.

_____ **21.** Which of the following is *not* a characteristic of the rehabilitation operations at a hazardous materials incident?
  A. Located in the warm zone
  B. Protected from the weather
  C. Easily accessible to EMS
  D. Free from exhaust fumes

_____ **22.** As soon as possible after a hazmat team member exits the hot zone, the EMT in the rehab operations should:
  A. have him drink a pint of water.
  B. remove his protective clothing.
  C. begin the decontamination process.
  D. reassess his vital signs.

_____ **23.** You are confronted with a patient at risk for causing secondary contamination in which treatment calls for irrigation with water. The hazmat team has not yet arrived. Which of the following actions is *not* recommended?
  A. Cut the patient's clothes off.
  B. Irrigate the patient with tepid water.
  C. Flush runoff water down the nearest drain.
  D. Use disposable equipment for treatment.

_____ **24.** Which of the following is *not* a feature of a good local disaster plan?
  A. All emergency responders should be familiar with the plan.
  B. The plan must be based on the actual availability of resources.
  C. The plan must be rehearsed to ensure it works correctly.
  D. The plan should be generic and meet national standards.

_____ **25.** Upon arrival of the first EMS unit at the scene of an MCI, the crew leader should do all of the following *except*:
  A. assume command.
  B. conduct a scene walk-through.
  C. call for backup.
  D. begin patient treatment.

_____ **26.** Which of the following is *not* a principle of good communication at an MCI?
  A. The person responsible for incident management should have a unique Command name.
  B. Responding units should be informed that a disaster plan is in effect.
  C. The majority of communications should be done via radio transmission.
  D. Communications between Command and sector officers should be face-to-face.

_____ **27.** If an MCI involves hazardous materials, an additional _____ sector is needed.
   A. hazmat
   B. extrication
   C. rehabilitation
   D. decontamination

_____ **28.** You are responding to a collision between a loaded school bus and a tractor trailer truck. You are being informed that the bus is on its side and there a number of injured children. You are quickly reviewing the roles of the management personnel at a major incident like this while en route. The individual at an MCI who is responsible for sorting and prioritizing patients is the _____ supervisor.
   A. triage
   B. treatment
   C. transportation
   D. extrication

_____ **29.** If children in the crash described in multiple-choice question 28 are assessed as having decreased mental status, they will be considered Priority:
   A. 1.
   B. 2.
   C. 3.
   D. 4.

_____ **30.** If children in the crash described in multiple-choice question 28 are assessed as having signs of shock, they will be considered Priority:
   A. 1.
   B. 2.
   C. 3.
   D. 4.

_____ **31.** If children in the crash described in multiple-choice question 28 are assessed as having multiple-bone or joint injuries, they will be considered Priority:
   A. 1.
   B. 2.
   C. 3.
   D. 4.

_____ **32.** The driver of the truck described in multiple-choice question 28 was assessed as having died at the MCI scene. The driver should be considered a Priority:
   A. 1.
   B. 2.
   C. 3.
   D. 4.

_____ **33.** The individual at the MCI described in multiple-choice question 28 who is responsible for maintaining a supply of vehicles and personnel at a location away from the incident site is the _____ supervisor.
   A. extrication
   B. transportation
   C. staging
   D. triage

_____ **34.** The individual at the MCI described in multiple-choice question 28 who is responsible for determining patient destinations and notifying the hospitals of the incoming patients is the _____ supervisor.
   A. triage
   B. treatment
   C. transportation
   D. extrication

_____ **35.** Patient transport decisions at the MCI described in multiple-choice question 28 will be based on all of the following _except_:
   A. priority.
   B. destination facilities.
   C. transportation resources.
   D. patient's family preferences.

_____ **36.** The characteristics of the rehabilitation area must include all of the following _except_:
   A. located in the warm zone.
   B. protected from weather as much as possible.
   C. large enough to accommodate multiple rescue crews.
   D. free from exhaust fumes.

_____ **37.** You have been assigned to the rehabilitation area at a hazardous materials incident. One of your responsibilities will be the medical monitoring of the hazmat team prior to and after working in their chemical-protective suits. One team member comes into your area and is anxious to get suited back up and go back to work. You take a set of vitals on him that reveal the following: respiratory rate of 20 and regular, heart rate of 120 and bounding, and blood pressure of 132/84 mmHg. What should you do next with this team member?
   A. Take his oral temperature.
   B. Let him suit back up after drinking some fluids.
   C. Have him sit for 15 more minutes.
   D. Tell him he is done for the day.

_____ **38.** Proper hydration is an important element in preventing heat stress and promoting optimal physical performance. Based on your role as defined in multiple-choice question 37, how much fluid would be reasonable to consume per hour during physical exertion?
   A. 2 gallons
   B. 1 gallon
   C. 2 quarts
   D. 1 quart

_____ **39.** Some services administer different fluids in their rehab sectors. What other fluid would be appropriate to offer the team members?
   A. Coffee that is cold or hot
   B. Tea that is cold or hot
   C. Soda or diet soda
   D. Watered-down sports drink

_____ **40.** You are the first unit arriving at the scene of a multiple-casualty incident (MCI). A train car derailed and there are injured people all over. Aside from confirming the incident and calling for additional help, what is one of the first steps to begin triage?
   A. Talk to each patient and assign her or him a triage tag.
   B. Use the PA system to instruct those who can walk to go to a specific location.
   C. Locate the dead and have them removed from the scene.
   D. Evaluate the mental status of each patient.

_____ **41.** You will be using the START system in the MCI described in multiple-choice question 40. This system utilizes each of the following parameters *except*:
   A. a pulse or circulation check.
   B. a respiration assessment.
   C. the mental status of the patients.
   D. the number of broken bones each patient has.

_____ **42.** When utilizing the START system, the amount of treatment provided prior to tagging the patients is limited to:
   A. splinting and applying a cervical collar.
   B. opening an airway and applying pressure on a bleeding wound.
   C. traction splinting and occlusive dressings.
   D. assisting patients in taking their own pain medications.

COMPLETE THE FOLLOWING

1. List the information you should be prepared to give when you call for assistance from CHEMTREC.

_____

_____

_____

_____

_____

2. List four characteristics of the rehabilitation operations at a hazardous materials incident.

A. _____

B. _____

C. _____

D. _____

COMPLETE THE CHART

Fill in the blanks to complete the chart.

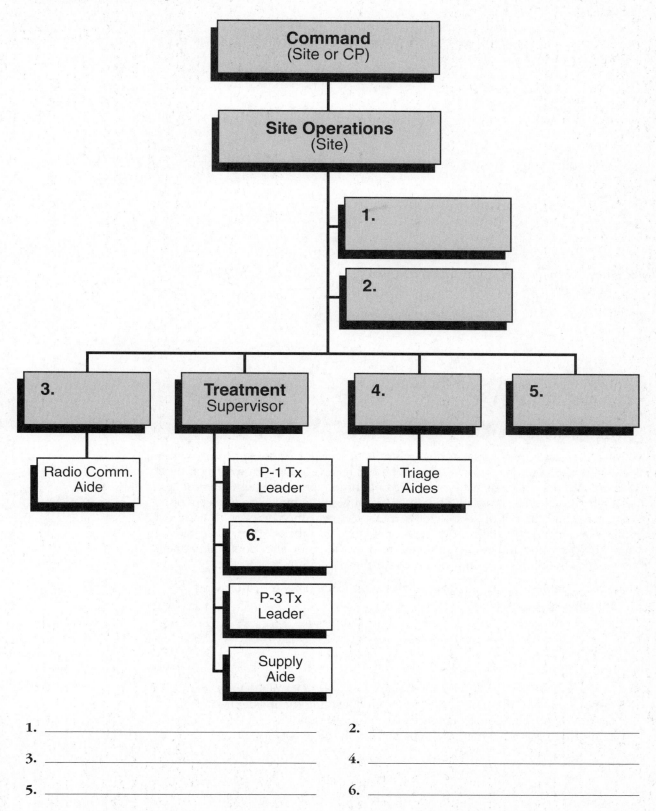

1. _____   2. _____

3. _____   4. _____

5. _____   6. _____

STREET SCENES DISCUSSION

Review the Street Scene on page 1036 of the textbook. Then answer the following questions.

1. For this call, would it have been appropriate to request a helicopter if it were available?

2. How could you find enough additional ambulances?

3. Suppose there was a bus involved at this scene and there were 20 low-priority patients. How can you transport them?

CASE STUDY

▶ THE SCHOOL BUS MCI

You are dispatched to a school bus collision in a major intersection in town. The dispatcher notifies you en route that he has received numerous calls on the collision, and the police as well as the fire department are en route. Callers state that a large truck collided at a high rate of speed with the bus in an intersection, overturning the bus full of schoolchildren. As you near the center of town, the traffic is backed up in both directions for about five blocks. The police have arrived on the scene and are beginning to reroute the traffic after confirming that there are many injured children on and near the bus.

1. What would be your initial role as the crew leader of the first-arriving ambulance at the scene?

2. **(A)** Which vest from the MCI kit should you wear? **(B)** What are your responsibilities? After declaring the MCI, confirming the incident with dispatch, and establishing contact with the police and fire officers, you begin to estimate the number of patients with the assistance of your two crew members.

3. What would be the most likely job to designate to one of your partners?

4. What are his or her specific functions?

You size up the situation and determine that there were 40 children on the bus, half of whom have numerous contusions and cuts and who are walking around the scene crying. You decide to designate a nearby store as the location for the Priority 3 patients. You have one of your partners make a PA announcement that the walking wounded should go to that location. In addition, you call for 10 ambulances and another school bus to respond.

5. Where would be the best place to stage the ambulances?

6. What should be the role of the crew leader on the first ambulance arriving at the staging area?

7. Should any ambulances report directly to the scene?

8. Are there any other sector supervisors needed at this time?

The fire department has cleared the bus for entry now that it is stabilized and no longer leaking any fuel. Inside are 15 patients who need to be removed from the bus. Many of the patients have head injuries, fractures, contusions, and glass cuts.

9. How should these patients be removed from the bus, if it is possible?

10. Once removed from the bus, where should the patients be taken?

Prioritize the patients described below into the following categories: Priority 1 (critical and unstable), Priority 2 (potentially unstable), Priority 3 (stable, walking wounded), Priority 4 (dead).

11. A 7-year-old female who complains of a swollen, deformed right lower arm and a contusion to the head with no loss of consciousness. She is alert and has vital signs that are normal for her age.

12. A 9-year-old male who has a seizure disorder and who has been unconscious since the collision. He has already had two observed grand-mal seizures without a lucid interval.

13. A 10-year-old male who was thrown through the front window of the bus because he was standing up talking to the bus driver. He was ejected from the vehicle; was found approximately 50 feet from the bus; and has a large contusion, depressed skull fracture, and no vital signs.

14. An 8-year-old female who has a bruise on the left upper quadrant and the forehead. She denies any loss of consciousness but is pale and clammy, and has a rapid heart rate for her age.

The treatment supervisor has set up a treatment area across the street from the collision in the gas station parking lot. He has set out a large yellow and a large red tarp. There is also a smaller black tarp inside the gas station for the Priority 4 patients. As the incident proceeds, you are able to obtain additional assistance from the firefighters at the scene for lifting the patients being removed from the bus and carried on backboards to the treatment area. Also, the area is becoming quite congested because a number of parents are arriving at the scene.

15. What is the best thing to do with the parents?

16. As a smooth flow of ambulances begins to arrive from the staging area, who should coordinate the destinations of the patient transports and communicate with the hospitals?

17. What might this person want to know immediately from the local hospitals?

18. Other than the bus that was ordered for the Priority 3 patients, is there any other form of transportation that should be considered for this incident?

19. How should the decision be made about who rides on the bus to a hospital?

20. As the incident is wrapped up, how could you, as Command, deal with the media and the emotional and physical needs of your personnel?

EMT SKILLS
PERFORMANCE CHECKLIST

▶ **ESTABLISHING COMMAND AT A MULTIPLE-CASUALTY INCIDENT (MCI) (PP. 1019–1026)**

❑ Perform a scene size-up.

❑ Locate the police and fire officers and establish a unified command post.

❑ Don the command vest.

❑ Notify the EMS dispatcher:

- Designate an EMS Operations Supervisor (as needed).
- Declare an MCI.
- Describe the extent of the incident.
- Characterize it as ongoing or contained.
- Give the approximate number of patients.
- Give the location of the command posts.
- Request the number of BLS and ALS units.

▶ **DESIGNATE A TRIAGE SUPERVISOR**

❑ Designate a staging supervisor and a location for staging, and notify the dispatcher to have all additional ambulances respond to staging.

❑ Request the dispatcher to roll call the local hospitals for bed availability.

❑ Designate the treatment supervisor and location for this area (as needed).

❑ Designate the transportation supervisor and location for this area (as needed).

❑ Consider the need for aeromedical evacuation and an appropriate landing zone near the scene.

❑ Consider the usefulness of a school bus to transport the "walking wounded," low-priority patients. Make sure that everyone on the bus is medically examined and that medical personnel also ride the bus.

❑ Consider the need for an extrication area (if one is not already established).

❑ Consider the need for a safety supervisor (as needed).

❑ Consider the need for rehabilitation operations for personnel.

❑ Keep the dispatcher and other service chiefs in close contact throughout the incident.

❑ Along with the police and fire officers, consider the need for a public information supervisor to work with the arriving media representatives.

40

Highway Safety and Vehicle Extrication

Standard: EMS Operations (Vehicle Extrication)

Competency: Applies fundamental knowledge of operational roles and responsibilities to ensure patient, public, and personnel safety.

OBJECTIVES

After reading this chapter you should be able to:

40.1 Describe the risks to EMS providers during highway emergency operations.

40.2 Given a variety of highway response scenarios, describe how to create as safe a work area as possible.

40.3 Discuss particular considerations in ensuring safety during night operations.

40.4 Describe the purposes and events of each of the ten phases of vehicle extrication and rescue operations.

40.5 In a rescue situation, recognize and manage hazards by wearing appropriate protective gear, safeguarding your patient, managing traffic, safely dealing with deployed air bags and energy-absorbing bumpers, managing spectators, and exercising safe practices around electrical hazards.

40.6 Describe actions taken at a rescue scene by those trained to do so regarding control of vehicle fires, stabilizing a vehicle, and gaining access to patients.

40.7 Given a variety of vehicle extrication and rescue scenarios, safely perform patient care and operational tasks as part of an emergency response team.

©2012 Pearson Education, Inc.
Emergency Care, 12th Ed.

MATCH TERMINOLOGY/ DEFINITIONS

A. When moving toward the rear of the vehicle, the second post you see, which supports the roof

B. Glass used in an automobile's side and rear windows designed to break into small, rounded pieces rather than sharp fragments

C. Named after a well-known consumer advocate, this casehardened pin is held by the cams of an automobile's doorlocking system

D. Three-part procedure used by rescue personnel to free a patient trapped in a vehicle

E. When a patient is pinned and requires assistance, sometimes mechanical, to free him

F. Cribbing or blocking a vehicle or structure to prevent further unintended, uncontrolled movement

G. Access that requires tools or special equipment to reach the patient

H. Post in front of the driver's compartment that supports the roof and windshield

I. Safety glass used in the windshields of automobiles, made of two sheets of plate glass bonded to a sheet of tough plastic

J. Blocks of hardwood, usually 4 × 4 × 18-inch or 2 × 4 × 18-inch, used to stabilize a vehicle

K. Process by which entrapped patients are rescued from vehicles, buildings, tunnels, or other places

_____ **1.** A post

_____ **2.** B post

_____ **3.** Complex access

_____ **4.** Cribbing

_____ **5.** Disentanglement

_____ **6.** Entrapment

_____ **7.** Extrication

_____ **8.** Laminated glass

_____ **9.** Nader pin

_____ **10.** Stabilization

_____ **11.** Tempered glass

MULTIPLE-CHOICE REVIEW

_____ **1.** Trench, dive, ice, and high-angle rescue is frequently carried out by:
   A. industrial rescue teams.
   B. specialty rescue teams.
   C. police rescue services.
   D. commercial rescue services.

_____ **2.** The phases of extrication include all of the following *except*:
   A. gaining access to the patient.
   B. defining patient care.
   C. disentangling the patient.
   D. sizing up the situation.

_____ **3.** On arrival at the scene of a motor vehicle crash, you and your crew ensure that the location is safe and find it will be necessary to size up the situation. An important part of a rescue scene size-up is:
   A. determining the extent of entrapment.
   B. starting IVs on the patient.
   C. removing shattered glass from around the patient.
   D. informing the patient about the extent of vehicle damage.

____ **4.** During size-up of a collision, you must be able to "read" a collision and develop an action plan based on your knowledge of rescue operations and your:
   A. previous experience at collision scenes.
   B. judgment of the extent of vehicle damage.
   C. estimate of the patient's condition and priority.
   D. evaluation of the resources available.

____ **5.** You are on the scene of a car that crashed into a bridge overpass abutment. The patient is entrapped and seriously injured. When developing an action plan for patient extrication, always keep in mind:
   A. the potential for observation by bystanders.
   B. that time is very critical to some patients' trauma management.
   C. the cost of further damage to the vehicle.
   D. the type of vehicle that is involved in the incident.

____ **6.** If a vehicle has an airbag that deployed, the manufacturer recommends:
   A. airing out the car for 15 minutes prior to treating the patient.
   B. placing masks on patients before treating.
   C. lifting the bag and examining the steering wheel and dash.
   D. using HEPA masks before gaining access.

____ **7.** The unsafe act that contributes most to collision scene injuries is failure to:
   A. eliminate or control hazards during operations.
   B. wear protective gear during rescue operations.
   C. recognize mechanisms of injury early on.
   D. select the proper tool for the task.

____ **8.** Every year, EMTs and rescuers are injured at the scene of collisions. Factors that may contribute to injuries of rescuers at a collision include all of the following *except*:
   A. careless attitude toward personal safety.
   B. a lack of skill in tool and equipment use.
   C. physical problems that impede strenuous effort.
   D. limiting the inner circle to rescuers who are in protective gear.

____ **9.** Good protective gear at the scene of a collision includes all of the following *except*:
   A. firefighter or leather gloves.　　　　**C.** steel toe, high-top work shoes.
   B. fire-resistant trousers or turnout pants.　　**D.** plastic "bump caps."

____ **10.** To ensure adequate eye protection at the collision scene, the EMT should wear _____ and protect the patient with a(n) _____.
   A. safety goggles with a soft vinyl frame; aluminized rescue blanket
   B. hinged plastic helmet shield; disposable paper blanket
   C. thermal mask or shield; lightweight vinyl-coated tarpaulin
   D. safety glasses with small lenses; wool blanket

____ **11.** During an extrication, an aluminized rescue blanket may be used to:
   A. maintain the rescuer's body heat.
   B. smother fire in the engine compartment.
   C. protect the patient from poor weather and flying particles.
   D. none of these.

____ **12.** The police have not arrived and you have positioned your ambulance to temporarily block the traffic till flares are set up. When using flares, the EMT should:
   A. watch for spilled fuel or other combustibles prior to igniting.
   B. throw them out of the moving vehicle to save time.
   C. use them as a traffic wand to divert traffic.
   D. always walk with oncoming traffic while positioning them.

©2012 Pearson Education, Inc.
Emergency Care, 12th Ed.

_____ **13.** When there is an electrical hazard, the safe zone:
  A. should be established as soon as the power company arrives.
  B. does not exist due to the numerous dangers of an electrical hazard.
  C. should be far enough away to ensure that an arcing wire does not cause injury.
  D. is located at least 10 feet from the ground gradient.

_____ **14.** As of 2009, federal highway standards have required that all emergency responders:
  A. take the incident command course.
  B. comply with NFPA 1500.
  C. wear ANSI safety vests when working in highway operations.
  D. don PPE prior to touching bleeding patients.

_____ **15.** If a vehicle collides with a broken utility pole with wires down, you should:
  A. ignore it because the vehicle will not conduct electricity.
  B. tell the vehicle's occupants to stay in the vehicle.
  C. immediately shut off the vehicle's ignition switch.
  D. don full protective gear and remove downed wires.

_____ **16.** In wet weather, a phenomenon known as _____ may provide your first clue that a wire is down.
  A. an arc   **C.** lightning
  B. ground gradient   **D.** flash point

_____ **17.** You are on the scene of a collision between a car and a utility pole. The pole is literally split in two and hanging by the wires. As you approach the vehicle, you feel a tingling sensation in your legs and lower torso. Which action should you take?
  A. Turn 180 degrees and shuffle with both feet together to safety.
  B. Turn 90 degrees and walk as quickly as possible to safety.
  C. Ask your partner for his hand and have him pull you to safety.
  D. Turn 180 degrees and crawl to safety.

_____ **18.** If there is a fire in the car's engine compartment and people are trapped in the vehicle, you should do all of the following _except_:
  A. quickly and carefully remove the patients.
  B. ensure that the fire department has been called.
  C. don protective gear and use your fire extinguisher.
  D. apply a short spine board to the driver right away.

_____ **19.** When a vehicle's hood is closed and there is an engine fire, you should do all of the following _except_:
  A. use emergency moves to remove occupants.
  B. let the fire department extinguish the fire.
  C. fully open the hood to extinguish the fire.
  D. let the fire burn under the closed hood.

_____ **20.** When a vehicle rolls off the roadway into a field of dried grass, it is possible that a fire may be caused by the:
  A. catalytic converter.
  B. leaking radiator fluid.
  C. ground gradient.
  D. airbag deployment.

_____ **21.** "Try Before You Pry" is the foundation for the _____ procedure.
  A. disentanglement
  B. stabilization
  C. simple access
  D. entanglement

_____ 22. You are on the scene of a two-car, high-speed, head-on collision The scene is safe and the traffic has been diverted by the police. Once the vehicle you were assigned to is stabilized and an entry point is gained, you should immediately do all of the following *except*:
   A. begin the primary assessment.
   B. crawl inside the vehicle.
   C. provide manual cervical stabilization.
   D. pull the patient out of the access hole.

_____ 23. On evaluation of the vehicle and once you have gained access to the second automobile in the crash described in multiple-choice question 22, you find an unconscious 25-year-old male patient who is in a sitting position behind the wheel with both his legs pinned. Which is the best approach to disentanglement of this patient?
   A. Displace the doors, cut the roof, and then displace the dash.
   B. Pull the dash, cut the doors, and then push the seat.
   C. Cut the roof, displace the doors, and then displace the dash.
   D. Cut the roof, displace the dash, and then displace the doors.

_____ 24. The decision is made to remove the roof of one of the vehicles from the crash described in multiple-choice question 22. Which of the following is *not* a reason for disposing of the roof to access a patient?
   A. It makes the entire interior of the vehicle accessible.
   B. It creates a large exit through which to remove a patient.
   C. It provides fresh air and helps cool off the patient.
   D. It helps to stabilize the vehicle quickly.

_____ 25. You are at the scene of a major car wreck where the driver has the dash on his lap. The extrication will involve displacing the dash and steering wheel. You notice that the airbag has not yet deployed. What should be done?
   A. Apply heat to the steering wheel.
   B. Drill a hole into the airbag module.
   C. Disconnect the battery cable.
   D. Displace the steering column.

COMPLETE THE FOLLOWING

1. List the ten phases of the extrication or rescue process.

   A. _____   F. _____

   B. _____   G. _____

   C. _____   H. _____

   D. _____   I. _____

   E. _____   J. _____

2. List the personal protective equipment that you should wear at a collision site where you will be providing patient care within the inner circle on a patient who is entrapped.

   A. _____

   B. _____

   C. _____

   D. _____

LABEL THE PHOTOGRAPHS

Label each procedure on the lines provided.

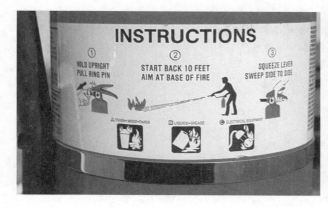

1. _____

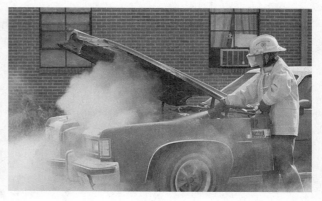

2. _____

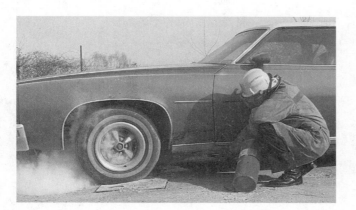

3. _____

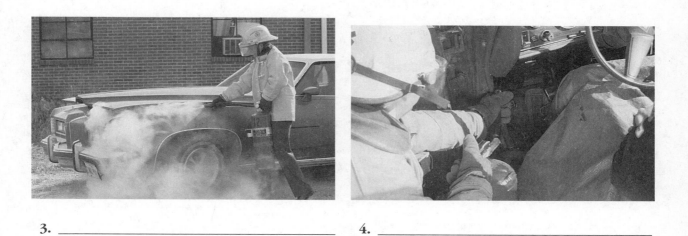

4. _____

5. _____

STREET SCENES DISCUSSION

Review the Street Scene on page 1062 of the textbook. Then answer the following questions.

1. Suppose the patient had been trapped under the dashboard. Would it make more sense to pop open the doors and then take off the roof? Or should the roof come off first?

2. What is the significance of a vehicle with 10 feet of intrusion?

3. Should ALS be requested for this patient?

41

EMS Response to Terrorism

Standard: EMS Operations (Terrorism and Disaster)

Competency: Applies fundamental knowledge of operational roles and responsibilities to ensure patient, public, and personnel safety.

OBJECTIVES

After reading this chapter you should be able to:

41.1   Define key terms introduced in this chapter.

41.2   Give examples of chemical, biological, radiological, nuclear, and explosive agents that may be used in terrorism incidents.

41.3   Describe the risks to first responders in terrorism incidents.

41.4   Discuss clues, such as occupancy or location, type of event, timing of events, and on-scene warning signs, that help with identification of suspicious events.

41.5   Given a scenario involving a terrorism incident, predict the types of harm that may occur.

41.6   Apply the principles of time, distance, and shielding to minimize exposure to harm from terrorism incidents.

41.7   Discuss types of harm and self-protection measures for each of the following:

a. Chemical incident
b. Biological incident
c. Radiological/nuclear incident
d. Explosive incident

41.8   Discuss how chemical and biological agents can be disseminated and weaponized.

41.9   Describe the characteristics associated with the following:

a. Chemical agents
b. Biological agents
c. Radiological/nuclear devices
d. Incendiary devices

41.10 Describe blast injury patterns and treatment for blast injuries.

41.11 Discuss strategy, tactics, and self-protection with regard to a terrorist incident.

MATCH TERMINOLOGY/ DEFINITIONS

A. Terrorism directed against the government or population without foreign direction

B. Roentgen equivalent (in) humans; a measure of radiation dosage

C. Spreading

D. The dose or concentration of an agent multiplied by the time, or duration

E. The movement of a substance through a surface or, on a molecular level, through intact materials

F. Pathways into the body, generally by absorption, ingestion, injection, or inhalation

G. Destructive devices, such as bombs, placed to be activated after an initial attack and timed to injure emergency responders who rush in to help care for those targeted by an initial attack

H. Terrorism that is foreign-based or directed

I. Contact with or presence of a material where it does not belong and that is somehow harmful to persons, animals, and/or the environment

J. Packaging or producing a material, such as a chemical, biological, or radiological agent, so that it can be used as a weapon, for example, by dissemination in a bomb detonation or as an aerosol sprayed over an area or introduced into a ventilation system

K. The unlawful use of force or violence against persons or property to intimidate or coerce a government, the civilian population, or any segment thereof, in furtherance of political or social objectives

L. Weapons, devices, or agents intended to cause widespread harm and/or fear in a population

M. Specific operational actions to accomplish assigned tasks

N. Able to move through the animal–human barrier; transmissible from animals to humans

O. Broad general plans designed to achieve desired outcomes

P. Abnormal constriction of the pupil

_____ **1.** Contamination

_____ **2.** Dissemination

_____ **3.** Domestic terrorism

_____ **4.** Exposure

_____ **5.** International terrorism

_____ **6.** Permeation

_____ **7.** Rem

_____ **8.** Routes of entry

_____ **9.** Secondary devices

_____ **10.** Strategies

_____ **11.** Tactics

_____ **12.** Terrorism

_____ **13.** Weaponization

_____ **14.** Weapons of mass destruction (WMD)

_____ **15.** Zoonotic

_____ **16.** Miosis

MULTIPLE-CHOICE REVIEW

_____ 1. In addition to armed attacks, the types of terrorism incidents may be remembered by the EMT using the acronym:
- **A.** OPQRST.
- **B.** CBRNE.
- **C.** CUPS.
- **D.** AVPU.

_____ 2. Environmental terrorists, survivalists, militias, and racial-hate groups are examples of:
- **A.** international terrorists.
- **B.** state-sponsored terrorist groups.
- **C.** domestic terrorists.
- **D.** religious freedom fighters.

_____ 3. The EMT should be alert to clues when on the scene of a suspicious incident. An acronym designed to help with this process is:
- **A.** CBRNE.
- **B.** TRACEM-P.
- **C.** SAMPLE.
- **D.** OTTO.

_____ 4. Potential high-risk targets of terrorists typically include:
- **A.** controversial businesses.
- **B.** infrastructure systems.
- **C.** public buildings.
- **D.** any of these.

_____ 5. Why is April 19 a day when the U.S. government stands at heightened security awareness for government facilities?
- **A.** It is the anniversary of the Pearl Harbor attack.
- **B.** It is the anniversary of the bombing of the Murrah building in Oklahoma City.
- **C.** It is the anniversary of the birth of the FBI.
- **D.** It is the anniversary of the Bay of Pigs incident.

_____ 6. Responding EMTs who arrive on the scene of an incident should watch for signs that they may be dealing with a suspicious incident. Examples of unexplained patterns of illness or deaths may include each of the following _except_:
- **A.** car crashes involving more than two patients with serious traumatic injuries.
- **B.** unexplained symptoms of skin or eye irritation.
- **C.** unexplained vapor clouds, mists, and plumes.
- **D.** unexplained signs of airway irritation.

_____ 7. The acronym TRACEM-P is designed to help rescuers understand the types of harm to which they can be exposed. What does the letter E refer to?
- **A.** "Emergency"
- **B.** "Environmental"
- **C.** "Biological/etiological"
- **D.** "Essential"

_____ 8. Danger from alpha particles, beta particles, or gamma rays is caused by _____ harm.
- **A.** chemical
- **B.** radiological
- **C.** biological/etiological
- **D.** mechanical

_____ 9. The major routes through which WMD agents can enter the body include each of the following _except_:
- **A.** absorption.
- **B.** ingestion.
- **C.** osmosis.
- **D.** inhalation.

_____ 10. The types of harm from radiological/nuclear incidents include radiological, chemical, and _____ harm.
- **A.** psychological
- **B.** mechanical
- **C.** thermal
- **D.** all of these

_____ 11. The primary harm from a nuclear explosion involves _____ harm.
- **A.** chemical
- **B.** mechanical
- **C.** psychological
- **D.** biological

_____ 12. The mainstays of self-protection at a radiological incident include all of the following *except*:
   A. time.   C. distance.
   B. Standard Precautions.   D. shielding.

_____ 13. You are on the scene where there is a suspicion that someone may have been exposed to anthrax. Which is the most lethal route of exposure to anthrax?
   A. Skin contact   C. Inhalation
   B. Ingestion   D. Injection

_____ 14. The _____ route of exposure is very effective with vesicants but less effective with many of the biological agents.
   A. dermal   C. airborne
   B. vector   D. bloodborne

_____ 15. Features that influence the potential for a biological agent's use as a weapon include:
   A. infectivity and virulence.   C. transmissibility and lethality.
   B. toxicity and incubation period. D. any of these.

_____ 16. The quality of being poisonous, especially the degree of strength of a toxic microbe or of a poison, is referred to as:
   A. infectivity.   C. virulence.
   B. toxicity.   D. transmissibility.

_____ 17. The relative ease with which an agent causes death in a susceptible population is referred to as the:
   A. stability of the product.   C. lethality of the agent.
   B. infectivity of the agent.   D. virulence of the virus.

_____ 18. Which virus did the World Health Organization declare eradicated worldwide in 1980 through immunization efforts?
   A. Polio   C. Viral hemorrhagic fever
   B. Encephalitis   D. Smallpox

_____ 19. Which of the following is *not* a common mechanism for performing decontamination?
   A. Demulsification   C. Disinfection
   B. Chemical reaction   D. Absorption and adsorption

_____ 20. A process that simply reduces the concentration of the contaminant is called:
   A. removal.   C. dilution.
   B. disposal.   D. emulsification.

_____ 21. You have responded to a building collapse. It is believed that the three-story office building was vacant at the time of the collapse. The fire department personnel believe there was an explosion that caused the front of the building to cave in. Of the following, each are types of harm, in addition to mechanical harm, that can result from an explosive incident *except*:
   A. thermal harm.   C. water damage.
   B. asphyxiation.   D. chemical hazards.

_____ 22. After the scene is safe at the scene described in multiple-choice question 21, you are called to the back of the building where you find an elderly man who lives in the alleyway there. He is coughing and complaining of breathing problems. It is obvious that he may have inhaled a large quantity of dust when the building collapsed. What is another danger to this patient?
   A. His skin may be very dirty or greasy.
   B. There are often toxic particles, such as asbestos, in the dust.
   C. The water he was drinking may be contaminated.
   D. He may be developing hypothermia.

_____ **23.** In recent years, investigations in the United States have uncovered groups manufacturing a chemical called _____, which is designed to interrupt the body's protein manufacturing process at the cellular level by _____.
  A. staphylococcal enterotoxin; causing extreme fat wasting
  B. botulinum; killing off the bone marrow
  C. ricin; altering the RNA needed for proper proteins
  D. trichothecene mycotoxins; eliminating absorbic acid

_____ **24.** You were called to the scene of a patient who is very weak and is complaining of a fever. He has a number of bruises, and the sclera of his eyes seem to be leaking blood from the tiny capillaries. He works in a lab and has been doing some "top secret" experiments recently. What could be the cause of this sickness?
  A. Smallpox   **C.** Encephalitis
  B. Rabies   **D.** A viral hemorrhagic fever

INSIDE/OUTSIDE: SLUDGEM

1. When a nerve agent acts on the parasympathetic nervous system, what is the enzyme that is usually inhibited by the nerve agent?

_____

2. What are the seven most common signs and symptoms that occur due to overstimulation of the parasympathetic nervous system?

  A. _____

  B. _____

  C. _____

  D. _____

  E. _____

  F. _____

  G. _____

COMPLETE THE FOLLOWING

1. List the four major routes of entry of poisons into the body.

  A. _____

  B. _____

  C. _____

  D. _____

2. List four broad classifications of chemical weapons.

A. _____

B. _____

C. _____

D. _____

STREET SCENES DISCUSSION

Review the Street Scene on page 1097 of the textbook. Then answer the following questions.

1. Why would you consider the organization a potential threat to emergency services personnel?

2. Is it unusual to find a motor vehicle collision in an isolated location such as the one in this scenario?

3. Is it an acceptable practice to stop and not proceed if the emergency services personnel feel they are in imminent danger?

4. What are some other examples of groups or types of domestic terrorists that have been identified?

Interim Exam 3

Use the answer sheet on pages 411–412 to complete this exam. It is perforated, so it can be removed easily from this workbook.

1. The circulation of blood throughout the body, filling the capillaries and supplying the cells and tissues with oxygen and nutrients, is called:
   A. physiology.
   B. perfusion.
   C. bleeding.
   D. metabolism.

2. You find a 19-year-old male trauma patient lying across the front seat of his sports car after a head-on collision. He is making gurgling sounds as he breathes. What should you do?
   A. Ventilate him.
   B. Suction the airway.
   C. Hyperextend the neck.
   D. Apply high-concentration oxygen.

3. Sometimes a _____ can act as a full-body splint when the critical trauma patient described in multiple-choice question 2 must be immobilized quickly.
   A. wheeled stretcher
   B. short KED
   C. warm blanket
   D. long backboard

4. On further examination of the patient in multiple-choice question 2, you note that the patient has two fractured femurs, a crushed pelvis, and a possible abdominal injury. You should:
   A. not apply a traction splint(s).
   B. consider the PASG if your protocol allows.
   C. set up an ALS intercept en route to the hospital.
   D. do all of these.

5. When you must minimize the scene care of a multiple-trauma patient, you can perform any of the following *except*:
   A. suction the airway.
   B. ventilate with a BVM.
   C. bandage all the lacerations.
   D. immobilize the cervical spine.

6. Even when you are trying to cut scene time for a multiple-trauma patient, the one thing you should *not* cut out is:
   A. applying a traction splint if needed.
   B. the secondary exam.
   C. scene safety.
   D. immobilization.

7. You are treating a 17-year-old male patient who fell from two stories and is in severe pain. Internal bleeding is not visible, so you must base the severity of blood loss on:
   A. signs and symptoms exhibited.
   B. what the patient tells you.
   C. the size of the contusion.
   D. advice from medical direction.

8. For the patient described in multiple-choice question 7, the factors on which severity of bleeding depends include all of the following *except*:
   A. the rate of bleeding and the amount of blood loss.
   B. the patient's age and weight.
   C. the ability of the patient's body to respond and defend against blood loss.
   D. the patient's history of diabetes.

9. Blood that oozes and is dark red is most likely from a(n):
   A. vein.
   B. capillary.
   C. artery.
   D. lymphatic vessel.

10. You are treating a 22-year-old female who slashed her wrist in an effort to end her life. The wound is spurting bright red blood, and she has decided to let you treat her. After trying direct pressure and elevation to control the bleeding, the next step would be to:
    A. apply a tourniquet to the leg.
    B. apply an air splint to the arm.
    C. press on the brachial artery.
    D. press on the femoral artery.

11. When other methods have failed to control bleeding for the patient in multiple-choice question 10, you should:
    A. apply the PASG.
    B. apply an air splint.
    C. press harder on the pressure point.
    D. apply a tourniquet.

12. Signs of internal bleeding include all of the following *except*:
    A. painful, swollen, or deformed extremities.
    B. a tender, rigid abdomen.
    C. vomiting bile.
    D. bruising.

13. Examples of penetrating trauma include all of the following *except* a
   A. handgun bullet wound.
   B. carving-knife wound.
   C. fall from a height.
   D. screwdriver stab wound.

14. Examples of blunt trauma include all of the following *except*:
   A. blast injuries.
   B. auto-pedestrian collisions.
   C. gunshot wounds.
   D. falls.

15. You are treating a 49-year-old male patient who was assaulted. You suspect he may have some internal bleeding. The signs and symptoms of internal bleeding are:
   A. the same as those of shock.
   B. identical to those of external bleeding.
   C. usually not present in elderly patients.
   D. easy to stabilize in the field.

16. Which of the following is *not* considered a type of shock?
   A. Hypovolemic
   B. Hydrophobic
   C. Cardiogenic
   D. Neurogenic

17. The point at which the body can no longer compensate for low blood volume is referred to as the:
   A. compensated phase of shock.
   B. anaphylactic phase of shock.
   C. decompensated phase of shock.
   D. terminal phase of shock.

18. What are the major components of the central nervous system?
   A. Cranial nerves
   B. Peripheral nerves
   C. Brain and spinal cord
   D. Vessels and support tissue

19. Which of the following is *not* a division of the nervous system?
   A. Central
   B. Peripheral
   C. Autonomic
   D. Voluntary

20. The skull is made up of the cranium and the facial bones. The cranium consists of the _____ areas of the skull.
   A. temporal, mandible, and maxilla
   B. frontal, parietal, and distal
   C. anterior, forehead, and lateral
   D. forehead, top, back, and upper sides

21. The bones forming the face include all of the following *except*:
   A. vertebrae.   C. mandible.
   B. zygomatic.   D. maxillae.

22. The brain and spinal cord are bathed in:
   A. cerebrospinal fluid.
   B. lymphatic fluid.
   C. synovial fluid.
   D. mucous secretion.

23. The spine is divided into sections called:
   A. joints.   C. coccygeal.
   B. vertebrae.   D. compartments.

24. The lumbar area of the spine includes _____ vertebrae.
   A. 3   C. 8
   B. 5   D. 12

25. A bacterial disease that can be used in an act of biological terrorism to inflict serious illness, severe diarrhea, dehydration, and electrolyte imbalances in its victims is:
   A. plague.   C. ricin.
   B. anthrax.   D. cholera.

26. A 22-year-old female struck her head and states that she feels groggy and has a headache. She most likely has:
   A. an abrasion.   C. a contrecoup.
   B. a concussion.   D. none of these.

27. A 50-year-old male driver who was involved in an automobile collision states that he did not lose consciousness. However, a bystander says that he ran to the car after the collision and tried to talk to the driver, but said that the driver "just sat there staring off into space for a few minutes." This patient may have any of the following *except*:
   A. contusion.
   B. concussion.
   C. coup injury.
   D. attention deficit.

28. A patient has some memory loss after a head injury. This is referred to as:
   A. bruising.
   B. amnesia.
   C. verbally responsive.
   D. "seeing stars."

29. A bruising of the brain occurs on the side of the injury. This is referred to as a(n) _____ injury.
   A. contrecoup   C. coup
   B. hematoma   D. epidural

©2012 Pearson Education, Inc.
Emergency Care, 12th Ed.

30. A collection of blood within the skull or the brain is called:
- **A.** a subdural hematoma.
- **B.** an epidural hematoma.
- **C.** an intracerebral bleed.
- **D.** any of these.

31. All of the following make a head injury worse *except*:
- **A.** limited room for expansion inside the skull.
- **B.** increased pressure in the skull.
- **C.** increased carbon dioxide level in the brain.
- **D.** decreased respiration leading to increased cellular perfusion.

32. An assessment strategy used to check an extremity for injury or paralysis in a conscious patient is:
- **A.** checking for a proximal pulse.
- **B.** assessing equality of strength.
- **C.** checking for foot wave.
- **D.** confirming sensitivity.

33. The time between exposure and the appearance of symptoms is referred to as the:
- **A.** toxicity period.
- **B.** incubation period.
- **C.** transmissibility time frame.
- **D.** infectivity window.

34. If a patient has a brain injury with a skull fracture, the patient's pupils tend to be:
- **A.** equal.
- **C.** constricted.
- **B.** dilated.
- **D.** unequal.

35. Which of the following describes the blood pressure and pulse for a patient with a traumatic brain injury?
- **A.** Decreased blood pressure, increased pulse
- **B.** Decreased blood pressure, decreased pulse
- **C.** Increased blood pressure, increased pulse
- **D.** Increased blood pressure, decreased pulse

36. Consider the possibility of a cranial fracture whenever you note:
- **A.** deep lacerations or severe bruises to the scalp or forehead.
- **B.** a deformed femur.
- **C.** facial deformity.
- **D.** blood or other fluids in the airway.

37. The spinal column is made up of _____ shaped bones.
- **A.** 33 regularly
- **B.** 33 irregularly
- **C.** 12 regularly
- **D.** 12 irregularly

38. Any blunt trauma above the clavicles may damage the _____ vertebrae.
- **A.** lumbar
- **C.** sacral
- **B.** cervical
- **D.** thoracic

39. Priapism is:
- **A.** a persistent erection of the penis.
- **B.** spasms of the hands and feet.
- **C.** apparent only in unconscious patients.
- **D.** uncontrolled muscle twitches of the thighs.

40. You are assessing a 22-year-old male who you suspect sustained a spine injury when he fell off the roof. Often with a cervical-spine injury, the patient in a supine position may have his arms:
- **A.** straight out at his side.
- **B.** stretched out above his head.
- **C.** down at his side.
- **D.** across his chest.

41. The EMT should consider that any injury of an elderly person could be a sign of:
- **A.** a severe fall.
- **B.** Alzheimer's disease.
- **C.** abuse or neglect.
- **D.** depression.

42. Geriatric patients usually have decreased elasticity of the lungs and decreased activity of cilia that result in:
- **A.** increased risk of heart attack.
- **B.** diminished activity and tolerance of physical stress.
- **C.** decreased ability to clear foreign substances from the lungs.
- **D.** decreased energy and tolerance of hot and cold.

43. Your patient is a 70-year-old male who was found confused and walking on the side of the highway. The loss of skin elasticity and shrinking of sweat glands in this geriatric patient can cause:
- **A.** diminished activity and tolerance of physical stress.
- **B.** decreased ability to clear foreign substances from the lungs.
- **C.** decreased energy and tolerance of hot and cold.
- **D.** thin, dry, wrinkled skin.

44. Diminished function of the thyroid gland is one of the effects of aging. This results in:
- **A.** thin, dry, wrinkled skin.
- **B.** decreased energy and tolerance of heat and cold.
- **C.** depression and loss of social support.
- **D.** decreased strength.

©2012 Pearson Education, Inc.
Emergency Care, 12th Ed.

Interim Exam 3 **403**

45. An elderly patient falls, which may indicate a more serious problem, such as:
   A. viral pneumonia.
   B. acute alcoholism.
   C. abnormal heart rhythm.
   D. severe depression.

46. An unstable object impaled in the cheek wall should be:
   A. stabilized from the outside.
   B. stabilized from the inside.
   C. pulled out if easily done.
   D. stabilized from the inside and the outside.

47. If possible, an 18-year-old male patient with facial fractures should be transported on a long spine board in the _____ position.
   A. supine
   B. Trendelenburg
   C. head-elevated
   D. prone

48. The pressure point for controlling bleeding from the leg is the:
   A. carotid artery.
   B. brachial artery.
   C. subclavian vein.
   D. femoral artery.

49. Care for an open wound includes all of the following except:
   A. picking embedded particles out of the cut.
   B. controlling bleeding.
   C. bandaging the dressing in place.
   D. cleaning the wound surface.

50. Your patient is a 55-year-old woman who called EMS because she has a nosebleed that has not stopped all afternoon. The best method for control of nasal bleeding is:
   A. packing the nose with cotton.
   B. pinching the nostrils together.
   C. packing the nose with gauze.
   D. applying pressure to the facial artery.

51. The first step in caring for possible internal bleeding—after ensuring respiration and circulation and controlling life-threatening external bleeding—is:
   A. administering liquids by mouth to the patient.
   B. applying a bulky dressing.
   C. treating for shock.
   D. placing the patient in a sitting position.

52. A razor blade cut is an example of a(n):
   A. incision.
   B. abrasion.
   C. contusion.
   D. laceration.

53. The injury in which flaps of skin and tissue are torn loose or pulled off completely is called a(n):
   A. laceration.
   B. amputation.
   C. incision.
   D. avulsion.

54. A 22-year-old female patient has an object impaled in the forearm. After the control of profuse bleeding, you should:
   A. remove the object.
   B. place a pressure dressing over the site.
   C. stabilize the object.
   D. apply firm pressure to a pressure point.

55. Which of the following is a sign of shock?
   A. High blood pressure
   B. Constricted pupils
   C. Slowed pulse rate
   D. Pale, cool, clammy skin

56. An object impaled in the eye should be:
   A. stabilized with gauze and protected with a disposable cup.
   B. removed carefully and a pressure dressing applied.
   C. shielded with a cup taped over the orbit.
   D. removed and a dressing applied with minimum pressure.

57. A lacerated eyelid or injury to the eyeball should be:
   A. flushed with water.
   B. covered with a cold pack.
   C. covered with folded 4 × 4s.
   D. covered with dark patches.

58. All open wounds to the chest should be considered:
   A. life threatening.
   B. potentially infectious.
   C. a low priority.
   D. an indication for PASG.

59. Before moving a 35-year-old supine male patient with possible spinal injuries onto a long spine board, you should always:
   A. align the teeth and tape the jaw in place.
   B. apply a short spine board.
   C. apply a rigid collar.
   D. secure a KED to the patient.

60. The initial effort to control bleeding from a severed neck artery should include:
   A. direct pressure or pinching.
   B. applying tape.
   C. pressure points.
   D. occlusive dressing.

61. The most reliable sign of spinal-cord injury in a conscious 30-year-old female patient is:
   A. pain without movement.
   B. paralysis of extremities.
   C. pain with movement.
   D. tenderness along the spine.

62. When caring for an open abdominal wound with evisceration:
   A. replace the organ but cover with occlusive material.
   B. replace the organ but cover with a bulky dressing.
   C. do not replace the organ but cover with occlusive material.
   D. do not replace the organ but cover with a moistened dressing.

63. A 35-year-old female patient who is in acute abdominal distress but denies any vomiting should be transported to the ED:
   A. in the Trendelenburg position with legs straight.
   B. in the coma position.
   C. face up with the knees bent.
   D. in the recumbent position with one knee bent.

64. When a joint is locked into position, the EMT should:
   A. pull traction on the extremity.
   B. straighten it.
   C. splint it in the position found.
   D. skip splinting and transport immediately.

65. A splint properly applied to an extremity should prevent all of the following *except*:
   A. circulation to the extremity.
   B. an open bone injury.
   C. motion of bone fragments.
   D. damage to muscles and blood vessels.

66. A fracture to the humerus shaft is best cared for by immobilizing with a(n):
   A. wrist sling.
   B. rigid splint or sling and swathe.
   C. air-inflated splint.
   D. sling and swathe.

67. A fracture to the proximal end of the humerus is best cared for by immobilizing with a(n):
   A. wrist sling and swathe.
   B. padded board, sling, and swathe.
   C. air-inflated splint.
   D. sling and swathe.

68. Your 40-year-old female patient fell backward onto her left elbow and heard a loud snap. She has a distal pulse and sensation. The best way to immobilize a fractured elbow when the arm is found in the bent position and there is a distal pulse is to:
   A. straighten the arm and apply an air-inflated splint.
   B. keep the arm in its found position and apply a short, padded board splint.
   C. keep the arm in its found position and apply an air-inflated splint.
   D. straighten the arm and apply a wire-ladder splint.

69. If a severe deformity exists or distal circulation is compromised when you are splinting, you should:
   A. push protruding bones back into place.
   B. align to anatomical position under gentle traction.
   C. immediately move the patient to a stretcher.
   D. immobilize in the position found.

70. The first step in immobilizing a fractured wrist with distal pulse is to:
   A. correct angulation of the wrist.
   B. secure a padded board splint to the wrist.
   C. place the broken hand in its position of function.
   D. tape the wrist.

71. A 40-year-old female patient with a fractured pelvis should be immobilized on an orthopedic stretcher or long spine board with:
   A. legs bound together with wide cravats.
   B. long padded boards secured down each side of the body.
   C. stabilizing sandbags placed between the legs.
   D. straps securing the torso and pelvis.

72. A fractured femur is best immobilized with a(n) _____ splint.
   A. long padded   C. rigid vacuum
   B. air-inflated   D. traction

73. Before immobilizing a fractured knee:
   A. assess distal circulation and sensory and motor function.
   B. straighten the angulation.
   C. apply firm traction.
   D. flex the leg at the knee.

74. The best method for immobilizing a suspected ankle fracture is a(n) _____ splint.
   A. traction
   B. padded board
   C. pillow splint
   D. air-inflated

75. A sprain is an injury in which:
  A. tendons are torn.
  B. ligaments are torn.
  C. cartilage is crushed.
  D. muscles spasm.

76. Which of the following is *not* true of open extremity injuries?
  A. The skin has been broken or torn.
  B. There is increased likelihood of infection.
  C. Definitive care is provided in the prehospital setting.
  D. Such injuries require surgery at the hospital.

77. Muscle is attached to bone by:
  A. cartilage.
  B. ligaments.
  C. smooth muscles.
  D. tendons.

78. A partial thickness burn involves the:
  A. epidermis.
  B. epidermis and dermis.
  C. epidermis, dermis, and subcutaneous layers.
  D. epidermis, dermis, and subcutaneous layers, and muscles.

79. The entire back of a 50-year-old female's right arm and her entire chest have been burned. What percentage of surface burn would you report?
  A. 13.5 percent   C. 27 percent
  B. 18 percent   D. 36 percent

80. A moderate burn involves:
  A. partial and full thickness burns of the face and hands.
  B. full thickness burns over less than 2 percent of the body surface.
  C. superficial burns covering more than 50 percent of the body surface.
  D. superficial burns covering less than 20 percent of the body surface.

81. Partial thickness burns cause:
  A. swelling and blistering.
  B. nerve damage.
  C. slight swelling.
  D. scarring.

82. A 40-year-old male patient is suffering from chemical burns to the skin caused by dry lime. After putting on PPE, your next step should be to:
  A. wash the area with running water.
  B. remove the lime with phenol.
  C. remove the lime with alcohol.
  D. brush away the lime.

83. Acid burns to the eyes should be flooded with water for at least _____ minute(s).
  A. 1   C. 10
  B. 5   D. 20

84. A method for estimating the extent of a burn is the:
  A. rule of nines.
  B. rule of percentages.
  C. rule of degree.
  D. burn assessment rule.

85. If a woman is having her first baby, the first stage of labor will usually last an average of _____ hours.
  A. 4
  B. 8
  C. 12
  D. 16

86. During the most active stage of labor, the uterus usually contracts every _____ minutes.
  A. 1 to 2
  B. 2 to 3
  C. 5 to 9
  D. 10 to 15

87. If the amniotic sac does not break during delivery, the EMT should:
  A. do nothing; it will break after birth.
  B. quickly remove it with sterile scissors.
  C. puncture it with a finger.
  D. transport the patient immediately.

88. To assist the mother in delivering the baby, gently:
  A. pull at the baby's shoulders.
  B. support the baby's head.
  C. rotate the baby to the left or right.
  D. push your gloved hand into the vagina.

89. After the delivery, which of the following should be done first?
  A. Clamp and cut the cord.
  B. Suction the baby's mouth and nose.
  C. Lay the baby on his back.
  D. Lift the baby by the feet and slap the buttocks.

90. Following delivery, if spontaneous respiration does not begin after suctioning the baby's mouth and nose, the EMT should first:
  A. begin mouth-to-mouth-and-nose resuscitation.
  B. apply mechanical resuscitation with 100 percent oxygen.
  C. vigorously rub the baby's back.
  D. transport immediately, administering 100 percent oxygen.

91. You are on the scene of a car crash. To assist with patient access, the EMT should initially do each of the following *except*:
    A. try opening each car door.
    B. roll down windows.
    C. ask the patient to unlock the doors.
    D. pull the patient out the side windows.

92. What dictates the specific technique used for spinal immobilization of a patient at a collision extrication?
    A. Requirements for speed of removal
    B. How many rescuers are available for removal
    C. Whether an airbag has deployed
    D. None of these

93. Which step in the phases of the rescue process is out of order?
    1. Sizing up the situation
    2. Gaining access
    3. Disentangling the patient
    4. Stabilizing the vehicle
    A. 1
    B. 2
    C. 3
    D. 4

94. Considerations for size-up of a collision include all of the following *except*:
    A. potential hazards.
    B. need for additional EMS units.
    C. number of patients involved.
    D. number of ambulances in the region.

95. To minimize injuries at a collision, the EMT should:
    A. use a limited number of tools.
    B. deactivate the safety guards on tools.
    C. wear highly visible clothing.
    D. wait until the police arrive on the scene.

96. The vehicle's catalytic converter can be a source of ignition at a collision because it:
    A. often emits sparks.
    B. is often over 1,200°F.
    C. may leak gasoline.
    D. pumps high-pressure fumes.

97. The three-step process of disentanglement described in the text includes all of the following *except*:
    A. opening the trunk and cutting the battery cable.
    B. creating exits by displacing doors and roof posts.
    C. disentangling occupants by displacing the front end.
    D. gaining access by disposing of the roof.

98. Which of the following is *true* about dealing with a collision vehicle's electrical system?
    A. It should be disabled by cutting a battery cable.
    B. If it must be disrupted, disconnect the ground cable from the battery.
    C. Cutting the battery cable can assist in rescue operations.
    D. Disconnecting the ground cable produces a spark that can ignite battery gases.

99. When positioning flares, use a formula that includes the stopping distance for the posted speed plus the:
    A. angle of the road.
    B. radius of the danger zone.
    C. reaction distance.
    D. margin of safety.

100. Once the vehicle has been stabilized, the *next* part of an extrication procedure for patient rescue is to:
    A. dispose of the vehicle's roof.
    B. displace the front end of the vehicle.
    C. displace doors and roof posts.
    D. do none of these.

101. The Emergency Medical Dispatcher (EMD) has told you the exact location of a collision, how many and what kinds of vehicles are involved, and any known hazards. What other information would you like the EMD to provide concerning this collision?
    A. How many persons are injured
    B. The direction designator
    C. How to contact the person who reported the collision
    D. The nature of the emergency

102. Which of the following is an *unnecessary* question for the Emergency Medical Dispatcher to ask when receiving a call for help?
    A. How old is the patient?
    B. What's the patient's gender?
    C. What's the patient's name?
    D. Is the patient conscious?

103. When operating a siren, be aware that:
    A. the continuous sound of a siren could worsen a patient's condition.
    B. all motorists will hear and honor your signal.
    C. the siren must be used continuously when carrying injured patients.
    D. it is necessary to pull up close to vehicles and sound the siren.

104. All of the following are factors that affect an ambulance's response to a scene *except*:
A. the day of the week.
B. the time of day.
C. detours.
D. danger zones.

105. If a patient develops cardiac arrest during transport, have the operator of the ambulance:
A. adjust the ambulance's speed.
B. stop the ambulance.
C. contact the hospital emergency department.
D. assist you with CPR.

106. When transferring a nonemergency patient to the emergency department personnel, you should:
A. wait for emergency staff to call for the patient.
B. off-load, wheel to the designated area, and stay with the patient.
C. check to see what is to be done with the patient.
D. off-load, wheel to the designated area, and leave the patient.

107. The last step when transferring a patient is to:
A. wait to help the emergency department staff.
B. transfer the patient's valuables.
C. obtain your release.
D. transfer patient information.

108. At the hospital, as soon as you are free from patient-care activities, you should:
A. notify dispatch you are back in service.
B. quickly clean the vehicle's patient compartment.
C. prepare the prehospital care report.
D. check on patient status with the emergency department.

109. Which of the following is *not* a biohazard?
A. Suction catheters
B. Contaminated dressings
C. Blood-soaked linen
D. Unopened gauze bandages

110. Which of the following is *not* a benefit of an EMS/hospital equipment exchange program?
A. Patients are not subjected to injury-aggravating movement.
B. Delay of the crew at the hospital is prevented.
C. Ambulances can return to quarters fully equipped.
D. Completeness and operability of equipment is ensured.

111. Vigorous cleaning of the ambulance while parked at the hospital is prevented or restricted by all of the following limitations *except*:
A. time.
B. equipment.
C. space.
D. law.

112. You have just assisted the mother in delivering a healthy newborn. The first clamp placed on the umbilical cord should be about _____ inches from the baby.
A. 2   C. 10
B. 5   D. 12

113. If bleeding continues from the umbilical cord after clamping and cutting, the EMT should:
A. clamp the cord again.
B. unclamp the cord and tie.
C. apply a sterile dressing.
D. transport the baby immediately.

114. Which of the following is the maximum amount of time the EMT should wait for the placenta to be delivered before transporting the mother and infant?
A. 20 minutes   C. 1 hour
B. 45 minutes   D. 2 hours

115. Delivery of the placenta is usually accompanied by the loss of no more than _____ of blood.
A. 500 cc   C. 800 cc
B. 600 cc   D. 1,000 cc

116. The first step to control vaginal bleeding after birth is to:
A. apply a pressure dressing.
B. position a sanitary napkin.
C. massage the uterus.
D. pack the vagina with sterile gauze.

117. Along with physical and mental fitness, ambulance operators should be able to:
A. move other vehicles off the roadway.
B. perform under stress.
C. always be up for a run.
D. justify feelings of superiority.

118. When driving an ambulance, you should realize that there are no state laws that grant the:
A. use of controlled additional speed.
B. passage through traffic signals.
C. privilege of special parking at the scene.
D. absolute right of way.

119. If, during birth, the umbilical cord presents first, you should:
   A. gently push the cord back into the vagina.
   B. gently push up on the baby's head or buttocks to keep pressure off the cord.
   C. gently push on the cervix.
   D. clamp and cut the cord.

120. If an arm presentation without a prolapsed cord is noted, the EMT should:
   A. reach up the vagina and turn the baby.
   B. do nothing; the delivery will be normal.
   C. transport immediately and provide O_2.
   D. insert a gloved hand and push back the vaginal wall.

121. A baby is considered premature if it weighs less than 5 pounds or is born before the _____ week of pregnancy.
   A. 35th   C. 37th
   B. 36th   D. 38th

122. Which of the following signs is *not* an indication that a child has an airway disease?
   A. Wheezing
   B. Breathing effort on exhalation
   C. Rapid breathing
   D. Lack of airway passage swelling

123. The soft spot on top of an infant's head is called a:
   A. contusion.   C. fontanelle.
   B. depression site.   D. suture.

124. After calming a snake-bite victim and treating for shock, you locate the fang marks. Next, you should:
   A. immobilize the affected extremity.
   B. conserve patient body heat.
   C. cleanse the wound site.
   D. apply a tourniquet to the extremity.

125. A 49-year-old male patient who was installing a new roof on a very hot day complains of severe muscle cramps in his legs and feels faint. You should move the patient to a cool place and begin care by:
   A. administering oxygen by nonrebreather.
   B. transporting the patient immediately.
   C. administering oxygen by nasal cannula.
   D. giving the patient water.

126. In cases of sudden infant death syndrome, the EMT should:
   A. hunt for evidence of child abuse.
   B. hold off on care and simply transport the body.
   C. declare the patient dead.
   D. provide resuscitation and transport to the hospital.

127. Which of the following might lead you to consider child abuse?
   A. Multiple skinned knees
   B. A burn from chewing an electric cord
   C. Injuries to the center of the back and upper arms
   D. Both ankles are sprained

128. Your patient was outdoors on a very cold, windy day chopping wood. You notice that he did not have gloves on or a hat. You suspect he may have frostbite. With frostbite, the:
   A. underlying tissues feel frozen to the touch.
   B. skin is commonly mottled and grayish blue.
   C. skin blisters and swells.
   D. affected area feels frozen, but only on the surface.

129. The initial sign of hypothermia is:
   A. shivering.
   B. numbness.
   C. drowsiness and slow breathing.
   D. white, waxy skin.

130. Extreme hypothermia is characterized by:
   A. unconsciousness and absence of discernible vital signs.
   B. shivering, numbness, and drowsiness.
   C. flaccid muscles.
   D. rapid breathing.

131. Common causes of shock in children include infections, trauma, blood loss, and:
   A. meningitis.   C. dehydration.
   B. heart failure   D. lack of insulin.

132. A sunken fontanelle may indicate:
   A. elevated intracranial pressure.
   B. hypertension.
   C. dehydration.
   D. fever.

133. Flowing oxygen over the face of a small child so it will be inhaled is referred to as the _____ technique.
   A. blow-by   C. supplemental
   B. rebreather   D. flow-by

134. A complication of a rapidly rising temperature in a child is often:
   A. hyperactivity.
   B. a seizure.
   C. vomiting.
   D. ringing in the ears.

135. A group of viral illnesses that results in inflammation of the larynx, trachea, and bronchi is called:
   A. meningitis.   C. asthma.
   B. anaphylaxis.   D. croup.

136. The strong, white, fibrous material covering the bones is called the:
   A. shell.
   B. perineum.
   C. marrow.
   D. periosteum.

137. The coming apart of a joint is referred to as a:
   A. fracture.
   B. sprain.
   C. dislocation.
   D. strain.

138. Overstretching or overexertion of a muscle is called a:
   A. strain.
   B. sprain.
   C. dislocation.
   D. fracture.

139. In a heat emergency, the patient with _____, dry skin requires rapid cooling and immediate transport.
   A. pale
   B. hot
   C. cool
   D. warm

140. As frostbite progresses and exposure continues, the skin turns from white and waxy to:
   A. blotchy and grayish yellow.
   B. pale and pinkish red.
   C. deep blue at the nose and cheeks.
   D. cherry red, except for the extremities.

141. To treat a patient with deep frostbite:
   A. immerse the limb in 105°F water and transport the patient.
   B. rub snow on the frozen area or apply cold packs if available.
   C. cover the frostbitten area, handle it as gently as possible, and transport the patient.
   D. protect the frostbitten area by keeping it cold and transport the patient.

142. Your patient fell onto his right leg. The indications for a traction splint are a painful, swollen, deformed mid-thigh with
   A. an open fracture of the lower leg.
   B. extensive blood loss and shock.
   C. no joint or lower leg injury.
   D. either ankle or knee involvement.

143. The level of training established by OSHA for those who actually plug, patch, or stop the release of a hazardous material is called:
   A. First Responder Awareness.
   B. First Responder Operations.
   C. Hazardous Materials Technician.
   D. Paramedic.

144. At a hazardous materials incident site, the "safe zone" should be located:
   A. downwind/downhill.
   B. downwind/same level.
   C. upwind/same level.
   D. upwind/downhill.

145. A resource that must be maintained at the work site by the employer and that must be available to all employees working with hazardous materials is called:
   A. NFPA 704.
   B. a Material Safety Data Sheet.
   C. the *Emergency Response Guidebook*.
   D. a shipping manifest.

146. The responsibilities of EMS personnel at a hazmat incident include caring for the injured and:
   A. staging personnel and equipment in the warm zone.
   B. monitoring and rehabilitating the hazmat team members.
   C. decontaminating those exiting the hot zone.
   D. notifying medical direction about the incident.

147. You are assigning triage tags to multiple patients at a bus crash. Categorizing a patient as Priority 1 at an MCI means that the patient:
   A. is serious but does not have life-threatening injuries or illness.
   B. has minor musculoskeletal or soft-tissue injuries.
   C. is dead or fatally injured.
   D. has treatable life-threatening illness or injuries.

148. The MCI supervisor responsible for communicating with the treatment areas to determine the number and priority of the patients in each respective treatment area is called the _____ supervisor.
   A. staging
   B. triage
   C. treatment
   D. transportation

149. A Priority 2 patient would be color-coded as _____ to identify his or her treatment priority at an MCI.
   A. black
   B. green
   C. yellow
   D. red

150. At an MCI, patients who are assessed as having minor injuries should be categorized as Priority:
   A. 1.
   B. 2.
   C. 3.
   D. 4.

Interim Exam 3 Answer Sheet

Fill in the correct answer for each item. When scoring, note that there are
150 questions valued at 0.666 points each.

1. [ ] A	[ ] B	[ ] C	[ ] D		36. [ ] A	[ ] B	[ ] C	[ ] D
2. [ ] A	[ ] B	[ ] C	[ ] D		37. [ ] A	[ ] B	[ ] C	[ ] D
3. [ ] A	[ ] B	[ ] C	[ ] D		38. [ ] A	[ ] B	[ ] C	[ ] D
4. [ ] A	[ ] B	[ ] C	[ ] D		39. [ ] A	[ ] B	[ ] C	[ ] D
5. [ ] A	[ ] B	[ ] C	[ ] D		40. [ ] A	[ ] B	[ ] C	[ ] D
6. [ ] A	[ ] B	[ ] C	[ ] D		41. [ ] A	[ ] B	[ ] C	[ ] D
7. [ ] A	[ ] B	[ ] C	[ ] D		42. [ ] A	[ ] B	[ ] C	[ ] D
8. [ ] A	[ ] B	[ ] C	[ ] D		43. [ ] A	[ ] B	[ ] C	[ ] D
9. [ ] A	[ ] B	[ ] C	[ ] D		44. [ ] A	[ ] B	[ ] C	[ ] D
10. [ ] A	[ ] B	[ ] C	[ ] D		45. [ ] A	[ ] B	[ ] C	[ ] D
11. [ ] A	[ ] B	[ ] C	[ ] D		46. [ ] A	[ ] B	[ ] C	[ ] D
12. [ ] A	[ ] B	[ ] C	[ ] D		47. [ ] A	[ ] B	[ ] C	[ ] D
13. [ ] A	[ ] B	[ ] C	[ ] D		48. [ ] A	[ ] B	[ ] C	[ ] D
14. [ ] A	[ ] B	[ ] C	[ ] D		49. [ ] A	[ ] B	[ ] C	[ ] D
15. [ ] A	[ ] B	[ ] C	[ ] D		50. [ ] A	[ ] B	[ ] C	[ ] D
16. [ ] A	[ ] B	[ ] C	[ ] D		51. [ ] A	[ ] B	[ ] C	[ ] D
17. [ ] A	[ ] B	[ ] C	[ ] D		52. [ ] A	[ ] B	[ ] C	[ ] D
18. [ ] A	[ ] B	[ ] C	[ ] D		53. [ ] A	[ ] B	[ ] C	[ ] D
19. [ ] A	[ ] B	[ ] C	[ ] D		54. [ ] A	[ ] B	[ ] C	[ ] D
20. [ ] A	[ ] B	[ ] C	[ ] D		55. [ ] A	[ ] B	[ ] C	[ ] D
21. [ ] A	[ ] B	[ ] C	[ ] D		56. [ ] A	[ ] B	[ ] C	[ ] D
22. [ ] A	[ ] B	[ ] C	[ ] D		57. [ ] A	[ ] B	[ ] C	[ ] D
23. [ ] A	[ ] B	[ ] C	[ ] D		58. [ ] A	[ ] B	[ ] C	[ ] D
24. [ ] A	[ ] B	[ ] C	[ ] D		59. [ ] A	[ ] B	[ ] C	[ ] D
25. [ ] A	[ ] B	[ ] C	[ ] D		60. [ ] A	[ ] B	[ ] C	[ ] D
26. [ ] A	[ ] B	[ ] C	[ ] D		61. [ ] A	[ ] B	[ ] C	[ ] D
27. [ ] A	[ ] B	[ ] C	[ ] D		62. [ ] A	[ ] B	[ ] C	[ ] D
28. [ ] A	[ ] B	[ ] C	[ ] D		63. [ ] A	[ ] B	[ ] C	[ ] D
29. [ ] A	[ ] B	[ ] C	[ ] D		64. [ ] A	[ ] B	[ ] C	[ ] D
30. [ ] A	[ ] B	[ ] C	[ ] D		65. [ ] A	[ ] B	[ ] C	[ ] D
31. [ ] A	[ ] B	[ ] C	[ ] D		66. [ ] A	[ ] B	[ ] C	[ ] D
32. [ ] A	[ ] B	[ ] C	[ ] D		67. [ ] A	[ ] B	[ ] C	[ ] D
33. [ ] A	[ ] B	[ ] C	[ ] D		68. [ ] A	[ ] B	[ ] C	[ ] D
34. [ ] A	[ ] B	[ ] C	[ ] D		69. [ ] A	[ ] B	[ ] C	[ ] D
35. [ ] A	[ ] B	[ ] C	[ ] D		70. [ ] A	[ ] B	[ ] C	[ ] D

71.	[ ] A	[ ] B	[ ] C	[ ] D		111.	[ ] A	[ ] B	[ ] C	[ ] D
72.	[ ] A	[ ] B	[ ] C	[ ] D		112.	[ ] A	[ ] B	[ ] C	[ ] D
73.	[ ] A	[ ] B	[ ] C	[ ] D		113.	[ ] A	[ ] B	[ ] C	[ ] D
74.	[ ] A	[ ] B	[ ] C	[ ] D		114.	[ ] A	[ ] B	[ ] C	[ ] D
75.	[ ] A	[ ] B	[ ] C	[ ] D		115.	[ ] A	[ ] B	[ ] C	[ ] D
76.	[ ] A	[ ] B	[ ] C	[ ] D		116.	[ ] A	[ ] B	[ ] C	[ ] D
77.	[ ] A	[ ] B	[ ] C	[ ] D		117.	[ ] A	[ ] B	[ ] C	[ ] D
78.	[ ] A	[ ] B	[ ] C	[ ] D		118.	[ ] A	[ ] B	[ ] C	[ ] D
79.	[ ] A	[ ] B	[ ] C	[ ] D		119.	[ ] A	[ ] B	[ ] C	[ ] D
80.	[ ] A	[ ] B	[ ] C	[ ] D		120.	[ ] A	[ ] B	[ ] C	[ ] D
81.	[ ] A	[ ] B	[ ] C	[ ] D		121.	[ ] A	[ ] B	[ ] C	[ ] D
82.	[ ] A	[ ] B	[ ] C	[ ] D		122.	[ ] A	[ ] B	[ ] C	[ ] D
83.	[ ] A	[ ] B	[ ] C	[ ] D		123.	[ ] A	[ ] B	[ ] C	[ ] D
84.	[ ] A	[ ] B	[ ] C	[ ] D		124.	[ ] A	[ ] B	[ ] C	[ ] D
85.	[ ] A	[ ] B	[ ] C	[ ] D		125.	[ ] A	[ ] B	[ ] C	[ ] D
86.	[ ] A	[ ] B	[ ] C	[ ] D		126.	[ ] A	[ ] B	[ ] C	[ ] D
87.	[ ] A	[ ] B	[ ] C	[ ] D		127.	[ ] A	[ ] B	[ ] C	[ ] D
88.	[ ] A	[ ] B	[ ] C	[ ] D		128.	[ ] A	[ ] B	[ ] C	[ ] D
89.	[ ] A	[ ] B	[ ] C	[ ] D		129.	[ ] A	[ ] B	[ ] C	[ ] D
90.	[ ] A	[ ] B	[ ] C	[ ] D		130.	[ ] A	[ ] B	[ ] C	[ ] D
91.	[ ] A	[ ] B	[ ] C	[ ] D		131.	[ ] A	[ ] B	[ ] C	[ ] D
92.	[ ] A	[ ] B	[ ] C	[ ] D		132.	[ ] A	[ ] B	[ ] C	[ ] D
93.	[ ] A	[ ] B	[ ] C	[ ] D		133.	[ ] A	[ ] B	[ ] C	[ ] D
94.	[ ] A	[ ] B	[ ] C	[ ] D		134.	[ ] A	[ ] B	[ ] C	[ ] D
95.	[ ] A	[ ] B	[ ] C	[ ] D		135.	[ ] A	[ ] B	[ ] C	[ ] D
96.	[ ] A	[ ] B	[ ] C	[ ] D		136.	[ ] A	[ ] B	[ ] C	[ ] D
97.	[ ] A	[ ] B	[ ] C	[ ] D		137.	[ ] A	[ ] B	[ ] C	[ ] D
98.	[ ] A	[ ] B	[ ] C	[ ] D		138.	[ ] A	[ ] B	[ ] C	[ ] D
99.	[ ] A	[ ] B	[ ] C	[ ] D		139.	[ ] A	[ ] B	[ ] C	[ ] D
100.	[ ] A	[ ] B	[ ] C	[ ] D		140.	[ ] A	[ ] B	[ ] C	[ ] D
101.	[ ] A	[ ] B	[ ] C	[ ] D		141.	[ ] A	[ ] B	[ ] C	[ ] D
102.	[ ] A	[ ] B	[ ] C	[ ] D		142.	[ ] A	[ ] B	[ ] C	[ ] D
103.	[ ] A	[ ] B	[ ] C	[ ] D		143.	[ ] A	[ ] B	[ ] C	[ ] D
104.	[ ] A	[ ] B	[ ] C	[ ] D		144.	[ ] A	[ ] B	[ ] C	[ ] D
105.	[ ] A	[ ] B	[ ] C	[ ] D		145.	[ ] A	[ ] B	[ ] C	[ ] D
106.	[ ] A	[ ] B	[ ] C	[ ] D		146.	[ ] A	[ ] B	[ ] C	[ ] D
107.	[ ] A	[ ] B	[ ] C	[ ] D		147.	[ ] A	[ ] B	[ ] C	[ ] D
108.	[ ] A	[ ] B	[ ] C	[ ] D		148.	[ ] A	[ ] B	[ ] C	[ ] D
109.	[ ] A	[ ] B	[ ] C	[ ] D		149.	[ ] A	[ ] B	[ ] C	[ ] D
110.	[ ] A	[ ] B	[ ] C	[ ] D		150.	[ ] A	[ ] B	[ ] C	[ ] D

BASIC CARDIAC LIFE SUPPORT REVIEW

Some EMT students learned cardiopulmonary resuscitation (CPR) before they began their EMT course. Others learn it in their EMT course. This section reviews the elements of CPR in accordance with the American Heart Association's 2010 Guidelines for Cardiopulmonary Resuscitation and Emergency Cardiovascular Care.

MATCH TERMINOLOGY/ DEFINITIONS

A. Providing artificial ventilations to a person who has stopped breathing or whose breathing is inadequate

B. Manual thrusts to the abdomen used to dislodge an airway obstruction

C. When breathing and heartbeat stop

D. Pulse felt between the groove of the Adam's apple and the muscles located along the side of the neck

E. Requirement that the amount of time you spend compressing the patient's chest should be the same as the time spent for release

F. Bulging of the stomach that may be caused by forcing air into the patient's stomach during rescue breathing

G. When brain cells die

H. Red or purple skin discoloration that occurs when gravity causes the blood to sink to the lowest parts of the body and collect there

I. Placing the patient on his side to allow for drainage from the mouth and to prevent the tongue from falling backward.

J. Maneuver that provides for maximum opening of the airway

K. Pulse measured by feeling the major artery of the arm; the absence of this pulse is used as a sign, in infants, that heartbeat has stopped and CPR should begin

L. Actions you take to revive a person—or at least temporarily prevent biological death—by keeping the person's heart and lungs working

M. Maneuver used to open the airway of a patient with a suspected spine injury

_____ **1.** Biological death

_____ **2.** Brachial pulse

_____ **3.** Cardiopulmonary resuscitation

_____ **4.** Carotid pulse

_____ **5.** Clinical death

_____ **6.** 50:50 rule

_____ **7.** Gastric distention

_____ **8.** Head-tilt, chin-lift maneuver

_____ **9.** Abdominal thrust

_____ **10.** Jaw-thrust maneuver

_____ **11.** Line of lividity

_____ **12.** Recovery position

_____ **13.** Rescue breathing

MULTIPLE-CHOICE REVIEW

_____ 1. Four to six minutes after a patient's breathing and heartbeat stop, the _____ cells will begin to die.
   A. heart
   B. brain
   C. liver
   D. kidney

_____ 2. Once clinical death occurs, how long does it usually take for biological death to occur?
   A. 4 minutes
   B. 6 minutes
   C. 8 minutes
   D. 10 minutes

_____ 3. In the CAB method of cardiopulmonary resuscitation, the "A" stands for:
   A. air flow.
   B. arterial pulse.
   C. airway.
   D. aorta.

_____ 4. In the CAB method of cardiopulmonary resuscitation, the "C" stands for:
   A. cardiac.
   B. compression.
   C. circulation.
   D. carotid.

_____ 5. To determine if an adult or a child (over a year old) is pulseless, the EMT should check for a pulse at the _____ artery.
   A. femoral
   B. brachial
   C. radial
   D. carotid

_____ 6. To determine pulselessness in an infant, the EMT should use the _____ artery.
   A. brachial
   B. carotid
   C. femoral
   D. apical

_____ 7. You are alone and do not have an AED. After determining unresponsiveness in an adult, the next thing you should do before starting CPR is:
   A. reposition the patient.
   B. activate EMS.
   C. establish an open airway.
   D. check for breathing.

_____ 8. When an unconscious patient's head flexes forward, the _____ could cause an airway obstruction.
   A. hypopharynx
   B. uvula
   C. tongue
   D. larynx

_____ 9. One of the best methods to relieve an airway obstruction due to the positioning of the patient's tongue is the _____ maneuver.
   A. jaw-thrust
   B. abdominal-thrust
   C. head-tilt, chin-lift
   D. jaw-lift

_____ 10. The head-tilt, chin-lift maneuver should _not_ be used on a:
   A. stroke victim.
   B. diabetic patient.
   C. diving accident victim.
   D. patient who had a seizure in bed.

_____ 11. The recommended maneuver for health care providers for opening the airway of a patient with possible cervical-spine injury is the _____ maneuver.
   A. jaw-thrust
   B. mouth-to-nose
   C. head-tilt, chin-lift
   D. jaw-lift

_____ 12. After opening the airway in a patient who requires rescue breathing, the EMT should inflate the patient's lung with:
   A. one quick, full breath.
   B. two breaths, 1 second each.
   C. one-half of a breath.
   D. four slow breaths.

©2012 Pearson Education, Inc.
Emergency Care, 12th Ed.

_____ **13.** You are treating a 55-year-old male who was found unresponsive by his wife. You have completed a set of compressions and now your initial two ventilations are not resulting in chest rise. Your next step is to:
  A. continue standard mouth-to-mask ventilations.
  B. administer oxygen.
  C. perform the steps of CPR.
  D. deliver four quick breaths.

_____ **14.** A common problem in the resuscitation of infants and children caused by improper head position or too quick ventilations is:
  A. spinal injury.   **C.** pulmonary trauma.
  B. gastric distention.   **D.** airway injury.

_____ **15.** Adult rescue breathing should be provided at a rate of _____ breaths per minute.
  A. 5–7   **C.** 15–20
  B. 10–12   **D.** 21–25

_____ **16.** Infants should be ventilated at the rate of one breath every _____ seconds.
  A. 3   **C.** 8
  B. 5   **D.** 10

_____ **17.** When you arrived on the scene, bystanders were already performing ventilations on the patient. If a patient has a distended abdomen due to air being forced into the stomach, the EMT should:
  A. manually press on the abdomen to relieve the distention.
  B. decrease the oxygen concentration being administered to the patient.
  C. be prepared to suction should the patient vomit.
  D. increase the force of the ventilation.

_____ **18.** Why is the recovery position used?
  A. It protects the airway and allows for drainage from the mouth.
  B. It forces the mouth to remain open at all times.
  C. It protects the patient's head during a seizure.
  D. It makes oxygen administration possible in the unconscious patient.

_____ **19.** When delivering chest compressions during CPR, which of the following is _not_ correct?
  A. Keep your elbows straight.
  B. Keep your hands on the sternum.
  C. Deliver compressions with a stabbing motion.
  D. Move from your hips.

_____ **20.** The adult CPR compression point is located on the middle of the _____, centered between the nipples.
  A. clavicle   **C.** ribs
  B. substernal notch   **D.** sternum

_____ **21.** Before beginning chest compressions, the health care provider assesses the patient's pulse for a maximum of _____ seconds.
  A. 10   **C.** 15
  B. 25   **D.** 20

_____ **22.** For an adult, the one-rescuer compression-to-ventilation ratio is:
  A. 5:1.   **C.** 15:2.
  B. 5:2.   **D.** 30:2.

_____ **23.** The adult CPR compression rate in one-rescuer CPR is at least _____ times a minute.
  A. 60   **C.** 100
  B. 80   **D.** 120

_____ 24. The adult CPR compression rate in two-rescuer CPR is at least
_____ times a minute when an advanced airway is in place.
A. 60   C. 100
B. 80   D. 120

_____ 25. The compression depth for an adult or older child should be:
A. at least 1 inch.
B. at least 2 inches.
C. one-third to one-half the depth of the chest.
D. one-half to three-fourths the depth of the chest.

_____ 26. The compression depth for an infant should be:
A. 1 to 1.5 inches.
B. 1.5 to 2 inches.
C. one-third to one-half the depth of the chest.
D. one-half to three-quarters the depth of the chest.

_____ 27. The compression-to-ventilation ratio for a young child or infant when there
are two rescuers should be:
A. 15:1.   C. 30:2.
B. 15:2.   D. 5:1.

_____ 28. The compression-to-ventilation ratio for a young child or infant when there is
only one rescuer doing the CPR is:
A. 15:1.   C. 30:2.
B. 15:2.   D. 5:1.

_____ 29. The compression rate when performing CPR on a 9-month-old infant is
at least _____ times a minute.
A. 70   C. 90
B. 80   D. 100

_____ 30. When opening the airway of a 9-month-old infant, use a:
A. full head-tilt method.   C. slight head-tilt.
B. jaw-thrust method.   D. neck hyperextension method.

_____ 31. With effective CPR, the patient's pupils may:
A. dilate.   C. assume a ground-glass appearance.
B. constrict.   D. begin to move.

_____ 32. CPR compressions are delivered to children:
A. in the same manner as they are delivered to adults.
B. with the fingertips of the index and middle fingers.
C. with the palm of one hand.
D. with the heel of one hand.

_____ 33. With the exceptions of defibrillation or advanced cardiac life support
measures to be initiated, CPR should not be interrupted for more than
_____ seconds.
A. a few   C. 15
B. 10   D. 20

_____ 34. If you are treating a 40-year-old female patient with a partial airway
obstruction, poor air exchange, and gray skin, you should:
A. wait for the patient to stop breathing, then ventilate.
B. treat the patient for a complete airway obstruction.
C. increase the delivered oxygen concentration.
D. do none of these.

_____ 35. Complete airway obstruction in a conscious patient is indicated by:
A. crowing sounds.   C. gurgling sounds.
B. an inability to speak.   D. snoring sounds.

_____ **36.** When you recognize complete airway obstruction in a conscious adult or child patient, you should immediately:
  A. place the patient in the supine position and check the pulse.
  B. deliver four back blows in rapid succession.
  C. deliver rapid abdominal thrusts until the obstruction is relieved.
  D. attempt to ventilate the patient.

_____ **37.** To deliver chest thrusts to an unconscious 35-year-old female patient, place the patient in the _____ position.
  A. upright   **C.** coma
  B. prone   **D.** supine

_____ **38.** You are treating an unresponsive 42-year-old male patient with a complete airway obstruction. You have been unsuccessful in your initial two attempts to ventilate the patient. Which is the correct sequence to continue your effort?
  A. Finger sweeps, back blows, adominal thrusts
  B. Abdominal thrusts, finger sweeps, back blows
  C. Ventilations, finger sweeps, adominal thrusts
  D. Chest compressions, look in mouth, ventilations

_____ **39.** When treating a woman in her eighth month of pregnancy and who has a complete airway obstruction, the EMT should:
  A. use abdominal thrusts.   **C.** use chest thrusts.
  B. only use the back blows.   **D.** start rescue breathing immediately.

_____ **40.** If a patient has a partial airway (mild) obstruction and is able to speak and cough forcefully, you should:
  A. perform abdominal thrusts.   **C.** perform the chest thrust.
  B. carefully watch the patient.   **D.** position the patient on the floor.

_____ **41.** A major difference between the adult and infant obstructed airway procedure is:
  A. chest thrusts are used with children only.
  B. back slaps are administered to infants.
  C. blind finger sweeps are not used with infants.
  D. the number of abdominal thrusts is greater in the adult.

_____ **42.** While you are trying to clear an adult's obstructed airway, the patient loses consciousness. You open the airway, look in the mouth, and attempt to ventilate. If this fails:
  A. deliver chest thrusts/compressions.
  B. retilt the head and again attempt to ventilate.
  C. deliver four back blows.
  D. attempt another finger sweep.

_____ **43.** You have been unsuccessful in initially ventilating an unconscious infant. You reposition the infant's head and attempt to ventilate again but are unsuccessful. Your next step is to perform:
  A. a series of chest thrusts.   **C.** abdominal thrusts.
  B. back blows and chest thrusts.   **D.** a tongue-jaw lift.

_____ **44.** Which of the following is _not_ a sign of choking in an infant?
  A. Ineffective cough   **C.** Wheezing
  B. Agitation   **D.** Strong cry

_____ **45.** In health care provider training, in respect to the procedure of CPR, children are treated as adult patients once they have reached:
  A. 8 years of age.
  B. puberty.
  C. 10 years of age.
  D. greater than 1 year of age.

COMPLETE THE FOLLOWING

1. List four of the five special circumstances in which CPR should *not* be initiated by the EMT even though the patient has no pulse.

   A._____

   B._____

   C._____

   D._____

2. Once the EMT has started CPR, list four situations in which CPR can be stopped.

   A._____

   B._____

   C._____

   D._____

3. List the information missing from the chart on the next page.

   A._____

   B._____

   C._____

   D._____

   E._____

   F._____

   G._____

Age	Adult Puberty and older	Child 1 to puberty	Infant Birth to 1 year
Compression depth	**(A)**	⅓ to ½ depth of the chest (2 inches)	⅓ to ½ depth of the chest (1½ inches)
Compression rate	At least 100/min	**(B)**	At least 100/min (newborn 120/min)
Each ventilation	1 second	**(C)**	1 second
Pulse check location	Carotid artery (throat)	**(D)**	Brachial artery (upper arm)
One-rescuer CPR compression-to-ventilation ratio	**(E)**	30:2	30:2
Two-rescuer compression-to-ventilation ratio	**(F)**	**(G)**	15:2

Answer Key

Note: Page numbers in parentheses ( ) refer to page numbers in the textbook where answers can be found or supported.

Chapter 1: Introduction to Emergency Medical Care

MATCH TERMINOLOGY/ DEFINITIONS

1. **(I)** Designated agent—an EMT or other person authorized by a Medical Director to give medications and provide emergency care (p. 16)

2. **(E)** Off-line medical direction—consists of standing orders issued by the Medical Director that allow EMTs to give certain medications or perform certain procedures without speaking to the Medical Director or another physician (p. 16)

3. **(H)** On-line medical direction—orders from the on-duty physician given directly to an EMT in the field by radio or telephone (p. 16)

4. **(A)** 911 system—a system for telephone access to report emergencies (p. 8)

5. **(C)** Medical direction—the oversight of the patient-care aspects of an EMS system by the Medical Director (p. 15)

6. **(D)** Medical Director—a physician who assumes the ultimate responsibility for the patient-care aspects of the EMS system (p. 15)

7. **(B)** Quality improvement—a process of continuous self-review with the purpose of identifying and correcting aspects of the system that require improvement (p. 19)

8. **(F)** Protocols—lists of steps, such as assessment and interventions, to be taken in different situations (p. 15)

9. **(G)** Standing order—a policy or protocol issued by a Medical Director that authorizes EMTs and others to perform particular skills in certain situations (p. 16)

MULTIPLE-CHOICE REVIEW

1. **(B)** In the 1790s, France began to transport wounded soldiers so they could be cared for by physicians away from the scene of the battle. (p. 5)

2. **(C)** In 1966, the National Highway Safety Act charged the United States Department of Transportation with developing EMS standards. (p. 6)

3. **(B)** Computerization is helpful, but it is not considered a major NHTSA EMS system assessment standard. (pp. 6–7)

4. **(C)** Specialty hospitals include: poison control centers, trauma centers, burn centers, and pediatric centers. Most hospitals have an emergency department. Correctional facilities and primary care centers are not considered EMS specialty care units. (p. 7)

5. **(A)** The U.S. Department of Transportation publishes curricula for the EMR, EMT, Advanced EMT, and EMT-Paramedic levels. (pp. 8–9)

6. **(C)** The EMT curriculum deals with basic assessment and care of the patient. The EMT course is not limited to immediate life-threatening care. Electrocardiograms are beyond the scope of the EMT curriculum, and advanced airway techniques are optional, not a major emphasis, in the EMT curriculum. (p. 9)

7. **(B)** The care provided by the EMT is based on assessment findings. It is not delayed until transportation, nor should it be guided by attorneys. EMTs do not make a diagnosis; rather, treatment is based on patient complaints. (p. 10)

8. **(A)** During the transfer of care, continuity of care can be improved by providing pertinent patient information to the hospital staff. This includes information on the patient's condition and observation of the scene. (p. 10)

9. **(D)** While patient advocacy—speaking up for your patient—is one of the important roles of the EMT, it is not your primary responsibility. Your first responsibility is keeping yourself safe. (p. 10)

10. **(A)** Good personality traits of the EMT include: pleasant, cooperative, resourceful, a self-starter, emotionally stable, able to lead, neat and clean, of good moral character, having respect for others, in control of personal habits, and controlled in conversation. (pp. 11–12)

11. **(D)** An EMT should be in control of personal habits such as smoking, drinking, and using inappropriate language in order to avoid contaminating the patient's wounds, making inappropriate decisions, and rendering improper care. (p. 11)

12. **(C)** Avoiding inappropriate conversation is paramount in protecting a patient's confidentiality. (p. 11)

13. **(C)** Continuing education includes attending conferences and watching training videos that further your education. Because procedures often change, rereading your old textbook cannot keep you up to date on these changes. (p. 12)

14. **(C)** By definition, quality improvement is a process of continuous self-review with the purpose of identifying and correcting aspects of the EMS system that require improvement. (p. 13)

15. **(B)** Additional ways of providing quality improvement are listed in the answer to multiple-choice question 16. (pp. 14–15)

16. **(C)** Participating in continuing education and keeping careful written documentation are just two of the ways EMTs can work toward quality care. Others include becoming involved in the quality improvement process, maintaining your equipment, and obtaining feedback from patients and the hospital staff. (pp. 14–15)

17. **(D)** Each EMS system should have a Medical Director to provide oversight of patient care procedures. (p. 16)

18. **(C)** As an EMT, you act as an extender, or designated agent, of the Medical Director. (p. 16)

19. **(D)** On-line medical direction involves talking to a physician over the telephone or radio. Off-line medical direction includes the physician developing protocols and policies, advising the EMS service, and reviewing quality assurance issues. (pp. 15–16)

20. (C) Oral glucose is one of the medications for which EMTs need on-line medical approval in order to administer it. (p. 16)

21. (B) New EMTs will see the transition of EMS from decisions based on traditions to decisions based on research. (pp. 16–17)

22. (C) EMTs should treat all patients in a nonjudgmental and fair manner. (p. 11)

23. (D) Evidenced-based patient-care decisions are based on forming a hypothesis, a review of the literature, and an evidence evaluation. (p. 16)

24. (B) Injury prevention for geriatric patients and campaigns to reduce tobacco use are examples of an EMT's role in public health. (p. 17)

COMPLETE THE FOLLOWING

1. The categories and standards of an EMS system established by the National Highway Traffic Safety Administration are: (any six) (pp. 6–7)
   - regulation and policy
   - resource management
   - human resources and training
   - trauma systems
   - public information and education
   - communications
   - transportation
   - facilities
   - evaluation
   - medical direction

2. Six types of specialty hospitals are: (p. 8)
   - trauma centers
   - burn centers
   - cardiac centers
   - poison control centers
   - stroke centers
   - pediatric centers

3. Four levels of EMS certification are: (pp. 8–9)
   - Emergency Medical Responder
   - EMT
   - Advanced EMT
   - EMT-Paramedic

STREET SCENES DISCUSSION

Scene safety, patient assessment (first), (and then) patient care, lifting and moving patients, and patient transport.

Chapter 2: The Well-Being of the EMT

MATCH TERMINOLOGY/ DEFINITIONS

1. **(C)** Contamination—the introduction of dangerous chemicals, disease, or infectious materials (p. 25)

2. **(E)** Pathogens—the organisms that cause infection, such as viruses and bacteria (p. 23)

3. **(F)** Multiple-casualty incident (MCI)—an emergency involving multiple patients (p. 38)

4. **(A)** Standard Precautions—a strict form of infection control based on the assumption that all blood and other body fluids are infectious (p. 23)

5. **(B)** Critical incident stress management (CISM)—a comprehensive system that includes education and resources to both prevent stress and deal with stress appropriately when it occurs (p. 39)

6. **(G)** Decontamination—the removal or cleaning of dangerous chemicals and other dangerous or infectious materials (p. 42)

7. **(H)** Hazardous-material incident—the release of a harmful substance into the environment (p. 41)

8. **(I)** Stress—a state of physical and/or psychological arousal to a stimulus (p. 36)

9. **(D)** Personal protective equipment (PPE)—equipment that protects the EMS worker from infection and/or exposure to the dangers of rescue operations (pp. 25–28)

MULTIPLE-CHOICE REVIEW

1. **(C)** To maintain a healthy lifestyle, the EMT should get at least 6 hours of sleep a day. (p. 23)

2. **(D)** By definition, a pathogen is an organism that causes infection, such as a virus or bacteria. (p. 23)

3. **(C)** Because the EMT cannot identify patients who carry infectious diseases just by looking at them, all body fluids must be considered infectious and Standard Precautions must be taken all the time. (p. 23)

4. **(C)** Standard Precautions involves handwashing, disposable gloves, and eye protection. A HEPA mask is used to protect against airborne particles that may cause TB. Leather gloves are helpful in a rescue to protect the EMT from cutting his or her hands but are not useful for Standard Precautions. (pp. 23–24)

5. **(B)** Surgical masks are routinely used for treating patients with a potential for blood or fluid spatter. If TB is suspected, a HEPA mask should be used. (p. 27)

6. **(A)** Whenever a mask is placed on a patient, the EMT needs to monitor the patient to ensure that respirations are adequate and the airway is open. Check often to ensure the patient doesn't vomit into the mask. If you think the patient has TB, you should wear a HEPA mask, not a surgical mask. (p. 27)

7. **(B)** In some states, keeping lists of certain types of patients, such as AIDS patients, may be a violation of the law. All other responses listed are ways to plan safety precautions. You never know which of your patients may have a communicable disease, so you need to treat them all as if they do and take Standard Precautions. (pp. 32–34)

8. **(C)** The purified protein derivative (PPD) (also known as TST) is a test for tuberculosis and is not a vaccine. (p. 35)

9. **(C)** The employee safety regulations come under the Occupational Safety and Health Administration (OSHA). The FDA regulates drugs and foods; the FCC regulates radio equipment; and the Public Health Service provides regulations and educational efforts to ensure that children are immunized, water is clean, and so on. (p. 31)

10. **(C)** Employers of EMTs must make available the hepatitis B vaccination series as outlined in the OSHA standards on bloodborne pathogens, which took effect in March 1992. Employers must also provide training and personal protective equipment. (pp. 31, 35)

11. **(B)** The Ryan White CARE Act provides two different systems for infectious disease exposure—airborne disease exposure and bloodborne disease exposure. Ensure that you understand these notification procedures because treatment must be timely in order to be effective. (pp. 32–33)

12. **(C)** The designated officer is responsible for gathering facts surrounding emergency responder airborne or bloodborne infectious disease exposures. Be sure you know who the designated officer is in your organization. (p. 32)

13. **(B)** It is safest to assume that any person with a productive cough may be infected with TB. The number of cases of

Chapter 2 (continued)

multidrug-resistant TB is rising, so you should learn to recognize situations in which the potential of TB exposure exists, as well as the signs and symptoms of TB patients. (pp. 34–35)

14. (C) The diseases H1N1, chicken pox, German measles, and whooping cough are all spread by the airborne route. (pp. 28–30)

15. (D) The well-being of the EMT involves understanding and dealing with job stress, ensuring scene safety, and taking Standard Precautions to avoid contracting diseases. (p. 22)

16. (B) An adult cardiac arrest is considered a routine EMS call. Calls involving a higher potential for causing excess stress on EMS providers include calls involving infants and children, elder abuse, death or injury of a coworker, plus severe injuries and MCIs. (p. 38)

17. (C) The warning signs that an EMT is being affected by stress include irritability with family, friends, and coworkers; inability to concentrate; changes in daily activities; difficulty sleeping or nightmares; loss of appetite; loss of interest in sexual activity; anxiety; indecisiveness; guilt; isolation; and loss of interest in work. (pp. 38–39)

18. (D) Talking about your feelings with your partners is healthy. (p. 39)

19. (C) By definition, a critical incident stress debriefing is a process in which a team of trained peer counselors and mental health professionals meets with rescuers and health care providers who have been involved in a major incident. (p. 39)

20. (D) All are true. Also the normal reactions to stress should be discussed, and follow-up should be arranged for those who may need it. (pp. 38–39)

21. (A) Most medical professionals and EMS leaders agree the best course of action for an EMT experiencing significant stress from a serious call is to seek help from a mental health professional with appropriate experience. (p. 39)

22. (C) The emotional stages that patients go through when they find out they are dying include denial, anger, bargaining, depression, and acceptance. (pp. 39–40)

23. (B) The emotional stages have differing duration and magnitude but generally occur in the following order: denial, anger, bargaining, depression, and acceptance. (pp. 39–40)

24. (B) All responses are correct except lying to the patient by saying everything will be all right when it will not. (p. 40)

25. (B) It is not an EMT's responsibility to respond to dangerous situations. Rather, you should retreat, radio to police for assistance, and reevaluate the scene once it has been secured by the police. (pp. 42–45)

26. (D) All of the stressors listed may affect the EMT. (p. 38)

27. (C) Hans Selye, MD, first coined the phrase *general adaptation syndrome* as the body's response to stress. (pp. 35–36)

28. (C) The three phases of general adaptation syndrome are: alarm, resistance, and exhaustion. (p. 36)

29. (B) Stress reactions occurring days, weeks, or even months after an incident are called post-traumatic stress reactions. (pp. 36–37)

30. (D) The CDC recommends the use of alcohol-based hand cleaners when soap and water are not available. (p. 26)

31. (C) The normal mode of transmission of the disease chickenpox (varicella) is by airborne droplets. (p. 29)

32. (A) Hepatitis is not thought to be spread by respiratory secretions or oral or nasal secretions as bacterial meningitis, pneumonia, or tuberculosis would be. (p. 29)

33. (B) Mothers are thought to be able to pass the disease AIDS to their unborn child. (p. 29)

34. (B) Selye described the stress triad as involving adrenal gland enlargement, bleeding gastric ulcers, and wasting of the lymph nodes. (pp. 36–37)

COMPLETE THE FOLLOWING

1. Types of calls with high potential of stress for EMS personnel include: (p. 38)
- MCIs
- infants and children
- severe injuries
- abuse and neglect
- death of a coworker

2. Signs and symptoms of stress include: (any five) (pp. 38–39)
- irritability with family, friends, and coworkers
- inability to concentrate
- changes in daily activities
- loss of interest in sexual activity
- anxiety
- isolation
- loss of interest in work
- loss of appetite
- difficulty sleeping

3. The critical elements of the infection control plan required by Title 29 Code of Federal Regulation 1910.1030 are: (any five) (p. 31)
- infection exposure control plan
- adequate education and training
- hepatitis B vaccination
- personal protective equipment (PPE)
- methods of control
- housekeeping
- labeling
- postexposure evaluation and follow-up

STREET SCENES DISCUSSION

1. Hepatitis B, C, or D, or HIV

2. AZT, safe sex with a condom, and regular blood tests

3. Yes, by being inoculated for hepatitis B, he may have prevented contraction of the disease.

4. Hepatitis B is a very hardy virus that kills approximately 200 health care workers each year.

Chapter 3: Lifting and Moving Patients

MATCH TERMINOLOGY/ DEFINITIONS

1. (A) Basket stretcher—stretcher, made of steel wire mesh and tubular steel rim or plastic and steel rim, used to transport patients from one level to another or over rough terrain (p. 62)

2. (H) Body mechanics—proper use of the body to facilitate lifting and moving and to prevent injury (p. 71)

©2012 Pearson Education, Inc.
Emergency Care, 12th Ed.

3. **(D)** Direct carry—method of transferring a patient from bed to stretcher in which two or more rescuers curl the patient to their chests, then reverse the process to lower the patient to the stretcher (p. 65)

4. **(M)** Direct ground lift—method of lifting and carrying a patient from ground level to a stretcher during which two or more rescuers kneel, curl the patient to their chests, stand, then reverse the process to lower the patient to the stretcher (p. 65)

5. **(K)** Draw-sheet method—method of transferring a patient from bed to stretcher by grasping and pulling the loosened bottom sheet of the bed (p. 65)

6. **(N)** Emergency move—removal of a patient from a hazardous environment in which safety is the first priority and spinal integrity is second priority (p. 52)

7. **(F)** Extremity lift—method of lifting and carrying a patient in which one rescuer slips her or his hands under the patient's armpits and grasps the wrists, while another rescuer grasps the patient's knees (p. 65)

8. **(O)** Log roll—procedure done by three or four rescuers that is designed to move a patient onto a long backboard without compromising spinal integrity (p. 55)

9. **(L)** Long axis—line that runs down the center of the body from the top of the head and along the spine (p. 55)

10. **(E)** Nonurgent move—patient move that may be made if speed is not a priority (p. 56)

11. **(I)** Power grip—gripping, with as much hand surface as possible, the object being lifted, with all fingers bent at the same angle (p. 50)

12. **(G)** Power lift—also called the squat-lift position; a lift is made from a squatting position, with the weight to be lifted close to the body, and with the EMT's feet apart and flat on the ground, body weight on or just behind the balls of the feet, and back locked in (p. 50)

13. **(C)** Scoop (orthopedic) stretcher—stretcher that splits in halves, which can be pushed together under the patient (p. 57)

14. **(B)** Stair chair—portable folding chair with wheels used to transport a patient in a sitting position up or down stairs (p. 57)

15. **(J)** Urgent move—patient move that should be done quickly yet without any compromise of spinal integrity (p. 52)

MULTIPLE-CHOICE REVIEW

1. **(C)** To ensure your own safety when lifting a patient, it is important to use your legs, not your back, to lift. Some EMTs use a soft back brace when they lift. These devices should be used only if your physician suggests you do so. When lifting, keep the weight as close to your body as possible. Consider the weight of the patient you are lifting: be realistic about your limitations and ask for help. (p. 50)

2. **(B)** Avoid twisting motions while you are lifting; such motions can lead to a back injury. When lifting a patient, you should communicate clearly and frequently with your partner and know your limitations. (p. 50)

3. **(A)** When lifting a cot or stretcher, use an even number of people so that the balance of the device is maintained. Your feet should be a comfortable distance apart so that you can maintain balance. If a third person is positioned on the heaviest side, he or she stands a greater chance of

being injured. If you must use only one hand to carry a piece of equipment, never compensate by using your back. (p. 58)

4. **(A)** When placing all fingers and the palm in contact with the object being lifted, you are using a power grip. A power lift involves squatting and using the legs. The lock grip and grip lift are inventive distracters for this question. (p. 50)

5. **(A)** When you must push an object, keep the line of pull through the center of your body by bending your knees. Also keep the weight as close to your body as possible, avoid pushing or pulling overhead, and keep elbows bent with arms close to your sides. (p. 50)

6. **(D)** The fact that the dispatcher has another, more serious call is not an appropriate reason to compromise the patient's spine. The situations in which an emergency move would be used include fire or danger of fire, explosives or other hazardous chemicals, and inability to protect the patient from other hazards at the scene. (p. 52)

7. **(C)** If the patient is on the floor or ground and the EMT has decided that an emergency move is appropriate, the patient can be moved by pulling on his or her clothing in the neck and shoulder area, which maintains some spinal integrity and doesn't require additional equipment or other rescuers. (p. 53)

8. **(B)** If the patient has an altered mental status, the EMT should consider an urgent move. The emergency move is used in situations where there is a real danger to the rescuer or the patient, such as a fire. (p. 52)

9. **(C)** When doing a log roll, lean from your hips and use your shoulder muscles to help with the roll. Also try to keep your back straight and position yourself right next to the patient. Maintaining spinal integrity is more important than speed. (p. 55)

10. **(A)** The final step in packaging a patient on a wheeled stretcher is securing the patient to the stretcher. The particulars about using towels under the head and top sheets are specific to the standard operating procedures of your service. Adjusting the back rest is optional and depends on the patient's condition. (pp. 56–59)

11. **(D)** If you are carrying a patient down stairs, when possible use a stair chair because it weighs less than a stretcher. Do not flex at the waist with or without bent knees. Both hands should be used to carry the stair chair. (p. 61)

12. **(B)** A patient that large will likely need to be transported on a stretcher designed to carry her weight, such as a bariatric stretcher. The other devices would be difficult at best. (p. 58)

13. **(A)** You have a patient positioned on a scoop-style stretcher and wish to lower the patient from a rooftop. You should place the stretcher and patient in a plastic basket stretcher. Make sure the basket is rated for the lift and you have the appropriate training in high-angle rescue techniques. It is not necessary to take the patient out of the scoop to place him into the wire basket. Never lower the patient in the scoop alone because this could lead to serious injury or death. (p. 62)

14. **(A)** To avoid trauma to an injured spine, the best patient-carrying device would be the long spine board for immobilization. Then place the patient on the wheeled stretcher to move him or her. (p. 65)

15. **(D)** The direct ground lift is an example of a nonurgent move for a patient who has no spine injury. (p. 65)

16. **(B)** Power lifters or weight lifters use the squat-lift, and EMTs should also try to use this technique for their own safety. (p. 50)

17. **(D)** Position your feet shoulder width and on firm, flat ground when lifting a patient. (p. 50)

18. **(B)** Do not compensate by leaning when lifting with one hand. (p. 50)

19. **(C)** A comfortable new device that can be used to transport a supine patient who has sustained a spinal injury is a vacuum mattress. The scoop, stairchair, and KED would *not* be used on a spinal-injured patient. (p. 62)

20. **(B)** When an EMT is using an air vacuum mattress, the patient is placed on the device and the air is withdrawn by the pump. The mattress will then form a rigid and conforming surface around the patient. These devices are new and rapidly expanding in usage. (p. 62)

COMPLETE THE FOLLOWING

1. Seven patient-carrying devices include: (pp. 57, 62)
   - wheeled ambulance stretcher
   - portable ambulance stretcher
   - stair chair
   - scoop stretcher
   - spine board
   - basket stretcher
   - flexible stretcher

2. Body mechanic principles include: (any four) (pp. 49–50)
   - Position your feet properly.
   - When lifting, use your legs, not your back, to do the lifting.
   - When lifting, never twist or attempt to make any moves other than the lift.
   - When lifting with one hand, do not compensate by leaning.
   - Keep the weight as close to your body as possible.
   - When carrying a patient on stairs, use a stair chair instead of a stretcher when possible.

3. The two types of stretchers are manual and power.

LABEL THE PHOTOGRAPHS (PP. 53–54)

1. Shoulder drag
2. Incline drag
3. Foot drag
4. Clothes drag
5. Firefighter's drag
6. Blanket drag
7. One-rescuer assist
8. Cradle carry
9. Pack strap carry
10. Piggy-back carry
11. Firefighter's carry
12. Two-rescuer assist

STREET SCENES DISCUSSION

1. You can try to use the vest-type immobilization device if she fits into it.

2. As long as the chest straps connect, the device should work to get her out of the car if you and your partners move her carefully. If the leg straps do not reach, you may need to omit them.

3. Obese people do not like to lie supine because it makes breathing difficult. Once she is on a long backboard, the vest can be loosened and 10-foot straps can be used around the long backboard to secure her chest, pelvis, and legs.

CASE STUDY: MORE THAN THE AVERAGE PATIENT

1. Normally a stair chair is used to remove patients on the second floor; however, considering the size of this patient and the fact that his back is hurting him, it makes sense to keep him in the supine position.

2. A direct ground lift with such a heavy patient would be dangerous to the EMT. A draw-sheet method lift would be more appropriate, especially if the sheet could be replaced with blankets and a number of sheets.

3. The decision to call the fire department to obtain more rescuers was a wise one because this is a very heavy patient.

4. A bariatric unit is designed to transport obese patients. These units have special stretchers rated for more weight and larger patients, as well as lifts and ramps to prevent the need for the EMTs to have to lift the stretcher into the ambulance.

5. A scoop stretcher has points to hold on to and is designed for smaller patients. The Reeves can be placed under an obese patient and has many hand holds for carrying. It can also slide on the floor or stairs if needed.

6. If the Reeves did not work, another option would be a plastic stokes basket provided that it is rated for the size and weight of the patient.

7. The highest priority is always the safety of the EMTs. Having a lot of help in this instance was a good thing so no rescuer went home with a back injury.

Chapter 4: Medical/Legal and Ethical Issues

MATCH TERMINOLOGY/ DEFINITIONS

1. **(M)** Abandonment—leaving a patient after care has been initiated and before the patient has been transferred to someone with equal or greater medical training (p. 83)

2. **(B)** Advance directive—a DNR order (p. 80)

3. **(L)** Confidentiality—the obligation not to reveal information obtained about a patient except to other health care professionals involved in the patient's care, or under subpoena, or in a court of law, or when the patient has signed a release of confidentiality (p. 83)

4. **(F)** Consent—permission from the patient for care or other action by the EMT (p. 76)

5. **(I)** Crime scene—the location where a crime has been committed or any place that evidence relating to a crime may be found (pp. 87–88)

6. **(K)** DNR order—a legal document, usually signed by the patient and his or her physician, that states that the patient has a terminal illness and does not wish to prolong life through resuscitative efforts (p. 80)

7. (D) Duty to act—an obligation to provide care to a patient (p. 83)

8. (E) Expressed consent—consent given by adults who are of legal age and mentally competent to make a rational decision in regard to their medical well-being (p. 76)

9. (G) Good Samaritan laws—a series of laws, varying in each state, designed to provide limited legal protection for citizens and some health care personnel who are administering emergency care (p. 83)

10. (O) HIPAA—a federal law protecting the privacy of patient-specific health care information and providing the patient with control over how this information is used and distributed (p. 84)

11. (A) Implied consent—the consent it is presumed that a patient or patient's parent or guardian would give if they could, such as for an unconscious patient or a parent who cannot be contacted when care is needed (p. 77)

12. (C) Liability—being held legally responsible (p. 78)

13. (J) Negligence—a finding of failure to act properly in a situation in which there was a duty to act, that needed care as would reasonably be expected of the EMT was not provided, and that harm was caused to the patient as a result (p. 81)

14. (N) Organ donor—a person who has completed a legal document that allows for donation of organs and tissues in the event of death (p. 85)

15. (H) Scope of practice—a set of regulations and ethical considerations that define the scope, or extent and limits, of the EMT's job (p. 75)

MULTIPLE-CHOICE REVIEW

1. (B) The collective set of regulations and ethical considerations governing the EMT's responsibilities is called the scope of practice. Duty to act is an obligation to provide care to the patient. Advance directives are the written and signed wishes of the patient in advance of any event where resuscitation might be undertaken. The Good Samaritan laws vary by state and often do not cover the EMT. (p. 75)

2. (B) Legislation that governs the skills and medical interventions that an EMT may perform not only differs from state to state, but may even vary from region to region within the state. (p. 75)

3. (C) Making the physical/emotional needs of the patient a priority is considered an ethical responsibility of the EMT. A legal responsibility would be ensuring that consent was gained prior to treating a patient. Advance directives involve orders on how a patient wants to be treated in the event that resuscitation is needed. Protocols are models of care that an EMT follows in treating patients. (p. 89)

4. (C) Applied consent is a meaningless term that is often put on exams to test the student's understanding of consent terminology. The types of consent include consent for a minor or child, consent for a mentally incompetent adult, expressed consent (see the answer for multiple-choice question 5), and implied consent (see the answer for multiple-choice question 6). (pp. 76–78)

5. (A) Expressed consent is obtained by informing an adult patient of a procedure you are about to perform and its associated risks, then gaining his or her permission to proceed. Negligence is a finding of failure to act properly in a situation where there was a duty to act. Implied consent is

defined in the answer for multiple-choice question 6, and applied consent is a meaningless term. (p. 82)

6. (C) Consent that is based on the assumption that an unconscious patient would approve the EMT's life-saving interventions is called implied consent. Expressed consent, negligence, and applied consent are explained in the answer for multiple-choice question 5. (p. 77)

7. (C) A patient refusal of medical aid or transport does not require any physician's signature. Your official record of a patient's refusal to accept medical aid must carefully and completely document the attempts you made to get the patient to accept care. Include the names of any witnesses to your attempts, and include the patient's "release" form with the patient's witnessed signature. (pp. 77–78)

8. (B) Forcing a competent adult patient to go to the hospital against his or her will may result in assault and battery charges against the EMT. You could also be charged with kidnapping the patient. Both implied consent and negligence are discussed in the answers to multiple-choice questions 5 and 6. (p. 78)

9. (C) All choices are correct except C. In all cases of refusal, you should advise patients to call back at any time if there is a problem or they wish to be cared for or transported. While there may be patients who legitimately refuse care, such as for minor wounds, patients with any significant medical condition should be transported to the hospital. (pp. 77–78)

10. (D) A DNR order is a physician's order to "do not resuscitate" a patient. This is also referred to as an advance directive. (p. 80)

11. (A) There are varying degrees of DNR orders, expressed through a variety of detailed instructions that may be part of the order, such as allowing for CPR only if cardiac or respiratory arrest was observed. Comfort care measures such as intravenous feeding, administering pain medications, and the long-term use of a respirator are part of a living will and are not part of a DNR order. These orders generally do not specify procedures that are improper, such as specifying that only 5 minutes of artificial respiration will be attempted. (pp. 80–81)

12. (B) In a hospital, long-term life-support and comfort care measures would consist of intravenous feeding and the use of a respirator. Once a patient is considered terminal, routine inoculations would not be needed. Infection control by the health care providers is a given. Documentation needs to be the same as it would be had the patient not had an advance directive. (p. 80)

13. (B) To prove negligence, an attorney must prove the EMT had a duty to the patient, failed to provide the standard of care or breached his or her duty, and that this failure, or breach, caused harm to the patient. (pp. 81–82)

14. (C) Termination of care of the patient without ensuring the continuation of care at the same level or higher is called abandonment. Always turn your patient over to a health care professional in the ED. Liability is being held legally responsible, battery is attacking someone physically, and a breach of duty is not acting when you have an obligation to act. (p. 83)

15. (D) Information considered confidential includes patient history gained through interview, assessment findings, and treatment rendered. The release of this information can cause embarrassment as well as potential harm to the patient. In the past, when the public was uninformed about the causes and consequences of AIDS, release of a patient's HIV positive status caused cross burnings and graffiti on the property of patients' homes. (p. 83)

16. **(D)** The only times an EMT may release confidential patient information is to inform other health care professionals who need to know the information to continue care; to report incidents required by state law, such as rape or abuse; and to comply with a legal subpoena. It is not your responsibility to release confidential patient information in an effort to protect the other victims of a motor vehicle collision. (p. 83)

17. **(D)** Medical identification insignia that indicate serious patient medical conditions come in the form of bracelets, necklaces, and cards because patients wear and/or carry these all the time and they are easily located. Patches are not forms of medical IDs. (p. 85)

18. **(B)** The patient is not dead yet, so treat the critical patient who has an organ donor card the same as any other patient and inform the ED physician. Withholding oxygen therapy from the critically ill patient will just speed his or her demise. (p. 85)

19. **(A)** At a crime scene, the EMT should avoid disturbing any evidence unless emergency care requires. The patient him- or herself provides valuable information. The position the patient is found in, the condition of the clothing, and injuries are all pieces of evidence. Do not move obstacles from around the patient to make more room to work; this may destroy evidence. Leave the search of the house for clues to the police. It is not your responsibility. (pp. 87–88)

20. **(B)** Commonly required reporting situations include sexual assault, domestic abuse, and child and elder abuse. A crime in a public place does not require the EMT to report the crime to the authorities. (p. 88)

21. **(C)** The extent (or limits) of the EMT's job is called the scope of practice (p. 75)

22. **(B)** The patient may not have a life-threatening injury but he was unconscious prior to your arrival and may not be mentally competent to refuse at this time based on all the alcohol he admits drinking within the last hour. (pp. 77–78)

23. **(C)** The federal law designed to protect patients' private medical information is the Health Insurance Portability and Accountability Act (HIPAA). (p. 84)

24. **(A)** It is always important to monitor the vital signs and mental status of any patient who is restrained. (p. 87)

25. **(B)** Dirt and carpet fibers are examples of microscopic evidence found at a crime scene. (p. 87)

COMPLETE THE FOLLOWING

1. For a patient to refuse care or transport, these four conditions must be fulfilled: (p. 78)
   - The patient must be mentally competent and oriented.
   - The patient must be fully informed.
   - The patient must sign a "release" form.
   - The patient must be of legal age or an emancipated minor.

2. Negligence, or failure to act properly, requires all of the following circumstances in order to be proven: (pp. 81–82)
   - The EMT had a duty to the patient.
   - The EMT did not provide the standard of care.
   - The actions of the EMT in not providing the standard of care caused harm to the patient.

3. Four examples of conditions that may be listed on a medical identification device (such as a necklace, bracelet, or card) include: (p. 85)
   - Heart conditions
   - Diabetes
   - Allergies
   - Epilepsy

STREET SCENES DISCUSSION

1. Not really. This is not a confidentiality issue. It is more of an ethical issue and a matter of professional behavior in any conversation you have about any patient's residence. If, however, there are hazards observed while treating the patient in his residence (e.g., fire hazards, uncaged dangerous animals, explosives, dangerous conditions to future responders as well as to the patient), you should seriously consider notifying the appropriate authorities in your community.

2. Yes, it is medical documentation. You can always write things that the patient says in quotes in the narrative section of the PCR, too.

3. The appropriate equipment for Standard Precautions would be gloves, and because the patient was vomiting, a mask and eye shield.

CASE STUDY: A WITNESSED COLLISION: FIRST ON THE SCENE

1. No, unless your state law requires you to stop. You should understand that once you do stop, however, you should not leave the patient except in the hands of another EMT or advanced EMT. Leaving a patient is considered abandonment, an example of "gross negligence."

2. Yes and no! Anyone can be sued. Most states do have some form of Good Samaritan laws or laws dealing specifically with EMS personnel that protects you in this situation, provided you do not render treatment that is grossly negligent.

3. Yes, in most states.

4. Nine-One-One (911).

5. A) What is the exact location of the sick or injured person?
   B) What is your call-back number?
   C) How old is the patient?
   D) What's the problem?
   E) What's the patient's sex?
   F) Is the patient breathing?

6. The police, the fire department, and the ambulance service.

7. Assign them to perform manual stabilization of the head and neck and to help with lifting the patient once the ambulance arrives.

8. The patient could have additional broken bones, internal bleeding, or a head or neck injury, to name a few.

9. No permission is needed because consent is implied when the patient is unconscious.

10. He could have a ruptured spleen, fractured ribs, and back and neck injuries, in addition to the obvious fractured leg.

11. Assign someone to lift the patient's injured leg and hold it as still as possible.

12. Yes, he is conscious and must give expressed consent.

13. No, not until you check with the EMT or paramedic in charge to be sure your assistance is no longer needed.

14. Gross negligence due to abandonment.

Chapter 5: Medical Terminology and Anatomy and Physiology

MATCH TERMINOLOGY/ DEFINITIONS

▶ PART A

1. **(K)** Abdominal quadrants—four divisions of the abdomen used to pinpoint the location of a pain or injury (p. 99)

2. **(N)** Acetabulum—the pelvic socket into which the ball of the proximal end of the femur fits to form the hip joint (p. 107)

3. **(P)** Acromioclavicular joint—the joint where the acromion and the clavicle meet (p. 107)

4. **(H)** Acromion process—the highest portion of the shoulder (p. 107)

5. **(M)** Aerobic metabolism—the conversion of glucose into energy by the use of oxygen (p. 120)

6. **(D)** Alveoli—the microscopic sacs of the lungs where gas exchange with the bloodstream takes place (p. 109)

7. **(J)** Anaerobic metabolism—the conversion of glucose into energy without the use of oxygen (p. 120)

8. **(B)** Anatomical position—the standard reference position for the body in the study of anatomy. In this position, the body is standing erect, facing the observer, with arms down at the sides and the palms of the hand forward. (p. 96)

9. **(E)** Anatomy—the study of body structure (p. 95)

10. **(A)** Anterior—the front of the body or body part (p. 96)

11. **(F)** Aorta—the largest artery in the body. It transports blood from the left ventricle to begin systemic circulation. (p. 114)

12. **(C)** Appendix—a small tube located near the junction of the small and large intestines in the right lower quadrant of the abdomen, the function of which is not well understood (p. 123)

13. **(O)** Arteriole—the smallest kind of artery (p. 113)

14. **(I)** Artery—any blood vessel carrying blood away from the heart (p. 113)

15. **(L)** Atria—the two upper chambers of the heart; the right atrium receives unoxygenated blood returning from the body and the left receives oxygenated blood returning from the lungs (p. 112)

16. **(G)** Automaticity—the ability of the heart to generate and conduct electrical impulses on its own (p. 109)

▶ PART B

1. **(O)** Autonomic nervous system—the division of the peripheral nervous system that controls involuntary motor functions (p. 122)

2. **(R)** Bilateral—on both sides (p. 130)

3. **(T)** Bladder—the round, saclike organ of the renal system used as a reservoir for urine (p. 130)

4. **(S)** Blood pressure—the pressure caused by blood exerting force against the walls of the blood vessels (p. 117)

5. **(N)** Brachial artery—artery of the upper arm; the site of the pulse checked on an infant in CPR (p. 130)

6. **(Q)** Bronchial—the two large sets of branches that come off the trachea and enter the lungs (p. 130)

7. **(P)** Calcaneus—the heel bone (p. 130)

8. **(M)** Capillary—a thin-walled, microscopic blood vessel where the oxygen/carbon dioxide and nutrient/waste exchange with the body's cells takes place (p. 115)

9. **(K)** Cardiac conduction system—a system of specialized muscle tissue that conducts electrical impulses that stimulate the heart to beat (p. 130)

10. **(H)** Cardiac muscle—specialized involuntary muscle found only in the heart (p. 131)

11. **(A)** Cardiovascular system—the system made up of the heart and the blood vessels (p. 112)

12. **(L)** Carotid arteries—the large neck arteries, one on each side of the neck, that carry blood from the heart to the head (p. 114)

13. **(G)** Carpals—the wrist bones (p. 131)

14. **(F)** Central nervous system (CNS)—the brain and spinal cord (p. 120)

15. **(D)** Central pulses—the carotid and femoral pulses, which can be felt in the central part of the body (p. 131)

16. **(J)** Circulatory system—see cardiovascular system (p. 112)

17. **(I)** Clavicle—the collarbone (p. 131)

18. **(B)** Coronary arteries—blood vessels that supply the muscle of the heart (p. 113)

19. **(E)** Cranium—the top, back, and sides of the skull (p. 131)

20. **(C)** Cricoid cartilage—the ring-shaped structure that forms the lower portion of the larynx (p. 131)

▶ PART C

1. **(G)** Dermis—the inner layer of the skin, rich in blood vessels and nerves, found beneath the epidermis (p. 124)

2. **(I)** Diaphragm—the muscular structure that divides the chest cavity from the abdominal cavity (p. 109)

3. **(N)** Diastolic blood pressure—the pressure in the arteries when the left ventricle is refilling (p. 117)

4. **(J)** Digestive system—system by which food travels through the body and is broken down into absorbable forms (p. 122)

5. **(D)** Distal—further away from the torso (p. 98)

6. **(L)** Dorsal—referring to the back of the body or the back of the hand or foot (p. 97)

7. **(K)** Dorsalis pedis—artery supplying the foot, lateral to the large tendon of the big toe (p. 131)

8. **(P)** Endocrine system—system of glands that produce chemicals called hormones that help to regulate many body activities and functions (p. 124)

9. **(M)** Epidermis—the outer layer of the skin (p. 123)

10. **(Q)** Epiglottis—a leaf-shaped structure that prevents food and foreign matter from entering the trachea (p. 109)

11. **(H)** Epinephrine—a hormone produced by the body; as a medication, it dilates respiratory passages and is used to relieve a severe allergic reaction (p. 131)

12. **(R)** Exhalation—a passive process in which the intercostal muscles and the diaphragm relax, causing the chest cavity to decrease in size and air to flow out of the lungs (p. 109)

13. **(T)** Femoral artery—the major artery supplying the leg (p. 131)

14. **(O)** Femur—the large bone of the thigh (p. 131)

15. **(S)** Fibula—the lateral and smaller bone of the lower leg (p. 131)

16. **(C)** Fowler position—a sitting position (p. 99)

17. **(F)** Gallbladder—a sac on the underside of the liver that stores bile produced by the liver (p. 131)

18. **(B)** Glottic opening—the proximal opening of the trachea (p. 109)

19. **(A)** Humerus—the bone of the upper arm, between the shoulder and the elbow (p. 131)

20. **(E)** Hypoperfusion—inadequate perfusion of the cells and tissues of the body caused by insufficient flow of blood through the capillaries (p. 131)

▶ **Part D**

1. **(F)** Hyoid bone—the free-floating bone in the neck that provides structure to the larynx (p. 109)

2. **(H)** Ilium—the superior and widest portion of the pelvis (p. 131)

3. **(J)** Inferior—away from the head; usually compared with another structure that is closer to the head (p. 98)

4. **(L)** Inhalation—an active process in which the intercostal muscles and the diaphragm contract, expanding the size of the chest cavity and causing air to flow into the lungs (p. 109)

5. **(N)** Insulin—a hormone produced by the pancreas or taken as a medication by diabetics (p. 131)

6. **(P)** Involuntary muscle—muscle that responds automatically to brain signals but cannot be consciously controlled (p. 131)

7. **(A)** Ischium—the lower, posterior portion of the pelvis (p. 131)

8. **(Q)** Joint—the point where two bones come together (p. 108)

9. **(I)** Kidney—organs of the renal system used to filter blood and regulate fluid levels in the body (p. 131)

10. **(R)** Large intestine—the muscular tube that removes water from waste products received from the small intestine and removes anything absorbed by the body toward excretion from the body (p. 131)

11. **(B)** Larynx—the voicebox (p. 131)

12. **(D)** Lateral—to the side, away from the midline of the body (p. 97)

13. **(T)** Ligament—tissue that connects bone to bone (p. 100)

14. **(K)** Liver—the largest organ of the body, produces bile to assist in breakdown of fats and assists in the metabolism of various substances in the body (p. 131)

15. **(S)** Lungs—the organs where exchange of atmospheric oxygen and waste carbon dioxide takes place (p. 109)

16. **(O)** Malleolus—protrusion on the side of the ankle (p. 131)

17. **(G)** Mandible—the lower jaw bone (p. 131)

18. **(M)** Manubrium—the superior portion of the sternum (p. 131)

19. **(C)** Maxillae—the two fused bones forming the upper jaw (p. 131)

20. **(E)** Medial—toward the midline of the body (p. 97)

▶ **Part E**

1. **(I)** Metacarpals—the hand bones (p. 131)

2. **(N)** Metatarsals—the foot bones (p. 131)

3. **(J)** Mid-axillary line—a line drawn vertically from the middle of the armpit to the ankle (p. 97)

4. **(P)** Mid-clavicular line—the line through the center of each clavicle (p. 97)

5. **(M)** Midline—an imaginary line drawn down the center of the body, dividing it into right and left halves (p. 97)

6. **(O)** Muscle—tissue that can contract to allow movement of a body part (p. 100)

7. **(R)** Musculoskeletal system—the system of bones and skeletal muscles that supports and protects the body and permits movement (p. 100)

8. **(F)** Nasal bones—the nose bones (p. 132)

9. **(T)** Nasopharynx—the area directly posterior to the nose (p. 132)

10. **(Q)** Nervous system—the system of brain, spinal cord, and nerves that governs sensation, movement, and thought (p. 120)

11. **(E)** Orbits—the bony structures around the eyes; the eye sockets (p. 132)

12. **(D)** Oropharynx—the area directly posterior to the mouth (p. 132)

13. **(C)** Palmar—referring to the palm of the hand (p. 132)

14. **(H)** Pancreas—a gland located behind the stomach that produces insulin and juices that assist in digestion of food in the duodenum of the small intestine (p. 132)

15. **(B)** Patella—the kneecap (p. 132)

16. **(A)** Pelvis—the basin-shaped bony structure that supports the spine and is the point of proximal attachment for the lower extremities (p. 132)

17. **(S)** Penis—the organ of male reproduction responsible for sexual intercourse and the transfer of sperm (p. 132)

18. **(K)** Perfusion—the supply of oxygen to and removal of wastes from the cells and tissues of the body as a result of the flow of blood through the capillaries (p. 117)

19. **(L)** Peripheral nervous system—the nerves that enter and leave the spinal cord and travel between the brain and organs without passing through the spinal cord (p. 120)

20. **(G)** Peripheral pulses—the radial, brachial, posterior tibial, and dorsalis pedis pulses, which can be felt at peripheral points of the body (p. 132)

▶ **Part F**

1. **(G)** Phalanges—the toe bones and finger bones (p. 132)

2. **(I)** Pharynx—the area directly posterior to the mouth and nose; it is made up of the oropharynx and the nasopharynx (p. 132)

3. **(N)** Physiology—the study of body function (p. 95)

4. **(D)** Plane—a flat surface formed when slicing through a solid object (p. 96)

5. **(J)** Plantar—referring to the sole of the foot (p. 132)

6. **(L)** Plasma—the fluid portion of the blood (p. 132)

7. **(P)** Platelets—components of the blood; membrane-enclosed fragments of specialized cells (p. 132)

8. **(K)** Posterior—the back of the body or body part (p. 96)

9. **(M)** Posterior tibial artery—artery supplying the foot, behind the medial ankle (p. 132)

10. **(H)** Prone—lying face down (p. 99)

11. **(Q)** Proximal—closer to the torso (p. 99)

12. **(T)** Pubis—the medial anterior portion of the pelvis (p. 132)

13. **(R)** Pulmonary artery—the vessels that carry blood from the right ventricle of the heart to the lungs (p. 114)

14. **(S)** Pulmonary veins—the vessels that carry oxygenated blood from the lungs to the left atrium of the heart (p. 114)

15. **(O)** Pulse—the rhythmic beats caused as waves of blood move through and expand the arteries (pp. 116–117)

16. **(F)** Radial artery—artery of the lower arm. It is felt when taking the pulse at the wrist (p. 115)

17. **(C)** Radius—the lateral bone of the forearm (p. 132)

18. **(A)** Recovery position—lying on the side (p. 99)

19. **(E)** Red blood cells—components of the blood that carry oxygen to and carbon dioxide away from the cells (p. 132)

20. **(B)** Renal system—the body system that regulates fluid balance and filtration of the blood (p. 124)

▶ **PART G**

1. **(L)** Reproductive system—the body system that is responsible for human reproduction (p. 127)

2. **(J)** Respiration—the process of moving oxygen and carbon dioxide between circulating blood and the cells (p. 111)

3. **(K)** Respiratory system—the system of nose, mouth, throat, lungs, and muscles that brings oxygen into the body and expels carbon dioxide (p. 109)

4. **(I)** Scapula—the shoulder blade (p. 132)

5. **(N)** Shock—hypoperfusion (p. 132)

6. **(H)** Skeleton—the bones of the body (p. 132)

7. **(M)** Skin—the layer of tissue between the body and the external environment (p. 123)

8. **(G)** Skull—the bony structure of the head (p. 132)

9. **(O)** Small intestine—the muscular tube between the stomach and the large intestine, divided into the duodenum, the jejunum, and the ileum, which receives partially digested food from the stomach and continues digestion (p. 132)

10. **(A)** Spleen—an organ located in the left upper quadrant of the abdomen that acts as a blood filtration system and a reservoir for reserves of blood (p. 132)

11. **(P)** Sternum—the breastbone (p. 132)

12. **(B)** Stomach—muscular sac between the esophagus and the small intestine where digestion of food begins (p. 132)

13. **(Q)** Subcutaneous layers—the layers of fat and soft tissue found below the dermis (p. 132)

14. **(C)** Superior—toward the head (p. 97)

15. **(S)** Supine—lying on the back (p. 99)

16. **(D)** Systolic blood pressure—the pressure created in the arteries when the left ventricle contracts and forces blood out into the circulation (p. 133)

17. **(R)** Tarsals—the ankle bones (p. 133)

18. **(E)** Tendon—tissue that connects muscle to bone (p. 133)

19. **(T)** Thorax—the chest (p. 106)

20. **(F)** Thyroid cartilage—the wing-shaped plate of cartilage that sits anterior to the larynx and forms the Adam's apple (p. 133)

▶ **PART H**

1. **(K)** Tibia—the medial and larger bone of the lower leg (p. 133)

2. **(G)** Torso—the trunk of the body; the body without the head and the extremities (p. 133)

3. **(L)** Trachea—the windpipe; the structure that connects the pharynx to the lungs (p. 109)

4. **(E)** Trendelenburg position—a position in which the patient's feet and legs are higher than the head (p. 100)

5. **(M)** Ulna—the medial bone of the forearm (p. 133)

6. **(C)** Urethra—connecting the bladder to the vagina or penis for excretion of urine (p. 133)

7. **(N)** Uterus—female organ of reproduction used to house the developing fetus (p. 133)

8. **(A)** Vagina—the female organ of reproduction used for both sexual intercourse and as an exit from the uterus for the fetus (p. 133)

9. **(O)** Valve—a structure that opens and closes to permit the flow of a fluid in only one direction (p. 133)

10. **(B)** Vein—any blood vessel returning blood to the heart (p. 115)

11. **(P)** Venae cavae—the superior vena cava and the inferior vena cava, which return blood from the body to the right atrium (p. 112)

12. **(D)** Ventilation—the process of moving gases (oxygen and carbon dioxide) between inhaled air and the pulmonary circulation of the blood (p. 109)

13. **(Q)** Ventral—referring to the front of the body (p. 133)

14. **(F)** Ventricles—the two lower chambers of the heart (p. 133)

15. **(R)** Venule—the smallest kind of vein (p. 133)

16. **(H)** Vertebrae—the 33 bones of the spinal column (p. 133)

17. **(S)** Voluntary muscle—muscle that can be consciously controlled (p. 133)

18. **(I)** White blood cells—components of the blood; white blood cells produce substances that help the body fight infection (p. 116)

19. **(T)** Xiphoid process—the inferior portion of the sternum (p. 133)

20. **(J)** Zygomatic arches—form the structure of the cheeks (p. 133)

21. **(X)** Combining form—roots that are combined in medical terms (p. 93)

22. **(Y)** Compound—two or more whole words combined (p. 93)

23. **(Z)** Prefix—used to modify or qualify a root word (p. 94)

24. **(W)** Root—foundation of a word (p. 93)

25. **(V)** Suffix—word ending that forms nouns, adjectives, and verbs (p. 94)

26. **(U)** Testes—the male organ that produces sperm (p. 133)

MULTIPLE-CHOICE REVIEW

1. **(C)** The abdomen is a cavity of the body containing hollow and solid organs. Body systems include: respiratory, cardiovascular, musculoskeletal, skin (integumentary), nervous, endocrine, and digestive. (p. 130)

2. **(B)** If a patient is lying on his or her left side, this position is called the recovery, or left lateral recumbent, position.

The Fowler position is sitting on a stretcher, supine is lying on the back, and prone is lying on the stomach. (pp. 99–100)

3. **(C)** When a patient who is having difficulty breathing is placed in a sitting-up position on a stretcher, this position is called Fowler. Lying on the stomach is prone; lying on the back is supine. Trendelenburg is defined in the answer for multiple-choice question 4. (p. 100)

4. **(D)** When a patient who is dizzy and passing out is placed in the "lying flat with the head lower than the legs" position by the EMT, this is called the Trendelenburg position. For an explanation of the other choices, see the answer for multiple-choice question 3. (p. 100)

5. **(B)** The musculoskeletal system has three main functions: It gives the body shape, provides for body movements, and protects vital internal organs. Body sensation is a function of the nervous system. The skin, or integumentary system, is the body's outer covering. The cardiovascular system, working along with the respiratory system, transports oxygen into the cells. (p. 100)

6. **(C)** The upper jaw is also called the maxillae. The way to remember which of the two jaw bones is which, maxillae or mandible, is to use the rhyme "the mandible is moveable." The orbits are the areas around the eyes, and the nasal bone protects the nose. (p. 131)

7. **(A)** The spinal column consists of the 7 cervical, 12 thoracic, 5 lumbar, 5 sacral, and 4 coccyx bones. (p. 106)

8. **(C)** An injury to the cervical spine may be fatal because control of the muscles for breathing arise from the spinal cord at this level. The lumbar region is also subject to injury because it is not supported by other parts of the skeleton. The thoracic spine, as well as the sacral spine and coccyx, are less easily injured. (p. 107)

9. **(A)** The patient who was run over by the truck may have broken his lower extremities. The bones in the lower extremities include: the femur, tibia, fibula, patella, tarsals, metatarsals, calcaneus, and phalanges. The ischium is a pelvic bone. The ulna and radius are bones in the forearm. The orbits are the areas around the eyes in the face. (p. 100)

10. **(A)** Bones in the upper extremities include the humerus, ulna, radius, carpals, metacarpals, and phalanges. The cervical bones are in the neck, and the tibia and calcaneus are in the lower extremities. (p. 100)

11. **(D)** The types of muscle tissue include voluntary, involuntary, and cardiac. Cardiac muscle has a specific quality called automaticity, or the ability to generate and conduct electrical impulses on its own. (p. 108)

12. **(A)** The type of muscle that allows body movement such as walking is called voluntary. Involuntary and cardiac muscles are described in the answers for multiple-choice questions 11 and 13. Smooth is the same as involuntary. (p. 108)

13. **(B)** Involuntary, or smooth, muscle is found in the blood vessels, gastrointestinal system, lungs, and urinary system and controls the flow of materials through these systems. The heart has a special type of muscle (cardiac), and the quadriceps and biceps have voluntary, or (skeletal) striated, muscle. (p. 108)

14. **(B)** The larynx is the structure in the throat that is commonly known as the voicebox. The pharynx is the area directly posterior to the mouth and nose, the trachea is the windpipe, and the sternum is the breastbone. (p. 131)

15. **(B)** The epiglottis is a leaf-shaped valve that prevents food and foreign objects from entering the trachea. The bronchi are the two major tubes that allow air to enter each of the two lungs. The pharynx and larynx are defined in the answer for multiple-choice question 14. (p. 131)

16. **(C)** The normal order of passage of oxygen from the environment to the lungs is through mouth and nose to the pharynx, through the larynx, through the trachea, into the bronchi, into the bronchioles, and then into the alveoli. Normally air does not go into the esophagus, which is a tube that brings food into the stomach. (p. 110)

17. **(C)** When the diaphragm and intercostal muscles relax, the size of the chest cavity decreases, causing exhalation. When the diaphragm contracts, it moves down, enlarging the chest cavity; the intercostal muscles pull the chest upward and outward to enlarge the cavity. This rapid pressure change accounts for air moving from the outside environment to fill the cavity. (p. 109)

18. **(D)** The difference between the adult airway and the pediatric airway is that all structures are smaller and more easily obstructed in a child. Actually, the adult's tongue takes up proportionately less space in the mouth than the child's. The trachea and cricoid cartilage is softer and more flexible in a child. (p. 111)

19. **(B)** The body system that is responsible for the breakdown of food into absorbable forms is called the digestive system. The nervous system controls the body, the endocrine system manages intricate functions such as insulin balance and hormone production, and the integumentary system covers the surface of the body. (p. 122)

20. **(C)** An organ that contains acidic gastric juices that begin the breakdown of food into components that the body will be able to convert to energy is the stomach. The other organs are parts of the digestive system, which handles the food once it is already broken down. (pp. 122–123)

21. **(B)** The major artery in the thigh is called the femoral artery. The carotid is in the neck, radial is in the wrist, and brachial is in the arm. (p. 131)

22. **(C)** The vessel that carries oxygen-poor blood from the portion of the body below the heart and back to the right atrium is called the inferior vena cava. The posterior tibial is a pulse that can be palpated on the posterior aspect of the medial malleolus. The internal jugular is a vein that drains blood from the head. The aorta is the largest artery, which carries oxygen-rich blood away from the left ventricle. (p. 133)

23. **(B)** The left atrium receives blood from the pulmonary veins (the only veins that contain oxygenated blood). The left atrium then pumps the blood into the left ventricle, where it is then pumped out to the rest of the body. (pp. 114–115)

24. **(C)** The fluid that carries the blood cells and nutrients is called plasma. Platelets are defined in the answer for multiple-choice question 25. Urine is a waste product of the body excreted by the kidneys and held in the urinary bladder prior to being excreted from the body. (p. 132)

25. **(B)** The blood component that is essential to the formation of blood clots is called platelets. Plasma is the fluid part of the blood that carries blood cells and nutrients. The white blood cells fight infection, and the red cells carry oxygen to or carbon dioxide away from tissues. (p. 132)

26. (A) The pressure on the walls of an artery when the left ventricle contracts is called the systolic pressure. The pressure upon relaxation is the diastolic pressure. Residual and arterial pressures are utilized in critical care monitoring. (p. 117)

27. (A) The two main divisions of the nervous system are the central and peripheral nervous systems. The bones, muscles, and spinal column are parts of the musculoskeletal system. The spinal cord and brain are major components of the central nervous system. (p. 120)

28. (D) Nerves that carry information from throughout the body to the brain are sensory nerves. The motor nerves allow for movement. Spinal nerves, along with the brain, are actually a part of the central nervous system. There is no specific category called cardiac nerves. (p. 120)

29. (C) One of the functions of the integumentary system is to protect the body from the environment, bacteria, and other organisms. Other functions of the skin include water balance, temperature regulation, excretion, and shock absorption. The respiratory system eliminates excess oxygen into the atmosphere. The nervous system regulates the diameter of the blood vessels in the circulation. The skin (integumentary system) prevents environmental water from entering the body. (p. 123)

30. (C) The system that secretes hormones, such as insulin and adrenaline, and that is responsible for regulating body activities is called the endocrine system. The skin provides covering, and the nervous system provides overall control. The gastrointestinal system digests food. (p. 122)

31. (B) No sensation and motor function in both of a patient's legs is referred to as paraplegia. This should be documented on the prehospital care report. Quadriplegia would be no sensation and motor function in all four extremities. (p. 120)

32. (D) A pulmonologist is a specialist in the care of lung disease. The other physicians are involved with other organs primarily. (p. 109)

COMPLETE THE FOLLOWING

1. Arteries in the body include: (p. 112)
- Coronary
- Aorta
- Pulmonary
- Carotid
- Femoral
- Brachial
- Radial
- Posterior tibial
- Dorsalis pedis

2. Functions of the skin include: (p. 123)
- Protection
- Water balance
- Temperature regulation
- Excretion
- Shock absorption

3. Definitions of the terms listed include the following: (pp. 97–98)

A) lateral—to the side, away from the midline of the body.

B) medial—toward the midline of the body.

C) proximal—closer to the torso.

D) distal—further away from the torso.

E) superior—toward the top or lower portion.

F) inferior—toward the bottom or upper portion.

INSIDE/OUTSIDE PRACTICAL PATHOPHYSIOLOGY

Elderly patients, females, and diabetics often have silent-MIs.

During a stress reaction, or compensation from blood loss, the brain tells the adrenal glands to secrete epinephrine and norepinephrine. The epi causes increased heart rate and the nor-epi causes vasoconstriction in the periphery, thus allowing more blood to stay in the vital organs.

The adrenal glands are part of the endocrine system.

The heart is an essential component of the cardiovascular system.

LABEL THE DIAGRAMS

▶ **ANATOMICAL POSTURES (P. 99)**

1. Supine

2. Prone

3. Recovery

▶ **ANATOMICAL POSITION (PP. 97–98)**

▶ **DIAGRAM 1**

1. Distal

2. Proximal

3. Midline

4. Mid-clavicular line

5. Medial

6. Lateral

7. Palmar

8. Left

9. Dorsal

10. Right

▶ **DIAGRAM 2**

11. Anterior (ventral)

12. Posterior (dorsal)

13. Superior

14. Mid-axillary line

15. Inferior

▶ **TOPOGRAPHY OF THE TORSO (P. 101)**

1. Scapular region

2. Lumbar region

3. Iliac crest

4. Pubis

5. Maxilla

6. Thorax region

7. Sternoclavicular joints

8. Suprasternal (jugular) notch

9. Mandible

10. Sternum

11. Diaphragm

12. Sacrum

STREET SCENES DISCUSSION

1. Manual stabilization is needed because the slightest movement of the neck could cause serious, permanent damage—or death—if in fact there is an actual injury to the child's spine.

2. As an EMT who was dispatched to the scene, you clearly have a duty to act. That means, yes, the driver of the truck is a patient in need of evaluation.

MATCH TERMINOLOGY/ DEFINITIONS

1. **(J)** Pathophysiology—the study of how disease processes affect function of the body (p. 137)

2. **(C)** Electrolyte—a substance that, when dissolved in water, separates into charged particles (p. 137)

3. **(R)** Metabolism—the cellular function of converting nutrients to energy necessary for cell function (p. 137)

4. **(P)** Aerobic metabolism—the cellular process where oxygen is used to metabolize glucose (pp. 137–138)

5. **(T)** Anaerobic metabolism—the cellular process where glucose is metabolized into energy without oxygen (p. 138)

6. **(O)** Patent—open, clear, and free from obstruction (p. 142)

7. **(N)** Tidal volume—the volume of air moved in or out during one cycle of breathing (p. 142)

8. **(Q)** Dead air space—air that occupies the space between the mouth and alveoli but does not actually reach the area of gas exchange (p. 142)

9. **(S)** Chemoreceptors—chemical sensors in the brain and blood vessels that identify changing levels of oxygen and carbon dioxide (p. 143)

10. **(U)** Plasma oncotic pressure—the pull exerted on water in and around the body cells into the bloodstream by large proteins in the plasma portion of the blood (p. 143)

11. **(K)** Hydrostatic pressure—the push of water out of the bloodstream as a result of the pressure within the vessel (p. 143)

12. **(B)** Cardiac output—the amount of blood ejected from the heart in 1 minute (HR × SV) (p. 147)

13. **(M)** Systemic vascular resistance—the pressure in the peripheral blood vessels that the heart must overcome to pump blood (p. 146)

14. **(V)** V/Q match—ventilation/perfusion match (p. 148)

15. **(I)** Perfusion—the constant supply of oxygen and nutrients to the cells by the flow of blood (p. 148)

16. **(G)** Dehydration—an abnormally low amount of water in the body (p. 149)

17. **(F)** Edema—swelling associated with the movement of water into the interstitial space (p. 150)

18. **(H)** Hypersensitivity—an exaggerated response by the immune system to a particular substance (p. 153)

19. **(L)** Stretch receptors—sensors in the blood vessels designed to identify internal pressure (p. 145)

20. **(D)** FiO_2—fraction of inspired oxygen; the concentration of oxygen in the air we breathe (p. 138)

21. **(E)** Minute volume—the volume of air moved in one cycle of breathing (p. 142)

22. **(A)** Stroke volume—the amount of blood ejected from the heart in one contraction (p. 146)

MULTIPLE-CHOICE REVIEW

1. **(C)** The study of how disease processes affect the function of the body is called pathophysiology. (p. 136)

2. **(B)** The nucleus contains the DNA. (p. 136)

3. **(A)** Water management influences the concentration of electrolytes. (p. 137)

4. **(B)** Lactic acids are formed during a crush injury. (p. 138)

5. **(A)** The patient must have a patent airway to allow movement of air in and out of the chest. (p. 142)

6. **(C)** The minute volume is the best assessment of the amount of air going into and out of the lungs each minute. (p. 142)

7. **(D)** All of the examples illustrate a decreased minute volume. (p. 142)

8. **(A)** The medulla controls the respirations. (p. 142)

9. **(B)** Respiration is activated by changing pressure within the thorax. Inhalation is an active process and exhalation is a passive process. (p. 142)

10. **(C)** The chemoreceptors in the brain and vascular space stimulate the respiratory system to increase the rate and/or tidal volume. (p. 142)

11. **(D)** Plasma oncotic pressure is a force exerted by large proteins in the blood and pulls water into the bloodstream. (p. 143)

12. **(B)** A dysfunctioning liver can produce a dehydrated patient with massive edema. (p. 150)

13. **(B)** The stretch receptors in certain blood vessels begin the process of blood vessel constriction due to the development of shock. (p. 145)

14. **(C)** The constriction of peripheral vessels can be a major risk factor for heart disease and stroke. (p. 146)

15. **(A)** Septic patients often have capillary permeability problems. (p. 150)

16. **(D)** The average person ejects approximately 60 ml of blood each contraction. This is the person's stroke volume. (p. 146)

17. **(B)** Contractility refers to the forceful squeezing of the heart muscle. (p. 146)

18. **(D)** The patient's stroke volume depends on the patient's afterload, contractility, and preload. (p. 146)

19. **(C)** On a moment's notice, the only way the patient can increase her or his cardiac output is by increasing her or his heart rate. (p. 147)

20. **(C)** When a cardiac patient has another heart attack and his cardiac output drops, this is often due to a decrease in the strength of contractions. (p. 147)

21. **(D)** Fluids in our bodies are distributed based on all the factors that were listed. (p. 150)

22. **(B)** A patient with severe vomiting and diarrhea may have a condition called dehydration. (p. 149)

23. **(D)** The signs of neurological impairment include: inability or difficulty speaking, visual or hearing disturbance, and weakness on one side of the body. (p. 151)

24. **(A)** Graves disease is an example of a condition where the glands of the body are producing too much hormone. (pp. 151–152)

25. **(B)** Nausea and vomiting are the most common disorders of the digestive system. (p. 152)

COMPLETE THE FOLLOWING

1. **A)** In the respiratory system: air must bring oxygen in and remove CO_2, there must be a significant minute volume, and the alveoli must be capable of exchanging gas.
   B) In the cardiovascular system: there must be enough blood, the heart must pump the blood, there must be pressure in the system to move blood between the cells and the alveoli, and the blood must be capable of carrying oxygen and CO_2.

2. A ventilation/perfusion match involves: (A) alveoli that have sufficient air, and (B) that air is matched with sufficient blood in the pulmonary capillaries.

3. Shock is defined as poor perfusion.

INSIDE/OUTSIDE PRACTICAL PHYSIOLOGY

During the fight-or-flight situation, the body:

1. constricts the blood vessels (in the periphery).
2. increases the heartbeat.
3. dilates the pupils.
4. begins to sweat (skin).
5. increases the respiratory rate and depth.

STREET SCENES DISCUSSION

1. No, letting a patient who you suspect has internal bleeding stand could cause him to pass out. Next time lift him to the stretcher!

2. With days of diarrhea, the patient becomes dehydrated from loss of the fluid part of his blood. Our bodies need food for energy. Going without eating for a couple of days is never a good thing.

3. An example of a severe GI problem would be a stomach ulcer, which can cause a hole in the wall of the stomach and lots of bleeding. This can be life-threatening if left unmanaged.

Chapter 7: Life Span Development

MATCH TERMINOLOGY/ DEFINITIONS

1. **(H)** Infancy—stage of life from birth to 1 year of age (p. 157)
2. **(P)** Moro reflex—when startled, an infant throws his arms out, spreads his fingers, then grabs with his fingers and arms (p. 158)
3. **(I)** Palmar reflex—when you place your finger in an infant's palm, he will grasp it (p. 159)
4. **(B)** Rooting reflex—when you touch a hungry infant's cheek, he will turn his head toward the side touched (p. 159)
5. **(A)** Sucking reflex—when you stroke a hungry infant's lips, he will start sucking (p. 159)
6. **(O)** Bonding—the sense that needs will be met (p. 160)

7. **(J)** Trust versus mistrust—concept developed from an orderly, predictable environment versus a disorderly, irregular environment (p. 160)
8. **(M)** Scaffolding—building on what one already knows (p. 160)
9. **(C)** Temperament—the infant's reaction to his environment (p. 160)
10. **(D)** Toddler phase—stage of life from 12 to 36 months (p. 160)
11. **(N)** Preschool age—stage of life from 3 to 5 years (p. 161)
12. **(K)** School age—stage of life from 6 to 12 years (p. 162)
13. **(E)** Adolescent—stage of life from 13 to 18 years (p. 163)
14. **(F)** Early adulthood—stage of life from 20 to 40 years (p. 164)
15. **(L)** Middle adulthood—stage of life from 41 to 60 years (p. 165)
16. **(G)** Late adulthood—stage of life from 61 years and older (p. 166)

MULTIPLE-CHOICE REVIEW

1. **(B)** The infant has a head that is equal to 25 percent of her total body weight. She is also primarily a nose breather at this age. (p. 158)
2. **(C)** The infant who has nasal congestion can get in trouble fast because she is a primary nose breather at this age. (p. 158)
3. **(D)** Infants get their immunity and antibodies from breastfeeding by their mother, vaccinations they receive, and beginning to produce their own antibodies. (p. 158)
4. **(A)** The Cushing reflex is not normally found in the infant. It may be found if the infant has a life-threatening brain injury. (p. 159)
5. **(B)** The sucking reflex occurs when a mother strokes the infant's lips, thus causing the baby to start sucking. (p. 159)
6. **(C)** Temperament is her reaction to the environment. (p. 160)
7. **(A)** Anxiety and insecurity are exhibited by the infant in a disorderly environment. This is the characteristic of trust versus mistrust. (p. 160)
8. **(C)** The child who is developing would be more, not less, susceptible to illness as she enters the toddler years. (p. 160)
9. **(A)** The adolescent years are the beginning of the self-destructive behaviors such as drinking alcohol, using tobacco products, and abusing drugs. (p. 163)
10. **(B)** The peak physical condition occurs between the ages of 19 and 26. (p. 165)
11. **(D)** The medical history that includes taking anti-cholesterol medications and lots of dieting to try to control weight gain is most likely to come from a patient in the middle adulthood years. (p. 165)
12. **(D)** Examples of the psychosocial challenges that a person may have to deal with in his or her late adulthood years include living environment, self-worth, financial burdens, and death and dying issues. (p. 166)
13. **(D)** The age of the patient may effect your assessment in each of the following ways: the parent or caregiver will need to help you when assessing an infant, the parent who is in late adulthood is likely to have a history of cardiovascular disorders, and the adolescent often experiments with alcohol and tobacco products. (p. 166)

14. (B) The EMT's ability to communicate with a younger patient is not likely to be disrupted by the fear of death or dying, as it might be with an older patient. (p. 167)

15. (B) Both males and females reach reproductive maturity during the adolescent years. (p. 164)

16. (B) Girls are usually finished growing by the age of 16. (pp. 163–164)

17. (C) Boys are usually finished growing by the age of 18. (p. 164)

18. (B) Serious family conflicts occur in some adolescents as the child strives for independence and the parents strive for more control. (p. 164)

19. (C) The leading cause of death in young adulthood is accidents. (p. 164)

20. (D) The experts believe that the highest levels of job stress occur in the young adult age group. (p. 165)

COMPLETE THE FOLLOWING

1. The eight stages of life discussed in the chapter include infancy, toddler, preschool age, school age, adolescence, early adulthood, middle adulthood, and late adulthood.

2. Examples of characteristics that appear in each of the following age groups:

A) 2 months—tracks objects with eyes; recognizes familiar faces.

B) 3 months—moves objects to mouth with hands; distinct facial expressions (smile, frown).

C) 4 months—drools without swallowing; begins to reach out to people.

D) 5 months—sleeps through the night without waking for feeding; discriminates between family and strangers.

STREET SCENES DISCUSSION

1. This patient is in the preschool age group.

2. Once it is clear that the patient has a pulse (you do not suspect a cardiac arrest), the priority for treatment is "A," airway; "B," breathing; and then "C," circulation (i.e., life-threatening bleeding and pulse/shock).

3. The second set of vitals is not normal for this patient and should lead you to believe there may be some life-threatening internal bleeding.

Chapter 8: Airway Management

MATCH TERMINOLOGY/ DEFINITIONS

1. (E) Airway—the passageway by which air enters or leaves the body; the structures of the airway are the nose, mouth, pharynx, larynx, trachea, bronchi, bronchioles, and alveoli (p. 173)

2. (C) Patent airway—an airway that is open and clear and will remain open and clear, without interference to the passage of air into and out of the lungs (p. 174)

3. (F) Head-tilt, chin-lift—a method of correcting blockage of the airway by the tongue by tilting the head back and lifting the chin; this method is indicated when no trauma, or injury, is suspected (p. 181)

4. (A) Jaw-thrust maneuver—a method for (means of) correcting blockage of the airway by moving the jaw forward without tilting the head or neck; this method is indicated when trauma, or injury, is suspected to open the airway without causing further injury to the spinal cord in the neck (p. 182)

5. (B) Oropharyngeal airway—a curved device inserted through the patient's mouth into the pharynx to help maintain an open airway (p. 183)

6. (H) Nasopharyngeal airway—a flexible breathing tube inserted through the patient's nose into the pharynx to help maintain an open airway (p. 183)

7. (D) Gag reflex—vomiting or retching that may result when something is placed in the back of the pharynx; this is tied to the swallow reflex (p. 184)

8. (G) Suctioning—use of a vacuum device to remove blood, vomitus, and other secretions or foreign materials from the airway (p. 188)

MULTIPLE-CHOICE REVIEW

1. (C) During breathing, for air to move into and out of the lungs the airflow must be unobstructed and move freely. (p. 174)

2. (D) Inhaled air can travel through the nasopharynx, the oropharynx, and the laryngopharynx. (pp. 174–175)

3. (B) The hypopharynx is also called the laryngopharynx. The other choices are structures of the lower airway (glottis and trachea) and the nose (nares). (p. 175)

4. (C) The leaf-like structure protecting the opening (glottic) of the trachea is the epiglottis. (p. 174)

5. (B) The lower airway is inferior to the larynx, so the bronchial passages or alveoli may be congested. The foreign body that gets ingested usually is in the upper airway. (p. 174)

6. (B) If the patient has an inadequate airway, he or she may have signs such as absent air movement; unusual hoarse or raspy quality to the voice; and abnormal sounds such as wheezing, crowing, and stridor. (p. 179)

7. (B) The child with an inadequate airway has retractions above the clavicles and between the ribs. (p. 179)

8. (D) Yes, it is significant that she is so short of breath that she is not moving enough air to speak in full sentences. (p. 179)

9. (D) The low volume and raspy tone could be due to airway swelling from the neck trauma. (p. 179)

10. (C) Children who are experiencing inadequate breathing often have nasal flaring when they breathe. (p. 179)

11. (D) An open airway is paramount because the patient who is not breathing deteriorates rapidly. This is a life-threatening situation. Open the airway, then clear the mouth and administer oxygen. (p. 180)

12. (B) Trauma victims require the jaw-thrust maneuver to open the airway. (p. 182)

13. (A) The jaw-thrust maneuver is the most appropriate method of opening the airway on a patient with suspected head, neck, or spine injury. (p. 182)

14. **(B)** With the patient in the supine position, the EMT should position him- or herself at the head of the patient to do airway maneuvers properly. (p. 180)

15. **(D)** Do not tilt or rotate the patient's head. All other choices are steps to perform the jaw-thrust maneuver. In addition, you will need to retract the patient's lower lip with your thumb to keep the mouth open. (p. 182)

16. **(B)** The jaw-thrust is used when you suspect possible neck, head, or spinal trauma. (p. 182)

17. **(C)** The OPA or NPA should be used to keep the tongue from blocking the airway. (p. 184)

18. **(C)** The gag reflex protects the glottic opening by causing the patient to vomit or retch when something is placed in the back of the conscious patient's throat. (p. 184)

19. **(A)** The proper sized OPA extends from the corner of the patient's mouth to the tip of the earlobe *or* the center of the mouth to the angle of the jaw. (p. 185)

20. **(A)** The OPA should be inserted upside down, with the tip toward the roof of the mouth, then flipped 180 degrees over the tongue in an adult patient. (p. 185)

21. **(B)** Insert the NPA with the bevel toward the nasal septum. Measure it from the patient's nostril to his or her earlobe. (p. 187)

22. **(D)** When inserting an NPA, use a water soluble lubricant such as Lubifax®, Surgilube®, or KY-Jelly®. (p. 187)

23. **(C)** Suctioning the airway removes blood, vomitus, and other secretions. Large particles (teeth and solid particles) should be removed using a finger sweep with a gloved finger. (p. 188)

24. **(A)** Any patient who might vomit requires the EMT to have a suction unit right at the patient's side. (p. 188)

25. **(C)** The Yankauer suction tip is a rigid device with a larger bore than most flexible catheters. It is usually not used with a responsive patient, although it certainly is possible. (p. 190)

INSIDE/OUTSIDE: THE SOUNDS OF A PARTIALLY OBSTRUCTED AIRWAY

1. Stridor is typically a high-pitched upper airway sound. (p. 179)

2. Hoarseness often develops due to a partial airway swelling, such as from a respiratory burn of the airway. (p. 179)

3. Snoring is a noise of the upper airway due to soft tissue creating impedance to the flow of air. (p. 179)

4. Liquids in the upper airway produce a gurgling sound. (p. 179)

COMPLETE THE FOLLOWING

1. The signs of inadequate airway are: (any six) (pp. 178–179)
   - No signs of breathing or air movements.
   - Evidence of foreign bodies in the airway, including blood, vomit, or objects such as broken teeth.
   - No air can be felt or heard at the nose or mouth, or the amount of air exchanged is below normal.
   - Inability to speak or difficulty speaking.
   - Unusual horse or raspy quality to the voice.
   - Chest movements are absent, minimal, or uneven.

- Movement associated with breathing is limited to the abdomen (abdominal breathing).
- Breath sounds are diminished or absent.
- Noises such as wheezing, crowing, stridor, snoring, gurgling, or gasping are heard during breathing. In children, there may be retractions (a pulling in of the muscles) above the clavicles and between and below the ribs.
- Nasal flaring (widening of the nostrils with respirations) may be present, especially in infants and children.

2. Identify five indications for using airway adjuncts. (any five) (p. 184)
   - Only use an OPA on patients who do not exhibit a gag reflex.
   - Open the patient's airway manually before using an adjunct device.
   - When inserting the airway, take care not to push the patient's tongue into the pharynx.
   - Have suction ready prior to inserting any airway.
   - Do not continue inserting the airway if the patient begins to gag.
   - When an airway adjunct is in place, you must maintain the head-tilt, chin-lift or jaw-thrust maneuver and monitor the airway.
   - After an airway adjunct is in place, continue to be ready to provide suction if the gag reflex returns.
   - If the patient regains consciousness or develops a gag reflex, remove the airway immediately.
   - Use infection control practices while maintaining the airway.

STREET SCENES DISCUSSION

1. An oropharyngeal airway (OPA). Try inserting one of the appropriate size (center of the mouth to angle of the jaw *or* corner of the mouth to the earlobe) starting upside down and then flipping it 180 degrees over the tongue into proper position.

2. Quickly turn the patient onto his side, remove the airway adjunct and BVM, and allow him to vomit. Make sure you clear out the airway so he does not aspirate vomitus into his lungs.

3. Yes, consider an ALS unit. If one is not on scene when you are ready to transport, arrange an intercept en route to the hospital. ALS providers can intubate the patient and administer medication as needed.

CASE STUDY: THE RAPIDLY CHANGING AIRWAY

1. The patient most likely has a lower airway partial obstruction. She is still moving air, but the wheezing is caused by air being forced through her narrowed bronchioles. She also speaks in short, choppy sentences, which is an indication of severe respiratory distress.

2. The short choppy sentences are an indication of severe shortness of breath or respiratory distress.

3. If she loses consciousness, insert an OPA as long as she does not have a gag reflex.

4. This is a medical patient and you have no evidence of head or neck trauma, so use the head-tilt, chin lift to position the airway.

Chapter 8 (continued)

5. The most common reason patients make a snoring noise is due to the partial obstruction of the tongue in the back of the throat. Reposition her airway so it is open all the way and the snoring should go away.

6. Gurgling sounds in the airway are usually due to fluid. Roll her to the side, scoop out any large particles, and then remove by suctioning out her airway.

Chapter 9: Respiration and Artificial Ventilation

MATCH TERMINOLOGY/ DEFINITIONS

▶ PART A

1. (I) Respiration—breathing (p. 201)

2. (J) Respiratory distress—increased work of breathing; a sensation of shortness of breath (p. 201)

3. (B) Respiratory failure—the reduction of breathing to the point where oxygen intake is not sufficient to support life (p. 201)

4. (A) Respiratory arrest—when breathing stops completely (p. 202)

5. (G) Minute volume—the amount of air breathed in during each respiration multiplied by the number of breaths per minute (p. 198)

6. (H) Dead space—areas of the lungs outside the alveoli where gas exchange with the blood does not take place (p. 199)

7. (C) Cyanosis—a blue or gray color resulting from lack of oxygen in the body (p. 206)

8. (D) Airway—the passageway by which air enters or leaves the body; the structures of the airway are the nose, mouth, pharynx, larynx, trachea, bronchi, and lungs (p. 194)

9. (F) Patent airway—an airway (passage from nose or mouth to lungs) that is open and clear and will remain open and clear, without interference to the passage of air into and out of the body (p. 194)

10. (E) Head-tilt, chin-lift maneuver—a means of correcting blockage of the airway by the tongue by tilting the head back and lifting the chin; used when no trauma, or injury, is suspected (p. 194)

▶ PART B

1. (I) Jaw-thrust maneuver—a means of correcting blockage of the airway by moving the jaw forward without tilting the head or neck; used when trauma, or injury, is suspected to open the airway without causing further injury to the spinal cord in the neck (p. 182)

2. (J) Ventilation—the breathing in of air or oxygen or providing breaths artificially (p. 198)

3. (B) Artificial ventilation—forcing air or oxygen into the lungs when a patient has stopped breathing or has inadequate breathing (p. 208)

4. (A) Pocket face mask—a device, usually with a one-way valve, to aid in artificial ventilation; a rescuer breathes through the valve when the mask is placed over the patient's face. It also acts as a barrier to prevent contact with a patient's breath or body fluids. It can be used with supplemental oxygen when fitted with an oxygen inlet. (pp. 210–212)

5. (G) Bag-valve mask—a handheld device with a face mask and self-refilling bag that can be squeezed to provide artificial ventilations to a patient. It can deliver air from the atmosphere or oxygen from a supplemental oxygen supply system. (pp. 214–216)

6. (H) Stoma—a permanent surgical opening in the neck through which the patient breathes (p. 215)

7. (C) Flow-restricted, oxygen-powered ventilation device (FROPVD)—a device that uses oxygen under pressure to deliver artificial ventilations. Its trigger is placed so that the rescuer can operate it while still using both hands to maintain a seal on the face mask. It has automatic flow restriction to prevent overdelivery of oxygen to the patient. (pp. 216–218)

8. (D) Automatic transport ventilator (ATV)—a device that provides positive pressure ventilations. It includes settings designed to adjust ventilation rate and volume, is portable, and is easily carried on an ambulance. (pp. 218–219)

9. (F) Oropharyngeal—a curved device inserted through the patient's mouth into the pharynx to help maintain an open airway (p. 183)

10. (E) Nasopharyngeal—a flexible breathing tube inserted through the patient's nose into the pharynx to help maintain an open airway (p. 183)

▶ PART C

1. (H) Gag reflex—vomiting or retching that results when something is placed in the back of the pharynx; this is tied to the swallow reflex (p. 184)

2. (F) Suctioning—use of a vacuum device to remove blood, vomitus, and other secretions or foreign materials from the airway (p. 188)

3. (D) Hypoxia—an insufficiency of oxygen in the body's tissues (p. 201)

4. (B) Oxygen cylinder—a cylinder filled with oxygen under pressure (pp. 225–227)

5. (A) Pressure regulator—a device connected to an oxygen cylinder to reduce cylinder pressure to a safe level for delivery of oxygen to a patient (pp. 225–227)

6. (C) Flowmeter—a valve that indicates the flow of oxygen in liters per minute (pp. 222–223)

7. (E) Humidifier—a device connected to the flowmeter to add moisture to the dry oxygen coming from an oxygen cylinder (p. 223)

8. (G) Nonrebreather mask—a face mask and reservoir bag device that delivers high concentrations of oxygen; the patient's exhaled air escapes through a valve and is not rebreathed (p. 229)

9. (I) Nasal cannula—a device that delivers low concentrations of oxygen through two prongs that rest in the patient's nostrils (p. 230)

10. (J) Venturi mask—a face mask and reservoir bag that delivers specific concentrations of oxygen by mixing oxygen with inhaled air (p. 231)

©2012 Pearson Education, Inc.
Emergency Care, 12th Ed.

MULTIPLE-CHOICE REVIEW

1. **(D)** During ventilation, the diaphragm and chest muscles contract and relax to change the pressure in the chest. Carbon dioxide exits (not enters) the body during expiration. (p. 198)

2. **(B)** Respiratory failure is inadequate breathing and is a precursor to respiratory arrest. The complete cessation of breathing is respiratory arrest. (p. 201)

3. **(C)** When breathing is limited to abdominal movement, the patient may not be breathing adequately. (p. 201)

4. **(D)** Signs of inadequate breathing in a child include cyanotic skin, lips, tongue, or earlobes; retractions between and below the ribs; and nasal flaring. (pp. 205–206)

5. **(B)** Breathing at a rate of 14 to 18 breaths per minute is normal and not a sign of inadequate breathing. (p. 206)

6. **(B)** All of the signs listed are found with inadequate breathing *except* air felt at the nose and mouth with exhalation, which is normal. (p. 206)

7. **(D)** Inadequate breathing in a young child includes less than 12 breaths per minute, more than 36 breaths per minute, and cyanosis of the lips and earlobes. (p. 206)

8. **(A)** A patient with respiratory failure would have mottled or blotchy skin color. (p. 206)

9. **(D)** Cyanosis can be checked by observing the patient's tongue, nail beds, and earlobes. (p. 206)

10. **(C)** One indication that a patient is experiencing inadequate breathing is that she talks in short, choppy sentences because she is out of breath. (p. 206)

11. **(D)** The first step to aid a patient who is not breathing is to open the airway. (p. 210)

12. **(B)** Narcotics can cause respiratory depression and lead to hypoxia. (p. 207)

13. **(B)** A normal breathing rate for an adult patient would be 12 to 20 per minute. (p. 206)

14. **(D)** If the patient is not breathing or breathing is inadequate, the EMT needs to provide positive pressure ventilation, artificial ventilation, and/or assistance with a BVM device. (p. 208)

15. **(A)** Hypothermia is not one of the normal side effects of positive pressure ventilation. (p. 208)

16. **(B)** Hyperventilation can lead to a lower BP, vasoconstriction, and limited flow to the brain as well as blowing off too much CO_2. (p. 208)

17. **(A)** If you have two rescuers to attend to the airway, the one rescuer using the BVM is the least effective method because you will tire and it is difficult to do a one-handed seal for a long time. (pp. 208, 214)

18. **(C)** A color change from cyanotic blue to pink is not a sign of inadequate ventilation. (p. 207)

19. **(B)** Ventilations should be delivered over 1 second. (p. 207)

20. **(B)** A BVM should have a non-jam valve with an oxygen inlet when used by EMS personnel. (p. 212)

21. **(A)** The BVM should be capable of withstanding cold temperatures. (p. 212)

22. **(D)** If the patient has suspected trauma, the jaw-thrust maneuver should be used and not the head-tilt, chin-lift maneuver. (p. 182)

23. **(D)** The BVM should be used with an oral airway. The reservoir bag and oxygen tank should always be used. (pp. 212–214)

24. **(D)** If the patient's chest does not rise and fall when ventilating, the EMT should reposition the head and reattempt ventilations, check for escape of air around the mask, and use an alternative method of artificial ventilation. (p. 208)

25. **(C)** If the patient has a stoma and needs ventilatory assistance, the best device to use is a BVM. (p. 215)

26. **(D)** The FROPVD should operate in both ordinary and extreme environmental conditions, have an audible alarm when the relief valve is activated, and have a trigger so two hands can be used to seal the mask. (pp. 216–217)

27. **(C)** The Sellick maneuver (cricoid pressure) is designed to reduce entry of air into the esophagus during ventilations. (p. 215)

28. **(B)** Use the ATV when you only have one EMT on the airway to do ventilations. (p. 208)

29. **(C)** When fully pressurized, an oxygen tank should have approximately 2,000 psi on the gauge. (p. 224)

30. **(B)** The portable oxygen cylinder that will last the longest in the field, of the choices listed, is the E tank. An M tank is not a portable tank. (p. 220)

31. **(A)** Prior to connecting the regulator to the oxygen supply cylinder, the EMT should remove the protective seal and then open the valve. (pp. 225–226)

32. **(C)** Humidified oxygen is not needed in adult patients being transported for a short distance. (p. 223)

33. **(A)** The concerns about dangers of giving too much oxygen to patients with COPD are invalid in the out-of-hospital setting when the patient is in respiratory distress. The priority always is to treat the respiratory distress with high-flow and high-concentration oxygen in the field. (p. 225)

34. **(D)** The best choice of the choices listed is a nonrebreather mask for the heart attack patient. (p. 219)

35. **(D)** The oxygen concentration of the nonrebreather mask is approximately 80 percent to 90 percent. (p. 229)

36. **(B)** The flow rate of a nonrebreather mask should be 12 to 15 liters per minute. Then adjust as the patient breathes so she or he does not overbreathe the bag. (p. 229)

37. **(C)** The oxygen concentration of a nasal cannula is between 24 percent and 44 percent. (p. 229)

38. **(B)** The patient has a decreased respiratory excursion due to the pain from the rib fractures. She may have a faster than normal rate, but the tidal volume is diminished, thus making her minute volume go down. The reduced minute volume is a serious life threat if it is not managed promptly. (p. 199)

39. **(D)** The anatomical dead space is the area in the lungs (trachea, bronchi, bronchioles) outside the alveoli where air exchange cannot take place. (p. 199)

40. **(C)** When assessing and managing the breathing of a child, remember that the trachea is softer and more flexible. (p. 233)

COMPLETE THE FOLLOWING

1. To determine signs of adequate breathing, the EMT should: (p. 201)
   A) look for adequate and equal expansion of both sides of the chest when the patient inhales.
   B) listen for air entering and leaving the nose, mouth, and the chest.
   C) feel for air moving out of the nose or mouth.
   D) check for typical skin coloration.
   E) note the rate, rhythm, quality, and depth of breathing typical for a person at rest.

2. To determine the signs of adequate artificial ventilation, the EMT should: (p. 201)
   A) watch the chest rise and fall with each ventilation.
   B) ensure that the rate of ventilation is sufficient (approximately 10 to 12 per minute in adults).

3. The patient may have inadequate artificial ventilation when the EMT notices that: (p. 202)
   A) the chest does not rise and fall with ventilations.
   B) the rate of ventilation is too fast or too slow.

INSIDE/OUTSIDE: RESPIRATORY DISTRESS TO RESPIRATORY FAILURE

1. The respiratory depth and rate will increase. (p. 205)
2. The blood vessels in the arms and legs will constrict. (p. 205)
3. The wheezes are due to bronchoconstriction and air being forced through narrowed passageways. (p. 205)
4. The patient often becomes anxious because of hypoxia of the brain. (p. 205)
5. When the patient gets tired, the chest muscles may no longer support the effort of breathing and this may be pre-respiratory arrest. Never a good sign. (p. 205)

STREET SCENES DISCUSSION

1. Use an OPA. Select the proper size (center of the mouth to the angle of the jaw *or* corner of the mouth to the earlobe), and then insert it upside down and flip it over the tongue, or insert it straight in with the help of a tongue depressor.
2. Roll the patient to the side, sweep out the mouth with your gloved finger, and then suction with a rigid tip such as a Yankauer.
3. For a patient in respiratory distress, it is always appropriate to call for ALS, for medications, for more help in assessment, and for additional hands should the situation change quickly.

CASE STUDY: THE COMPLICATED AIRWAY: THE SELF-INFLICTED SHOOTING

1. Open the airway by jutting the jaw and pulling the tongue forward out of the throat.
2. A) Yes, the patient needs to be suctioned.
   B) The maximum time is about 15 seconds per attempt. Keep in mind, however, that you must adequately clear the airway so he does not aspirate any blood. If the patient is in cardiac arrest, the maximum time is reduced to about 10 seconds.
3. Yes, an oral or nasal airway would be helpful to this patient.
4. A bag-valve mask should be used to assist this patient's ventilations.
5. A) Use 12 to 15 liters per minute.
   B) Use it but do not rely solely on it because the patient may have poor perfusion, and the device may have an inaccurate reading.
6. A) A full D tank has about 350 liters in it.
   B) A pressure of 2,000 to 2,200 pounds per square inch (psi).
   C) It takes about 19 to 20 minutes to run the tank down to 200 psi (which is 10 percent left in the tank). Let's say that the full tank has 350 liters. By subtracting 10 percent ($350 - 35 = 315$) and then dividing 315 by 15 liters per minute, you are left with 21. Just to be on the safe side, round down 1 minute because you never know for sure that the tank actually had every bit of the 2,200 psi when you began. There is also a formula in the text that some EMTs may use, but it is not easily done in your head!
7. A) Do not exceed 15 seconds.
   B) You are removing oxygen when you suction the patient.
   C) A rigid Yankauer suction tip is most appropriate in this patient.
8. A) This patient is a high priority.
   B) His complicated airway is the major problem, making him a priority patient.
   C) He should be transported right away.
   D) Take him to a trauma center if there is one in your region.
9. ALS may be helpful for fluid infusion en route to the hospital, advanced airway procedures, and more trained hands to manage the patient.
10. If you heard bubbling around the mask, suction and reassess your mask seal.

Interim Exam 1

1. **(C)** Most EMT courses today are based on models developed by the United States National Highway Transportation Safety Administration (NHTSA). The American Red Cross (ARC) is involved in disaster relief and basic first aid and CPR training. The American Heart Association (AHA) is involved in basic and advanced cardiac life support as well as cardiovascular research. The National Institutes of Health (NIH) provides grants for health research. (p. 6)
2. **(D)** Being pleasant, cooperative, sincere, and a good listener inspires confidence in patients and bystanders. Do not put patient safety above your own, and do not lie to the patient by telling him or her everything is all right. (p. 11)
3. **(C)** Negligence is a failure to act properly in a situation in which there was a duty to act, needed care as would reasonably be expected of the EMT was not provided, and harm was caused to the patient as a result. Abandonment means you left the patient in no one's care. Breach of promise is a distracter. (p. 81)
4. **(D)** For a patient to refuse care or transport, he or she must be mentally competent, oriented fully, and informed of potential consequences of refusing care. Document the refusal on a release form. (p. 76)

5. (B) In the case of an unconscious patient, consent may be assumed. This is known as implied consent. *Triage* is a French word that means "to sort." Immunity is a protection from liability. Applied is a distracter. (p. 76)

6. (D) Even though the child's injury is not described as life threatening, parental consent is still required. A minor cannot give expressed consent. Only life-threatening situations involve implied consent. (p. 77)

7. (C) Good Samaritan laws, which are found in a number of states, grant immunity from liability to off-duty rescuers who act in good faith to provide care to the level of their training. (p. 83)

8. (A) Entering hazmat scenes with SCBA is not the responsibility of an EMT. Protecting yourself and others, recognizing potential problems, and notifying the hazardous-materials response team are the responsibilities of an EMT at a hazardous-materials incident. (p. 41)

9. (B) The form of infection control based on the presumption that all body fluids are infectious is called Standard Precautions. An infectious disease is a reason to take Standard Precautions. (p. 23)

10. (D) The distance that the object is to be carried is a consideration when planning to lift, but it is not as important as the other factors. (p. 50)

11. (C) Use the leg muscles. Do not twist or use your back muscles while lifting; both actions may cause injury. (p. 50)

12. (C) Use the stair chair whenever possible, especially one with the tracks on it. (p. 58)

13. (C) Keep your arms bent, *not* fully extended, when pushing or pulling objects. (p. 50)

14. (D) Unconsciousness is not a reason to use an emergency move. Use an urgent move for an unconscious patient. (p. 52)

15. (A) The greatest danger of an emergency move is that a spinal injury may be aggravated. (p. 52)

16. (B) This is an extremity lift. The draw-sheet method involves a sheet. The direct ground lift requires lifting the patient from a supine position onto the rescuer's knees and then to the stretcher. The direct carry involves two rescuers lifting and curling the patient into their chests, then returning to a standing position, and then walking together with the patient. (p. 66)

17. (B) When moving a patient from the ambulance stretcher to the hospital stretcher, you probably will use the modified draw-sheet method. (p. 66)

18. (A) The EMTs should move to opposite sides of the stretcher to load it into the ambulance. (p. 59)

19. (B) Patients without spinal injury or fractures can be moved to a stretcher or stair chair via the extremity lift. A slide transfer is from a bed to a bed. Chair lift and indirect carry are distracters. (p. 65)

20. (A) Drags are used only for emergencies because they do not protect the neck and spine. (p. 52)

21. (B) Use an even number of rescuers to lift patient-carrying devices. Odd numbers will create an imbalance. (p. 58)

22. (B) To control the patient's airway and bleeding, use an urgent move, the rapid extrication procedure. Taking time to apply a short backboard may cause a deadly delay in removing the patient. (p. 52)

23. (D) The piggyback carry requires that the patient be conscious so she can hold on to the rescuer. (p. 65)

24. (C) The firefighter's carry is generally done in one sweeping motion. (p. 54)

25. (C) A flexible stretcher is used in narrow hallways or restricted areas to remove a patient without spinal injuries. (p. 57)

26. (B) Carefully drag the patient's clothing, trying to minimize further spinal injury. The other moves would not be used on a patient with a spinal injury. (p. 53)

27. (C) If the patient has no spinal injury and there are no space restrictions, then move the patient on the wheeled-ambulance stretcher. (p. 56)

28. (D) Proper personal protective equipment can prevent injuries to you and your crew. (p. 43)

29. (A) When a threat presents itself, retreat to a safe area. (p. 44)

30. (B) Eustress is positive stress. Distress is negative, can be cumulative, and may require a critical incident debriefing. (pp. 36–37)

31. (C) When responding to a violent situation, observation begins when you enter the neighborhood or immediate area of the scene. (p. 44)

32. (B) One crew member should always carry a portable radio to enable her or him to call for police assistance. (p. 44)

33. (B) Quickly control bleeding. Then have the dog locked in another room so it doesn't try to protect its owner by attacking you. (p. 44)

34. (C) Treat life-threatening problems and transport a patient who refuses care and then becomes unconscious. (p. 77)

35. (B) An advance directive is the expressed wishes of the patient or family in writing. If one of these documents is signed and at the patient's side, it can simplify resuscitation situations. (p. 80)

36. (C) The oral wishes of the patient's family are not a reason to withhold medical care. (p. 80)

37. (D) Providing care within the scope of your practice, using proper documentation, and being courteous and respectful can prevent lawsuits. (p. 78)

38. (D) If you are proven negligent, you may be required to pay for the patient's lost wages, medical expenses, and pain and suffering. Generally, insurance costs would not be your responsibility. (pp. 81–82)

39. (D) The skin, not the musculoskeletal system, regulates body temperature. The musculoskeletal system gives the body shape, protects internal organs, and provides for body movement. (p. 102)

40. (C) The superior portion of the sternum is called the manubrium. (p. 106)

41. (B) The protrusion on the inside of the ankle is called the medial malleolus. The lateral malleolus is on the outside of the ankle. (p. 107)

42. (B) Automaticity is the ability of the heart to generate and conduct electrical impulses on its own. (p. 109)

43. (A) The autonomic nervous system, a division of the peripheral nervous system, controls involuntary motor functions. (p. 12)

44. (B) The anatomical position is a standard reference position for the body in which the body is standing erect, facing the observer. The arms are down at the sides, and the palms of the hands are facing forward. (p. 97)

45. (A) See the answer for multiple-choice question 44. (p. 97)

46. (D) Plantar refers to the sole of the foot. (p. 107)

47. (C) The zygomatic bones are the cheekbones. (p. 106)

48. (D) The heart is superior to, or above, the stomach. (p. 97)

49. (B) Knees are proximal, or closer, to the torso compared to the toes. The toes are distal, or farther away, from the torso than are the knees. (p. 97)

50. (C) Supine means lying on the back. Prone means lying face down. (p. 99)

51. (C) The abdomen is divided into four parts, or quadrants. (p. 99)

52. (A) The torso consists of the abdomen, pelvis, and thorax. (p. 133)

53. (A) The heart is located in the center of the thoracic cavity. There is no such thing as the cardiac cavity. (p. 106)

54. (C) The structure that divides the chest from the abdominal cavity is the diaphragm. (p. 99)

55. (C) The kneecap is the patella. The ilium is a pelvic bone, the malleolus is in the ankle, and the phalanges are fingers and toes. (p. 101)

56. (C) The cranium is the skull minus the facial bones. (p. 106)

57. (A) The acromion process of the scapula is the highest portion of the shoulder. (p. 107)

58. (C) Good Samaritan laws provide some limited immunity to EMS personnel in some states. (p. 83)

59. (B) Unconsciousness in adults or children allows implied consent, thus allowing for care to begin. (p. 77)

60. (C) For negligence, three actions must be proved: the EMT had a duty to act, the EMT breached that duty, and this breach of duty caused harm (physical or psychological) to the patient. (p. 81)

61. (B) Lying on the stomach face down is a prone position, recovery is on the side, and supine is lying face up. Coma is a distracter. (p. 99)

62. (C) Patients who are dying over a period of time go through the following stages, in this order: denial, anger, bargaining, depression, and then acceptance. (p. 40)

63. (B) The National Registry of Emergency Medical Technicians has established professional standards for EMS since 1970. (p. 6)

64. (D) Most patients are transported by ground ambulance. (p. 6)

65. (B) EMT-Intermediates are trained to start IVs, perform advanced airway procedures, and administer some medications beyond the EMT. (p. 9)

66. (B) Quality improvement is a continuous self-review of the EMS system or service. (p. 13)

67. (B) The Medical Director assumes the ultimate responsibility for the patient-care aspects of the EMS system. (p. 15)

68. (A) A common cause of lawsuits against EMS agencies is patients who refuse care. (p. 77)

69. (D) The scope of practice defines the legal limits of the EMT's job. (p. 75)

70. (A) Decisiveness is *not* a sign of stress. (pp. 38–39)

71. (D) Most motor vehicle collisions don't result in excessive stress reactions. (p. 38)

72. (B) Increasing consumption of fatty foods is the wrong reaction to stress. (p. 39)

73. (A) If you want to reduce stress, request a change in shift or work location. Increasing your workload in any way will further increase your stress level. (p. 39)

74. (D) The integumentary system protects the body from the environment, bacteria, and other organisms. (p. 104)

75. (C) After a major EMS incident, stress is normal and expected. (p. 39)

76. (B) The five stages of grief include a stage where the patient may retreat to a world of his or her own. This is called depression. (pp. 39–40)

77. (B) A crushing injury causes anaerobic metabolism and will increase the production of lactic acids at the cellular level. (p. 137)

78. (C) A disease spread by exposure to an open wound or sore of an infected individual is caused by a bloodborne pathogen. (p. 33)

79. (D) Hepatitis is an infection that causes inflammation of the liver. (p. 23)

80. (C) Airborne diseases are spread by inhaling or absorbing droplets from the air through the eyes, nose, or mouth. (p. 33)

81. (D) The hepatitis B virus kills approximately 200 health workers every year in the United States. (p. 31)

82. (B) Assume that a patient with a productive cough has TB. (p. 34)

83. (D) HIV is not an airborne disease; it is a bloodborne disease. (p. 29)

84. (C) There is about a 30 percent chance of spreading hepatitis B with an infected needle. (pp. 28–29)

85. (A) There is about a 0.5 percent chance of spreading HIV with an infected needle. (p. 29)

86. (C) To protect yourself from TB, take Standard Precautions and wear a HEPA or N-95 respirator. A surgeon's mask will not protect you from this airborne disease. (p. 27)

87. (A) Use a pocket mask with one-way valve when you are confronted with a nonbreathing patient and you are alone. The bag-valve mask needs two rescuers in order to be used effectively. You do not blow directly into the ET tube or the one-way valve. (p. 27)

88. (C) Handwashing after each patient contact is an effective method of infection control and will reduce others' exposure risks. (p. 26)

89. (B) The Ryan White CARE Act establishes procedures for emergency response workers to find out if they have been exposed to life-threatening infectious diseases. OSHA does not require this. There is no such thing as an AIDS protection act. (p. 32)

90. (A) OSHA 1910.1030 requires an exposure control plan and annual training. (p. 31)

91. (D) The OSHA regulation requires that every employer of EMTs provide hepatitis B vaccination. Insurance or annual physicals are not required. (p. 31)

92. (D) Engineering controls to prevent spread of infectious diseases include all those listed. (p. 31)

93. (C) The OSHA bloodborne pathogen standard does not address the use of HEPA respirators because they are used for an airborne disease (e.g. TB). (p. 31)

94. **(B)** High-risk locations for TB do not include day-care centers because children are not prone to TB. (p. 34)

95. **(D)** Avoid approaching a scene with your lights and sirens on because this attracts a crowd, which you wish to avoid. (p. 42)

96. **(A)** Notify police immediately if there may be any weapons at the scene. The police are responsible for weapons control; your responsibility is patient care. (p. 42)

97. **(A)** Respiratory failure is the reduction of breathing to the point where oxygen intake is not sufficient to support life. Respiratory support is what you provide. Respiratory arrest is when breathing stops. Anoxic metabolism occurs in the absence of breathing. (p. 201)

98. **(C)** Cyanosis, or blue or gray skin, is *not* a sign of adequate breathing. (p. 201)

99. **(B)** Widening of the nostrils with respirations is called nasal flaring. Increased breathing rate is hyperventilation. Wheezes are a musical tone caused by spasms of the small airways. (p. 179)

100. **(B)** Blue or gray skin is called cyanosis. Anemia is a disease in which the patient has too few red blood cells. (p. 205)

101. **(C)** Inability to speak in full sentences is a sign of shortness of breath. Snoring is a noise made from a partial airway obstruction caused by the tongue. (p. 206)

102. **(B)** EMTs do not routinely insert ET tubes. All other answers listed are principal procedures used by the EMT to treat life-threatening respiratory problems. (p. 207)

103. **(A)** The tongue causes most airway problems. (p. 183)

104. **(D)** If the unconscious patient is found at the bottom of a stairwell, you will need to assume a neck or spine injury and use the jaw-thrust maneuver. (pp. 181–182)

105. **(B)** The one-rescuer bag-valve mask is the least effective in creating a seal, so it would be the last choice. (p. 207)

106. **(C)** A ventilation rate that is too fast or too slow may result in inadequate artificial ventilation. (p. 208)

107. **(A)** The standard respiratory fitting on a bag-valve mask is 15/22 mm. (p. 213)

108. **(D)** A bag-valve mask should not have a pop-off valve. (pp. 212–213)

109. **(C)** The proper bag-valve mask oxygen flow rate is 15 liters per minute. (p. 213)

110. **(B)** The most recent American Heart Association's guidelines now state that ventilation (i.e., mouth-to-mask, bag mask, or other forms of ventilation with or without supplementary oxygen) should involve sufficient ventilation volume to achieve visible chest rise. (p. 213)

111. **(C)** The first step in artificial ventilation of a stoma breather is to clear any mucus or secretions that may be obstructing the stoma. (pp. 215–216)

112. **(A)** The audible alarm on the flow-restricted, oxygen-powered ventilation device should go off when the relief valve is activated but not when ventilation is activated. (p. 216)

113. **(B)** The oropharyngeal and nasopharyngeal airways are the most common airway adjuncts. (p. 183)

114. **(D)** Use an oropharyngeal airway on all unconscious patients with no gag reflex. Airway usage is not restricted to only medical or only trauma patients. (p. 183)

115. **(C)** When suctioning a patient, never suction for longer that 15 seconds. You do not *hypo*ventilate, but do *hyper*ventilate the patient prior to and after suctioning.

Always wear eye protection and a mask when suctioning. Suction on the way out. (p. 188)

116. **(C)** The emergency situation in which there is a failure of the cardiovascular system to provide sufficient blood to all the vital tissues is called shock. (p. 202)

117. **(C)** Insufficiency in the supply of oxygen to the body's tissues is called hypoxia. Anoxia means no oxygen is being supplied to the cells. No-oxia is a distracter. Cyanosis is a result of hypoxia. (p. 201)

118. **(A)** Change the oxygen cylinder before the pressure gauge reads 200 psi at the lowest, otherwise you may damage the inside of the tank. (p. 220)

119. **(C)** Store cylinders in a cool, dry area, *not* in a warm, humid room. (p. 222)

120. **(A)** Use a nonrebreather mask for high-concentration oxygen delivery to the breathing patient. EMTs do not use partial rebreather masks in the field. A nasal cannula is a low-concentration device. (p. 229)

121. **(B)** The concentration of oxygen administered by a nasal cannula is between 24 and 44 percent. (p. 229)

122. **(B)** Do not remove the dentures unless they are loose. Dentures allow for an improved seal between the patient's face and mask. (p. 232)

123. **(A)** A child's mouth and nose are smaller and more easily obstructed than an adult's. The child's chest wall is softer. The trachea is narrower, so it is more easily obstructed. (p. 193)

124. **(A)** Respiratory arrest is complete breathing stoppage. (p. 202)

125. **(C)** The flow-restricted, oxygen-powered ventilation device is usually not used in children. Other devices listed are. (p. 218)

126. **(A)** A flowmeter allows the control of oxygen in liters per minute. A humidifier helps prevent the oxygen from being so dry. A reservoir is used on the BVM to increase the oxygen concentration. (pp. 222–223)

127. **(B)** The constant flow selector valve flowmeter allows for the control of the flow of oxygen in liters per minute in stepped increments. The Bourdon gauge and pressure compensated flowmeters are adjustable without stepped increments. (p. 223)

128. **(A)** Some systems use oxygen humidification to prevent drying out the patient's mucous membranes. Humidifiers are usually not used in systems with short transports and, unless they are disposable, may actually increase the potential for infection spread. (p. 223)

129. **(C)** Patients in the end stage of a respiratory disease are often on hypoxic drive. Carbon dioxide drive is the normal drive mechanism for healthy people. (p. 225)

130. **(D)** COPD is chronic obstructive pulmonary disease. (p. 225)

131. **(D)** With an air mattress, the patient is placed on the device and the air is withdrawn by the pump. The mattress then forms a rigid and conforming surface around the patient. These devices are new and are rapidly expanding in use. (p. 62)

132. **(C)** The body system that is responsible for the breakdown of food into absorbable forms is called the digestive system. The nervous system controls the body, the urinary system eliminates the liquid wastes from the bladder, and the integumentary system covers the surface of the body. (p. 122)

133. **(C)** A stress reaction that involves either physical or psychological behavior manifested days or weeks after an incident is called a post-traumatic stress disorder. Acute is based on a specific incident and occurs right after that incident. Burnout is an expression for a rescue worker who has become uncaring and completely disinterested, and cumulative stress is based on many incidents over a long period of time. (pp. 36–37)

134. **(B)** An agency privacy officer is required by the Health Insurance Portability and Accountability Act (HIPPA). NFPA sets firefighting standards and electrical codes, the Ryan White Law deals with communicable diseases and notification of emergency services personnel. The Privacy Control Act of 2002 does not pertain. (p. 84)

135. **(D)** Twelve breaths per minute times 500 mL of air per breath = 6,000 ml per minute in the adult patient. (p. 142)

136. **(C)** Dehydration can be caused by loss of fluids for multiple days, which can occur with severe diarrhea and vomiting. (p. 149)

137. **(A)** When a patient is short of breath, he or she often speaks in short, choppy sentences. (p. 201)

138. **(B)** Young infants breathe primarily through their noses and they are unable to blow their noses on their own, so nasal congestion can be a major problem. (p. 158)

139. **(B)** When the mother strokes the infant's lips and the baby starts sucking, this nervous system reflex is known as the sucking reflex. (p. 159)

140. **(C)** The adolescent years are the beginning of self-destructive behaviors. (p. 163)

141. **(D)** The leading cause of death in the young adult years is accidents. (p. 165)

142. **(D)** The family conflict of control versus independence becomes an issue with adolescents in some cases. (p. 163)

143. **(B)** Girls are usually finished growing by the age of 16. (p. 163)

144. **(B)** When an elderly patient sits forward with her elbows outward (tripod position) and speaks in short, choppy sentences, she most likely has breathing difficulties. (p. 201)

145. **(B)** The proper way to open the airway of a patient who you do not suspect has neck trauma is to use the head-tilt, chin-lift maneuver. The modified jaw thrust and the head-tilt, neck-lift have not been taught since early 2000. (p. 181)

146. **(C)** Measure the NPA from the tip of the nose to the earlobe, or measure the diameter of the patient's smallest finger. Insert in the right nares with the open side of the bevel facing the nasal septum. (p. 183)

147. **(C)** Respiratory distress leads to respiratory failure, which in turn leads to respiratory arrest if it is not treated appropriately. (p. 201)

148. **(D)** The patient may have any of those signs listed except air that can be felt at the nose or mouth on exhalation, which would be normal and not considered a sign of inadequate breathing. (p. 201)

149. **(B)** The normal breathing rate for an adult is 12 to 20 per minute. (p. 203)

150. **(D)** If the patient's breathing becomes inadequate, it may become necessary for the EMT to assist ventilations with a BVM or positive pressure ventilator or to provide artificial ventilations. (p. 203)

Chapter 10: Scene Size-Up

MATCH TERMINOLOGY/ DEFINITIONS

1. **(G)** Scene size-up—steps taken by an ambulance crew when approaching the scene of an emergency call: checking scene safety; taking Standard Precautions; noting the mechanism of injury or nature of the patient's illness; determining the number of patients; and deciding what, if any, additional resources to call for (p. 245)

2. **(D)** Danger zone—the area around the wreckage of a vehicle collision or other incident within which special safety precautions should be taken (p. 248)

3. **(C)** Mechanism of injury—a force or forces that may have caused injury (p. 262)

4. **(A)** Penetrating trauma—injury caused by an object that passes through the skin or other body tissues (p. 262)

5. **(B)** Blunt-force trauma—injury caused by a blow that does not penetrate the skin or other body tissues (p. 262)

6. **(E)** Index of suspicion—awareness that there may be injuries (p. 262)

7. **(F)** Nature of the illness—what is medically wrong with the patient (p. 262)

MULTIPLE-CHOICE REVIEW

1. **(A)** The EMT approaches the scene and surveys to determine if there are any threats to his or her safety. Next, the safety of the patient and the EMT's crew members are of concern. (p. 248)

2. **(D)** A size-up needs to be an ongoing process and not just confined to the beginning of the call because things often change and can make the scene hazardous. (pp. 247–248)

3. **(B)** Always conduct your own size-up and do not rely on that of other agencies solely. (pp. 247–248)

4. **(D)** At the scene of a traffic collision, just in case there is a fuel leak, do not automatically park your vehicle downhill from the scene. (p. 248)

5. **(A)** Always watch and listen for signals from other emergency service providers who are on the scene before you arrive. (p. 248)

6. **(B)** When there are no apparent hazards, the danger zone should extend at least 50 feet in all directions from the wreckage. (p. 248)

7. **(C)** When a collision vehicle is on fire, consider the danger zone to extend at least 100 feet in all directions. (p. 248)

8. **(A)** It is essential that the EMT do a good scene size-up to identify the potential for a violent situation. It may take some time to identify the name and amount of toxic substances as well as the number of patients, and their diagnoses may not be made until the patients are in the ED. (p. 250)

9. **(D)** The equipment and/or supplies used for Standard Precautions by the EMT during scene size-up includes eye protection, face mask or eyeshield, and disposable gloves. (p. 252)

10. **(B)** The key element of Standard Precautions is always to have the PPE readily available. You do not always wear protective clothing; you wear it as needed. (p. 252)

©2012 Pearson Education, Inc. *Emergency Care, 12th Ed.*

11. **(B)** Injuries to bones and joints are usually associated with falls and vehicle collisions. (p. 252)

12. **(C)** The MOI helps the EMT predict injuries and injury patterns. (p. 252)

13. **(C)** The law of inertia states that a body in motion will remain in motion unless acted upon by an outside force. (p. 254)

14. **(A)** When a patient who was not restrained takes the "up-and-over" pathway, he or she is likely to sustain head and neck injuries. (p. 254)

15. **(C)** The brake pedal is not a likely cause of injury for the patient in multiple-choice question 14. (p. 257)

16. **(C)** When a patient has knee, leg, and hip pain from a car crash, it is likely she or he was involved in a head-on, down-and-under MOI. (p. 254)

17. **(D)** For an unrestrained occupant or driver, the roll-over is a very serious collision. (p. 257)

18. **(D)** A flat rear tire is not a MOI, although it could have caused an incident. (p. 257)

19. **(A)** A severe fall for an adult is over 15 feet or three times the adult's height. (p. 258)

20. **(A)** In a penetrating injury limited to the penetrated area and without broader injury due to cavitation in the wound, the injury is usually due to a low-velocity (less than 200 feet/second) injury. (pp. 258–259)

21. **(C)** The pressure wave around the bullet's tract through the body is called cavitation. (p. 259)

22. **(C)** An injury that does not penetrate the skin is a blunt-force trauma. (p. 259)

23. **(B)** In the situation where you and your partner are treating a 350-pound male. (p. 260)

24. **(A)** If your eyes begin to tear, there is a possibility that you might be exposed to something in the air. It is best to evacuate the patients from that area of the building and call the fire department to help identify the potentially toxic substance. (p. 260)

25. **(B)** If there are more patients than you can handle, immediately call for additional EMS resources. (p. 260)

26. **(B)** When arriving at the scene of a collision, the EMT should don head protection, a bunker coat, and a reflective vest. (p. 252)

27. **(C)** If once you arrive you perceive that you are confronted by danger, retreat to a safe location and ask for the police to respond and secure the scene. (p. 252)

28. **(A)** One of the most important parts of the incident command/management system is the need for all personnel to follow the instructions of the person in change and not "freelance." (p. 248)

COMPLETE THE FOLLOWING

1. The five signals that violence may be a danger on your call include:
   A) fighting or loud voices.
   B) weapons visible or in use.
   C) signs of alcohol or other drug use.
   D) unusual silence.
   E) knowledge of prior violence.

2. The guidelines for establishing a danger zone include the following:
   A) When there are no apparent hazards, consider the danger zone to extend at least 50 feet in all directions from the wreckage.
   B) When fuel has been spilled, consider the danger zone to extend a minimum of 100 feet in all directions from the wreckage.
   C) When a collision vehicle is on fire, consider the danger zone to extend at least 100 feet in all directions, even if the fire appears small or limited to the engine compartment.
   D) When wires are down, consider the danger zone as the area in which people or vehicles might be contacted by energized wires if the wires pivot around their points of attachment.
   E) When a hazardous material is involved, check the ERG for suggestions about where to park or ask the Incident Commander to request advice from CHEMTREC.

3. Five types of motor vehicle collisions and common injury patterns for each type would be the following:
   A) Head-on collision—up-and-over, causing head and neck and chest injuries, and the down-and-under pathway, causing knee, leg and hip injuries.
   B) Rear-end collisions—commonly cause head and neck injuries.
   C) Side-impact collisions—cause lateral injuries to the neck as well as the head, chest, abdomen, pelvis, and thighs being struck directly.
   D) Roll-over collisions—are very serious and may involve ejections or partial ejections.
   E) Rotational impact collisions—cause multiple injury patterns as the vehicle spins around the point of impact.

STREET SCENES DISCUSSION

1. If the driver of the truck tells you the truck is overturned and leaking a hazardous product, you should begin to establish a danger zone, call for additional help, identify the product, refer to the ERG for appropriate perimeter distance, and stay away from the spilled product.

2. If the driver has a weapon and is intoxicated, he can be harmful to you or himself. Retreat to a safe location and notify the police immediately.

Chapter 11: The Primary Assessment

MATCH TERMINOLOGY/ DEFINITIONS

1. **(C)** ABCs—airway, breathing, and circulation (p. 266)

2. **(F)** AVPU—a memory aid for classifying a patient's levels of responsiveness, or mental status (p. 272)

3. **(D)** Chief complaint—in emergency medicine, the reason EMS was called, usually in the patient's own words (p. 271)

4. **(A)** General impression—impression of the patient's condition that is formed on first approaching the patient, based on the patient's environment, chief complaint, and appearance (p. 267)

5. **(G)** Interventions—actions taken to correct a patient's problem (p. 286)

6. **(B)** Mental status—level of responsiveness (p. 272)

7. **(E)** Primary assessment—the first element in assessment of a patient; steps taken for the purpose of discovering and dealing with any life-threatening problems (p. 266)

8. **(H)** Priority—the decision regarding the need for immediate transport of the patient versus further assessment and care at the scene. (p. 286)

MULTIPLE-CHOICE REVIEW

1. **(D)** The assessment of blood pressure is not part of the primary assessment. It is part of taking vital signs. (p. 267)

2. **(D)** The patient's past medical history is *not* part of the general impression. (p. 267)

3. **(B)** Drug-use paraphernalia may give clues about the cause of the patient's problem and would be part of the environment in which you found the patient. (pp. 267, 270)

4. **(B)** The chief complaint is the patient's own words about why the ambulance was called. (pp. 271–272)

5. **(D)** When forming a general impression, always look, listen, and smell. Note the patient's age and sex and look at the patient's position. Listen for sounds such as moaning or gurgling. Smell for hazardous fumes, urine, feces, vomitus, or decay. (p. 267)

6. **(B)** Rubbing the patient's sternum briskly is the most common way to determine the patient's level of responsiveness. Ammonia inhalants can cause injury. Placing the patient's hands in water doesn't work. Pressing on the person's nail beds is a way of assessing capillary refill. (pp. 272, 274)

7. **(D)** AVPU stands for "alert, verbal, painful stimuli, unresponsive." (p. 272)

8. **(C)** See the answer for multiple-choice question 7. (p. 272)

9. **(B)** See the answer for multiple-choice question 7. (p. 272)

10. **(B)** The unresponsive patient will be a higher priority and in need of quicker transport. The jaw-thrust maneuver is usually not used on responsive patients unless they have head, neck, or spinal injuries. (p. 278)

11. **(D)** If a patient is not alert and her breathing rate is slower than 8, provide positive pressure ventilations with 100 percent oxygen. (pp. 270–271)

12. **(B)** An alert patient with a breathing rate faster than 24 warrants high-concentration oxygen via nonrebreather. (pp. 270–271)

13. **(D)** The circulation assessment includes evaluating pulse, skin (condition, color, and temperature), and bleeding. The blood pressure is a vital sign taken moments after the primary assessment. (p. 278)

14. **(D)** Good circulation exhibits in the skin as warm, dry, and normal in color provided the assessment is not complicated by the environment in which you find the patient (e.g., rain or cold). (p. 278)

15. **(C)** Poor circulation exhibits as cool, pale, and moist skin. Increased perfusion and high blood pressure may show as flush-colored skin. Cold exposure exhibits as red in the early stages, and then pale to cyanotic in prolonged cases. (p. 278)

16. **(A)** To evaluate skin color or the presence of jaundice or cyanosis on a dark-skinned patient, look at the lips or nail beds. (p. 278)

17. **(C)** If even one large vessel or several smaller ones are bleeding, a patient can lose enough blood in a minute or two to die. Severe blood loss is life threatening. (p. 278)

18. **(B)** Any life threats observed during the primary assessment should be treated immediately. (pp. 266–267)

19. **(D)** High-priority conditions include poor general impression, unresponsive, responsive but not following commands, difficulty breathing, shock, complicated childbirth, chest pain with systolic blood pressure less than 100, uncontrolled bleeding, severe pain anywhere. (pp. 278–279)

20. **(C)** Uncomplicated childbirth is not a priority. See the answer for multiple-choice question 19. (pp. 278–279)

21. **(C)** You should consider administering oxygen by nonrebreather mask. The nasal cannula is too little, bag-valve mask ventilations are not needed, and the paper bag trick is dangerous and can lead to hypoxia. (p. 280)

22. **(A)** In the adult trauma patient, capillary refill is no longer used as an indicator of poor perfusion because it is a poor and unreliable indicator. It is still useful in the child. (p. 283)

23. **(C)** The steps of the primary assessment are designed to be followed in order. (p. 267)

24. **(B)** If you suspect that the patient is lifeless, the approach changes to a C-A-B approach in which you assess the circulation first because the absence of circulation means chest compressions need to be started right away. (pp. 265–267)

COMPLETE THE FOLLOWING

1. The six steps of the primary assessment are listed below. (p. 267)
   - Form a general impression
   - Assess mental status
   - Assess airway
   - Assess breathing
   - Assess circulation
   - Determine priority

2. State what the letters in AVPU stand for. (p. 272)
   A = "alert"—awake and oriented (person, place, and day)
   V = "verbal"—responds to verbal stimuli
   P = "painful"—responds to painful stimuli
   U = "unresponsive"—does not respond to any stimuli

3. List five high-priority conditions. (any five) (p. 279)
   - Poor general impression
   - Unresponsive
   - Responsive but not following commands
   - Difficulty breathing
   - Shock
   - Complicated childbirth
   - Chest pain with systolic pressure less than 100
   - Uncontrolled bleeding
   - Severe pain anywhere

STREET SCENES DISCUSSION

1. The airway is always the highest priority. Suction the patient's airway while maintaining spinal stabilization. Once the airway is clear, administer high-concentration oxygen.

2. This patient is a high priority. ALS would be helpful for intubation and another set of trained hands.

3. Even though the patient seems to be okay, it is always a good idea for the patient to be checked in the hospital due to the potential for aspiration or damage to the structures of the airway.

©2012 Pearson Education, Inc.
Emergency Care, 12th Ed.

CASE STUDY: CAR-BIKE COLLISION ON MAIN STREET USA

1. Attend to the scene size-up and other safety issues.

2. Primary assessment or primary survey

3. The mechanism of injury or MOI

4. You were not there to see what happened, so the bystander's information is very helpful in determining the MOI.

5. Determine the mental status using AVPU.

6. Alert because Tony knows his name, where he is, and the day of the week (oriented to person, place. and day).

7. The primary assessment is always done in order so essential steps are not missed. If a life threat is identified, the EMT manages it and moves on to the next step.

8. The C step (or "circulation") includes assessment of the pulse (present and/or within normal range), the external bleeding, and the skin CTC (color, temperature, and condition).

9. To be safe it would be best to make Tony a priority patient because he may have some internal bleeding in addition to the fractured clavicle due to the fact that he was moving along when he crashed. Moving while injured is considered a significant mechanism of injury.

Chapter 12: Vital Signs and Monitoring Devices

MATCH TERMINOLOGY/ DEFINITIONS

PART A

1. **(L)** Auscultation—when a stethoscope is used to listen for characteristic sounds (p. 302)

2. **(C)** Blood pressure—force of blood against the walls of the blood vessels (p. 299)

3. **(J)** Brachial artery—major artery of the arm (p. 294)

4. **(B)** Bradycardia—a slow pulse; any pulse rate below 60 beats per minute (p. 293)

5. **(D)** Carotid pulse—the pulse felt along the large artery on either side of the neck (p. 294)

6. **(N)** Constrict—get smaller (p. 298)

7. **(M)** Dilate—get larger (p. 298)

8. **(A)** Diastolic blood pressure—the pressure remaining in the arteries when the left ventricle of the heart is relaxed and refilling (p. 299)

9. **(E)** Palpation—touching or feeling; a pulse or blood pressure may be palpated with the fingertips (p. 302)

10. **(H)** Pulse—the rhythmic beats felt as the heart pumps blood through the arteries (p. 291)

11. **(I)** Pulse quality—the rhythm (regular or irregular) and force (strong or weak) of the pulse (p. 294)

12. **(F)** Pulse rate—the number of pulse beats per minute (p. 293)

13. **(K)** Pupil—the black center of the eye (p. 298)

14. **(O)** Radial pulse—the pulse felt at the wrist (p. 294)

15. **(G)** Reactivity—in the pupils of the eyes, reacting to light by changing size (p. 298)

PART B

1. **(B)** Respiratory quality—normal or abnormal (shallow, labored, noisy) character of breathing (p. 295)

2. **(A)** Respiratory rate—number of breaths taken in 1 minute (p. 295)

3. **(E)** Respiratory rhythm—the regular or irregular spacing of breaths (p. 296)

4. **(F)** Oxygen saturation—the ratio of the amount of oxygen present in the blood to the amount that could be carried, expressed as a percentage (p. 307)

5. **(G)** Sign—an indication of a patient's condition that is objective, or can be observed by another person; an indication that can be seen, heard, smelled, or felt by the EMT or others (p. 290)

6. **(I)** Sphygmomanometer—the cuff and gauge used to measure blood pressure (p. 301)

7. **(H)** Symptom—an indication of a patient's condition that cannot be observed but rather is subjective or is something felt and reported by the patient (p. 322)

8. **(D)** Systolic pressure—the pressure created when the heart contracts and forces blood out into the arteries (p. 299)

9. **(C)** Tachycardia—a rapid pulse; any pulse rate above 100 beats per minute (p. 293)

10. **(M)** Blood pressure monitor—machine that automatically inflates a blood pressure cuff and measures blood pressure (p. 302)

11. **(L)** Pulse oximeter—an electronic device for determining the amount of oxygen carried in the blood, known as the oxygen saturation or SpO_2 (p. 307)

12. **(J)** Vital signs—outward signs of what is going on inside the body, including respirations; pulse; skin color, temperature, and condition (plus capillary refill in infants and children); pupils; and blood pressure (p. 291)

13. **(K)** Brachial pulse—the pulse felt in the upper arm (p. 294)

MULTIPLE-CHOICE REVIEW

1. **(D)** Pulse oximetry is not officially considered a vital sign. The respiratory rate and quality, skin color and condition, and the pulse rate and quality are all vital signs. (p. 291)

2. **(B)** A sign that gives important information about the patient's condition but is *not* considered a vital sign is the mental status. All other signs listed are vital signs. (p. 291)

3. **(B)** Vital signs should be recorded as they are obtained to prevent you from forgetting them and to note the time they were taken. The vitals can change quickly as the patient's condition changes. They are taken at least twice to develop trends in vital signs. The first measurements you take are called baseline vital signs. (p. 312)

4. **(D)** A pulse rate that exceeds 100 beats per minute is called tachycardia. See Table 12-1 for normal pulse rates and possible causes of change in pulse quality. (p. 293)

5. **(D)** Based upon the pulse alone, a sign that something may be seriously wrong with a patient could be a sustained rate below 48 beats per minute, a sustained rate above 126 beats per minute, and/or a rate above 150 beats per minute. (p. 293)

6. **(B)** In addition to the answer for multiple-choice question 5, another serious indicator found in the pulse may be an irregular rhythm. An athlete with a pulse of 50 is not

unusual because aerobic training will lower the at-rest pulse. Exercise normally increases the pulse rate. (p. 294)

7. **(C)** The quality of the pulse includes determining the rhythm and force. (p. 294)

8. **(C)** A patient described as having a thready pulse has a weak pulse. See Table 12-1. (p. 294)

9. **(C)** The normal pulse rate for a school-age child (6–10 years) is 70 to 110. See Table 12-1. (p. 293)

10. **(A)** The normal pulse rate for an adult is 60 to 100. See Table 12-1. (p. 293)

11. **(B)** The pulse at the thumb side of the wrist is referred to as the radial pulse. The femoral pulse is in the thigh. The carotid pulse is in the neck. The brachial pulse is in the arm. (p. 294)

12. **(C)** When assessing the carotid pulse, the EMT should be aware that excessive pressure can slow the heart, especially in older patients. Never assess the carotid pulses on both sides at the same time. (p. 294)

13. **(C)** The number of breaths a patient takes in one minute is called the respiratory rate. (p. 295)

14. **(A)** The respiratory rate is classified as normal, slow, or rapid. The respiratory *quality* is classified as normal, shallow, labored, or noisy. The pulse force is classified as weak, thready, or full. (p. 295)

15. **(C)** If the EMT is treating a patient with a sustained respiratory rate above 24 or below 8 breaths per minute, high-concentration oxygen must be administered. Also be prepared to assist ventilations. (p. 295)

16. **(B)** The normal respiration rate for an adult at rest is 12 to 20. See Table 12-2. (p. 295)

17. **(C)** The normal respiration rate for a toddler (1–3 years of age) is 20 to 30. See Table 12-2. (p. 296)

18. **(A)** Shallow breathing occurs when there is only slight movement of the chest or abdomen. Stridor or grunting on expiration indicates an airway obstruction. The chest muscles normally expand fully with each breath. (p. 295)

19. **(B)** Many resting people breathe more with their diaphragm than with their chest muscles. (p. 295)

20. **(D)** Delayed capillary refill is *not* a sign of labored breathing. When a patient has labored breathing, he or she may have an increase in the work of breathing, use of accessory muscles, nasal flaring, and retractions above the collarbones. (p. 295)

21. **(C)** A harsh, high-pitched sound heard on breathing when a patient has labored breathing is called crowing. Nasal flaring, grunting, and gurgling are signs of upper airway problems. (p. 295)

22. **(C)** When the quality of a patient's respirations is abnormal due to something blocking the flow of air, this is referred to as noisy breathing. Sounds to be concerned with are snoring, wheezing, gurgling, and crowing. (p. 295)

23. **(A)** A sound made by the patient that usually indicates the need to suction the airway is called gurgling. Crowing and stridor are upper airway noises. Wheezing is usually an indication of a lower airway problem. (p. 295)

24. **(B)** The best places to assess skin color in adults are the inside of the cheek and the nail beds as well as the inside of the lower eyelids. (pp. 297–298)

25. **(C)** Blood loss, shock, hypotension, or emotional distress may result in pale skin. Jaundiced skin is due to liver abnormalities. See Table 12-3. (p. 297)

26. **(D)** A patient with a lack of oxygen in the red blood cells resulting from inadequate breathing or heart function will exhibit cyanotic skin. Pink skin is normal, pale skin is due to shock, and flushed skin is a result of hypertension. See Table 12-3. (p. 297)

27. **(D)** The skin of a patient who has liver abnormalities may appear jaundiced, or yellowish. See Table 12-3. (p. 297)

28. **(B)** Cold, dry skin is frequently associated with exposure to cold. Shock and anxiety would result in skin that is cool and clammy. See Table 12-4. (p. 297)

29. **(A)** Hot, dry skin is frequently associated with high fever or heat exposure. See Table 12-4. (p. 297)

30. **(B)** A diabetic patient uses a blood sugar monitoring device called a glucose meter or glucometer. (p. 309)

31. **(C)** Diabetic patients check their blood sugar with a glucose meter, and the device reports milligrams of glucose per deciliter of blood. (p. 309)

32. **(B)** If a patient is in direct sunlight or very bright conditions, the EMT should test the pupils by covering the patient's eyes for a few moments, then uncovering one eye at a time. (p. 298)

33. **(D)** A patient in shock does not normally have unequal pupils. The pupils may be unequal due to stroke, head injury, or eye injury. See Table 12-5. (p. 300)

34. **(B)** Fright, blood loss, drugs, and treatment with eye drops may cause the patient's pupils to become dilated. Constricted pupils are often due to narcotics. Unequal pupils are addressed in the answer for multiple-choice question 33. (p. 300)

35. **(A)** When the left ventricle of the heart relaxes and refills, the pressure in the arteries is called the diastolic pressure. (p. 299)

36. **(B)** The pulse oximeter should be used with patients complaining of respiratory problems. It is inaccurate with hypothermic or shock patients, and it may produce falsely high readings in patients with carbon monoxide poisoning. (p. 307)

37. **(A)** The pulse oximeter is helpful because it encourages you to be more aggressive about providing oxygen therapy. (p. 307)

38. **(C)** The oximeter produces falsely high readings in patients with carbon monoxide poisoning. (p. 307)

39. **(B)** Chronic smokers may have a pulse oximeter reading that is higher than it actually is. (p. 307)

40. **(C)** The normal pulse oximeter reading for a healthy person should be between 95 percent and 100 percent. (p. 307)

41. **(C)** Feel the patient's skin with the back of the hand to determine the patient's skin temperature. (p. 305)

42. **(B)** The normal blood glucose reading should be 60 to 80 mg/dl. (pp. 309–312)

43. **(A)** The systolic blood pressure is created when the heart contracts. (p. 299)

44. **(C)** When the environment is noisy, as it would be in crowed bar, a BP can be taken by palpation without a stethoscope. This reveals only the systolic reading. (p. 302)

45. **(C)** The limit below which hypotension is considered serious in an adult patient is 90 mmHg. (pp. 299–300)

46. **(D)** The assessment of a patient with an altered mental status can easily involve all the devices listed. (p. 291)

©2012 Pearson Education, Inc.
Emergency Care, 12th Ed.

COMPLETE THE FOLLOWING

1. The five vital signs are: (p. 291)
   - pulse
   - respiration
   - skin (temperature, color, and condition)
   - pupils
   - blood pressure

2. The potential causes of each condition are listed below: (p. 301)

   A) High blood pressure—medical condition, exertion, fright, emotional distress, or excitement

   B) Low blood pressure—athlete or other person with normally low blood pressure; blood loss; late sign of shock

   C) Cool, clammy skin—sign of shock, anxiety

   D) Cold, moist skin—body is losing heat

   E) Cold, dry skin—exposure to cold

   F) Hot, dry skin—high fever; heat exposure

   G) Hot, moist skin—high fever; heat exposure

LABEL THE DIAGRAM (P. 294)

1. Carotid
2. Brachial
3. Radial
4. Femoral
5. Pedal

STREET SCENES DISCUSSION

1. No. The patient had a chief complaint of abdominal pain, which cannot be diagnosed and treated in the field, especially in an elderly patient.

2. Normal ranges for an adult are respirations between 12 and 20, pulse between 60 and 100, systolic blood pressure between 90 and 150, and diastolic blood pressure between 60 and 90. Pulse ox readings between 95 and 100 are considered normal.

3. Yes, as you would any information pertinent to the patient's current condition. (Black, tarry stools often indicate bleeding into the intestines or lower gastrointestinal tract.)

CASE STUDY: CALL FOR A "MAN DOWN"

1. In the primary assessment, the EMT determines the mental status and checks the airway, breathing, and circulation, then prioritizes the patient.

2. Gurgling means there is fluid in the upper airway, so you should have your sucking unit and rigid tip Yankauer ready to go.

3. He can talk to you and answer questions but he is *not* oriented to person, place, and day, so he is V, for "verbal."

4. Normal vitals for a young adult would be a respiration of 12 to 20 and regular, a pulse rate of 60 to 100 and regular, and a BP of 120/80.

5. If the patient is a diabetic with an altered mental status, check the blood sugar level with the glucometer.

6. Yes, in most EMS systems.

7. Every 5 minutes because an altered mental status is unstable. If he becomes alert, every 15 minutes would be fine.

©2012 Pearson Education, Inc.
Emergency Care, 12th Ed.

MATCH TERMINOLOGY/ DEFINITIONS

1. **(E)** Colostomy—a surgical opening in the wall of the abdomen with a bag in place to collect excretions from the digestive system (p. 336)

2. **(A)** Crepitation—the grating sensation or sound or feeling of broken bones rubbing together (p. 332)

3. **(F)** DCAP-BTLS—a memory aid to remember deformities, contusions, abrasions, punctures/penetrations, burns, tenderness, lacerations, and swelling, which are symptoms of injury found by inspection or palpation during patient assessment (p. 320)

4. **(L)** Detailed physical exam—an assessment of the head, neck, chest, abdomen, pelvis, extremities, and posterior of the body to detect signs and symptoms of injury (p. 342)

5. **(K)** Distention—a condition of being stretched, inflated, or larger than normal (p. 336)

6. **(I)** Focused history and physical exam—the step of patient assessment that follows the primary assessment (p. 320)

7. **(J)** Ileostomy—see colostomy (p. 336)

8. **(H)** Jugular vein distention—bulging of the neck veins (p. 334)

9. **(B)** Paradoxical motion—movement of part of the chest in the opposite direction to the rest of the chest during respiration (p. 335)

10. **(C)** Priapism—persistent erection of the penis that can result from spinal cord injury and some medical problems (p. 337)

11. **(D)** Rapid trauma assessment—quick assessment of the head, neck, chest, abdomen, pelvis, extremities, and posterior body to detect signs and symptoms of injury (p. 332)

12. **(M)** Stoma—a permanent surgical opening in the neck through which the patient breathes (p. 335)

13. **(G)** Tracheostomy—a surgical incision in the neck held open by a metal or plastic tube (p. 335)

14. **(N)** Trauma patient—a patient suffering from one or more physical injuries (p. 316)

MULTIPLE-CHOICE REVIEW

1. **(C)** The EMT inspects and palpates each body part during the focused physical exam. He does not auscultate, or listen to, every body part, nor does he percuss, or tap, to elicit a tone from each body part. (p. 342)

2. **(B)** The reason the ambulance was called is the chief complaint. (p. 344)

3. **(D)** The history of the present illness or injury for a trauma patient includes the direction and strength of the force, actions taken to prevent or minimize injury, and equipment used to protect the patient. (p. 317)

4. **(C)** The physical exam includes inspection, auscultation, and palpation. (p. 342)

5. **(A)** Punctures/penetrations. (p. 321)

6. **(C)** Swelling. (p. 321)

7. **(B)** A deformity is an abnormally shaped body part. A hematoma is a collection of blood under the skin. A fracture is a broken bone. Crepitation is the sound or feel of broken bones rubbing against each other. (p. 329)

8. **(B)** Burns involve reddened, blistered, or charred-looking areas. An abrasion is a scrape, a laceration is a cut, and a contusion is a bruise. (p. 320)

9. **(C)** Tenderness is usually not evident until you palpate the patient. Pain is usually present even without applying pressure, or palpation, at least until another stronger pain source overrides it. (p. 320)

10. **(A)** Capillaries bleeding under the skin is called swelling. Punctures, lacerations, and abrasions are types of soft-tissue injuries. (p. 320)

11. **(A)** If the mechanism of injury exerts great force on the upper body, a cervical collar would be appropriate. In addition, apply a cervical collar if there is any soft-tissue damage to the head, face, or neck from trauma; if there has been a blow above the clavicles (collarbones); if the trauma patient has an altered mental status; or if injury cannot be ruled out—even if the MOI is not known. (p. 322)

12. **(A)** Any blow above the clavicles may damage the cervical spine. (p. 322)

13. **(B)** Experienced EMTs refer to soft collars as "neck warmers" because that is about all they are good for. Soft collars are inappropriate for field use because of their inability to provide rigid support. (p. 322)

14. **(B)** A cervical collar that is the wrong size may make breathing more difficult or obstruct the airway. The collar does not cause the spine injury, although mishandling it may do so. (p. 322)

15. **(D)** Cervical immobilization is based on the trauma patient's level of responsiveness, MOI, and location of injuries. (p. 322)

16. **(C)** A sign is an objective finding you can see, hear, or feel when examining the patient. (p. 320)

17. **(C)** A roll-over collision, a motorcycle collision, a pedestrian struck by a vehicle, and an adult who fell more than *three times* his or her height (which often involves a spine injury) are significant MOIs. (p. 326)

18. **(B)** When a patient is unrestrained in the front seat of an auto involved in a collision, the tell-tale sign is a spider-web crack in the windshield. This is also a sign that the patient went "up and over" to sustain the injury, rather than "down and under," which would present with leg injuries. (p. 326)

19. **(C)** Airbags minimize lacerations caused by the head striking the windshield. However, airbags can hide signs that could help you predict the severity of injuries caused by the collision. Be sure to move the collapsed bag and examine the steering wheel, which may give clues to the extent of the impact on the patient's chest. (p. 330)

20. **(C)** When assessing the head of an adult, look for wounds and deformities and listen for crepitation, the sound or feel of broken bones rubbing against each other. (p. 332)

21. **(A)** When assessing the adult female's neck, look for wounds and deformities and observe for jugular vein distention (JVD). (p. 334)

22. **(B)** Neck veins should be flat and not visible when a patient is sitting up. Flat neck veins in a patient who is lying down, however, may be a sign of blood loss. (p. 334)

23. **(B)** When assessing the chest of an adult patient, in addition to looking for crepitation and wounds, inspect/palpate for paradoxical motion, movement of part of the chest in the opposite direction from the rest of the chest. This is a sign of serious injury because it indicates a great deal of force was applied to the patient's chest. (p. 328)

24. **(B)** When assessing the adult's abdomen, in addition to looking for wounds and deformities, check to see if the patient has a colostomy and/or ileostomy, a surgical opening in the wall of the abdomen with a bag in place to collect excretions from the digestive system. (p. 328)

25. **(C)** When assessing the adult male patient's pelvis, in addition to checking for wounds, deformities, and tenderness, check for priapism (persistent erection of the penis), a sign of a potential spinal cord injury. (p. 329)

26. **(D)** When examining a patient, remember to tell the patient what you are going to do, assume spinal injury, and try to maintain eye contact. (p. 320)

27. **(B)** Critical trauma patients do not always have a detailed physical exam, especially on the scene. Performing a detailed physical exam is always a lower priority than addressing life-threatening problems. (p. 332)

28. **(B)** The detailed physical exam is usually done en route to the ED, as compared to the rapid trauma assessment. (p. 342)

29. **(B)** The final step of the detailed physical exam is to make sure you have notified the ED. (p. 342)

30. **(C)** A bruise behind the ear is called Battle's sign, which is indicative of a basilar skull fracture. (p. 334)

31. **(C)** Blood in the anterior chamber (front) of the eye tells you the eye is bleeding inside and that the patient's eye has sustained significant force. (p. 333)

32. **(B)** Clear fluid draining from the ears and nose is called cerebrospinal fluid. Mucous fluid lines the respiratory tract. Lymph bathes the cells and circulates throughout the body. Synovial fluid is in the joints. (p. 333)

33. **(D)** You do *not* look for crepitation. The other choices are specific to the mouth. (p. 332)

34. **(C)** The detailed physical exam is not designed for a medical patient because there are usually few signs that an EMT can find in the physical exam of a medical patient that are significant or about which the EMT can or should do anything. (p. 342)

35. **(D)** The safest and best thing to do for a patient who could be either medical or trauma is to assess for primary survey problems first. (p. 318)

COMPLETE THE FOLLOWING

1. The components of the focused history and physical exam for a trauma patient are as follows: (p. 327)
   - First take Standard Precautions.
   - Reconsider the mechanism of injury.
   - Continue manual stabilization of the head and neck.
   - Consider requesting for ALS personnel.
   - Reconsider transport decision.
   - Reassess mental status.
   - Perform a rapid trauma assessment.

©2012 Pearson Education, Inc.
Emergency Care, 12th Ed.

2. The areas assessed and what you are looking for in the rapid trauma assessment include: (p. 332)

A) Head—wounds, deformities, tenderness, plus crepitation.

B) Neck—wounds, deformities, tenderness, plus JVD and crepitation (then apply cervical collar).

C) Chest—wounds, deformities, tenderness, plus crepitation, paradoxical motion, and breath sounds (absent, present, equal).

D) Abdomen—wounds; deformities; tenderness; plus firm, soft, and distended.

E) Pelvis—wounds, deformities, tenderness, with gentle compression for tenderness or motion.

F) Extremities—wounds; deformities; tenderness; plus distal circulation, and sensory and motor function.

G) Posterior—wounds, deformities, tenderness. (To examine posterior, roll patient using spinal precautions.)

3. Examples of significant injuries or signs of significant injuries include: (p. 326)

▶ **SIGNIFICANT MECHANISMS OF INJURY**

A) Unresponsive or altered mental status

B) Airway that is not patent.

C) Respiratory compromise.

D) Pallor, tachycardia, and other signs of shock.

E) Penetrating wound of the head, neck, chest, or abdomen (e.g., stab and gunshot wound).

LABEL THE PHOTOGRAPHS

1. Head

2. Face

3. Ears

4. Eyes

5. Nose

6. Mouth

7. Neck

8. Chest

9. Abdomen

10. Pelvis

11. Upper extremities

12. Lower extremities

COMPLETE THE CHART

1. Crepitation

2. JVD

3. Crepitation

4. Paradoxical motion

5. Crepitation

6. Breath sounds

7. Firmness

8. Softness

9. Distention

10. Pain

11. Tenderness

12. Distal pulse

13. Distal motor function

14. Distal sensation

STREET SCENES DISCUSSION

1. If assessment reveals respirations less than 12, greater than 28, or very shallow, you should immediately use the BVM to assist ventilation.

2. Yes, call for ALS. A patient with an open chest wound needs advanced care. If possible, arrange for ALS to intercept you en route to the hospital.

3. Emergency care priorities would be to maintain the airway and adequate ventilation of the patient.

4. If the patient is injured on the left side of the chest, at the mid-clavicular line and at nipple level, a lung and the heart may be injured.

CASE STUDY: MOTORCYCLE MISHAP

1. Standard Precautions—protect yourself from the blood and other body fluids found on the patient.

2. Scene safety—most notably the traffic.

3. Mechanism of injury—a two-vehicle collision.

4. The number of patients.

5. Forming a general impression helps you to determine how serious the patient's condition is, which helps you set priorities for care and transport. The general impression is based on an immediate assessment of the environment and the patient's chief complaint and appearance. It gives you an idea of the sex and age of the patient, what happened and why EMS was called, whether the patient is injured or ill, and the severity of the patient's condition.

6. One of your partners should be holding manual stabilization of the patient's head and neck.

7. The patient appears to be "alert," or A on the AVPU scale.

8. His broken legs may not be the worst problem, and you must assess him for life-threatening injuries first.

9. The primary assessment for Tony should consist of forming a general impression, assessing mental status (both of which you have already done), assessing his ABC (airway, breathing, and circulation), and determining priority.

10. Signs of developing shock make Tony a high-priority patient.

11. Call for ALS right away. If they are not there by the time Tony is packaged, then try to arrange a quick meeting en route to the hospital. But do not delay transport waiting for an ALS unit to arrive.

12. Wounds, deformities, and tenderness.

13. *S*igns and symptoms, *A*llergies, *M*edications, *P*ertinent past medical history, *L*ast oral intake, *E*vents leading up to incident.

14. Assess respirations, pulse, blood pressure, skin (color, condition, temperature), and pupils.

15. A detailed physical exam of Tony would include an assessment of everything examined in the rapid trauma assessment, plus the face, ears, eyes, nose, and mouth.

Chapter 14: Assessment of the Medical Patient

MATCH TERMINOLOGY/ DEFINITIONS

1. **(I)** Chief complaint—the reason why EMS was called, usually in patient's own words (p. 356)

2. **(G)** Medical patient—a patient with one or more medical diseases or conditions (p. 351)

3. **(H)** Onset of pain—description of how fast or slow the pain came on and what the patient was doing when the pain started (p. 356)

4. **(E)** OPQRST—a memory device for the questions asked to get a description of the present illness (p. 356)

5. **(F)** Pertinent past history—history relating to the patient's chief complaint (p. 356)

6. **(C)** Provocation of pain—description of what makes the pain worse, such as sitting, standing, or eating certain foods (p. 356)

7. **(B)** Quality of pain—description of the pain, such as stabbing, crampy, dull, or sharp (p. 356)

8. **(A)** Radiation of pain—description of where pain is located and where it spreads to (p. 356)

9. **(D)** Severity of pain—description of how bad the pain is, often described on a scale of 1 to 10 (p. 356)

MULTIPLE-CHOICE REVIEW

1. **(D)** The rapid trauma exam is not used on a responsive medical patient. (p. 354)

2. **(B)** OPQRST is a memory aid to help the EMT remember questions that expand on the history of the present illness. The letters in the memory aid stand for "onset, provokes, quality, radiation, severity, and time." (p. 356)

3. **(B)** Something that triggers the pain is what provokes it. Onset is when the pain started. Quality is a description of the type of pain. Radiation is where the pain is located and where it spreads. (p. 356)

4. **(B)** "How bad is the pain?" is a severity question usually evaluated on a scale of 1 to 10. (p. 356)

5. **(C)** T stands for "time" (the time the pain started). The temperature is not relevant to this patient, and the tibia is the bone in the front of the lower leg. (p. 356)

6. **(A)** Vomiting is a sign of various medical illnesses. (p. 360)

7. **(B)** The additional information being provided is called the pertinent past history. (p. 357)

8. **(C)** "How have you felt today?" is a question about the events leading up to the illness. (p. 357)

9. **(B)** Patients with specific chief complaints and a known history may mean the EMT has to ask additional questions pertinent to the complaint. (p. 357)

10. **(C)** When a medical patient complains of difficulty breathing but does not have a prescribed medication for this condition, you should generally transport the patient to the hospital. (p. 360)

11. **(B)** The main difference in approach to the focused history and physical exam for the responsive versus the unresponsive patient is that the unresponsive patient will be given a rapid physical exam first. The responsive patient would get the OPQRST questions first. Bystanders and family are more important if the patient is unresponsive because they must supply information about the patient when he or she is unable to do so. (p. 362)

12. **(D)** An unresponsive patient would be unable to answer the SAMPLE history questions. (p. 363)

13. **(B)** Check the medical patient's extremities for sensation and motor function as well as pulse. The capillary refill is used only in the assessment of a child or infant. (p. 362)

14. **(C)** The "Vial of Life" sticker could mean that there are additional clues to the patient's medical history in the refrigerator. (p. 365)

15. **(D)** Most regions include the oxygen saturation in the vital signs of an adult patient. (p. 364)

16. **(B)** The highest priority in terms of patient assessment is the primary assessment because it identifies the life threats. (p. 351)

COMPLETE THE FOLLOWING

1. The components of a focused history and physical exam for an unresponsive medical patient include: (p. 363)
   - Rapid physical exam
   - Baseline vital signs
   - Past medical history
   - Interventions and transport

2. Assess the following seven areas during your rapid physical exam of the medical patient: (p. 362)
   - Head
   - Neck
   - Chest
   - Abdomen
   - Pelvis
   - Extremities
   - Posterior

COMPLETE THE CHART (P. 357)

1. Signs and symptoms
2. Allergies
3. Medications
4. Pertinent past history
5. Last meal
6. Events leading up to illness
7. Onset
8. Provokes
9. Quality
10. Radiation
11. Severity
12. Time

STREET SCENES DISCUSSION

1. A patient with breathing difficulty who speaks in short, choppy sentences may be breathing inadequately.

2. No. If there are no chest sounds during an asthma attack, the patient may not be moving enough air.

3. The term for lung sounds described as "noisy, like a whistling sound" is *wheezing*. A wheeze is a musical tone caused by air being forced through constricted air passageways. This is due to bronchoconstriction and the build-up of mucus.

4. Yes. If the patient has a prescribed inhaler, you may be able to assist the patient in taking the medication. This may be done only after consultation with medical direction, often during transportation to the hospital.

5. An SpO_2 of 96 percent means that the hemoglobin is saturated at 96 percent with oxygen. This is an acceptable reading.

Chapter 15: Reassessment

MATCH TERMINOLOGY/ DEFINITIONS

1. **(B)** Reassessment—a procedure for detecting changes in patient's condition; it involves four steps: repeating the primary assessment, repeating and recording vital signs, repeating the focused assessment, and checking interventions (p. 372)

2. **(A)** Trending—changes in a patient's condition over time, such as slowing respirations or rising pulse rate, that may show improvement or deterioration, and that can be shown by documenting repeated assessments (p. 375)

©2012 Pearson Education, Inc.
Emergency Care, 12th Ed.

MULTIPLE-CHOICE REVIEW

1. **(D)** It is important to observe and re-observe the patient. Therefore, in the reassessment, you need to repeat key elements of assessment procedures already performed in order to detect any changes in patient condition. (p. 375)

2. **(C)** The reassessment must never be omitted or skipped unless life-saving interventions prevent the EMT from doing it. Frequently, one partner can perform the reassessment while the other performs the interventions. (p. 375)

3. **(D)** Use a quiet, reassuring voice when talking to the child. Also maintain eye contact. Try to stay on the same level as the child or close to or at eye level. Raising your voice or towering over the patient will just scare a child. (p. 372)

4. **(D)** The reassessment does not involve repeating all interventions because some interventions may be adequate or are ongoing. However, it does involve evaluating the adequacy of your interventions more objectively and adjusting them as necessary. The ongoing assessment does include repeating the primary assessment for life threats, the focused assessment, and the vital signs. (p. 372)

5. **(B)** The sequence for performing the reassessment is: repeat the primary assessment, reassess vital signs, repeat the focused assessment, and check interventions. (p. 373)

6. **(D)** Applying a cervical collar is part of the rapid trauma assessment, not the primary assessment. When repeating the primary assessment, make sure that you reestablish patient priorities, monitor skin color and temperature, and maintain an open airway. (p. 372)

7. **(D)** The onset of shock is signaled by a rapid pulse and cool, clammy, and pale skin. This is a life threat and should be watched for continually and treated immediately. (p. 375)

8. **(C)** The mental status of an unresponsive child or infant can be checked by shouting (verbal stimulus) or by flicking the feet (painful stimulus). The parent can also be helpful by explaining how the child normally behaves. A sternal rub or pin to the foot is too aggressive and may injure the child. (p. 373)

9. **(B)** An example of checking interventions during the reassessment of a medical patient is ensuring adequacy of oxygen delivery. Taking a blood pressure is obtaining a vital sign and is not an intervention. Bandaging and applying a tourniquet are treatments. (p. 374)

10. **(C)** Frequent reassessment establishes trends, or changes over time, that the EMT needs to pay attention to. You may need to institute new treatments or adjust treatments you have already started based on these trends. (p. 375)

11. **(C)** The best way to determine if the patient is improving or deteriorating is to do frequent reassessments. (p. 375)

12. **(B)** Stable and 15 minutes. If the patient is stable, reassessment of vitals should be every 15 minutes. If the patient is not stable, the reassessment should be every 5 minutes. (p. 376)

13. **(A)** 5 minutes and unstable. See the answer for multiple-choice question 12. (p. 376)

14. **(C)** You should repeat the primary assessment whenever you believe there may have been a change in the patient's condition. This will help you determine if the patient needs to be reprioritized. (p. 372)

15. **(B)** Gurgling sounds in a patient's airway indicate the patient needs to be suctioned immediately. (p. 373)

16. **(B)** The patient with multiple fractures and splints applied must have these interventions reassessed en route to make sure the splints are not too tight. (p. 374)

COMPLETE THE FOLLOWING

1. The six steps involved in repeating the primary assessment are: (p. 372)
   - Reassess mental status.
   - Maintain an open airway.
   - Monitor breathing for rate and quality.
   - Reassess the pulse for rate and quality.
   - Monitor skin color and temperature.
   - Reestablish patient priorities.

2. The three steps for checking interventions are: (p. 374)
   - Ensure adequacy of oxygen delivery and artificial ventilation.
   - Ensure management of bleeding.
   - Ensure adequacy of other interventions.

STREET SCENES DISCUSSION

1. In a stroke patient, if there is any paralysis, the patient may not be able to clear and maintain her own airway.

2. The sense of hearing is one of the last senses to go. So be very careful what you say because the patient often can hear and understand you.

Chapter 16: Critical Thinking and Decision Making

MATCH TERMINOLOGY/ DEFINITIONS

1. **(E)** Critical thinking—an analytical process that can help someone think through a problem in an organized and efficient manner (p. 383)

2. **(D)** Diagnosis—a description or label for a patient's condition that assists a clinician in further evaluation and treatment. (p. 383)

3. **(B)** Differential diagnosis—a list of potential diagnoses compiled early in the assessment of the patient. (p. 383)

4. **(A)** EMS diagnosis/EMT diagnosis—a description or label for a patient's condition, based on the patient's history, physical exam, and vital signs, that assists the EMT in further evaluation and treatment. An EMS diagnosis is often less than a traditional medical diagnosis. (p. 383)

5. **(C)** Red flag—a sign or symptom that suggests the possibility of a particular problem that is very serious. (p. 384)

MULTIPLE-CHOICE REVIEW

1. **(D)** The conclusion that an EMT makes about a patient's condition after assessing the patient is called: presumptive diagnosis, EMS diagnosis, and EMT diagnosis. (p. 383)

2. **(C)** Critical thinking is the analytical process that assists the EMT in reaching a field diagnosis. (p. 382)

3. **(B)** The approach that clinicians use to arrive at a diagnosis includes gathering information, considering the possibilities, and reaching a conclusion. (p. 385)

4. **(C)** The differential diagnosis is a list of conditions that may be the cause of the patient's condition today. (p. 386)

5. **(A)** A red flag is a sign or symptom that suggests the possibility of a particular problem that is very serious. (p. 384)

6. **(D)** When a highly experienced physician comes to a diagnosis, he or she most likely used heuristics, pattern recognition, and shortcuts. (p. 386)

7. **(A)** The traditional approach to diagnosis involves narrowing down a long list of possibilities. (p. 384)

8. **(D)** Common heuristics or biases include illusory correlation, availability, representativeness, overconfidence, confirmation bias, anchoring and adjustment, and self-satisfying. (pp. 387–388)

9. **(B)** Specifically looking for evidence that supports the diagnosis you already have in mind is called a confirmation bias. (p. 388)

10. **(B)** When a patient does not fit the classic pattern, the EMT has to be careful not to make a representativeness error or give in to bias. (p. 388)

11. **(D)** Availability is the urge to think of things because they are more easily recalled, often due to recent exposure. (p. 388)

12. **(B)** Illusory correlation is when we draw conclusions about the world because of how something else works, implying one causes the other. (p. 388)

13. **(A)** Stopping the search for a diagnosis too soon can lead to missing out on the secondary diagnosis. (p. 388)

14. **(C)** Understanding the limitations of people and technology is a good first step in thinking like a highly experienced physician. (p. 390)

15. **(D)** The EMT who wants to think like a highly experienced physician should try to learn from others as well as organize data in his or her head, reflect on what he or she has learned, and realize that no one strategy works for everything. (p. 390)

16. **(B)** You should ask the patient about prior history with the rash or uticaria and not assume there is a correlation (illusionary) between the hives and this patient going into anaphalactic shock. Some patients will tell you, for example, that they always have a stress reaction to public speaking that causes the rash to appear. To find this out, you must get a history! (p. 388)

COMPLETE THE FOLLOWING

1. The eight ways in which an EMT can learn to think like a highly experienced physician are: (p. 390)
   A) Learn to love ambiguity.
   B) Understand the limitations of technology and people.
   C) Realize that no one strategy works for everything.
   D) Form a strong foundation of knowledge.
   E) Organize the data in your head.
   F) Change the way you think.
   G) Learn from others.
   H) Reflect on what you have learned.

STREET SCENES DISCUSSION

1. If, when you tested Mr. Ronson's blood sugar, the reading was within the normal range, the potential causes of his condition today would have been narrowed down a bit (no longer hypoglycemia) but still a serious concern.

2. Just because a patient exhibits a good Cincinnati Prehospital Stroke Scale score and does not actually complain of chest pain, you still need to keep "possible stroke or TIA" and "possible heart attack" on the list of potential problems Mr. Ronson is having today. As you learn more about these specific diseases later in the textbook, this need will become clearer to you.

3. If the patient were to become unconscious, you would need to position him properly so his airway is open and rapidly assess his carotid pulse. If you suspect a cardiac arrest, chest compressions would need to be started immediately.

4. If Mr. Ronson had a good gag reflex, and because he is a diabetic, it would have been appropriate to let him drink some juice with sugar in it or consider oral glucose per your local protocols (with a low blood sugar reading).

Chapter 17: Communications and Documentation

MATCH TERMINOLOGY/ DEFINITIONS

1. **(E)** Base station—a two-way radio at a fixed site such as a hospital or dispatch center (p. 395)

2. **(C)** Cell phone—a phone that transmits through the air instead of over wires so that the phone can be transported and used over a wide area (p. 395)

3. **(D)** Mobile radio—a two-way radio that is used or affixed in a vehicle (p. 395)

4. **(F)** Portable radio—a handheld, two-way radio (p. 395)

5. **(B)** Repeater— a device that picks up signals from lower-power radio units, such as mobile and portable radios, and retransmits them at a higher power; it allows low-power radio signals to be transmitted over longer distances (p. 395)

6. **(G)** Watt—the unit of measurement of the output of a radio (p. 395)

7. **(A)** Drop report (or transfer report)—an abbreviated form of the PCR that an EMS crew can leave at the hospital when there is not enough time to complete the PCR before leaving (p. 407)

MULTIPLE-CHOICE REVIEW

1. **(B)** EMS has progressed over the years due to the development of radio links among dispatchers, mobile units, and hospitals. (p. 395)

2. **(D)** The components of a communications system include the base station, mobile units, portable radios, repeaters, and cellular phones. (p. 395)

3. **(C)** A device that picks up a lower-power signal and then retransmits it at a higher power is called a repeater. Often when you are inside a residence or at the scene, it may be

necessary for the low-power radio to transmit to the repeater in the ambulance and then be retransmitted at a higher power so it will go further. (p. 395)

4. **(A)** The Federal Communications Commission (FCC) is responsible for approving communications and maintaining order on the airwaves. The FAA is the Federal Aviation Administration. FEMA is the Federal Emergency Management Agency. DOT is the Department of Transportation. (p. 396)

5. **(C)** The purposes of always following the general principles of radio transmission is to allow all persons to use the frequencies and to prevent delays. EMTs *should* request a repeat of orders from medical direction if they are unclear. The EMT should *not* use codes but communicate in plain English. (p. 397)

6. **(C)** Of the items listed, their correct sequence in a medical radio report is unit identification and level of provider, chief complaint, major past illness, and emergency medical care given. (p. 398)

7. **(B)** The reason the ambulance was called is the chief complaint. EMTs do not make diagnoses. (p. 398)

8. **(D)** The fact that a patient's abdomen feels rigid during palpation is a pertinent finding from the physical exam and is reported to the hospital. (p. 399)

9. **(C)** Updating the physician on the patient's mental status is a way of telling him or her how the patient is responding to the emergency medical care that was given. (p. 399)

10. **(A)** Whenever the EMT requests an order for medical direction over the radio, it is good practice to repeat the physician's order back word for word, question inappropriate orders, and speak slowly and clearly. (p. 397)

11. **(B)** Always question the physician about an order over the radio that you think is inappropriate or that you do not understand. The physician may have misinterpreted or misunderstood your communication. (p. 397)

12. **(B)** Crossing your arms and looking down at the patient sends the message, "I am not really interested." Be aware of the nonverbal messages you may send by your body position and posture. (pp. 401–402)

13. **(D)** If it is determined that a patient has a broken leg, tell the patient the truth in a calm voice and gentle manner. (p. 402)

14. **(A)** When treating a toddler, kneel down at the child's level to talk. Do not stare at the child. Never lie by saying you know his or her parents if you actually do not. The child will figure out that you are lying and will not trust you. (p. 404)

15. **(C)** The prehospital care report (PCR) serves as a legal document as well as an aid for research, education, and administrative efforts. EMTs do not routinely report all calls to the local police department. Because call information is confidential, it would never be used as a press release or as a receipt for the patient. (p. 404)

16. **(B)** The written PCR record provides a means for the emergency department staff to review the patient's prehospital care. (p. 407)

17. **(C)** The copy of the PCR left at the hospital should become part of the patient's permanent hospital record. (p. 407)

18. **(C)** A complete and accurate PCR will be your best recollection of the call. (p. 408)

19. **(D)** The person who completed a PCR may be called to court to testify about the call in a criminal proceeding, the

care provided to the patient, and the call in a civil proceeding. (p. 408)

20. **(B)** The routine review of PCRs for conformity to current medical and organizational standards is a process called quality improvement. (p. 408)

21. **(B)** Each individual box on a PCR is called a data element. The narrative is a written description. A key punch is used to input data into a computer. (pp. 408–409)

22. **(C)** The patient's Social Security number is not part of the minimum data set. It may be collected as part of insurance information. According to NHTSA, the minimum data set on a PCR should include respiratory rate and effort; skin color and temperature; times of incident, dispatch, and arrival at the patient; and capillary refill for patients less than 6 years old. (p. 409)

23. **(B)** Dispatch time is considered run data. (p. 409)

24. **(A)** Examples of patient data on a PCR would be date of birth and age. The other information is included elsewhere on the form. (p. 409)

25. **(C)** Experienced EMTs consider a good PCR as one that paints a picture of the patient. Attempting to identify symptoms the patient may have overlooked is falsification. (pp. 410–411)

26. **(B)** The statement "The patient has a swollen, deformed extremity" on the narrative portion of the PCR is an example of objective information. This means it is observable, measurable, or verifiable. Subjective information is information from an individual point of view. Pertinent negatives are examination findings that are negative (things that are *not* true) but are important to note. Nonstandard abbreviations should be avoided on PCRs. (pp. 410–411)

27. **(C)** Objective information is factual and need not be put in quotation marks. Subjective statements that are from an individual's point of view and that include opinions or actual statements made by bystanders, the patient, or a police officer should be in quotation marks. (p. 410)

28. **(B)** In the narrative section of a PCR, the EMT should include pertinent negatives. Do not write your personal conclusions about the situation or use the radio codes for each treatment. The vital signs and times they are taken are recorded in a different section, along with additional objective information. (pp. 410–411)

29. **(C)** Medical abbreviations should be used only if they are standardized to ensure that everyone who reads them will understand them. They are not used solely to save space in the narrative section of a PCR, to replace all words you cannot spell, or to ensure correct interpretation by physicians. (p. 411)

30. **(D)** When a patient refuses transport and before the EMT leaves the scene, he or she should document assessment findings and care given; try again to persuade the patient to go to a hospital; and ensure that the patient is able to make a rational, informed decision. (pp. 412–413)

31. **(D)** EMTs do not make a diagnosis. When completing a PCR on a patient refusal, the EMT should document that she was willing to return if the patient changed his mind, a complete patient assessment, and that alternative methods of care were offered. (pp. 412–413)

32. **(A)** If the EMT forgot to administer a treatment that is required by a state protocol, he or she should document on the PCR only treatment actually given. Never fill the form

out with excuses. Recording that the patient was given the forgotten treatment would be falsification. (p. 413)

33. **(A)** Falsification of information on a prehospital care report (PCR) may lead to suspension or revocation of your license or certification. (p. 413)

34. **(B)** To correct an error discovered while writing out a PCR, the EMT should draw a single horizontal line through the error, initial it, and write the correct information. Scribbling on the form is sloppy. You should be using a ballpoint pen to fill out the report; pencil and other erasures may be looked upon by others as an attempt to cover up a mistake in patient care. (pp. 415–416)

35. **(C)** If information was omitted on a PCR, the EMT should add a note with the correct information and the date, and initial it. It usually is not necessary to notify the Medical Director in this situation. (p. 415)

36. **(A)** An example of an instance in which it would *not* be unusual for the EMT to obtain only a limited amount of information is a multiple-casualty incident. An interhospital transfer and a child abuse call would probably be thoroughly documented with pertinent information. (p. 416)

37. **(A)** Special situation reports are used to document events that should be reported to local regulatory authorities. They must be accurate, neat, and submitted in a timely manner. They are reserved for special instances such as exposure to infectious disease, injury to EMTs, hazardous scenes, child or elder abuse, etc. (p. 417)

38. **(B)** Ambulance services are required by the Health Insurance Portability and Accountability Act (HIPAA) to take certain steps to safeguard patient confidentiality. The other federal agencies listed (OSHA, NHTSA, and U.S. DOT) do not regulate patient rights and confidentiality. (p. 411)

39. **(A)** An example of a method that an ambulance service would use to safeguard patient confidentiality includes requiring employees to place completed PCRs in a locked box. It would be inappropriate to use a patient's last name on the radio or review PCRs during QA meetings with a patient's name still on them. (p. 411)

40. **(D)** The policy an ambulance service develops concerning patient rights and confidentiality must take into consideration state regulations, local regulations, and HIPAA. (p. 411)

COMPLETE THE FOLLOWING

1. Examples of components of a communications system include: (p. 395)
   - **A)** base station radio.
   - **B)** mobile radio.
   - **C)** portable radio.
   - **D)** cell phones.
   - **E)** repeaters.

2. Interpersonal communications guidelines to use when dealing with patients, families, friends, and bystanders include the following: (pp. 401–403)
   - **A)** Use eye contact.
   - **B)** Be aware of your position and body language.
   - **C)** Use language the patient can understand.
   - **D)** Be honest.
   - **E)** Use the patient's proper name.
   - **F)** Listen.

3. Patient data on a PCR includes: (pp. 409–410)
   - **A)** the patient's name, address, date of birth, age, and sex.
   - **B)** billing and insurance information.
   - **C)** nature of the call.
   - **D)** mechanism of injury (MOI).
   - **E)** location where the patient was found.
   - **F)** treatment administered before arrival of EMTs.
   - **G)** signs and symptoms, including baseline and subsequent vital signs.
   - **H)** SAMPLE history.
   - **I)** care administered to and effect on the patient.
   - **J)** changes in condition throughout the call.

STREET SCENES DISCUSSION

1. Complete documentation is the best defense. Changes need to be made to all the copies of an incident report at the time of the changes.

2. Have the patient sign a refusal of treatment after discussing its importance.

3. The medical/legal view is that poor documentation equals poor assessment and/or care.

CASE STUDY:

1. You may have already used a mobile radio and a portable radio.

2. The reason why the ambulance was called in the patient's own words is called the chief complaint, or, in this case, for a car crash.

3. Initially your partner or some other EMS provider should manually stabilize the patient's head and neck.

4. No.

5. Based on the MOI, frontal striking a tree with lots of damage to the vehicle, and the fact that the patient did strike his head, you should talk him into being seen in the ED.

6. If you can't convince him, and your partner can't convince him, try your supervisor or your Medical Director on the radio or cell phone or a police officer.

7. Based on the information we have, the medical radio report would at least say:

   This is unit number XXX.
   This is EMT XXX.
   I have an ETA of XXX.
   En route to your facility with a 28-year-old male.
   He was involved in a single car crash with significant damage to the front of his vehicle.
   He is alert and states, "I was tired and may have fallen asleep at the wheel." He denies any loss of consciousness but does have a laceration on his forehead, which has stopped bleeding.
   He denies any major illness or other medical history.
   We have his head bandaged; he is immobilized with a collar, KED, and long board; and we have no requests for orders.
   He is resting comfortably at this point.

8. Additional information you have found out since the radio report and any changes in the patient's condition, as well as more detailed information you may not want to take the time to transmit over the radio.

MATCH TERMINOLOGY/DEFINITIONS

1. **(H)** Activated charcoal—a powder, usually premixed with water, that will adsorb some poisons and help prevent them from being absorbed by the body (p. 427)

2. **(E)** Aspirin—a medication used to reduce the clotting ability of blood to prevent and treat clots associated with myocardial infarction (p. 426)

3. **(L)** Contraindication—specific signs or circumstances under which is it not appropriate and may be harmful to administer a drug to a patient (p. 432)

4. **(F)** Epinephrine—a drug that helps to constrict the blood vessels and relax passages of the airway; it may be used to counter a severe allergic reaction (p. 429)

5. **(A)** Indications—specific signs or circumstances under which it is appropriate to administer a drug to a patient (p. 432)

6. **(B)** Inhaler—a spray device with a mouthpiece that contains an aerosol form of a medication that a patient can spray directly into his airway (p. 428)

7. **(M)** Nitroglycerin—a drug that helps to dilate the coronary vessels that supply the heart muscle with blood (p. 429)

8. **(D)** Oral glucose—medication given by mouth to treat an awake patient (who is able to swallow) with an altered mental status and a history of diabetes (p. 426)

9. **(G)** Oxygen—a gas commonly found in the atmosphere; it is used as a drug to treat any patient whose medical or traumatic condition may cause him to be hypoxic (p. 426)

10. **(C)** Pharmacology—the study of drugs, their sources, characteristics, and effects (p. 425)

11. **(I)** Pharmacodynamics—the study of the effects of medications on the body (p. 434)

12. **(K)** Side effect—any action of a drug other than the desired action (p. 432)

13. **(J)** Untoward effect—an effect of a medication in addition to its desired effect that may be potentially harmful to the patient (p. 432)

MULTIPLE-CHOICE REVIEW

1. **(D)** The study of drugs and their effects is called pharmacology. Anatomy is the study of the structure of the body. Physiology is the study of the functions of the body. Medicinology is a distracter. (p. 425)

2. **(A)** Medications that are routinely carried on the EMT-level EMS unit are aspirin, oral glucose, and oxygen. The patients may carry nitroglycerin, epinephrine, and prescribed inhalers. (pp. 426–427)

3. **(C)** An EMT-B administers aspirin to promote less clotting during a potential MI. (p. 426)

4. **(B)** A history of a GI bleed would be a contraindication to the administration of aspirin in the field. (p. 426)

5. **(B)** The brain is very sensitive to low levels of sugar in the blood, which may be caused by poorly managed diabetes; this can be a cause of a diabetic patient's altered mental status. (p. 426)

6. **(A)** Oral glucose is given between the patient's cheek and gum because this area contains many blood vessels that allow absorption and because it is easier for the patient to swallow the medication. (p. 426)

7. **(C)** Examples of medications that the patient may have in his possession that the EMT may assist the patient in taking under the appropriate circumstances are epinephrine (Epi-Pen®), a prescribed inhaler (bronchodilator), nitroglycerin, and aspirin. Patients do not generally carry home oxygen with them. EMTs do not assist patients in the administration of glucose injections, anticonvulsants, anti-inflammatories, insulin, or antihypertensives. (pp. 428–430)

8. **(C)** Patients who have a medical history of asthma, emphysema, and chronic bronchitis may carry a bronchodilator. (pp. 428–429)

9. **(C)** The drug nitroglycerin is used to dilate the coronary vessels. It is not used to constrict or dilate the peripheral vessels. (p. 429)

10. **(C)** The comprehensive government publication listing all drugs in the United States is called the *U.S. Pharmacopoeia*. (p. 431)

11. **(B)** The name that the manufacturer uses in marketing a drug is called the trade name. The generic name is used more generally by all manufacturers. (p. 431)

12. **(D)** A circumstance in which a drug should not be used because it may cause harm to the patient or offer no effect in improving the patient's condition or illness is called a contraindication. An indication is a specific sign or circumstance under which it is appropriate to administer a drug. An adverse reaction is usually not known in advance. Side effects, although not desirable, are not a reason to withhold a medication (e.g., headache from nitroglycerin). (p. 432)

13. **(A)** An action of a drug that is other than the desired action is called a side effect. See the answer for multiple-choice question 12. (p. 432)

14. **(D)** Prior to administering a medication to a patient, you must know the route of administration, proper dosage, and the actions the medication will take. You should know the generic name but you are not expected to know the chemical name. (p. 433)

15. **(B)** Drugs prescribed for pain relief are called analgesics. See Table 18–1. (p. 436)

16. **(D)** Drugs prescribed to reduce high blood pressure are called anti-hypertensives. See Table 18–1. (p. 436)

17. **(C)** Drugs prescribed for heart rhythm disorders are called antiarrhythmics. See Table 18–1. (p. 436)

18. **(B)** Drugs prescribed to relax the smooth muscles of the bronchial tubes are called bronchodilators. See Table 18–1. (p. 436)

19. **(C)** Drugs prescribed for prevention and control of seizures are called anticonvulsants. See Table 18–1. (p. 436)

20. **(A)** Drugs prescribed to help regulate the emotional activity of the patient to minimize the peaks and valleys in her or his psychological and emotional state are called antidepressants. See Table 18–1. (p. 436)

21. **(C)** Administering tiny aerosol particles to treat a disease, such as asthma, in a patient is considered the inhaled route of administration. (pp. 433–434)

Chapter 18 (continued)

22. (B) If you understood pharmacodynamics, you would understand the relationship between age and weight and dose, as well as the fact that the geriatric patient takes longer to eliminate medications, so they stay in his or her body longer. (p. 434)

COMPLETE THE FOLLOWING

1. The six medications an EMT can administer or assist a patient in taking are: (pp. 426–429)
   A) aspirin (ASA)
   B) prescribed inhalers
   C) oral glucose
   D) nitroglycerin (nitro)
   E) oxygen
   F) epinephrine auto-injectors (Epi-Pen® or Twin-Ject®)

Also activated charcoal in some EMS systems.

2. The five "rights" to adhere to when administering a medication are: (p. 433)
   A) The right patient.
   B) The right dose.
   C) The right medication.
   D) The right route.
   E) The right time to administer the medication.

STREET SCENES DISCUSSION

1. A side effect of nitroglycerin is a drop in blood pressure. If this should occur, you may need to lay the patient down and raise the legs as you call medical direction again for advice.

2. The patient expects the nitroglycerin to relieve his pain by dilating the coronary arteries, which supply the heart muscle with blood.

3. Yes, they are: "He denies any radiation down his arm or toward his jaw. He also denies any relief with the brief wait while sitting."

Chapter 19: Respiratory Emergencies

MATCH TERMINOLOGY/ DEFINITION

1. **(C)** Bronchoconstriction—blockage of the bronchi that lead from the trachea to the lungs (p. 461)
2. **(D)** Exhalation—another term for expiration (p. 445)
3. **(E)** Expiration—a passive process in which the intercostal muscles and the diaphragm relax, causing the chest cavity to decrease in size and force air from the lungs (p. 445)
4. **(B)** Inhalation—another term for inspiration (p. 445)
5. **(A)** Inspiration—an active process in which the intercostal muscles and the diaphragm contract, expanding the size of the chest cavity and causing air to flow into the lungs (p. 444)

MULTIPLE-CHOICE REVIEW

1. **(C)** The diaphragm separates the chest from the abdomen. The intercostal muscles are between the ribs. The sternocleidomastoid muscle is in the neck. The inguinal muscle is at the base of the abdomen. (p. 444)
2. **(B)** Expiration is a passive process in which the intercostal (rib) muscles and the diaphragm relax, causing the chest cavity to decrease in size and forcing air from the lungs. (p. 445)
3. **(C)** Although rhythm must be observed, it is not included under the *quality* of breathing. Quality includes breath sounds (diminished, unequal, or absent?), chest expansion (inadequate or unequal?), and depth of respirations (labored, increased respiratory effort, use of accessory muscles?). (p. 446)
4. **(C)** An unresponsive patient with shallow breaths and gasping with only a few breaths per minute is clearly breathing inadequately. You must provide artificial ventilation with supplemental oxygen, preferably via pocket face mask. (p. 446)
5. **(B)** Accessory muscles, such as those in the neck and abdomen, assist in breathing, especially when a patient is having difficulty breathing. Subdiaphragmatic is a location below the diaphragm. Smooth muscles line blood vessels. Extra muscles are an inventive distracter. (p. 451)
6. **(D)** Blue-colored skin (cyanosis) that feels clammy and cool is usually a sign of inadequate breathing. (p. 451)
7. **(A)** Snoring and gurgling sounds usually indicate a partially obstructed airway. Wheezing can be a sign of anything from airway obstruction to bronchoconstriction. Sniffling is usually from a runny nose. Whistling or grunting is a distracter. (p. 450)
8. **(C)** Respiratory conditions account for a large percentage of deaths in infants and children. Motor vehicle collisions cause child deaths, but not as high a percentage as respiratory conditions. Heart attacks are more rare in children. Infections are common in infants, but are less so in children. (p. 449)
9. **(D)** The cricoid cartilage of infants and children is less developed and less rigid than is an adult's. (p. 449)
10. **(B)** Infants and children depend more heavily on the diaphragm for breathing because the chest wall is softer. They do not inhale twice the air, and they may grunt only when they are in respiratory distress. (p. 449)
11. **(D)** Signs of inadequate breathing in infants and children include nasal flaring (widening of the nostrils), grunting, seesaw breathing, and retractions. Lip quivering is a distracter. (p. 449)
12. **(C)** It is not enough to simply make sure the patient is breathing. The patient must be breathing *adequately*. (p. 445)
13. **(A)** In order of preference, the procedure for providing assisted ventilation is as follows: 1. Pocket face mask with supplemental oxygen; 2. Two-rescuer BVM with supplemental oxygen; 3. Flow-restricted, oxygen-powered ventilator; 4. One-rescuer BVM with supplemental oxygen. (p. 448)
14. **(D)** If you are unsure about whether a patient needs artificial ventilation, you should provide artificial ventilation. (p. 448)

©2012 Pearson Education, Inc.
Emergency Care, 12th Ed.

15. **(B)** Artificially ventilate at a rate of 10–12 breaths per minute for an adult and 12–20 breaths per minute for infants and children, according to American Heart Association standards. (p. 448)

16. **(C)** See the answer for multiple-choice question 15. (p. 448)

17. **(C)** A low pulse in infants and small children in the setting of a respiratory emergency usually means trouble. In infants and children with respiratory difficulties, you may observe a slight increase in pulse early, but soon the pulse will drop significantly. (p. 449)

18. **(B)** Increase the force of ventilations for any patient—adult, child, or infant—if the chest does not rise and fall with each artificial ventilation, or the pulse does not return to normal. If the chest still does not rise, check that you are maintaining an open airway. (p. 448)

19. **(B)** When assessing the breathing of an adult, all of the following are important observations for the EMT to make: positioning, anatomy such as the barrel chest, color (i.e., pale, cyanotic, or flushed skin). (p. 450)

20. **(D)** Patients with lower airway obstruction may be wheezing, increase their breathing effort upon exhalation, and breathe rapidly without stridor. Their skin may be pale or blue, but not yellow. Yellow skin is an indication of liver abnormalities. (p. 452)

21. **(C)** A patient with breathing difficulty frequently speaks in short, choppy sentences. The other choices are distracters. (p. 450)

22. **(B)** In a tripod position, the patient is leaning forward with hands resting on the knees or table. The recovery position is lying on the side, which allows fluid to drain from the mouth. Supine with knees flexed is helpful with abdominal pain. (p. 451)

23. **(D)** Headache and vomiting are *not* commonly associated with breathing difficulties. Crowing, retractions, an increased pulse, and coughing are all common signs associated with breathing difficulty. Restlessness, shortness of breath, and chest tightness are common symptoms of patients with breathing difficulty. (p. 451)

24. **(B)** If a patient is suffering from breathing difficulty and is breathing adequately, administer oxygen via nonrebreather mask. The BVM and pocket mask are for patients in severe distress. (p. 448)

25. **(C)** If a patient is experiencing breathing difficulty and is breathing adequately, it is usually best to place him in the sitting-up position. (p. 448)

26. **(C)** Patients diagnosed with obstructive sleep apnea often sleep with a CPAP device. (p. 453)

27. **(C)** When giving a medication by an inhaler, a syringe is not needed. The patient must be alert and cooperative, and the right dose of unexpired medication must be given. (p. 462)

28. **(A)** Prior to coaching the patient in the use of an inhaler, first shake it vigorously. It is not necessary to test the unit by spraying it into the air. (p. 464)

29. **(B)** To ensure that the most medication is absorbed when using an inhaler, encourage the patient to hold the breath as long as possible so the medication can be absorbed by the lungs. Unless the medication is held in the lungs, it will have minimal or no value. (p. 464)

30. **(B)** CPAP blows oxygen or air continuously at a low pressure into the airway in an effort to push fluid out of the alveoli and back into the capillaries. (pp. 453–454)

31. **(C)** A physician realizes that his patient may become anxious and use the inhaler improperly. To help improve the volume of the medication that the patient is able to self-administer when in distress, the physician may prescribe a spacer device. (p. 462)

32. **(B)** Advair is not considered a medication that would be used in an emergency to reverse airway constriction because it is used to prevent attacks by reducing inflammation. The others—Ventolin, Proventil, and albuterol—are used in emergency situations. (p. 462)

33. **(D)** When assessing the lungs of a patient in respiratory distress, you hear a fine bubbling sound upon inspiration. This sound is caused by fluid in the alveoli and is called crackles. (p. 452)

34. **(C)** A side effect of CPAP can be gastric distention. (pp. 453–454)

35. **(B)** If there is no improvement using CPAP and the patient's mental status is diminishing, the EMT should remove the CPAP and ventilate the patient with a BVM. (pp. 453–454)

36. **(B)** Asthma is a chronic respiratory disease that has episodic exacerbations. (p. 457)

37. **(A)** The thin runner is most likely to have sustained a spontaneous pneumothorax by bursting a bleb on the wall of his lung. (pp. 458–459)

38. **(C)** CPAP can be very helpful with the patient who is alert and complaining of the signs and symptoms of acute pulmonary edema. (p. 453)

39. **(D)** Deep vein thrombosis after sitting for a long period of time from an international flight can lead to a pulmonary embolism. (p. 459)

40. **(A)** The disease epiglottitis used to be prominent in children but has been virtually eliminated due to infant inoculations. Today we see adult patients who were not vaccinated to prevent the disease. (pp. 459–460)

COMPLETE THE FOLLOWING

1. EMT observations of the patient with difficulty breathing should include: (p. 450)
   A) altered mental status, including restlessness, anxiety, or depressed LOC
   B) unusual anatomy (i.e., barrel chest)
   C) the patient's position (i.e., tripod, feet dangling)
   D) work of breathing
   E) pale, cyanotic, or flushed skin color
   F) pedal edema
   G) sacral edema
   H) noisy breathing

2. Vital sign changes for the patient with difficulty breathing can include: (any four) (p. 446)
   • increased pulse rate
   • decreasing pulse rate (especially in infants and children)
   • changes in breathing rate (above or below normal levels)
   • changes in breathing rhythm
   • hypertension or hypotension
   • oxygen saturation reading less than 95 percent

3. The common abnormal lungs sounds include: (p. 452)
   A) Wheezes: high-pitched sounds that will seem almost musical in nature. The sound is created by air moving through narrowed air passages in the lungs. It can be heard in a variety of diseases but is common in asthma and sometimes in chronic obstructive lung diseases such as

Chapter 19 (continued)

emphysema and chronic bronchitis. Wheezing is most commonly heard during expiration.

B) Crackles (rales): As the name indicates, a fine crackling or bubbling sound heard upon inspiration. The sound is caused by fluid in the alveoli or by the opening of closed alveoli. Some people refer to crackles as rales.

C) Rhonchi: lower-pitched sounds that resemble snoring or rattling. They are caused by secretions in larger airways as might be seen with pneumonia or bronchitis or when materials are aspirated (breathed) into the lungs. The difference between crackles and rhonchi is not always obvious and is somewhat subjective. However, rhonchi generally are louder than crackles.

D) Stridor: a high-pitched sound that is heard on inspiration. It is an upper airway sound indicating partial obstruction of the trachea or larynx. Stridor is usually audible without a stethoscope.

4. Pulse Oximeter Readings (p. 451)
Oxygen should be administered to all patients with respiratory distress regardless of their oxygen saturation readings. The oximeter reading in a normal, healthy person is typically
   A) 95 percent to 99 percent. An oximeter reading below
   B) 95 percent indicates hypoxia.

LABEL THE DIAGRAMS (P. 445)

1. Relaxation
2. Contraction (inspiration begins)
3. Inspiration
4. Relaxation (passive expiration begins)

STREET SCENES DISCUSSION

1. Anything related to the patient's respiratory condition is pertinent to the current problem. Document it!
2. Yes.
3. As you learned in Chapter 8, the procedures for airway evaluation, opening the airway, and artificial ventilation are best carried out with the patient lying supine, or flat on the back. However, if the patient must sit, sit her up on the stretcher, lay her head back, and work with her breathing efforts. This takes patience and practice.

CASE STUDY: THE 3 A.M. CALL: DAD SIMPLY CANNOT BREATHE

1. As you approach the patient, your Standard Precautions should include disposable gloves.
2. A HEPA mask or N-95 should be used if you suspect the patient may have a fever, cough, and possibly active TB.
3. Awake and alert patients who have breathing difficulty usually find the Fowler or semi-Fowler position most comfortable.
4. Patients who talk in short, choppy sentences usually have severe respiratory distress.
5. The initial oxygen administration should be given using a nonrebreather mask.

6. If the patient is breathing too fast, too slow, or too shallow, the bag-mask device would be more appropriate.
7. Albuterol is given, with medical direction approval, by inhaling two puffs through the patient's MDI.
8. No, the patient's family member's medicine is not prescribed for him. Use only the patient's prescribed medicine(s).
9. Yes, a spacer can be used, and some patients are more comfortable with the device attached to their MDI.
10. Expect to see tachycardia, slight tremors, and some anxiety from the medication.

Chapter 20: Cardiac Emergencies

MATCH TERMINOLOGY/ DEFINITIONS

PART A

1. **(D)** Acute coronary syndrome—a blanket term used to represent any symptoms related to lack of oxygen (ischemia) in the heart muscle (p. 471)
2. **(G)** Acute myocardial infarction (AMI)—the condition in which a portion of the myocardium dies as a result of oxygen starvation; often called a heart attack by laypersons (p. 480)
3. **(F)** Angina pectoris—pain in the chest, occurring when the blood supply to the heart is reduced and a portion of the heart muscle is not receiving enough oxygen (p. 479)
4. **(E)** Aneurysm—the dilation, or ballooning, of a weakened section of the wall of an artery (p. 478)
5. **(H)** Bradycardia—when the heart rate is slow, usually below 60 beats per minute (p. 472)
6. **(I)** Cardiovascular system—the heart and the blood vessels (p. 470)
7. **(A)** Congestive heart failure (CHF)—the failure of the heart to pump efficiently, leading to excessive blood or fluids in the lungs, the body, or both (p. 481)
8. **(C)** Coronary artery disease (CAD)—diseases that affect the arteries of the heart (p. 478)
9. **(B)** Dyspnea—shortness of breath; labored or difficulty breathing (p. 471)
10. **(J)** Dysrhythmia—a disturbance in heart rate and rhythm (p. 479)

PART B

1. **(B)** Edema—swelling resulting from a build-up of fluid in tissues (p. 481)
2. **(J)** Embolism—blockage of a vessel by a clot or foreign material brought to the site by the blood current (p. 478)
3. **(D)** Nitroglycerin—a medication that dilates the blood vessels (p. 476)
4. **(H)** Occlusion—blockage, as of an artery by fatty deposits (p. 478)
5. **(E)** Pedal edema—accumulation of fluid in the feet and ankles (p. 481)
6. **(C)** Pulmonary edema—accumulation of fluid in the lungs (p. 481)

7. **(I)** Pulseless electrical activity (PEA)—a condition in which the heart's electrical rhythm remains relatively normal, yet the mechanical pumping activity fails to follow the electrical activity, causing cardiac arrest (p. 487)

8. **(A)** Sudden death—a cardiac arrest that occurs within 2 hours of the onset of symptoms; the patient may have no prior symptoms of CAD (p. 480)

9. **(F)** Thrombus—a clot formed of blood and plaque attached to the inner wall of an artery or vein (p. 478)

10. **(G)** Ventricular fibrillation (VF)—a condition in which the heart's electrical impulses are disorganized, preventing the heart muscle from contracting normally (p. 487)

11. **(L)** Ventricular tachycardia (V-Tach)—a condition in which the heartbeat is quite rapid; if rapid enough, it will not allow the heart's chambers to fill with enough blood between beats to produce blood flow sufficient to meet the body's needs (p. 487)

12. **(K)** Asystole—a condition in which the heart has ceased generating electrical impulses (p. 487)

MULTIPLE-CHOICE REVIEW

1. **(C)** ACS, acute coronary syndrome, is a term that refers to a problem with the heart when it is not getting enough oxygen. A period of time when the heart stops is cardiac arrest. (p. 471)

2. **(C)** Tearing pain is usually the result of a dissecting aortic aneurysm. Chest pain from the heart is normally described as crushing pain, dull, squeezing, or a heavy sensation. (p. 478)

3. **(A)** The pain or discomfort from a heart problem commonly radiates to the arms and jaw. It may also radiate down to the upper abdomen. (p. 472)

4. **(C)** In addition to chest pain or discomfort, the patient with cardiac compromise will also complain of dyspnea. The patient with gastrointestinal distress will complain of diarrhea. Cardiac compromise patients usually have a sudden onset of sweating, *not* shivering. A headache is a side effect of nitroglycerin. (p. 472)

5. **(C)** Patients with heart problems may complain of pain in the center of the chest, mild chest discomfort, and difficulty breathing. They do not have sudden onset of sharp abdominal pain. (p. 472)

6. **(B)** If the heart is beating too fast or too slow, the patient with cardiac compromise may also lose consciousness. This is due to an inadequate supply of oxygenated blood to the brain. (p. 479)

7. **(C)** The signs and symptoms of an acute coronary syndrome do not include sharp pain in the lower abdomen combined with a fever. (p. 471)

8. **(C)** The patient with an acute coronary syndrome should be administered high-concentration oxygen; the nasal cannula does not provide high-concentration oxygen. (p. 471)

9. **(A)** The "position of comfort" for a patient who is having chest pain is typically sitting up. Patients who are hypotensive (systolic blood pressure less than 90) will usually feel better lying down because this position allows more blood flow to the brain. (p. 472)

10. **(C)** A patient with prescribed nitroglycerin should be given or assisted in taking nitroglycerin (up to three doses). Vital signs and chest pain should be reassessed after each dose. If this patient's blood pressure falls below 100 systolic, then treat for shock and transport promptly. (p. 476)

11. **(B)** You should consider using nitroglycerin when the patient is carrying his own nitro and has crushing chest pain. A side effect of nitro is a headache. Nitro is *not* given to unconscious patients or to those who are hypotensive, below 100 systolic. (p. 476)

12. **(C)** The role of medical direction in the treatment of an acute coronary syndrome patient is authorizing the EMT to assist the patient in taking prescribed nitroglycerin. (p. 476)

13. **(C)** To give nitroglycerin, the patient's blood pressure must *not* be lower than 100 systolic. Medical direction should authorize the administration of nitroglycerin, and the patient's physician should have prescribed it. (p. 476)

14. **(C)** The maximum number of doses of nitro routinely given in the field is three. (p. 476)

15. **(C)** If, after administering three doses of nitroglycerin, the patient's blood pressure falls below 100 systolic, you should treat for shock and transport promptly. (p. 476)

16. **(A)** Nitroglycerin is contraindicated for a patient who has a head injury. (p. 476)

17. **(C)** When considering administering aspirin to a cardiac patient, pay attention to allergies, asthma history, and if the patient is already taking anti-clotting meds. Viagra is relevant to nitro and not ASA. (p. 477)

18. **(C)** After administering nitro, it is important to reassess the vital signs. It is not necessary to lay the patient down unless his blood pressure drops. Continue the oxygen administration. (p. 476)

19. **(D)** The majority of cardiovascular emergencies are *not* a result of complications of cardiovascular surgery. Rather, they are a result of changes in the inner walls of arteries or problems with the heart's electrical and mechanical functions. (p. 478)

20. **(A)** When the body is subjected to exertion or stress, the heart rate normally increases. It would be unusual for the heart to stop with normal exertion. (p. 478)

21. **(B)** Coronary artery disease (CAD) is a result of the build-up of fatty deposits on the inner walls of the arteries. (p. 478)

22. **(D)** Risk factors for acute coronary syndrome include lack of exercise, cigarette smoking, and obesity; other risk factors include heredity, age, hypertension, and elevated blood levels of cholesterol and triglycerides. (p. 478)

23. **(C)** Hypertension as well as smoking and diet are risk factors that can be modified to reduce the risk of coronary artery disease. Unfortunately, a patient cannot change his or her age or heredity factors. (p. 478)

24. **(A)** The reason an emergency occurs in most cardiac-related medical emergencies is due to reduced blood flow to the myocardium. This may in turn cause cardiac arrest, loss of consciousness, or breathing difficulty. (p. 478)

25. **(B)** Angina pectoris means, literally, a pain in the chest. (p. 479)

26. **(B)** Nitroglycerin is administered to the patient with chest pain because it dilates the blood vessels and decreases the work of the heart. A drop in blood pressure is a side effect of nitro. Nitro should not be administered to unconscious patients. (p. 476)

27. **(B)** A condition in which a portion of the myocardium dies as a result of oxygen starvation is known as acute myocardial infarction. A coronary occlusion occurs when the coronary artery is completely blocked. Myocardial starvation is a distracter. (p. 480)

28. **(C)** Cardiac arrest occurring within 2 hours of the onset of cardiac symptoms is referred to as sudden death. (p. 480)

29. **(B)** Unfortunately, nearly 25 percent of the patients who experience a cardiac arrest within 2 hours of the onset of symptoms have no previous history of cardiac problems. (p. 480)

30. **(B)** The weak spots that begin to dilate form a condition called an aneurysm. (p. 478)

31. **(B)** Congestive heart failure is a condition in which excessive fluids build up in the lungs and/or other organs. An infection in the heart is a distracter. A chronic lung condition that requires a low concentration of oxygen administration is COPD. (p. 481)

32. **(B)** Damage to the left ventricle and blood backing up into the lungs usually present in the form of pulmonary edema. Pedal edema is the accumulation of fluid in the feet or ankles. Fibrinolytics are medications that dissolve blood clots. Diaphoresis is profuse sweating. (p. 481)

33. **(D)** The chain of survival does not include prevention. The elements of the chain of survival include early access, early CPR, early defibrillation, early advanced care, and early post-resuscitative care. (pp. 482–483)

34. **(C)** This patient has many of the signs and symptoms of CHF; he may also be experiencing left heart failure due to the blood-tinged sputum from acute pulmonary edema. (p. 481)

35. **(B)** CPR training by heart specialists is unnecessary in order to decrease the time it takes to start CPR on a cardiac arrest victim. Frankly, the bystanders are the first key personnel in saving the patient. (p. 483)

36. **(A)** The typical cardiac arrest victim is a male in his sixties. (p. 484)

37. **(D)** The most common witness to a cardiac arrest is a female in her sixties. (p. 484)

38. **(D)** Early defibrillation is the single most important factor in determining survival from cardiac arrest. If the time from the call to the arrival of the defibrillator is longer than 8 minutes, virtually no one survives cardiac arrest. (p. 484)

39. **(B)** See the answer for multiple-choice question 38. (p. 484)

40. **(B)** If the EMT is treating a cardiac arrest patient and there is no ALS unit in the community, the EMT should then package quickly and transport to the closest hospital while administering high-quality CPR throughout the call. To call for ALS from another town and wait for their arrival would take too much time. Do not delay on the scene until the patient regains a pulse. Transport with high-quality CPR! (p. 484)

41. **(D)** The EMT does not need to know how to administer epinephrine via IV or ET tube to manage a patient in cardiac arrest. Epinephrine administration, by the EMT, is designed for allergic or anaphylactic patients. (p. 484)

42. **(D)** When using a fully automated defibrillator, it is unnecessary to press the button to deliver the shock. This is because a *fully* automated defibrillator delivers the shock automatically once enough energy has been accumulated. (p. 486)

43. **(B)** The primary electrical disturbance resulting in cardiac arrest is ventricular fibrillation. (p. 484)

44. **(A)** The shockable rhythms include: ventricular fibrillation, ventricular tachycardia, and pulseless ventricular tachycardia. Asystole and PEA are not considered shockable rhythms. (p. 487)

45. **(A)** A nonshockable rhythm that can be the result of a terminally sick heart or severe blood loss is called pulseless electrical activity. (p. 487)

46. **(C)** A nonshockable rhythm that is commonly called flatline is named asystole. This condition is called flatline because the wavy line displayed on an ECG when there is electrical activity goes flat with asystole. (p. 487)

47. **(B)** When the AED is analyzing the patient's heart rhythm, the EMT must avoid touching the patient. If you are touching the patient, there can be interference from the electrical impulses of your heart and from movement of the patient's muscles. This can fool the AED's computer into believing there is a shockable rhythm when there really isn't one, or vice versa. Also, it's possible a shock could be delivered to you if you are touching the patient, and this shock could injure you. (p. 488)

48. **(D)** The AED should routinely be used on patients with shockable rhythms. If the patient is an adult, child, or infant, proceed with the AED. Always continue high-quality CPR and transport per local medical direction. (p. 488)

49. **(C)** The AED pads are first attached to the cables. Then the pad attached to the red cable is placed over the left lower ribs. The pad attached to the white cable is placed in the angle between the sternum and the right clavicle. (p. 488)

50. **(C)** If the patient has a pulse and is breathing adequately after the first shock, give high-concentration oxygen via nonrebreather mask and then transport. (p. 488)

51. **(B)** After three shocks, each separated by 2 minutes of high-quality compressions, the EMT should transport the patient unless local protocol says otherwise. Termination of an arrest can be done only with the approval of medical direction. (p. 488)

52. **(A)** Defibrillation comes first! Don't hook up oxygen or do anything that delays analysis of the rhythm or defibrillation. (p. 488)

53. **(D)** A patient with an implanted defibrillator can be defibrillated immediately. Emergency care, CPR, and defibrillation for this patient are the same as for other cardiac patients. A trauma patient with severe blood loss should not be defibrillated. If a patient is soaking wet or is touching anything metallic that another person is touching, you could receive a shock. Move these patients before defibrillating. (p. 495)

54. **(A)** If it is necessary to remove a nitro patch to defibrillate a patient, you should wear gloves to prevent the nitro from being absorbed into your skin. Do not use alcohol to cleanse the patient's skin; this could burn the patient's skin during defibrillation. (p. 495)

55. **(C)** If a patient has a cardiac pacemaker and needs to be defibrillated, the EMT should place the pad several inches away from the pacemaker battery. If you do not do this, you could damage the pacemaker with the AED shock. You cannot change the AED's power setting. EMTs do not remove pacemakers; this involves surgery. (p. 495)

COMPLETE THE FOLLOWING

1. The chain of survival includes: (p. 483)
   A) Early access
   B) Early CPR
   C) Early defibrillation
   D) Early advanced care
   E) Early post-resuscitation care

STREET SCENES DISCUSSION

1. Cardiac patients can deteriorate very quickly. This is usually due to fluid in the lungs, intense chest pain, or dysrhythmia. Each of these problems can be monitored and managed by advanced life support (ALS) personnel, so call for them early.

2. Give the patient (or help the patient take) nitroglycerin if all of the following conditions are met: she complains of chest pain, she has a history of cardiac problems, her physician has pre-scribed nitroglycerin (NTG), she has the nitroglycerin with her, her systolic blood pressure is greater than 90 mmHg, medical direction authorizes administration of the medication.

3. If the AED does not shock a pulseless patient, it means the patient does not have a shockable rhythm. Be sure to start immediately high-quality CPR compressions with as little interruption as possible.

4. This patient is in critical condition, so she is a high priority. Vital signs should be taken every 5 minutes on a critical patient.

Chapter 21: Diabetic Emergencies and Altered Mental Status

MATCH TERMINOLOGY/ DEFINITIONS

1. .(B) Diabetes mellitus—also called sugar diabetes or just diabetes, the condition brought about by decreased insulin production or the inability of the body cells to use insulin properly (p. 508)

2. (G) Epilepsy—a medical condition that causes seizures; with proper medication, many of these patients no longer have seizures (p. 518)

3. (A) Glucose—a form of sugar that provides the body's basic source of energy (p. 507)

4. (H) Hyperglycemia—high blood sugar (p. 509)

5. (F) Hypoglycemia—low blood sugar (p. 508)

6. (C) Insulin—a hormone produced by the pancreas or taken as a medication by many diabetics (p. 508)

7. (I) Seizure—a sudden change in sensation, behavior, or movement; the most severe form produces violent muscle contractions called convulsions (p. 516)

8. (E) Status epilepticus—a prolonged seizure, or when a person suffers two or more convulsive seizures without regaining full consciousness (p. 519)

9. (J) Stroke—a condition of altered function caused when an artery in the brain is blocked or ruptured, disrupting the supply of oxygenated blood or causing bleeding into the brain (p. 520)

10. (D) Syncope—fainting (p. 524)

MULTIPLE-CHOICE REVIEW

1. (C) The relationship of glucose to insulin is often described as a lock-and-key mechanism. For sugar to enter the body's cells, insulin must be present. The relationship is not oppositional, synergistic, or antagonistic. (p. 508)

2. (A) The condition brought about by decreased insulin production is known as diabetes mellitus. Hypotension is low blood pressure resulting from hypoperfusion, or shock, or other causes. Hypoglycemia is low blood sugar. A cerebrovascular accident occurs when an artery in the brain is blocked or ruptured. (pp. 508–509)

3. (C) The most common medical emergency for the diabetic patient is called hypoglycemia. (p. 508)

4. (A) When a diabetic overexercises or overexerts, a medical condition called hypoglycemia can develop because sugars in the body are used faster than normal. Hyperglycemia (high blood sugar) occurs because the diabetic does not produce enough natural insulin, which is needed to pass sugar from the blood into the cells. Acute pulmonary edema is fluid in the lungs, which is usually the result of left heart failure. (pp. 508–509)

5. (B) Potential causes of hypoglycemia: the patient may have taken too much insulin by mistake, the patient has been vomiting, or the patient has been fasting. A person does not lower sugar in the blood by eating a box of candy; this increases the blood sugar level. (p. 509)

6. (A) If sugar is not replenished quickly, the hypoglycemic patient may have permanent brain damage. (p. 509)

7. (C) The clues that a patient is a diabetic include a medical identification bracelet, the presence of insulin in the refrigerator, and information provided by family members. The fact that the patient eats low-fat food would have no effect on the patient's condition. (p. 510)

8. (B) In all patients with an altered mental status, always consider an airway or breathing problem first causing hypoxia. (p. 507)

9. (D) An intoxicated appearance and uncharacteristic behavior are typical of diabetic emergency. (p. 514)

10. (B) Diabetics often present the EMT with cold, clammy skin; anxiety; and combativeness. It is unusual for them to have a decreased heart rate. (p. 514)

11. (A) For the EMT to consider administering oral glucose, the patient must have altered mental status, have a history of diabetes, and be awake enough to swallow. Oral glucose is not administered to the patient with an absent gag reflex or to a patient with a seizure history who is not a diabetic. (p. 512)

12. (C) If you reassess a patient to whom you have adminis-tered oral glucose and note the patient's condition has not improved, you should consult medical direction about whether to administer more glucose. (p. 512)

13. (C) The recovery position prevents aspiration of fluids or stomach content into the lungs. The position is used for all non-spine-injured patients who are unresponsive or have an altered mental status. (p. 519)

14. (C) Children are less likely to eat correctly and are more active; as a result, they are more likely to exhaust blood sugar levels. Thus, children are more at risk for developing hypoglycemia. (p. 511)

15. (C) A sudden change in mental status may indicate an alteration in the patient's blood sugar level. (p. 509)

16. (B) Before and after administering oral glucose, make sure you document the mental status of the patient. Increasing the oxygen flow rate is not necessary because it should remain at 15 liters per minute by nonrebreather mask. The glass of water is not needed. (p. 512)

17. (D) One trade name of oral glucose is Insta-glucose. D_5W is an intravenous solution of dextrose in water. Lactose is another form of sugar, and insulin is a hormone produced by the pancreas to help the body break down sugar. (p. 515)

18. (D) Before deciding that a patient who is very confused and disoriented has a behavioral problem, the EMT should consider a potential head injury, a brain tumor, and hypoxia. There is no such thing as an allergy to glucose. (p. 506)

19. (B) Diabetics routinely test the level of sugar in their blood using a glucose meter. (p. 511)

20. (D) Complications of diabetes include: kidney failure, heart disease, and blindness. (p. 513)

21. (C) The reading on the glucose meter is reported in milligrams of glucose per deciliter of blood. (pp. 511–513)

22. (D) A diabetic with a sugar level below 80 is considered hypoglycemic. (p. 513)

23. (A) A diabetic with a sugar level above 120 is considered hyperglycemic. (p. 513)

24. (C) The most common cause of seizures in adults is not taking prescribed anti-seizure medication. (p. 517)

25. (A) Seizures are commonly caused by high fever, brain tumor, and infection. They are not generally a result of cold exposure. (p. 517)

26. (A) Idiopathic seizures occur spontaneously, have an unknown cause, and often start in childhood. Seizures in children who frequently have them are rarely life threatening, but you should treat seizures in an infant or child as if they are life threatening. (p. 517)

27. (A) Convulsive seizures may be seen with epilepsy or hypoglycemia. They are not seen with asthma, AMI, pulmonary embolism, or anaphylaxis. (p. 517)

28. (B) The best known condition that results in seizures is epilepsy. (p. 517)

29. (A) Not all seizures are alike. The type of seizure that most people associate with epilepsy and seizure disorders is called a generalized tonic-clonic seizure. The patient falls to the floor and has severe convulsions. (p. 517)

30. (D) The family's reaction to the seizure (e.g., they called 911 or were frightened by the seizure) is not important to emergency care. When obtaining the medical history of a seizure patient, find out how long the seizure lasted, what the patient did after the seizure, and what the patient was doing prior to the seizure. (p. 518)

31. (C) If a seizure patient becomes cyanotic, provide artificial ventilations with supplemental oxygen. Sometimes a seizure patient can stop breathing during the seizure. (p. 519)

32. (B) If you arrive on the scene of a seizure patient and notice that a bystander has placed a tongue blade in the corner of the patient's mouth, you should carefully remove the object from his mouth. Any object in the patient's mouth could cause an airway obstruction. Then begin oxygen administration. (p. 519)

33. (A) A seizure normally lasts about 1 to 3 minutes. Longer seizures (more than 5 to 10 minutes) are considered status epilepticus (p. 518)

34. (B) When a patient has two or more back-to-back seizures without regaining consciousness (or a seizure that lasts over 5 to 10 minutes), this is called status epilepticus. The treatment involves ALS medications, so either call an ALS unit or quickly get the patient to the ED. Status asthmaticus is a continuous asthmatic attack. Convulsions are uncontrolled muscular movements. (p. 519)

35. (D) If you suspect a conscious patient has had a stroke, transport in the semi-Fowler position and maintain the airway. These patients often vomit. If a suspected stroke patient was *unconscious*, you should transport in the recovery position. (p. 520)

36. (B) When a stroke patient has difficulty saying what he is thinking, even though he clearly understands you, he is experiencing expressive aphasia. (p. 520)

37. (C) When the patient can speak clearly but cannot understand what you are saying, she is experiencing receptive aphasia. (p. 520)

38. (D) A common sign of a stroke is headache. (p. 520)

39. (D) Signs and symptoms of a stroke include: vomiting, seizures, and loss of bladder control. (p. 520)

40. (B) When a patient has many of the signs and symptoms of a stroke that resolve completely in less than 24 hours, he or she experienced a transient ischemic attack (TIA). (pp. 520–521)

41. (C) The medical term for fainting is a syncopal episode. A stroke or CVA is a disruption to the blood supply to a portion of the brain, which causes cell damage. Treatment of syncope includes both oxygen administration and the Trendelenburg position. Hyperglycemia that lasts for a long period of time may cause a coma, but it doesn't cause a coma that occurs suddenly. (p. 524)

42. (B) Lightheadedness or dizziness is often due to poor perfusion to the brain. This is corrected by placing the patient in the supine position, administering oxygen, and increasing the volume as needed. (p. 524)

INSIDE/OUTSIDE: HYPOGLYCEMIA (P. 509)

1. Blood vessels constrict, the heart pumps faster and harder, and breathing accelerates.

2. Confusion, stupor, unconsciousness, and seizures are common.

INSIDE/OUTSIDE: HYPERGLYCEMIA (P. 510)

1. Systemic dehydration and potential hypovolemic shock develop.

2. The production of ketones can result in the fruity or acetone smell on the breath of the diabetic patient.

INSIDE/OUTSIDE: TONIC CLONIC SEIZURE (P. 517)

1. The tonic phase causes the body to become rigid, stiffening for no more than 30 seconds. Breathing may stop and the patient might bite his or her tongue and become incontinent.

2. The clonic phase involves the body jerking about violently for no more than 1 to 2 minutes. The patient may foam at the mouth and drool. His or her face and lips may become cyanotic.

3. The postictal phase is when the convulsions stop; the patient may be drowsy and very tired during this period.

COMPLETE THE FOLLOWING

1. The signs and symptoms of a diabetic emergency include: (any six) (pp. 510–511)
   - Rapid onset of altered mental status
   - Intoxicated appearance, staggering, slurred speech, and unconsciousness
   - Elevated heart rate
   - Cold, clammy skin
   - Hunger
   - Seizures
   - Uncharacteristic behavior
   - Anxiety
   - Combativeness

2. *Hyper*glycemia occurs because the diabetic does not produce enough natural insulin, which is needed to pass sugar out of the blood and into the cells. It usually involves a situation in which the diabetic has: (p. 509)
   A) not taken enough insulin to make up for the deficiency in natural insulin.
   B) forgotten to take his insulin.
   C) overeaten.
   D. an infection that has upset his insulin/glucose balance.

3. The five categories of causes for dizziness and syncope include:
   A) Hypovolemic
   B) Metabolic and structural
   C) Environmental/toxicological
   D) Cardiovascular
   E) Other causes

STREET SCENES DISCUSSION

1. They should be told how important it is that the patient eats because the oral glucose will wear off. Follow your agency's policy on refusals and involve medical direction as needed. Tell the patient and his friend not to hesitate to call EMS again if there is any change in the patient's mental status.

2. Too much exercise for the amount of sugar taken in, too much insulin, or vomiting a meal could also cause hypoglycemia.

3. If medical direction permits it, you could have tried giving the patient some orange juice with a teaspoon of sugar in it.

CASE STUDY: CALL FOR A MAN DOWN

1. Use the head-tilt, chin-lift maneuver.

2. Use the BVM and assist ventilations with 100 percent oxygen.

3. It could have been due to a seizure, no access to a bathroom, and intoxication.

4. Seizure patients take dilantin, so he could have a history of seizures.

5. No, that would be jumping to a conclusion. It is a likely cause, but you need to investigate further.

6. The oxygen is for potential hypoxia. The vitals are a baseline to compare the next set to and may help determine if there is internal bleeding. The blood sugar test helps to determine if the altered mental status is due to hypoglycemia.

7. Hypoglycemia.

8. Type II diabetes develops in later life due to the pancreas no longer being able to supply enough insulin. Only some type II diabetics take insulin injections. Most can control their diet and take oral meds—Things this patient seems to have difficulty doing!

Chapter 22: Allergic Reaction

MATCH TERMINOLOGY/ DEFINITIONS

1. **(C)** Allergen—something that causes an allergic reaction (p. 531)

2. **(F)** Allergic reaction—an exaggerated immune response (p. 531)

3. **(B)** Anaphylaxis—a severe or life-threatening allergic reaction in which the blood vessels dilate, causing a drop in blood pressure, and the tissues lining the respiratory system swell, interfering with the airway (p. 531)

4. **(E)** Auto-injector—a syringe preloaded with medication that has a spring-loaded device that pushes the needle through the skin when the tip of the device is pressed firmly against the body (p. 536)

5. **(D)** Epinephrine—a hormone produced by the body; as a medication, it constricts blood vessels and dilates respiratory passages and is used to relieve severe allergic reactions (p. 536)

6. **(A)** Hives—red, itchy, possibly raised blotches on the skin that often result from an allergic reaction (p. 534)

MULTIPLE-CHOICE REVIEW

1. **(C)** An exaggerated response of the body's immune system to any substance is called an allergic reaction. Vasoconstricting is the constriction of the vessels. A syncopal episode is when the patient passes out momentarily. (p. 531)

2. **(D)** Allergic reactions are sometimes treated as a high priority because they can cause airway obstruction. In anaphylaxis (a severe allergic reaction), exposure to the allergen causes blood vessels to dilate rapidly, which in turn causes a drop in blood pressure. Many tissues swell, including those that line the respiratory system. This swelling can obstruct the airway, leading to respiratory failure. Vomiting and hives are not life threatening. Most patients can tolerate a rapid pulse for a short while. (p. 536)

3. **(C)** The first time a person is exposed to an allergen, the person's immune system forms antibodies, which are an attempt by the body to "attack" the foreign substances (allergens). (p. 533)

4. **(A)** The second time a person is exposed to an allergen, the body reactions may include dilation of the blood vessels, massive swelling, and difficulty breathing. (p. 533)

5. **(D)** Red fruits and vegetables are not common causes of allergic reactions. Causes include: hornet stings, eggs and milk, poison ivy, and penicillin. (p. 531)

6. **(C)** Peanuts are not actually nuts, like almonds and walnuts; they are legumes. (p. 531)

7. **(B)** Hives are not a *respiratory* sign or symptom but are an effect of an allergic reaction on the skin. The respiratory signs and symptoms of anaphylactic shock include rapid breathing, cough, and stridor, as well as tightness in the throat or chest, labored or noisy breathing, hoarseness or loss of voice, and wheezing. (p. 534)

8. **(D)** The effects of an allergic reaction on the cardiac system could include increased heart rate and decreased blood pressure. (p. 534)

9. **(C)** To be considered a severe allergic reaction, a patient must have signs and symptoms of shock and/or respiratory distress. (p. 535)

10. **(B)** After administering epinephrine, the EMT should reassess the patient after 2 minutes. Do not decrease the oxygen and do not allow the patient to remain at home. (p. 536)

11. **(B)** If a patient has no history of allergies and is having her first allergic reaction, you should treat for shock and transport immediately. (p. 536)

12. **(A)** If a patient has an epinephrine auto-injector, besides helping administer the medication, you should always ask if the patient has any spare auto-injectors for the trip to the hospital just in case you need to contact medical direction again for permission to administer another dose of epinephrine to the patient. (p. 541)

13. **(B)** The location for injection with the auto-injector is the lateral mid-thigh. Injecting epinephrine in the back could cause a pneumothorax. Injection into the buttocks would require too much medication and take too long to act. (p. 538)

14. **(B)** The adult epinephrine auto-injector contains 0.3 mg and the child's contains 0.15 mg, or half the adult dose. The child dose is indicated for children weighing less than 66 pounds. (p. 540)

15. **(B)** Children commonly outgrow allergies as they mature. Infants rarely experience anaphylaxis; anaphylactic reactions are common in *older* children. Parents frequently can provide useful medical history. (p. 542)

16. **(B)** Compared to anaphalaxis, a simple allergic reaction would have local swelling. All the comparisons between anaphalaxis and a simple allergic reaction are shown in Table 22–1. (p. 536)

INSIDE/OUTSIDE

1. During the release of histamine, the following five reactions occur inside the body: (p. 533)
   A) Blood vessel dilation
   B) Decrease in the ability of capillaries to contain fluid
   C) Bronchoconstriction
   D) Production of thick mucus in the lungs
   E) Irritatated nerve endings

2. During the release of histamine, the following four signs can be observed outside the body: (p. 533)
   A) Flushed skin   C) Hives or uticaria
   B) Swelling   D) Wheezing and stridor

COMPLETE THE FOLLOWING

1. The signs and symptoms of allergic reaction or anaphylactic shock can include: (any ten) (p. 534)
   - Itching
   - Hives
   - Flushing
   - Swelling of the face, especially the eyes and lips
   - Warm, tingling feeling in the face, mouth, chest, feet, and hands
   - Feeling of tightness in the throat or chest
   - Cough
   - Rapid breathing
   - Labored breathing/tripod position
   - Noisy breathing
   - Hoarseness
   - Muffled voice
   - Loss of voice entirely
   - Stridor
   - Wheezing
   - Increased heart rate
   - Decreased blood pressure
   - Itchy, watery eyes
   - Headache
   - Runny nose
   - Sense of impending doom
   - Altered mental status
   - Flushed, dry skin or pale, cool, clammy skin
   - Nausea or vomiting
   - Vital signs change to: increased pulse, increased respiration, and decreased blood pressure

2. The important thing to recognize in any presentation is the presence of either respiratory distress or signs and symptoms of shock. (p. ???)

LABEL THE DIAGRAMS (P. 532)

1. Insect bites or stings

2. Food

3. Plants

4. Medications

STREET SCENES DISCUSSION

1. Yes, it would be appropriate, but only with medical direction's permission. It should be injected into the thigh.

2. Yes, it would be appropriate. If ALS will not be on the scene momentarily, then you could plan for an intercept en route.

3. Your priorities would be the patient's ABCs and defibrillation.

CASE STUDY: THE LAKEFRONT EMERGENCY

1. No, there is only one patient.

2. Yes, to the scene, or at least an intercept en route to the hospital due to the breathing difficulty.

3. Because she has breathing difficulty and cannot inhale deeply enough to speak for normal time periods.

4. She is alert and oriented.

©2012 Pearson Education, Inc.
Emergency Care, 12th Ed.

5. The sound is most likely a wheeze, which can be caused by asthma, upper airway obstruction, anaphylaxis, or right heart failure (cor pulmonale).

6. The posture or position of the patient, such as an upright tripod position; intercostal separation or retractions; accessory muscle use; cyanosis; and others.

7. This patient should be given oxygen by a nonrebreather mask at 15 liters per minute.

8. This is a high-priority patient due to her breathing difficulty, and she should be transported rapidly.

9. The position of comfort is generally best. But if she is able to breathe adequately, lay her down to improve her dizziness.

10. SAMPLE (signs and symptoms, allergies, medications, past medical history, last intake, and events leading up to illness).

11. **A.** Epinephrine.
    B) It would be appropriate to assist her with her epinephrine auto-injector (EpiPen®).

12. **A.** You must call medical direction for permission to administer epinephrine to the patient.
    B) Make sure the epinephrine auto-injector is prescribed to the patient, is not expired, and is clear.

13. **A.** Chief complaint is breathing difficulty with chest pain.
    B) OPQRST findings, vital signs, SAMPLE findings.
    C) Treatment given thus far (e.g., oxygen, positioning, epinephrine auto-injector per medical direction).

14. The paramedic would establish an IV, administer saline or Ringer solution, evaluate the need for airway or breathing management, and assess the need for additional epinephrine or other medications such as Benadryl.

Chapter 23: Poisoning and Overdose Emergencies

MATCH TERMINOLOGY/ DEFINITIONS

1. **(D)** Absorbed poisons—poisons that are taken into the body through unbroken skin (p. 548)

2. **(H)** Activated charcoal—a substance that adsorbs many poisons and prevents them from being absorbed by the body (p. 551)

3. **(P)** Antidote—a substance that will neutralize a poison or its effects (p. 553)

4. **(K)** Delirium tremens (DTs)—a severe reaction that can be part of alcohol withdrawal, characterized by sweating, trembling, anxiety, and hallucinations (p. 562)

5. **(I)** Dilution—thinning down or weakening by mixing with something else (p. 552)

6. **(E)** Downers—depressants, such as barbiturates, that depress the central nervous system, often used to bring on a more relaxed state of mind (p. 564)

7. **(M)** Hallucinogens—mind-affecting or mind-altering drugs that act on the central nervous system to produce excitement and distortion of perceptions (p. 565)

8. **(F)** Ingested poisons—poisons that are swallowed (p. 547)

9. **(L)** Inhaled poisons—poisons that are breathed in (p. 547)

10. **(J)** Injected poisons—poisons that are inserted through the skin, for example, by needle, snake fangs, or insect stinger (p. 548)

11. **(G)** Narcotics—a class of drugs that affects the nervous system and changes many normal body activities. Their legal use is for relief of pain; illicit use is to produce an intense state of relaxation. (p. 564)

12. **(A)** Poison—any substance that can harm the body by altering cell structure or functions (p. 546)

13. **(N)** Toxin—a poisonous substance secreted by bacteria, plants, or animals (p. 546)

14. **(B)** Uppers—stimulants, such as amphetamines, that affect the central nervous system to excite the user (p. 563)

15. **(O)** Volatile chemicals—vaporizing compounds, such as cleaning fluid, that are breathed in by an abuser to produce a "high" (p. 565)

16. **(C)** Withdrawal—state in which a patient's body reacts severely when deprived of an abused substance (p. 562)

MULTIPLE-CHOICE REVIEW

1. **(B)** Empty pill bottles or containers are a good environmental clue of poisoning. Just because a patient has vomited, has an altered level of responsiveness, or has a headache does not necessarily indicate poisoning. (p. 549)

2. **(A)** A poison is any substance that can harm the body, sometimes seriously enough to create a medical emergency. (p. 564)

3. **(C)** Although some of the over 1 million cases of poisoning in the United States each year result from murder or suicide attempts, most poisonings are accidental and involve young children. (p. 546)

4. **(B)** A substance secreted by plants, animals, or bacteria that is poisonous to humans is called a toxin. A narcotic is a drug that relieves pain; a drug is a chemical used to treat illness. (p. 546)

5. **(D)** Due to the poisons they produce, plants or fungi such as mistletoe, mushrooms, rubber plants, and holly can be dangerous to humans or pets. (p. 546)

6. **(B)** Botulism is a deadly disease caused by a toxin produced by bacteria. HIV is a virus. Steroids and penicillin are medications that, when used properly, are not deadly. (p. 546)

7. **(B)** Reactions to poisons are most serious in the ill and the elderly. (p. 546)

8. **(B)** Poisons interfere with, but do *not* enhance, the normal biochemical processes in the body. Poisons damage the body by destroying skin and other tissues, overstimulating (or depressing) the central nervous system, and displacing oxygen on the hemoglobin. (p. 547)

9. **(D)** Excretion is not a route of entry to the body but rather is a route of exit. Poisons enter the body through inhalation, ingestion, injection, and absorption. (p. 548)

10. **(C)** Carbon monoxide, chlorine, and ammonia are examples of inhaled poisons. (pp. 556–557)

11. **(A)** Insecticides and agricultural chemicals can be absorbed through the skin. Carbon monoxide and ammonia are inhaled. Insect stings and snake bites are injected. Aspirin and LSD are ingested. (p. 548)

12. **(B)** The venom of a snake bite is an injected poison. (p. 548)

13. **(A)** It is important to determine the time a poison was ingested because different poisons act on the body at different rates. The other answer choices are incorrect statements. (p. 547)

14. (B) If you suspect poisoning by ingestion, first ensure that a child has a patent airway, then ask the parent for the child's weight because the effects of most chemicals are weight dependent. (p. 549)

15. (B) The most common results of poisoning by ingestion are nausea and vomiting. All the other answers are plausible but not the most common. (p. 549)

16. (C) Activated charcoal is used to prevent poisons from being absorbed by the body. It does not speed up the digestion of most chemicals; rather, it prevents digestion. It does not dilute the poison or act as an antidote. (p. 551)

17. (D) The oral medication syrup of ipecac is no longer used by EMTs because it removes only about one-third of the stomach contents, it is slow to work, and the patient could get aspiration pneumonia if his or her mental status diminished and then he or she was to vomit. (pp. 551–552)

18. (C) The decision about when to use activated charcoal is best made with medical direction or poison control center consultation. It is not necessary to wait until the patient gets to the emergency department. The patient's family physician need not be consulted. (pp. 550–551)

19. (D) Activated charcoal is not routinely used with ingestion of caustic substances, strong acids, or strong alkalis. (pp. 550–551)

20. (B) Venom is an injected poison from a snake bite or other animal. Examples of caustic substances include lye, toilet bowl cleaner, and oven cleaner. (p. 559)

21. (A) A patient who continues to cough violently after a gasoline ingestion should not be given activated charcoal because he may aspirate the gasoline into his lungs. (p. 551)

22. (C) When a physician orders dilution of an ingested substance, you can use either water or milk. A cola drink will burn the stomach as well as produce gas from the carbonation. Coffee has caffeine in it, which will speed up the heart. (pp. 552–553)

23. (C) The most common inhaled poison is carbon monoxide. Carbon dioxide is a colorless gas that we exhale. Nitrogen is a gas that makes up about 79 percent of the air. Phosgene is a nerve gas. (pp. 556–557)

24. (A) If you smell an unusual odor as you approach a patient who has passed out while cleaning a large tank, you should stand back and attempt to learn more about the chemical involved. This action will also prevent you or your crew from being overcome by the chemical. (pp. 554–555)

25. (B) The principal prehospital treatment of a patient who has inhaled poison is administering high-concentration oxygen. (p. 555)

26. (C) Besides motor vehicle exhaust, you might also find carbon monoxide around an improperly vented wood-burning stove. Malfunctioning oil-, gas-, and coal-burning furnaces and stoves can also be sources of carbon monoxide. (pp. 556–557)

27. (B) Carbon monoxide affects the body by preventing the normal carrying of oxygen by the red blood cells. It does not cause severe respiratory burns or airway swelling, nor does it stimulate the central nervous system to decrease oxygen consumption. (pp. 556–557)

28. (D) Cherry-red lips are *not* typically seen. A conscious patient who you suspect has carbon monoxide poisoning may exhibit cyanosis, altered mental status, and dizziness. (p. 557)

29. (A) If a patient has been contaminated by poisonous powder, you should brush off as much of the powder as possible, then irrigate after determining that the powder does not react with water. (p. 560)

30. (B) The strong smell of rotten eggs is most likely due to a mixture producing hydrogen sulfide, which can be deadly. (p. 558)

31. (A) Acetone breath is not seen with alcohol abuse but is with diabetes. Do not confuse the odor of alcohol on the breath with acetone breath. (p. 562)

32. (C) Sweating, trembling, anxiety, and hallucinations found in the patient suffering from alcohol withdrawal are called delirium tremens. (p. 562)

33. (B) The patient who has mixed alcohol and other drugs will exhibit with depressed vital signs. (pp. 561–563)

34. (B) When interviewing an intoxicated patient, do not begin by asking if he has taken any drugs because the patient may think you are accusing him of a crime. (p. 561)

35. (A) Drugs that stimulate the nervous system to excite the user are called uppers. (p. 563)

36. (B) Tranquilizers or sleeping pills are examples of downers. (p. 564)

37. (B) Drugs that have a depressant effect on the central nervous system are called downers. (p. 564)

38. (C) Drugs capable of producing stupor or sleep that are often used to relieve pain are called narcotics. Narcotics also depress the respiratory system. (p. 564)

39. (D) Mind-altering drugs that act on the nervous system to produce an intense state of excitement or distortion of the user's perceptions are called hallucinogens. (p. 565)

40. (C) Hallucinogens are a class of drugs that have few legal uses and are dissolved in the mouth. In illegal forms, they are usually found as a colored dot on a piece of paper or in sugar cubes. (p. 565)

41. (B) Cleaning fluid, glue, and model cement are examples of volatile chemicals. Diuretics are medications that tend to increase the flow of urine in order to eliminate excess body fluids. (p. 565)

42. (A) A patient who has overdosed on an upper may have signs and symptoms such as excitement, increased pulse and breathing rates, dilated pupils, and rapid speech. (p. 563)

43. (B) A patient who has overdosed on a downer may have signs and symptoms such as sluggishness, sleepiness, and lack of coordination of body and speech. (p. 564)

44. (C) A patient who has overdosed on a hallucinogen may have signs and symptoms such as a fast pulse rate, dilated pupils, and a flushed face, and may be "seeing" or "hearing" things. (p. 565)

45. (D) A patient who has overdosed on a narcotic may have signs and symptoms such as reduced pulse rate and rate and depth of breathing, constricted pupils, and sweating. (p. 564)

INSIDE/OUTSIDE

1. The patient who overdoses on acetaminophen is likely to have irreparable liver damage on the "inside." (p. 554)

2. The patient who overdoses on acetaminophen is likely to experience loss of appetite, nausea, and vomiting during the first 4 to 12 hours on the outside." (p. 554)

COMPLETE THE FOLLOWING

1. If you suspect poisoning, document the following information: (p. 549)

   A) Route of poisoning
   B) Substance
   C) Amount
   D) Time

   E. Interventions
   F. Patient's weight
   G. Effects of poisoning
   H. Effects of treatment

2. The signs and symptoms of alcohol abuse include: (any six) (p. 562)
   - Odor of alcohol on a patient's breath or clothing
   - Swaying and unsteadiness of movement
   - Slurred speech
   - A flushed appearance to the face
   - Nausea or vomiting
   - Poor coordination
   - Slowed reaction time
   - Blurred vision
   - Confusion
   - Hallucinations
   - Lack of memory
   - Altered mental status

3. The phone number for the poison control center is 1–800-222-1222. (p. 559)

LABEL THE DIAGRAMS (P. 548)

1. Inhalation
2. Injection
3. Ingestion
4. Absorption

COMPLETE THE CHART (P. 565)

1. Upper
2. Narcotic
3. Mind-altering
4. Mind-altering
5. Volatile chemical
6. Downer
7. Downer
8. Upper
9. Upper
10. Downer
11. Mind-altering
12. Mind-altering
13. Mind-altering
14. Narcotic
15. Volatile chemical
16. Mind-altering
17. Narcotic
18. Narcotic
19. Downer
20. Narcotic
21. Downer
22. Mind-altering
23. Narcotic
24. Volatile chemical
25. Volatile chemical

STREET SCENES DISCUSSION

1. No, do not give activated charcoal to any patient with an altered mental status.

2. Your highest priority should be to keep the patient's airway clear and patent.

3. It is necessary to take the oil to the hospital so that hospital chemists can identify the substance that was ingested.

CASE STUDY: NOT A FUN PARTY FOR EVERYONE!

1. The first priority is to make sure the airway is open and clear.

2. The raspy cough and gurgling may indicate fluid in the airway and she needs to be suctioned.

3. If ALS is available, they should be called.

4. This is a high-priority call.

5. Rule out aspiration of a foreign substance.

6. This is a critical patient and she should be taken right to the ED.

7. Neither syrup of ipecac nor activated charcoal would be indicated due to the depressed mental status of the patient. The patient could regurgitate and possibly aspirate the stomach contents.

Chapter 24: Abdominal Emergencies

MATCH TERMINOLOGY/ DEFINITIONS

1. **(D)** Parietal pain—a localized intense pain from the peritoneum, which lines the abdominal cavity (p. 574)

2. **(E)** Peritoneum—the abdominal cavity (parietal) and covering of the organs with it (visceral) (p. 572)

3. **(A)** Referred pain—pain that is felt in a location other than where the pain originates (p. 574)

4. **(B)** Tearing pain—sharp pain that feels as if the body tissues are being torn apart (p. 574)

5. **(C)** Visceral pain—a poorly localized, dull, or diffuse pain that arises from the abdominal viscera (p. 574)

MULTIPLE-CHOICE REVIEW

1. **(B)** The membrane that covers the abdominal organs is called the visceral peritoneum. (p. 572)

2. **(C)** The organs outside the peritoneum that are found between the abdomen and the back are in the retroperitoneal space. (p. 572)

3. **(D)** Pain originating from an organ in the abdomen is called visceral. (p. 574)

4. **(D)** Pain from an organ is often described as intermittent, dull, achy, or diffuse. (p. 572)

5. **(C)** A patient with colicky pain is often experiencing visceral pain from a hollow organ in the abdomen. (p. 574)

6. **(B)** It is common for the patient who has a gallbladder attack to complain of pain in his right shoulder blade because nerve pathways from the gallbladder return to the spinal cord by way of shared pathways with the shoulder. (p. 575)

7. **(A)** If the patient has a chief complaint of abdominal discomfort, the last oral intake would be an important part of the SAMPLE history to ask because the food eaten may have been spoiled. (p. 580)

8. **(B)** An EMT who asks a young adult female patient who is complaining of abdominal discomfort where she is in her menstrual cycle is doing this to begin to focus on the possibility of an ectopic pregnancy. (p. 580)

9. **(A)** Palpate the painful quadrant of the abdomen last. (p. 581)

10. **(B)** When managing a patient who has a complaint of abdominal pain and has no difficulty breathing, yet has signs consistent with shock or hypoperfusion, the EMT should administer 10–15 lpm oxygen by nonrebreather mask. (pp. 583–584)

11. **(C)** The tearing sensation in the back, in the absence of any trauma, is most likely from an abdominal aortic aneurysm (AAA). (pp. 575–576)

12. **(B)** When a patient has sudden epigastic pain radiating to the shoulder, consider AMI. If it is associated with eating, especially fried foods, consider gallstones or cholecystitis. (p. 575)

13. **(D)** A patient writhing in pain or doing the uncomfortable dance due to back pain is most likely suffering from kidney stones or renal colic. (p. 577)

14. **(B)** The key points here are that the patient is young, most likely healthy, and participating in gym, and he may have injured himself lifting something very heavy. This is most likely a hernia. (pp. 576–577)

15. **(C)** Weakness; dizziness; and dark, tarry-looking diarrhea are often an indication of a bleeding stomach ulcer and a patient in shock. (p. 575)

COMPLETE THE FOLLOWING

1. List four solid structures (organs) of the abdomen. (p. 571)
   A) Liver   C) Spleen
   B) Kidney   D) Pancreas

2. List six hollow structures (organs) of the abdomen. (p. 571)
   A) Appendix   D) Stomach
   B) Large intestine E) Bladder
   C) Small intestine F) Gallbladder

3. When doing an assessment on a female patient with a chief complaint of abdominal pain, what five questions are important to ask? (p. 580)
   A) Where are you in your menstrual cycle?
   B) Is your period late?
   C) Do you have bleeding from the vagina now that is not menstrual bleeding?
   D) If you are menstruating, is the flow normal?
   E) Have you had this pain before?

LABEL THE DIAGRAM (P. 571)

▶ **SOLID ORGANS**
   A) Spleen
   B) Liver
   C) Pancreas
   D) Kidneys

▶ **HOLLOW ORGANS**
   A) Stomach
   B) Gallbladder
   C) Duodenum
   D) Large intestine
   E) Small intestine
   F) Bladder

STREET SCENES DISCUSSION

1. If the patient was 25 years old instead of 72 years old, you should definitely consider a complication of early pregnancy or an ectopic pregnancy, both of which can be life threatening to the patient and fetus.

2. If, when examining the patient's abdomen, you noticed that she has a pulsating mass and she complains of a tearing sensation in her abdomen radiating into her back, there is a good chance she may have an abdominal aortic aneurysm (AAA). This is a high priority because the patient will die if it bursts.

3. If the patient suddenly begins to complain of pain in the epigastric area and breaks out in a cold sweat, think acute myocardial infarction (AMI) and treat for it!

Chapter 25: Behavioral and Psychiatric Emergencies and Suicide

MATCH TERMINOLOGY/ DEFINITIONS

1. **(B)** Behavior—the manner in which a person acts (p. 588)

2. **(D)** Behavioral emergency—when a patient's behavior is not typical for the situation; when the patient's behavior is unacceptable or intolerable to the patient, his family, or the community; or when the patient may harm himself or others (p. 588)

3. **(A)** Excited delirium—bizarre and/or aggressive behavior, shouting, paranoia, panic, violence toward others, insensitivity to pain, unexpected physical strength, and hyperthermia, usually associated with cocaine or amphetamine use (p. 595)

4. **(C)** Positional asphyxia—inadequate breathing or respiratory arrest caused by a body position that restricts breathing (p. 597)

MULTIPLE-CHOICE REVIEW

1. **(D)** Differing lifestyles are not a *physical* cause of altered behavior. The behaviors of persons from other cultures and with different lifestyles may seem unusual to you but might be quite normal to the person performing them. (p. 589)

2. **(C)** Hypoactivity is a distracter and an incorrect response. Altered behavior ranging from irritability to altered mental status can be due to lack of oxygen (hypoxia), head trauma, or hypoglycemia. (p. 591)

3. **(C)** To calm a patient who is experiencing a stress reaction, you should explain things to the patient honestly. Do not lie because this will lead to mistrust of anything you say or do. Quick movements not only confuse but will scare the patient, not calm him. You, not the patient, should control the situation. Quickly restraining the patient will not calm him and should be used only as a last resort. (p. 590)

4. **(B)** Rather than having a neat appearance, a patient experiencing a behavioral emergency is more likely to have an unusual appearance, disordered clothing, or poor hygiene. In addition, he may exhibit panic and anxiety; agitated or unusual activity, such as repetitive motions; and unusual speech patterns, such as pressured-sounding speech. (p. 591)

5. **(B)** When you are called to care for a patient who has attempted suicide or is about to attempt suicide, your first concern must be your own safety. Once you ensure your safety, treat the patient as you would other patients. (pp. 593–594)

6. **(A)** Of the age groups listed, the highest suicide rates occur at ages 15–25. The other group with a high suicide rate consists of those over 40. Also, suicides among the elderly are increasing. (pp. 592–593)

7. **(C)** Most suicidal patients will not deny suicidal thoughts but rather will express them and tell others they are considering suicide. Take all threats of suicide seriously. Examples of a self-destructive activity include a defined lethal plan of action that has been verbalized, giving away personal possessions, and previous suicide threats. (pp. 592–593)

8. **(C)** A patient who has made the decision to commit suicide may actually appear to be coming out of depression, or improving. The fact that the decision has been made and an end is in sight can cause this apparent improvement. (p. 593)

9. **(D)** Stay out of kitchens when dealing with an aggressive patient. Kitchens are filled with dangerous weapons. Stay in a safe area until the police can control the scene. When assessing an aggressive patient for a possible threat to you or your crew, determine the patient's history of aggressive behavior, and pay attention to the patient's vocal activity (is he shouting at you?) and the patient's posture (watch body language). (pp. 594–595)

10. **(A)** If a patient stands in a corner of the room with fists clenched, screaming obscenities, you should request police backup and keep the doorway in sight. Raising your voice or challenging him could force a confrontation. Explaining that you would respond to the situation in the same way is simply being dishonest. (pp. 594–595)

11. **(B)** The family's ability to pay for services is not a consideration in evaluating whether to restrain a patient. Use of reasonable force to restrain a patient should involve an evaluation of the patient's size and strength, the mental state of the patient, and the available methods of restraint. (p. 595)

12. **(A)** The use of force by an EMT is allowed in most states in order to defend against an attack by an emotionally disturbed patient. While the police do not need to be present, it is very desirable to involve them. The fact that a patient has been drinking or refuses care does not take away his decision-making rights. (p. 595)

13. **(D)** Four rescuers, not two, should be used to secure a disturbed patient. This allows one rescuer to control each limb. Monitor all restrained patients carefully. (p. 596)

14. **(D)** Apply a surgical mask, but ensure that the patient is not likely to vomit or does not have breathing difficulties before applying. Placing the patient in a prone position may limit, but will not eliminate, the patient's ability to spit. Never place roller gauze or tape over a patient's mouth due to the risk of aspiration. (p. 596)

15. **(C)** When a patient is a danger to himself and others and needs to be transported against his will, the EMT should contact the police for assistance. Most states have a legal provision that allows such a patient to be transported and gives this authority to law enforcement personnel. Know your laws on treating patients without consent. (pp. 595–596)

INSIDE/OUTSIDE (P. 592)

1. The purpose of a neurotransmitter is to help the electrical impulses travel from one neuron across the synapse to the next nerve cell.

2. Medications such as Prozac®, Paxil®, and Zoloft® are in a class of medication called serotonin selective reuptake inhibitors (SSRIs). These medications are used to treat depression and other mental disorders by elevating the patient's mood. This is done by preventing the reuptake of the neurotransmitter serotonin.

COMPLETE THE FOLLOWING

1. Risk factors for suicide include the following: (p. 593)
   A) Depression
   B) High current or recent stress levels
   C) Recent emotional trauma
   D) Age (high rates at ages 15 to 25 and over 40)
   E) Alcohol and drug abuse
   F) Threats of suicide
   G) Suicide plans
   H) Previous attempts or suicide threats; history of self-destructive behavior
   I) Sudden improvement from depression

2. When a patient acts as if he may hurt himself or others, you should take the following precautions: (pp. 593–594)
   A) Do not isolate yourself from your partner or other sources of help.
   B) Do not take any action that may be considered threatening by the patient.
   C) Always be on the watch for weapons.

3. The behaviors you can expect to see in an aggressive or hostile patient include the following: (p. 594)
   A) Responds to people inappropriately
   B) Tries to hurt himself or others
   C) May have a rapid pulse and breathing
   D) Usually displays rapid speech and rapid physical movements
   E) May appear anxious, nervous, "panicky"

CASE STUDY: TODAY IS NOT THE DAY TO DIE

1. Take Standard Precautions and then, after ensuring the airway is open and breathing is adequate (the patient is talking to you), control the bleeding with a pressure bandage.

2. Apply direct pressure, then elevation and a pressure bandage. If this does not work, it may be necessary to consider the need for a tourniquet or pressure point depending on your local Medical Director's policies.

3. The oozing is probably coming from a capillary, and the flowing is probably venous. Arteries often will spurt at least till the systolic BP drops.

4. Yes, definitely, and document the answer on the PCR in "quotes."

5. Explain to him why it is essential that he needs to be taken to the hospital to deal with the wounds.

6. With enough help (one per extremity and one for the head) and with care to avoid hurting the rescuers and the EMS providers.

STREET SCENES DISCUSSION

1. Restraint is the responsibility of law enforcement. However, while law enforcement officers call and wait for backup, you may offer your assistance. Remember: Never assist unless there are sufficient personnel to do the job. You must be able to ensure your own safety and the safety of the patient. If you do assist, make certain the restraints used are humane.

2. The most humane form of restraint is a roller bandage or a sheet and tape. Leather restraints are also helpful. Metal and plastic handcuffs cut and rip the skin and should not be carried by EMTs.

3. No, you may need to convince the patient that taking vital signs is part of your normal routine, but do not skip them. Remember: There could be more than just a behavioral problem.

Chapter 26: Hematologic and Renal Emergencies

MATCH TERMINOLOGY/ DEFINITIONS

1. **(D)** Anemia—lack of a normal number of red blood cells in the circulation (p. 603)

2. **(C)** Continuous ambulatory peritoneal dialysis (CAPD)—a gravity exchange process for peritoneal dialysis in which a bag of dialysis fluid is raised above the level of an abdominal catheter to fill the abdominal cavity and lowered below the level of the abdominal catheter to drain the fluid out (p. 609)

3. **(B)** Continuous cycle-assisted peritoneal dialysis (CCPD)—a mechanical process for peritoneal dialysis in which a machine fills and empties the abdominal cavity of dialysis solution (p. 609)

4. **(E)** Dialysis—the process by which toxins and excess fluid are removed from the body by a medical system independent of the kidneys (p. 607)

5. **(A)** End-stage renal disease (ESRD)—irreversible renal failure to the extent that the kidneys can no longer provide adequate filtration and fluid balance to sustain life; survival with ESRD usually requires dialysis (p. 607)

6. **(J)** Exchange—one cycle of filling and draining the peritoneal cavity in peritoneal dialysis (p. 609)

7. **(I)** Peritonitis—bacterial infection within the peritoneal cavity (p. 611)

8. **(G)** Renal failure—loss of the kidneys' ability to filter the blood and remove toxins and excess fluid from the body (p. 607)

9. **(F)** Sickle cell anemia (SCA)—an inherited disease in which a genetic defect in the hemoglobin results in abnormal structure of the red blood cells (p. 603)

10. **(H)** Thrill—a vibration felt on gentle palpation, like the vibration that typically occurs within an arterial-venous fistula (p. 608)

MULTIPLE-CHOICE REVIEW

1. **(B)** Nephrology is the medical specialty that deals with the kidneys. (p. 602)

2. **(A)** The removal of oxygen from the cells is not a function of the blood; the blood brings oxygen to the cells. (pp. 602–603)

3. **(C)** The medical specialty concerned with blood disorders is called hematology. (p. 602)

4. **(C)** The white blood cells are a critical component of the blood and a critical component in the body's response to infection. (p. 602)

5. **(B)** The component of the blood that is designed to aggregate as a response to a bleeding injury is the platelets. (p. 602)

6. **(B)** The liquid in which the blood cells and platelets are suspended is called the plasma. (p. 603)

7. **(B)** The patient is a male, so it is not due to a menstrual period in this patient. A slow GI bleed could be the cause of a chronic anemia. (p. 603)

8. **(C)** Patients with sickle cell anemia often damage their spleen and may need to have it removed. The pain in the arms, legs, and abdomen is likely due to a sickle cell crisis. (pp. 603–605)

9. **(D)** Complications of a sickle cell crisis can include destruction of the spleen, acute chest syndrome, and priapism. (p. 605)

10. **(D)** The emergency treatment of the patient having a sickle cell crisis includes high-flow supplemental oxygen, monitoring for a high fever, and treating for shock if it develops. (p. 605)

11. **(B)** The patient with a long history of poorly controlled diabetes and hypertension is likely to die from an acute coronary syndrome, a stroke, or renal failure. (p. 607)

12. **(A)** When a patient has been trapped in a building for several days, he may sustain dehydration, shock, and acute renal failure. Chronic renal failure does not come on suddenly. (p. 607)

13. **(C)** Dialysis is the process by which an external medical system independent of the kidneys is used to remove toxins and excess fluid from the body. (p. 607)

14. **(C)** The kidney patient who goes to the clinic three times a week is likely getting hemodialysis. (pp. 607–608)

15. **(A)** A thrill is a vibration that can be palpated at the fistula in the arm of the dialysis patient. (p. 608)

16. **(D)** The symptoms that the patient may exhibit include shortness of breath; fluid in the lungs; and swollen ankles, hands, and face. (p. 610)

17. **(A)** The most commonly transported organ(s) are the kidneys. (p. 611)

18. **(A)** Development of an aortic aneurism is not a typical complication of dialysis. (p. 610)

COMPLETE THE FOLLOWING

1. List the two types of peritoneal dialysis. (p. 609)
   A) Continuous ambulatory peritoneal dialysis (CAPD)
   B) Continuous cycle-assisted peritoneal dialysis (CCPD)

2. What is the difference between the two types of peritoneal dialysis? (p. 609)

A) CAPD is the most common type. The fluid is left in the peritoneal cavity by clamping the catheter for 4 to 6 hours, and the patient repeats the exchange several times a day.
B) CCPD uses the same type of peritoneal catheter as is used in CAPD, but rather than using a gravity exchange, a machine is used to fill and empty the abdominal cavity with dialysis fluid three to five times during the night while the person sleeps. In the morning, the last fill remains in the abdomen with a dwell time that lasts the entire day.

STREET SCENES DISCUSSION

1. If the assessment of the patient shows that the blood glucose was 68 mg/dl, you will need to consider contacting medical control for consideration of glucose administration as well as contact ALS.

2. If the patient had a facial droop and weakness on the right side of the body, you should consider a potential stroke. It would make a lot of sense to administer oxygen, monitor the airway very closely, and transport to a stroke center.

3. If the patient had obvious pulmonary edema and red, frothy sputum, the patient is a high priority and may need Fowler position, oxygen administration, possibly BVM assist, and potentially CPAC and ALS.

Interim Exam 2

1. (D) The primary assessment includes assessing the airway, mental status, and circulation, as well as breathing. Blood pressure is a vital sign taken during the focused history and physical exam. (p. 265)

2. (B) Evaluating extremity mobility is not part of the primary assessment. Determining patient priority, forming a general impression, and assessing breathing are all part of the primary assessment. (p. 265)

3. (B) Environmental clues during the general impression of a child include recognizing that the child is holding pieces of a toy (perhaps he or she swallowed one of the pieces). Vital signs and associated signs or symptoms such as nausea are not part of the general impression. (p. 267)

4. (C) The patient's position, age, sex, sounds he or she is making, and smells from the environment are part of the general impression. Vital signs are not. (p. 267)

5. (B) Assessing mental status is the step of the primary assessment that comes after the general impression. (p. 265)

6. (C) AVPU stands for *A*lert, response to *V*erbal stimulus, response to *P*ainful stimulus, *U*nresponsive. (p. 272)

7. (B) See the answer for multiple-choice question 6. (p. 272)

8. (D) The lowest and most serious mental status is U, or unresponsive. (p. 272)

9. (B) If a patient's level of responsiveness is lower than Alert, you should at least administer high-concentration oxygen by nonrebreather mask. Consider this patient a high-priority transport. (p. 272)

10. (C) If a patient is talking or crying, assume an open airway. This condition may change, however, so you need to monitor the patient. (p. 272)

11. (C) If the patient is not alert and his or her breathing rate is slower than 8 breaths per minute, use a bag-valve mask to assist the ventilations. (p. 271)

12. (B) Pale and clammy skin indicates poor circulation, or shock. (p. 271)

13. (A) A patient who gives a poor general impression is a *high* priority. (p. 267)

14. (B) The patient whose only complaint is nausea and vomiting is not generally considered a high priority. (p. 278)

15. (A) The primary assessment varies depending on the age of the patient and whether there is a medical or trauma problem. The medical history does not change the primary assessment. (p. 274)

16. (C) The capillary refill test is used to evaluate the circulation of infants and children but is no longer advocated as an effective, reliable test for adults. (p. 283)

17. (B) Check the mental status of an unconscious infant by talking to the infant and flicking the infant's feet. The sternal rub would be too aggressive and could cause injury. (p. 283)

18. (B) A fever and a rash are not generally considered high priority. However, don't forget to take Standard Precautions and consider the need for a mask when treating such conditions. (p. 278)

19. (A) The difference between the general impression steps for a medical patient and those of a trauma patient is the need to provide manual stabilization of the head if you suspect spine injury in the trauma patient. (p. 280)

20. (C) Documenting examination findings that are negative (things that are not true) is called documenting a pertinent negative. (p. 411)

21. (D) When writing the PCR narrative section, do not state your personal opinion of the patient's condition. Only relevant facts, not subjective statements, should be documented. (pp. 410–411)

22. (B) An important concept of EMS documentation is "if it is not written down, you did not do it." The presumption is that, at the time of the incident, you had the opportunity to document everything that you observed and treated. (p. 411)

23. (A) If a patient does not wish to go to the hospital, document with a refusal-of-care form. Be sure to consult medical direction whenever there is a patient refusal. (pp. 412–413)

24. (B) Failure to perform an important part of patient assessment or care is an error of omission. Errors of commission are performing actions that are wrong or improper. (p. 413)

25. (C) Making up vitals is falsification and could endanger the patient's care. (pp. 413–415)

26. (C) An objective statement describes something that is measurable, observable, or verifiable, such as vital signs. (pp. 410–411)

27. (A) Stating that "the patient is alert and oriented" is an example of objective information that you observe but the patient does not tell you. (pp. 410–411)

28. (D) Statements from patients, bystanders, or family should be put in quotes on the PCR. (pp. 410–411)

29. (A) Statements about the rudeness of the family members are usually not relevant or needed on the PCR. (pp. 410–411)

30. (A) After establishing unresponsiveness in the primary assessment, proceed to open the airway. (p. 267)

31. (A) The term *sixth sense* refers to an EMT's clinical judgment, which is developed with experience. (p. 272)

32. (B) The vital signs are pulse; respirations; blood pressure; pupils; and skin condition, color, and temperature. (p. 291)

33. (B) The normal adult pulse rate at rest is between 60 and 100. (p. 293)

34. (D) The initial pulse rate for patients 1 year and older is normally taken at the radial pulse. (p. 294)

35. (D) A weak and thin pulse force is described as thready. (p. 294)

36. (B) Normal adult at-rest respiration rates vary from 12 to 20 breaths per minute. (p. 296)

37. (D) Crowing is a noisy, harsh sound heard during inhalation that indicates a partial airway obstruction. A gurgling sound is caused by fluid in the airway, which requires suctioning. (pp. 295–296)

38. (C) The systolic blood pressure is the arterial pressure created when the left ventricle of the heart contracts. (p. 299)

39. (B) Diastolic blood pressure is the arterial pressure created by relaxation and refilling of the left ventricle of the heart. (p. 299)

40. (B) Using a stethoscope along with a sphygmomanometer to take the blood pressure is a technique called auscultation. (pp. 301–303)

41. (A) Determining blood pressure by palpation is not as accurate as the auscultation method. This procedure is used when there is lots of noise around a patient. It is documented as the systolic reading. (pp. 304–305)

42. (A) Information that you see, hear, feel, and smell is a sign and can be measured. Information the patient tells you is a symptom. (p. 321)

43. (B) When you ask the patient, "Have you recently had any surgery or injuries?" you are inquiring about the patient's pertinent past history. (pp. 356–357)

44. (A) When you ask the patient, "Are you on birth control pills?" you are inquiring about the patient's medications. This may give some clues about the patient's present problem. (pp. 356–357)

45. (C) An acronym used to remember what questions to ask about the patient's present problem and past history is SAMPLE. AVPU is the level of responsiveness, PEARL is the status of the pupils, and DCAP-BTLS helps remind the EMT what to look for in a soft-tissue exam. (p. 356)

46. (D) When conducting a patient interview on an adult patient, the EMT should position himself close to the patient, identify himself, reassure the patient, and gently touch the patient's shoulder or rest a hand over the patient's. It is necessary to ask the patient's age. (pp. 401–402)

47. (D) Normal diastolic pressures range from 60 to 90 mmHg. (p. 301)

48. (C) Using the formula presented in the text, a 36-year-old man would have an estimated systolic blood pressure of 136 mmHg (100 + age). (p. 301)

49. (B) Using the formula presented in the text, a 26-year-old woman would have an estimated systolic blood pressure of 116 mmHg (90 + age). (p. 301)

50. (A) The stethoscope should *not* be placed under the cuff and then inflate the cuff when evaluating the blood pressure because it may give a false reading. (p. 302)

51. (C) When taking a patient's blood pressure, the stethoscope is placed over the brachial artery. The femoral artery is in the leg. (p. 302)

52. (C) The mechanism of injury (MOI) is the best indication of potential injury. (p. 326)

53. (B) When there are no apparent hazards at the scene of a collision, the danger zone should extend 50 feet in all directions from the wreckage. (p. 248)

54. (C) In the up-and-over (head-on) injury pattern, the patient is most likely to sustain head injuries. Chest and neck injuries are also common. Leg, knee, and hip injuries are usually the result of a down-and-under injury pattern. (pp. 254–256)

55. (C) A keen awareness that there may be injuries based on the mechanism of injury (MOI) is called index of suspicion. (p. 253)

56. (C) The purpose of the primary assessment is to discover and treat life-threatening conditions. (p. 267)

57. (C) The first step in the physical exam of *any* trauma patient is to reconsider the mechanism of injury (MOI). (pp. 327–330)

58. (C) The A in DCAP-BTLS stands for "abrasions." (p. 320)

59. (D) Clues to determining the patient's need for a cervical collar include mechanism of injury (MOI), level of responsiveness, and location of injuries. The breathing rate will not assist in determining the need for a cervical collar. (p. 253)

60. (B) The rapid assessment evaluates areas of the body where the greatest threats to the patient may be. (pp. 332–340)

61. (A) The detailed (secondary) exam is most often performed on the trauma patient with a significant mechanism of injury (MOI). (p. 316)

62. (A) To obtain a history of a patient's present illness, ask the OPQRST questions. These questions focus on the chief complaint and potential causes. (p. 354)

63. (C) The P in OPQRST stands for "provokes," which refers to questions such as "Can you think of anything that might have triggered this pain?" (p. 354)

64. (A) The correct order of the steps in the focused history and physical exam of the unresponsive medical patient is conduct a rapid physical exam, obtain baseline vital signs, gather the history of the present illness (OPQRST) from bystanders and family, and gather a SAMPLE history from bystanders and family. (p. 363)

65. (C) For a stable patient, the EMT should perform the reassessment every 15 minutes. For an unstable patient, the EMT should perform the reassessment every 5 minutes. (p. 376)

66. (A) During the reassessment, whenever you believe there may have been a change in the patient's condition, you should repeat the primary assessment. (p. 376)

67. (D) Cool, clammy skin most likely indicates shock. Exposure to cold causes dry, cold skin. Fever results in clammy and warm or hot skin. (p. 297)

68. (D) As an EMT, your overriding concern at all times is your own safety. Certainly your crew's safety is a priority, but your personal safety *must* come first. (p. 244)

69. (A) During the detailed (secondary) physical exam of the head of a trauma patient, inspect the ears and nose for blood or clear fluids. (p. 332)

70. (C) Infants and young children under the age of 8 are abdominal breathers. (p. 882)

71. (B) Repeaters are devices used when radio transmissions must be carried over long distances. (p. 395)

72. **(C)** If possible, position yourself at or below the patient's eye level. This position will be less threatening to the patient. (pp. 401–403)

73. **(B)** The first item given to the hospital in your medical radio report to the receiving facility is your unit identification/level of provider. (p. 398)

74. **(D)** The patient's attitude is not an essential component of the verbal report to the receiving hospital. (pp. 398–400)

75. **(C)** Medical radio reports should paint a picture of the patient's problem in words. (pp. 398–400)

76. **(D)** Always question orders from medical direction that you do not understand. (pp. 398–400)

77. **(A)** Medications that are carried on the ambulance and that EMTs can administer include activated charcoal, oxygen, oral glucose, and aspirin. Nitroglycerin, epinephrine, and the prescribed inhaler are medications that the EMT may assist the patient with administration. (pp. 425–427)

78. **(D)** Any action of a drug other than the desired action is called a side effect. (p. 432)

79. **(D)** Administering a drug subcutaneously means that the drug is injected under the skin. (p. 434)

80. **(D)** Infants and children depend more on the diaphragm for respiration than adults do. (p. 881)

81. **(A)** The order of preference for the steps in providing artificial ventilation are pocket face mask with supplemental oxygen; two-person bag-valve mask with supplemental oxygen; flow-restricted, oxygen-powered ventilator; and one-person bag-valve mask with supplemental oxygen. (p. 208)

82. **(B)** The adequate rate of artificial ventilation for a nonbreathing adult patient is 10–12 breaths per minute. (p. 206)

83. **(C)** The adequate rate of artificial ventilation for a nonbreathing infant or child patient is 12–20 breaths per minute. (p. 206)

84. **(A)** If an unresponsive adult makes snoring or gurgling sounds, he or she most likely has a serious airway problem requiring immediate intervention. (p. 203)

85. **(D)** The skin of a patient with inadequate breathing may be blue (or pale) in color and will feel cool and clammy. (p. 203)

86. **(C)** If a patient is experiencing breathing difficulty but is breathing adequately, it is usually best to place him in a position of comfort. This is generally a sitting-up position. (p. 203)

87. **(D)** The cause of adult chest pain due to a decreased blood supply to the heart is angina pectoris. Arrhythmia is an irregular heart rhythm. (p. 479)

88. **(C)** Most heart attacks are caused by narrowing or occlusion of a coronary artery. The coronary arteries supply the heart muscle with blood. (p. 480)

89. **(D)** Acute myocardial infarction is the condition in which a portion of the heart muscle dies because of oxygen starvation. (p. 480)

90. **(B)** An irregular or absent heart rhythm is called arrhythmia. (pp. 486–487)

91. **(A)** A pulse slower than 60 beats per minute is called bradycardia. (p. 502)

92. **(C)** An at-rest heart beat faster than 100 beats per minute is referred to as tachycardia. (p. 503)

93. **(A)** Congestive heart failure is the condition caused by excessive fluid build-up in the lungs and/or other organs and body parts because of inadequate pumping of the heart. (p. 502)

94. **(D)** A conscious patient with a possible heart attack is best placed in the position of comfort. For ease of breathing, this is usually a sitting position. (pp. 472–475)

95. **(A)** A diabetic found with a weak, rapid pulse and cold, clammy skin who complains of hunger pangs is probably suffering from hypoglycemia. Hyperglycemic patients often have warm, red, dry skin and an acetone breath. (pp. 516–524)

96. **(B)** In hyperglycemia, the patient's breath smells like acetone. (pp. 507–511)

97. **(A)** A conscious, hypoglycemic patient who is able to swallow is frequently administered oral glucose, with permission given by medical direction or standing orders. (pp. 513–516)

98. **(C)** If you cannot administer glucose to the diabetic patient because she is not awake enough to swallow, you should treat her like any other patient with altered mental status. Secure the airway, provide artificial ventilations if necessary, and be prepared to perform CPR if needed. (pp. 513–516)

99. **(C)** The first time a person is exposed to an allergen, the person's immune system forms antibodies. (pp. 531–532)

100. **(C)** To be considered a severe allergic reaction, a patient must have signs and symptoms of shock or respiratory distress. (p. 533)

101. **(B)** If a patient has no history of allergies and is having his first allergic reaction, you should treat for shock and transport immediately. (pp. 535–538)

102. **(C)** Carbon monoxide, chlorine, and ammonia are examples of inhaled poisons. (p. 547)

103. **(A)** It is important for the EMT to determine when the ingestion of a poison occurred because different poisons act on the body at different rates. (p. 549)

104. **(B)** The principal prehospital treatment of a patient who has inhaled poison is administering high-concentration oxygen. (pp. 554–556)

105. **(B)** If mixing alcohol and other drugs, patients exhibit with depressed vital signs. (pp. 561–563)

106. **(D)** Activated charcoal is contraindicated for patients who have ingested alkalis, gasoline, or acids. (pp. 550–553)

107. **(C)** Most cases of poisoning involve young children. (pp. 546–547)

108. **(C)** Poisons that are swallowed are ingested poisons. (p. 549)

109. **(B)** A gravity exchange process for peritoneal dialysis in which a bag of dialysis fluid is raised above the level of an abdominal catheter to fill the abdominal cavity and lowered below the level of the abdominal catheter to drain the fluid out is called continuous ambulatory peritoneal dialysis. (pp. 608–609)

110. **(C)** The dialysis patient who has extreme abdominal pain and a fever, and has not been feeling well since she got home from the clinic, could be developing peritonitis. (p. 610)

111. **(D)** A thrill is common in the arm used for dialysis. It is a vibration felt on palpation, which typically occurs within an arterial-venous fistula. (p. 608)

112. **(B)** Common presentations of patients experiencing psychiatric emergencies include panic or anxiety, suicidal or self-destructive behavior, and unusual speech patterns (i.e., too rapid or pressured-sounding speech). (pp. 590–591)

113. **(A)** Emergency care of a patient having a behavioral or psychiatric emergency includes each of the following: encourage the patient to discuss what is troubling him or her, do not lie to the patient, and be prepared to spend time talking to the patient. It is best to limit the physical contact with these patients. (p. 592)

114. **(A)** In a limited number of situations, you may have to utilize force. The use of force by an EMT is allowed when the EMT needs to defend him- or herself against an attack by an emotionally disturbed patient. (pp. 595–597)

115. **(B)** The organs found outside the peritoneum that are found between the abdomen and the back are in the retroperitoneal space. (pp. 572–573)

116. **(C)** The spleen is located in the upper left abdominal quadrant. (p. 572)

117. **(D)** Your 60-year-old male may have an abdominal aortic aneurysm if he tells you that he has a tearing sensation going into the middle of his back, no back problems, and a history of hypertension. (p. 573)

118. **(B)** The patient probably has a bleeding ulcer if he tells you that he has a history of alcoholism; stomach pains; weakness and dizziness, vomiting; and a very dark, foul-smelling diarrhea all day. (pp. 574–577)

119. **(D)** Your first step when called to care for any attempted suicide victim is to ensure your own safety. This may mean waiting for police assistance, depending on the circumstances of the suicide attempt. (pp. 593–594)

120. **(C)** If you are unable to perform normal assessment and care procedures because the patient is aggressive and hostile, you should seek advice from medical direction. (p. 594)

121. **(B)** The EMT is allowed to use reasonable force to defend against attack by an emotionally disturbed patient. (pp. 595–597)

122. **(A)** EMTs do not normally administer fluids to patients unless they have received special training. (pp. 385–386)

123. **(C)** When a patient presents with more than one condition or a familiar condition but under unusual circumstances, the EMT should assess the patient as usual and then seek advice if necessary. (pp. 15–16)

124. **(A)** When a patient tells you that he has a disease with which you are unfamiliar, it is best to respond by saying, "I'm not familiar with that disease. Could you tell me more about it?" (pp. 15–16)

125. **(C)** When a patient has two or more medical conditions that are presenting symptoms at the same time, it is a good idea to consult with medical direction for advice. (pp. 15–16)

126. **(D)** The patient with slurred speech may have had a cardiovascular accident, an overdose, or a seizure. (pp. 520–522)

127. **(C)** Patients who have had a seizure generally do not have chest pain. (pp. 516–527)

128. **(A)** A patient who is vomiting coffee-ground-like material probably has internal bleeding (i.e., GI bleed). (pp. 574–577)

129. **(D)** A wheeze is a common breathing sound found in patients having an asthma attack, allergic reaction, or bronchospasm. (p. 452)

130. **(B)** There is no specific EMT intervention for the patient with abdominal pain (aside from oxygen administration). (pp. 583–584)

131. **(C)** The EMT has been trained to cool down and apply oxygen to the patient suspected of having hyperthermia. (p. 816)

132. **(D)** The conclusion that an EMT makes about a patient's condition after assessing the patient is called presumptive diagnosis, EMS diagnosis, and EMT diagnosis. (p. 382)

133. **(C)** Critical thinking is the analytical process that assists the EMT in reaching a field diagnosis. (p. 382)

134. **(B)** The approach that clinicians use to arrive at a diagnosis includes gathering information, considering the possibilities, and reaching a conclusion. (pp. 384–385)

135. **(C)** The differential diagnosis is a list of conditions that may be the cause of the patient's condition today. (p. 386)

136. **(A)** A red flag is a sign or symptom that suggests the possibility of a particular problem that is very serious. (p. 384)

137. **(D)** When a highly experienced physician comes to a diagnosis, he or she most likely used heuristics, pattern recognition, and shortcuts. (p. 386)

138. **(A)** The traditional approach to diagnosis involves narrowing down a long list of possibilities. (p. 387)

139. **(D)** Common heuristics or biases include illusory correlation, availability, representativeness, overconfidence, confirmation bias, anchoring and adjustment, and self-satisfying. (pp. 386–388)

140. **(B)** Specifically looking for evidence that supports the diagnosis you already have in mind is called a confirmation bias. (p. 388)

141. **(B)** When a patient does not fit the classic pattern, the EMT has to be careful not to display representativeness error or bias. (pp. 388–390)

142. **(D)** Availability is the urge to think of things because they are more easily recalled, often due to recent exposure. (pp. 388–390)

143. **(B)** Illusory correlation is when we draw conclusions about the world because of how something else works, implying one causes the other. (pp. 388–390)

144. **(A)** Stopping the search for a diagnosis too soon can lead to missing out on the secondary diagnosis. (pp. 388–390)

145. **(B)** You are treating a respiratory patient who is conscious, alert, and in severe distress. He took an albuterol treatment prior to your arrival on the scene and at this point, you have been administering CPAP for about 10 minutes. With the mental status rapidly diminishing in this patient who is already on CPAP, you should remove the CPAP and ventilate the patient with a BVM device. (pp. 453–455)

146. **(C)** This was a long flight and the patient may have a pulmonary embolism based on the history of smoking and DVT and the shortness of breath. (p. 459)

147. **(A)** They both have numerous stings, but the daughter is experiencing the signs of an anaphylactic reaction compared to the simple allergic reaction the father is

having. The daughter will most likely have hypotension, which is a critical sign. (p. 535)

148. **(B)** She may have attempted suicide by mixing chemicals to produce hydrogen sulfide. CO is odorless. CO_2 and cyanide do not smell like rotten eggs. (pp. 553–554)

149. **(B)** The white blood cells are the cells that are critical in the body's response to infection and acting as the mediators of the body's immune response. (pp. 602–603)

150. **(A)** The complications of sickle cell disease can include each of the following: destruction of the spleen, acute chest syndrome, priapism, and stroke. (pp. 604–605)

Chapter 27: Bleeding and Shock

MATCH TERMINOLOGY/ DEFINITIONS

▶ PART A

1. **(J)** Arterial bleeding—bleeding from an artery, which is characterized by bright red blood and as rapid, profuse, and difficult to control (p. 620)

2. **(A)** Brachial artery—the major artery of the upper arm (p. 115)

3. **(C)** Capillary bleeding—bleeding that is characterized by a slow, oozing flow of blood (p. 617)

4. **(H)** Cardiogenic shock—lack of perfusion brought on not by blood loss, but by inadequate pumping action of the heart; it is often the result of a heart attack or congestive heart failure (p. 633)

5. **(B)** Compensated shock—when the patient is developing shock but the body is still able to maintain perfusion (p. 633)

6. **(E)** Decompensated shock—when the body can no longer compensate for low blood volume or lack of perfusion; late signs such as decreasing blood pressure become evident (p. 633)

7. **(I)** Femoral artery—the major artery supplying the thigh (p. 115)

8. **(G)** Hemorrhage—bleeding, especially severe bleeding (p. 619)

9. **(D)** Hemorrhagic shock—shock resulting from blood loss (p. 633)

10. **(F)** Hypoperfusion—inability of the body to adequately circulate blood to the body's cells to supply them with oxygen and nutrients (p. 619)

▶ PART B

1. **(F)** Hypovolemic shock—shock resulting from blood or fluid loss (p. 633)

2. **(E)** Irreversible shock—when the body has lost the battle to maintain perfusion to vital organs; even if adequate vital signs return, the patient may die days later due to organ failure (p. 633)

3. **(C)** Neurogenic shock—hypoperfusion due to nerve paralysis resulting in the dilation of blood vessels that increases the volume of the circulatory system beyond the point where it can be filled (p. 633)

4. **(I)** Perfusion—the supply of oxygen to and removal of wastes from the cells and tissues of the body as a result of the flow of blood through the capillaries (p. 619)

5. **(G)** Pressure dressing— a bulky dressing held in position with a tightly wrapped bandage to apply pressure that helps control bleeding (p. 625)

6. **(D)** Pressure point—a site where a main artery lies near the surface of the body and directly over a bone; pressure on such a point can stop distal bleeding

7. **(H)** Shock—the inability of the body to adequately circulate blood to the body's cells and thus supply them with oxygen and nutrients (p. 619)

8. **(A)** Tourniquet—a device used for bleeding control that constricts all blood flow to and from an extremity (p. 627)

9. **(B)** Venous bleeding— bleeding from a vein, which is characterized by dark red or maroon blood and is a steady flow that is easy to control (p. 621)

MULTIPLE-CHOICE REVIEW

1. **(B)** Blood that has been depleted of oxygen and loaded with carbon dioxide empties into the veins, which carry it back to the heart. (p. 618)

2. **(A)** Cells and tissues of the brain, spinal cord, and kidneys are the most sensitive to inadequate perfusion. (p. 619)

3. **(B)** The use of Standard Precautions is essential whenever bleeding is discovered or anticipated. (p. 623)

4. **(C)** Bleeding is classified as arterial, venous, and capillary. There is no category called cellular bleeding. (p. 620)

5. **(B)** Arterial bleeding is often rapid and profuse. Blood in arteries is maintained under high pressure by thick, muscular walls. For this reason, arterial hemorrhage is *more* difficult to control. Clot formation is also difficult because of this pressure. (p. 620)

6. **(B)** A steady flow of dark red or maroon blood is a result of venous bleeding. Deoxygenated blood travels back to the heart through veins. (p. 621)

7. **(C)** Bleeding described as oozing is usually a result of capillary bleeding. (p. 621)

8. **(B)** A large bleeding vein in the neck that sucks in debris or an air bubble (embolism) can cause heart stoppage or damage to the brain or lungs. Cover it with an occlusive dressing immediately. An evisceration occurs when an organ or part of an organ protrudes through a wound opening. (p. 621)

9. **(D)** Sudden blood loss of 1,000 cc in an adult is considered serious. This is double the amount that a blood donor gives. (p. 621)

10. **(D)** Sudden blood loss of 500 cc in a child is considered serious. (p. 621)

11. **(D)** Sudden blood loss of 150 cc in a 1-year-old infant is considered serious. (p. 621)

12. **(D)** The body's natural responses to bleeding are constriction of the injured blood vessel(s) and clotting. However, a serious injury may prevent effective clotting and thus allow continued bleeding. (p. 621)

13. **(B)** Do not wait for signs and symptoms of shock to appear before beginning treatment. Any patient with a significant amount of blood loss should be treated to *prevent* the development of shock. Many signs and symptoms of shock appear late in the process. (pp. 624–625)

14. **(D)** The major methods used to control external extremity bleeding include direct pressure, elevation, and application of a tourniquet. Vessel clamps are used in surgery. (p. 623)

15. **(B)** Administering supplemental oxygen improves oxygenation of the tissues. Blood loss decreases perfusion, which means that less oxygen is delivered to the tissues. Supplemental oxygen increases the oxygen saturation of the blood still present in the circulatory system. (p. 623)

16. **(C)** The most common and effective way to control severe external bleeding is by using a tourniquet. (p. 627)

17. **(C)** The initial, or first, dressing should not be removed from a bleeding wound because it is a necessary part of clot formation. Removing it may destroy developing clots or cause further injury. (p. 625)

18. **(B)** After controlling bleeding from an extremity using a pressure bandage, check the distal pulse to make sure the bandage is not too tight. If administering oxygen, use a nonrebreather mask at 15 liters per minute. (p. 625)

19. **(D)** Elevation is used to assist in bleeding control for the following reasons: it slows bleeding, raises the limb above the heart, and helps to reduce blood pressure in the limb. Actually, shock speeds up the pulse. (p. 626)

20. **(C)** It is inappropriate to use elevation to assist in bleeding control if you suspect musculoskeletal injuries because you could further injure the patient. (p. 626)

21. **(B)** A bleeding injury on the head should be controlled with direct pressure and not a tourniquet. (p. 630)

22. **(D)** Use of direct pressure may not be effective if the wound is bleeding profusely from an artery. (p. 625)

23. **(A)** An air splint is most effective for controlling venous and capillary bleeding. It is not usually effective for arterial bleeding, at least not until the arterial pressure has decreased below that of the pressure in the splint. An air splint may be used to maintain pressure on a bleeding wound *after* other manual methods have already controlled the bleeding. (p. 629)

24. **(D)** Do not insert the ice directly into the wound. When applying cold to a bleeding area, wrap the ice pack/cold pack in a cloth or towel. Do not apply directly onto the skin, and do not leave the ice pack/cold pack in place for more than 20 minutes. (p. 629)

25. **(B)** Some "experts" agree that the pneumatic antishock garment is useful for controlling bleeding from areas the garment covers. It is contraindicated for penetrating chest trauma and the patient in cardiogenic shock. Always check with your service Medical Director before implementing a PASG use protocol (p. 629)

26. **(A)** Bleeding from a clean-edged amputation is usually cared for initially with a pressure dressing because injured blood vessels seal themselves shut as a result of spasms produced by the muscular walls of the vessels. (p. 627)

27. **(C)** Rough-edged amputations, usually produced by crushing or tearing injuries, often bleed heavily because the nature of the injury does not allow for vasoconstriction. Bleeding from these wounds is difficult to control and, in some isolated cases, requires the use of a tourniquet. (p. 627)

28. **(A)** Once a tourniquet is in place, it must not be removed or loosened unless ordered by medical direction. Do not loosen because toxins will flow into the bloodstream. Never

cover the extremity because you must visually monitor the wound site and the effectiveness of the tourniquet. (p. 628)

29. **(C)** A blood pressure cuff can be used as a tourniquet if it is inflated to 150 mmHg or more. (p. 628)

30. **(D)** Allow the drainage of CSF to flow freely. The head injury has resulted in increased pressure within the skull, which is forcing fluid out of the cranial cavity. Do not attempt to stop this bleeding or fluid loss; this may increase the pressure in the skull. (p. 630)

31. **(B)** The medical term for a nosebleed is epistaxis. (p. 630)

32. **(D)** A cold pack applied to the bridge of the nose, by itself, will not control bleeding. To stop a nosebleed, place the patient in a sitting position, leaning forward; apply direct pressure by pinching the nostrils; and keep the patient calm. Try to avoid having the patient swallow blood. (p. 630)

33. **(A)** The leading cause of internal injuries and bleeding is blunt trauma. (p. 630)

34. **(A)** A blast injury is *not* usually considered penetrating trauma unless the blast propels sharp, flying objects that penetrate the patient. (pp. 630–631)

35. **(B)** Bradycardia and a flushed face are not commonly associated with internal bleeding. Signs of internal bleeding include vomiting a coffee-ground-like substance; dark, tarry stools; and a tender, rigid, or distended abdomen. (p. 631)

36. **(D)** A laceration to the forearm would be considered external, not internal, bleeding. A patient who has internal bleeding may have painful, swollen, or deformed extremities (from bleeding within the limb); signs and symptoms of shock; or bright red blood in the stool. (p. 630)

37. **(C)** Inadequate perfusion is referred to as shock or hypoperfusion. (p. 619)

38. **(D)** An isolated injury to the head does not commonly produce shock because there is not enough room within the adult skull to permit enough bleeding to cause shock. Shock may develop from pump failure, lost blood volume, or dilated blood vessels. (p. 633)

39. **(D)** Hypovolemic (hemorrhagic) shock caused by uncontrolled bleeding is the type of shock most often seen by EMTs. (p. 633)

40. **(C)** The heart attack patient is in shock as a result of pump failure, not as a result of the other mechanisms described. (p. 633)

41. **(C)** Neurogenic shock may result from the uncontrolled dilation of blood vessels due to nerve paralysis caused by spinal cord injuries. It takes time (such as the patient who was in his vehicle for hours after the injury) to lose the vascular tone in the legs and for vasodilation to occur. Septic shock may also result in the massive dilation of blood vessels. (p. 633)

42. **(A)** Shock in a patient whose body is still able to maintain perfusion to the vital organs is called compensated shock. (p. 633)

43. **(D)** Early signs of shock that show the body is compensating are increased heart rate; increased respirations; pale, cool skin; and *increased* capillary refill time in infants and children. (p. 633)

44. **(D)** The condition when the body has lost the battle to maintain perfusion to the organ systems is called irreversible shock. (p. 633)

45. **(A)** The patient in shock feels nauseated because blood flow is diverted from the digestive system to the vital

organs. Digestion of food is not a priority for the patient in shock. (p. 633)

46. **(C)** The pulse of a patient in shock increases in an attempt to pump more blood. (p. 634)

47. **(D)** A drop in blood pressure is a late sign of shock. The falling blood pressure signifies that the patient has entered the decompensated stage of the shock process. (p. 634)

48. **(D)** Additional signs of shock may include thirst, dilated pupils, and cyanosis around the lips and nail beds. The shock patient presents with pale, cool, clammy skin, *not* flushed, warm skin, because blood is quickly directed away from the skin and sent to organs such as the heart and brain. (p. 634)

49. **(B)** The EMT should be especially careful when evaluating pediatric shock patients because they may have very few signs until a large percentage of their blood volume (approximately 50 percent) is lost. There is no problem with giving them high-concentration oxygen. (p. 634)

50. **(A)** The concept of a "platinum 10 minutes" is the optimum on-scene time limit when treating a trauma patient. (p. 635)

INSIDE/OUTSIDE (P. 633)

1. The blood vessels constrict in the skin, kidneys, and gastrointestinal tract in response to the norepinephrine secreted by the adrenal glands.

2. When blood vessels constrict in the kidneys, the patient produces less urine to prevent the loss of additional fluid.

3. Blood vessel constriction in the GI tract causes the stomach to try to empty its contents, and the patient may become nauseated and vomit.

COMPLETE THE FOLLOWING

1. The major types of shock include: (p. 633)
   A) Hypovolemic
   B) Cardiogenic
   C) Neurogenic

2. The signs and symptoms of shock include: (any six) (p. 634)
   • Altered mental status
   • Pale, cool, clammy skin
   • Nausea and vomiting
   • Vital sign changes such as increased pulse, decreased blood pressure, and increased respirations
   • Thirst
   • Dilated pupils
   • Cyanosis
   • Delayed capillary refill in children

STREET SCENES DISCUSSION

1. The rib cage protects the stomach, spleen, liver, gallbladder, pancreas, and parts of the intestine.

2. Yes. If available, ALS should be requested to intercept if it is not on scene when you are ready to transport.

3. Changes to mental status due to hypoperfusion or internal bleeding are indicators that the patient may be decompensating. In this case, the patient needs surgery right away to stop the blood loss.

CASE STUDY: CONVENIENCE STORE SHOOTING

1. It ensures that the shooter is no longer on the scene.

2. Safety issues, number of patients, the need for additional resources.

3. Internal and external bleeding is present. He is going into decompensated shock, which is demonstrated by the fast, weak radial pulse. Estimate his blood pressure at less than 90 systolic.

4. He is in decompensating hypovolemic, or hemorrhagic, shock from blood loss.

5. His brain interprets his blood loss (fluid) as "low fluid volume." Therefore, he asks for fluids. In this case, it is too late to restore his fluid volume by asking him to drink fluids. He needs IV fluids and whole blood in the trauma center.

6. Bullet fragments can easily ricochet into the chest. (Always listen to the lung sounds of a trauma patient to prevent missing potential injuries to the lungs.)

7. Use a nonrebreather mask at 15 liters per minute. Monitor his ventilations closely in case you need to switch to a BVM.

8. Call for ALS immediately. If ALS has not arrived when you are ready to transport, arrange an intercept en route to the hospital.

9. A "platinum 10 minutes" on the scene.

10. A "golden hour" from the time of the injury to the surgery.

11. Insert an oral airway if he has no gag reflex. Switch to assisted ventilations if required. When the paramedics arrive, he should have an advanced airway inserted.

12. That's controversial and depends on your local protocols. Because he has internal bleeding and no penetrating chest wound or pulmonary edema, some protocols would allow PASG use.

13. Because this patient is being ventilated (at this time), he is considered critical. And in fact, he is in decompensated shock and moving to irreversible shock.

14. Administer two large-bore IVs of normal saline or Ringer solution, insert an advanced airway, monitor ECG, consider PASG, and administer assisted ventilations.

15. Review your sample radio report with your instructor.

Chapter 28: Soft-Tissue Trauma

MATCH TERMINOLOGY/ DEFINITIONS

▶ PART A

1. **(N)** Abrasion—a scratch or scrape (p. 646)

2. **(O)** Amputation—the surgical removal or traumatic severing of a body part, usually an extremity (p. 648)

3. **(H)** Avulsion—the tearing away or tearing off of a flap of skin or other soft tissue; this term may also be used for an eye pulled from its socket or a tooth dislodged from the gums (p. 648)

4. **(C)** Bandage—any material used to hold a dressing in place (p. 672)

5. **(F)** Closed wound—an internal injury in which there is no open pathway from the outside (p. 644)

6. **(M)** Contusion—a bruise (p. 645)

7. **(J)** Crush injury—an injury caused when force is transmitted from the body's exterior to its internal structures: Bones can be broken; muscles, nerves, and tissue can be damaged; and internal organs can rupture, causing internal bleeding (p. 645)

8. **(L)** Dermis—the inner layer of the skin found beneath the epidermis; it is rich in blood vessels and nerves (p. 643)

9. **(I)** Dressing—any material used to cover a wound in an effort to control bleeding and help prevent further contamination (p. 672)

10. **(B)** Epidermis—the outer layer of the skin (p. 642)

11. **(G)** Full thickness burn—a burn in which all the layers of the skin are damaged; also called a third-degree burn. There are usually areas of the skin that are charred black or areas that are dry and white. (p. 661)

12. **(A)** Hematoma—a swelling caused by the collection of blood under the skin or in damaged tissues as a result of an injured or broken blood vessel (p. 645)

13. **(D)** Laceration—a cut (p. 647)

14. **(K)** Occlusive dressing—any dressing that forms an airtight seal (p. 674)

15. **(E)** Open wound—an injury in which the skin is interrupted, exposing the tissue beneath (p. 646)

▶ **PART B**

1. **(E)** Partial thickness burn—a burn in which the epidermis is burned through and the dermis is damaged; also called a second-degree burn. Burns of this type cause reddening, blistering, and a mottled appearance. (p. 660)

2. **(H)** Pressure dressing—a dressing applied tightly to control bleeding (p. 674)

3. **(F)** Puncture wound—an open wound that tears through skin and destroys underlying tissues. A penetrating puncture wound can be shallow or deep. A perforating puncture wound has both an entrance and an exit wound (p. 647)

4. **(B)** Rule of nines—a method for estimating the extent of a burn. For an adult, each of the following areas represents 9 percent of the body surface: the head and neck, each upper extremity, the chest, the abdomen, the upper back, the lower back and buttocks, the front of each lower extremity, and the back of each lower extremity. The remaining 1 percent is assigned to the genital region. (p. 662)

5. **(C)** Rule of palm—a method for estimating the extent of a burn. The palm of the patient's hand, which equals about 1 percent of the body's surface area, is compared with the patient's burn to estimate its size. (p. 663)

6. **(G)** Subcutaneous layers—the layers of fat and soft tissues found below the dermis (p. 644)

7. **(D)** Superficial burn—a burn that involves only the epidermis, the outer layer of the skin; also called a first-degree burn. It is characterized by reddening of the skin and perhaps some swelling. An example is a sunburn. (p. 660)

8. **(A)** Universal dressing—a bulky dressing (p. 672)

MULTIPLE-CHOICE REVIEW

1. **(C)** The teeth, bones, and cartilage are *not* considered soft tissue. The soft tissues of the body include skin, blood vessels, fatty tissues, muscles, fibrous tissues, nerves, glands, and membranes. (p. 642)

2. **(D)** Blood insulation is a distracter. The functions of the skin include protecting the body by providing a barrier to germs, debris, and unwanted chemicals; shock (impact) absorption; and temperature regulation. (p. 642)

3. **(D)** Epithelial cells comprise the tissue that covers the respiratory tract. The layers of the skin are the epidermis, dermis, and subcutaneous layers. (p. 643)

4. **(A)** The layer of the skin called the epidermis is composed of dead cells, which are rubbed off or sloughed off and are replaced continuously. (p. 642)

5. **(B)** Specialized nerve endings in the skin layer called the dermis are involved with the senses of touch, cold, heat, and pain. (p. 643)

6. **(C)** Shock absorption and insulation are major functions of the subcutaneous layers of the skin. (p. 644)

7. **(C)** Wounds that usually result from the impact of a blunt object are called closed. Wounds resulting from stabbings, lacerations, and perforations are open wounds. (pp. 644–645)

8. **(B)** A closed wound that involves tissue damage and a collection of blood at the injury site is called a hematoma. A contusion is relatively minor. See the answer for multiple-choice questions 9 for crush injury. A penetration is a puncture wound. (p. 645)

9. **(C)** A soft-tissue injury caused by a force that can cause rupture or bleeding of internal organs is called a crush injury. (p. 645)

10. **(C)** An open wound is an injury in which the skin is interrupted, exposing the tissues underneath. See the answer for multiple-choice question 9 for crush injury. See the answer for multiple-choice question 8 for hematoma. (p. 646)

11. **(B)** A minor ooze of blood from capillary beds is from an injury called an abrasion. An amputation occurs when an extremity or digit is cut off or torn off completely. A laceration is a cut, and a puncture is a penetration or hole made with a sharp object. (p. 646)

12. **(C)** A cut caused by a sharp-edged object such as a razor blade or broken glass is called a laceration. See the answer for multiple-choice question 11 for abrasion. See the answer for multiple-choice question 13 for puncture. See the answer for multiple-choice question 14 for avulsion. (p. 647)

13. **(B)** When a sharp, pointed object passes through the skin or other tissue, a puncture wound has occurred. (p. 647)

14. **(A)** The tip of the nose is cut or torn off, which is called an avulsion. Attempt to preserve any avulsed part because it may be possible to restore the part surgically or to use it for skin grafts. (p. 648)

15. **(A)** The priority when treating severe open wounds is to control bleeding. While cleaning the wound, preventing contamination, and bandaging are important;\ it is necessary to first control bleeding by direct pressure (with elevation if necessary). (p. 646)

16. **(D)** Care for a laceration includes checking the pulse distal to the injury. Also check sensory and motor function. The patient may need stitches, plastic surgery, or a tetanus shot at the hospital, so do not put on butterfly bandages and release the patient. Never pull apart the edges of a laceration. (pp. 651–652)

17. **(D)** Various types of guns fired at close range can cause burns around the entry wound, injection of air into the tissues (causing severe damage), and damage to underlying tissue. The patient could present with a contusion if he or she was wearing a bulletproof vest, which spreads the energy of the impact. The patient would not have cold damage from a shooting injury (pp. 650–651)

18. **(A)** Never remove an impaled object. Care in the field for a patient with an impaled object includes stabilizing the object and leaving the object in place (unless it is impaled in the cheek). The bleeding control should be around the base of the glass, but do not press directly on the glass. Also do not leave it unstabilized and simply transport; it must be stabilized at the scene to avoid further damage to the hidden tissues and vessels (pp. 653–654)

19. **(C)** Never apply pressure to the object; rather, stabilize it with a bulky dressing. An impaled object may be plugging bleeding from a major artery while it is in place. To remove it may cause severe bleeding. Removal could also cause further injury to nerves, muscles, and other soft tissue. (p. 654)

20. **(A)** To control profuse bleeding resulting from an impaled object, position your gloved hands on either side of the object and exert downward pressure. Be careful not to push the actual object in any further. (p. 654)

21. **(A)** If you can see both ends of the object impaled in the cheek, pull it out in the direction it entered the cheek. However, never twist the object. If it is impaled into a deeper structure, stabilize it. The object may go into the oral cavity and create an airway obstruction or bleeding into the mouth, which may interfere with breathing or cause nausea or induce vomiting. (p. 654)

22. **(C)** If a patient has an impaled object in the eye, your care should include use of 4 × 4s to stabilize the object and a paper cup to cover the impaled object. Make sure to cover the uninjured eye. Never use plastic foam cups as the particles may flake into the eye. (p. 656)

23. **(D)** In cases where an avulsed flap of tissue has been torn loose but not off, the EMT should fold the skin back to its normal position, clean the wound surface, control bleeding, and dress the wound. Do not tear off the remainder of the flap. (p. 657)

24. **(C)** Amputated parts should be treated by placing them in a plastic bag and then on top of a sealed bag of ice. Do not put the part directly on ice or in dry ice. Follow local protocols with regard to use of saline. (p. 657)

25. **(C)** When treating an amputation, be sure to place a snug pressure dressing over the stump. A tourniquet should be used only if other methods fail. The amputated part should not be placed directly on ice nor should ice be used on the stump. (p. 657)

26. **(B)** When treating an amputation, whenever possible transport the patient and the amputated body part in the same ambulance. This will avoid delays and possibly save the person's limb. (p. 657)

27. **(A)** An air bubble sucked into a large vein in the neck is called an air embolus. The "bends," or decompression

sickness, involves nitrogen bubbles in the joints that do not enter the body through an external opening. (p. 652)

28. **(A)** The treatment of neck vein injury is aimed at preventing an embolus, preventing shock, and stopping bleeding. Do not compress the neck because you can injure the trachea or compress the arteries. (p. 651)

29. **(D)** To treat a neck laceration, the EMT should use an occlusive dressing to ensure material is not sucked into the wound. Do not use an ACE bandage because it could restrict breathing and arterial flow in the neck. (p. 651)

30. **(B)** When applying pressure to a neck wound, be sure you do not compress both carotids at the same time. This could cut off the blood supply to the brain and cause a stroke or other brain injury. (p. 651)

31. **(A)** Blast injuries are usually a mixture of open and closed injuries and can be very serious. (p. 650)

32. **(C)** The driver of the motor vehicle pitched forward after a head-on collision and struck the chest on the steering column, which is called a compression injury. The heart can be severely squeezed, the lungs can rupture, and the sternum and ribs can fracture. (p. 645)

33. **(A)** Blast injuries can include primary lacerations and abrasions, secondary projectile injuries, and tertiary injuries from air injection into the skin. (p. 650)

34. **(C)** An injury that has both an entrance and an exit is called a perforating puncture wound. (p. 647)

35. **(D)** Burn injuries often involve structures below the skin, such as muscles, nerves, bones, and blood vessels. (p. 661)

36. **(B)** In addition to physical damage caused by burns, patients often suffer emotional and psychological problems due to the lengthy recovery process and possibility of permanent disfigurement. (p. 659)

37. **(A)** When caring for a burn patient, think beyond the burn. Was there a possible medical emergency that caused the burn or did the burn aggravate an existing injury? (p. 659)

38. **(A)** When caring for burn patients, do not neglect assessment in order to begin burn care. A decision to transport immediately would be based on other injuries found. (p. 667)

39. **(D)** At normal temperature, distilled water is not a chemical that can burn a patient. Examples of agents causing burns are AC current, hydrochloric acid, and dry lime. (p. 660)

40. **(A)** A burn that involves only the epidermis is called a superficial burn. Epi thickness is a distracter. (p. 660)

41. **(B)** A burn that results in deep, intense pain, blisters, and mottled skin is called a partial thickness burn. (p. 660)

42. **(C)** To distinguish between a partial thickness burn and a full thickness burn, look for dry and white areas, which indicate a full thickness burn. Charred black or brown areas are also indicative of full thickness burns. (p. 660)

43. **(B)** Electrical burns are of special concern because they pose a great risk of severe internal injuries. Chemical burns may remain on the skin and continue to burn for hours. Radiation burns may cause the patient to lose his hair over time. (p. 660)

44. **(C)** Chemical burns are of special concern because they may remain on the skin and continue to burn for hours. Superheated gases are usually present in a room with a fire in which the ceiling temperature is very hot. Electrical burns may travel from one extremity to the other and pose a great potential for internal injury. (p. 660)

45. **(D)** Burns to the face are of special concern because they may involve airway injury. They may also involve eye injury. (p. 665)

46. **(C)** One of the types of burns that can interrupt circulation to distal tissues is a circumferential burn. The resulting encircling scarring tends to limit normal functions. (p. 665)

47. **(B)** You are treating an adult patient who has partial thickness burns to the entire left arm (9), chest (9), face, and neck (4½). The size of the burn area is 22.5 percent. (p. 663)

48. **(D)** You are treating an adult patient who has partial thickness burns totally covering the legs (18 + 18), chest (9), and abdomen (9). The size of the burn area is 54 percent. (p. 663)

49. **(A)** A burn the size of five palms would cover approximately 5 percent of the body surface area. (p. 663)

50. **(B)** The age of the patient is an important factor in burns. Patients under 5 and over 55 years of age have the most severe responses to burns. They also have a greater risk of death from burns. (p. 664)

51. **(A)** A partial thickness burn that involves less than 15 percent of the body surface is classified as a minor burn. (p. 665)

52. **(B)** A partial thickness burn that involves between 15 and 30 percent of the body surface area is classified as a moderate burn (p. 665)

53. **(C)** A partial thickness burn that involves more than 30 percent of the body surface area is classified as a critical burn (p. 665)

54. **(D)** Partial thickness burns on the wrist would not be considered critical unless the hand was involved. Critical burns include circumferential burns, moderate burns in an infant or elderly patient, and burns complicated by musculoskeletal injuries. (p. 665)

55. **(B)** A partial thickness burn that involves between 10 and 20 percent of the body surface area of a child under 5 years of age is classified as a moderate burn (p. 665)

56. **(C)** A full thickness burn to the front of the right forearm would not be considered a critical burn because it is only a small percentage of the body surface area. (p. 665)

57. **(A)** If a patient has a partial thickness burn to the entire back, the patient should be wrapped in a dry, sterile burn sheet. (p. 667)

58. **(B)** The primary care for a patient with a chemical burn is to wash away the chemical with flowing water. (pp. 667–668)

59. **(C)** You are treating a patient who was burned. The patient is having visual difficulties, is restless and irritable, has an irregular pulse rate, and has muscle tenderness. This patient probably has an electrical burn or potentially a near strike from lightning. (p. 670)

60. **(A)** If dry lime is the burn agent, brush it from the patient's skin and then flush with water. (p. 668)

61. **(A)** An occlusive dressing is used to form an airtight seal. (p. 652)

INSIDE/OUTSIDE (P. 669)

1. Because the alkali burn generally causes more damage to the cells and takes more water to neutralize.

2. Hydrofluoric acid is the exception to the rule; it is very dangerous because it penetrates very deep into the tissue.

COMPLETE THE FOLLOWING

1. The types of burns include the following: (p. 660)
   A) Thermal
   B) Chemical
   C) Electrical

2. The parts of the adult body that account for 9 percent each in the rule of nines are as follows: (pp. 662–663)
   A) Head and neck **E)** Upper back
   B) Each upper extremity **F)** Lower back and buttocks
   C) Chest **G)** Front of each lower extremity
   D) Abdomen **H)** Back of each lower extremity

3. The signs and symptoms of an electrical injury include: (any five) (p. 670)
   - Burns where energy enters and exits
   - Disrupted nerve pathways displayed as paralysis
   - Respiratory difficulties or respiratory arrest
   - Irregular heartbeat or cardiac arrest
   - Muscle tenderness with or without muscular twitching
   - Elevated blood pressure or low blood pressure with signs and symptoms of shock
   - Restlessness or irritability if conscious, or loss of consciousness
   - Visual difficulties
   - Fractured bones and dislocations from severe muscle contractions or from falling
   - Seizures

LABEL THE DIAGRAM (P. 661)

1. Superficial
2. Partial thickness
3. Full thickness
4. Skin reddened
5. Blisters
6. Charring

STREET SCENES DISCUSSION

1. Apply direct pressure as you elevate the arm. If that doesn't control the bleeding, hold a pressure point until the bleeding stops. Then firmly wrap the wound with a pressure bandage.

2. If the patient has an impaled object, do not attempt to remove it. Instead, stabilize the object in place with bulky dressings, applying pressure around the glass as each layer is positioned. Then secure the dressings in place with adhesive strips or tape. Be careful not to move the piece of glass.

3. If the patient already has low blood pressure, she is in very serious condition and needs rapid transport. Administer high-concentration oxygen, place her in a Trendelenburg position, keep her warm, and arrange for an ALS intercept en route to the hospital if possible.

Chapter 29: Chest and Abdominal Trauma

MATCH TERMINOLOGY/ DEFINITIONS

1. **(K)** Closed wound—an internal injury with no open pathway from the outside (p. 680)

2. **(J)** Dressing—any material (preferably sterile) used to cover a wound that will help control bleeding and help prevent additional contamination (p. 683)

3. **(H)** Evisceration—an intestine or other internal organ protruding through a wound in the abdomen (p. 688)

4. **(G)** Flail chest—fracture of two or more adjacent ribs in two or more places that allows for free movement of the fractured segment (p. 680)

5. **(D)** Occlusive dressing—any dressing that forms an airtight seal (p. 683)

6. **(C)** Open wound—an injury in which the skin is interrupted, exposing the tissue beneath (p. 683)

7. **(A)** Paradoxical motion—movement of ribs in a flail segment that is opposite to the direction of movement of the chest cavity (p. 680)

8. **(B)** Pneumothorax—air in the chest cavity (p. 683)

9. **(E)** Sucking chest wound—an open chest wound in which air is "sucked" into the chest cavity (p. 682)

10. **(I)** Tension pneumothorax—a type of pneumothorax in which air that enters the chest cavity is prevented from escaping (p. 683)

11. **(F)** Universal dressing—a bulky dressing (p. 677)

MULTIPLE-CHOICE REVIEW

1. **(D)** The chest can be injured from blunt trauma, penetrating trauma, and compression. (p. 680)

2. **(C)** By definition, a flail chest is two or more ribs fractured in two or more places, thus creating a free-floating segment of ribs. (p. 680)

3. **(B)** A patient with a flail segment or flail chest will have paradoxical respiration, where the segment moves opposite to the direction of the rest of the uninjured chest wall. (p. 680)

4. **(B)** When the delicate pressure balance within the chest cavity is compromised, initially the lung on the injured side will collapse. The patient will limit chest expansion due to the pain involved in breathing. (p. 682)

5. **(C)** A chest cavity open to the atmosphere is referred to as a sucking chest wound. A hemothorax is a condition in which the chest cavity fills with blood. (p. 682)

6. **(B)** Binding the chest will make it even harder for the patient to breathe. The treatment for an open chest wound includes maintaining an open airway, administering high-concentration oxygen, and sealing the open wound. (p. 683)

7. **(D)** When air becomes trapped in the chest cavity, it will *not* increase the ventilatory volume of the chest. Trapped air in the chest can put pressure on the unaffected lung and heart, reduce cardiac output, and affect oxygenation of the blood. (p. 683)

8. **(D)** The signs and symptoms of a pneumothorax or tension pneumothorax include tracheal deviation to the uninjured side, distended neck veins, and uneven chest wall movement. The depth of respiration is *not* increased. (p. 685)

9. **(B)** Coughed-up frothy blood is *not* a sign of traumatic asphyxia. The signs and symptoms include distended neck veins; head, neck, and shoulders that appear dark blue; and bloodshot and bulging eyes. (p. 686)

10. **(C)** When taping a four-sided occlusive dressing in place, have the patient forcefully exhale as you tape. The highest priority, however, is to get the dressing in place because the injury is life threatening and not all patients are conscious and able to follow your instructions. (p. 683)

11. **(B)** An open wound to the abdomen that is so large and deep that organs protrude is called an evisceration. (p. 688)

12. **(D)** Contusions over the upper ribs are signs of chest injury but not abdominal injuries. The signs of an abdominal injury include lacerations and puncture wounds to the lower back, large bruises on the abdomen, and indications of developing shock. (p. 687)

13. **(B)** Partially digested blood that is vomited looks like coffee grounds. (p. 687)

14. **(C)** Headache is not normally a symptom of an abdominal injury. The symptoms of an abdominal injury include cramps, nausea, and thirst. Patients may also experience pain that is initially mild and then rapidly becomes intolerable. (p. 687)

15. **(B)** Consider positioning the patient with an abdominal injury supine, with legs flexed at the knees. This position relaxes the abdominal muscles and reduces pain. (p. 691)

16. **(C)** When covering an exposed abdominal organ, the EMT should apply a sterile, saline-moistened dressing directly over the wound site before applying an occlusive dressing. Do not use aluminum foil because it can cut eviscerated organs. (p. 691)

17. **(D)** When a normally healthy teenager is struck in the chest, near the heart, and drops suddenly, often in cardiac arrest, his condition is caused by *commotio cordis*. (p. 687)

18. **(C)** The treatment of an evisceration should *never* include replacing or touching the exposed organ. This could cause serious damage to the part and increase the chance of infection. (p. 692)

INSIDE/OUTSIDE (P. 691)

1. Yes, especially with bullet tumble or secondary bullet fragments or bones (ribs) heading into the chest or abdomen.

2. Yes, depending on the location of the lungs in the chest because they take up a lot more room on inspiration, and the liver and spleen might have been missed with the large, inflated lungs. On the other hand, if the lungs were deflated due to exhalation, the liver and spleen would become more prominent targets.

COMPLETE THE FOLLOWING

1. Explain the following injuries:
   A) Commotio cordis—when someone gets hit in the center of the chest, the result is usually a bruise or even a fracture. In this case, the impact occurs at a vulnerable point in the cardiac cycle, causing the patient to go into ventricular fibrillation. (p. 687)
   B) Cardiac tamponade—when an injury to the heart causes blood to flow into the surrounding pericardial sac. (p. 686)
   C) Traumatic asphyxia—sudden compression of the chest, which causes the sternum and ribs to exert severe pressure on the heart and lungs, forcing blood out of the right atrium and into the jugular veins of the neck. (p. 686)
   D) Hemothorax—blood within the chest cavity, outside the lung. (p. 685)
   E) Pneumothorax—air within the chest cavity, outside the lung. (p. 685)

STREET SCENES DISCUSSION

1. If the patient slashed her abdomen, the EMT should lay her down, bandage the wound with an occlusive dressing, treat for shock with oxygen, and keep the patient warm. If ALS is available, call them and alert the hospital while en route.

2. If the patient gets dizzy and pale, she most likely lost a lot of blood internally, so treat her as described in the answer to Street Scenes Discussion question 1.

3. If the patient has a penetrating chest injury, apply an occlusive dressing as soon as possible. Seal all four corners, but if she gets a lot worse quickly, open up one side of the dressing or "burb" the dressing. Treat for shock, administer oxygen, and monitor the ventilatory volume for the need to support or assist with a BVM. Call ALS and, of course, notify the hospital while en route.

4. Seal that hole right away. If the hole is bigger than the glottic opening, no air will go in the glottic opening.

Chapter 30: Musculoskeletal Trauma

MATCH TERMINOLOGY/ DEFINITIONS

1. **(P)** Angulated fracture—fracture in which the broken bone segments are at an angle to each other (p. 706)

2. **(R)** Bones—hard but flexible living structures that provide support for the body and protection to vital organs (p. 696)

3. **(I)** Cartilage—tough tissue that covers the joint ends of bones and helps to form certain body parts such as the ear (p. 702)

4. **(Q)** Closed extremity injury—an injury to an extremity with no associated opening in the skin (p. 706)

5. **(S)** Comminuted fracture—a fracture in which the bone is broken in several places (p. 706)

6. **(T)** Compartment syndrome—injury caused when tissue such as blood vessels and nerves are constricted within a space as from swelling or from a tight dressing or cast (p. 708)

7. **(E)** Crepitus—a grating sensation or sound made when fractured bone ends rub together (p. 708)

8. **(B)** Dislocation—the disruption or "coming apart" of a joint (p. 706)

9. **(H)** Extremities—the portions of the skeleton that include the clavicles, scapulae, arms, wrists, and hands (upper extremities) and the pelvis, thighs, legs, ankles, and feet (lower extremities) (p. 696)

10. **(G)** Fracture—any break in a bone (p. 706)

11. **(O)** Greenstick fracture—an incomplete fracture (p. 706)

12. **(L)** Joints—places where bones articulate, or meet (p. 696)

13. **(N)** Ligaments—connective tissues that connect bone to bone (p. 702)

14. **(K)** Manual traction—the process of applying tension to straighten and realign a fractured limb before splinting; also called tension (p. 710)

15. **(A)** Muscles—tissues or fibers that cause movement of body parts and organs (p. 702)

16. **(C)** Open extremity injury—an extremity injury in which the skin has been broken or torn through from the inside by an injured bone or from the outside by something that has caused a penetrating wound with associated injury to the bone (p. 706)

17. **(M)** Sprain—the stretching and tearing of ligaments (p. 706)

18. **(J)** Strain—muscle injury resulting from overstretching or overexertion of the muscle (p. 706)

19. **(F)** Tendons—tissues that connect muscle to bone (p. 702)

20. **(D)** Traction splint—a splint that applies constant pull along the length of a lower extremity to help stabilize the fractured bone and to reduce muscle spasm in the limb; this type of splint is used primarily on femoral shaft fractures (p. 705)

MULTIPLE-CHOICE REVIEW

1. **(B)** As we age, our bones become deficient in calcium. (p. 698)

2. **(C)** The strong, white, fibrous material covering the bones is called the periosteum. (p. 698)

3. **(B)** In children, the majority of the long bone growth occurs in the growth plate (located at the ends of bones). Fractures in this area can be very serious and can lead to the shortening of a limb. (p. 702)

4. **(D)** Musculoskeletal injuries are caused by indirect, direct, and twisting forces. (p. 702)

5. **(B)** Fractures of the femur typically cause a 2-pint blood loss over the first 2 hours. If there are additional complications, such as an artery laceration, blood loss could be more severe. Blood loss from a fracture of the tibia or fibula would be about 1 pint, and a pelvic fracture would cause a 3- to 4-pint loss. (p. 705)

6. **(C)** The death rate from closed fracture of the femur dropped from 80 to 20 percent in the post–World War I period due to the invention of the traction splint. The PASG was used extensively in the Vietnam War. (p. 705)

7. **(C)** The bone marrow is where the red blood cells are produced. (p. 701)

8. **(C)** The stretching or tearing of ligaments is called a sprain. A strain is caused by overstretching or overexertion of the muscle. (p. 706)

9. **(B)** A break in the continuity of the skin of a painful, swollen, deformed extremity is considered an open bone or joint injury. A simple fracture and a closed fracture have no break in the skin. Grating is not a type of fracture. (p. 706)

10. **(C)** Proper splinting of a possible closed fracture is designed to prevent closed injuries from becoming open ones. (p. 711)

11. **(C)** The signs and symptoms of a bone or joint injury include grating (crepitus), swelling, and bruising. If shock develops, vomiting may occur. (p. 708)

12. **(A)** When a joint is locked into position, the EMT should splint the joint in the position found. Do *not* disregard splinting; it is not necessary to transport immediately unless the patient is a high priority for some other reason. If this is the case, then a long backboard would be used as a splint. (p. 712)

13. (C) The procedure, which is done at least twice whenever a splint is applied, is assessment for circulation, and for sensation and motor function distal to the injury. Once traction is applied, it is not reapplied. (p. 708)

14. (B) The treatment of a painful, swollen extremity (possible fracture) includes these steps: take Standard Precautions, splint the injury, elevate the extremity, and apply a cold pack. Do not elevate the extremity until it is splinted. (p. 710)

15. (C) Multiple fractures, especially of the femur, can cause life-threatening external and internal bleeding. (p. 705)

16. (A) Applying a cold pack to a possible fracture will help to reduce the swelling. It does not stop bleeding from the bone, nor does it stop all pain and discomfort. Do not use a pressure bandage at the site of a fracture because it may damage the bone ends. (p. 708)

17. (D) If the primary assessment of a patient with a musculoskeletal injury reveals the patient is unstable, do *not* take time to splint each individual injury. It is not in the patient's best interest to waste the precious early minutes treating minor injuries. (p. 707)

18. (D) A splint properly applied to a closed bone injury should help prevent damage to muscles, nerves, or blood vessels caused by broken bones, as well as prevent an open bone injury and motion of bone fragments. The splint should not prevent circulation to the extremity. (p. 711)

19. (D) Complications of bone injuries include excessive bleeding, increased pain from movement, and paralysis of the extremity. Distal sensation may be diminished but not increased. (p. 712)

20. (C) The objective of realignment is to assist in restoring circulation and to fit the extremity into a splint. (p. 710)

21. (A) If there is a severe deformity of the distal extremity or it is cyanotic or pulseless, the EMT should align with gentle traction before splinting. A pillow splint should not be used for alignment. If you delay splinting until en route to the hospital, the circulation to the extremity could be hindered. (p. 710)

22. (A) The types of splints generally carried by EMTs include rigid, formable, and traction. (p. 710)

23. (D) Rigid splints are seldom used to immobilize joint injuries in the position found, except for triangulation. Formable splints, such as the Sam Splint®, are used for this purpose. (p. 710)

24. (C) Traction splints are used specifically for fractures of the mid-shaft femur. (p. 705)

25. (D) When splinting, the EMT should immobilize the injury site and joints above and below. Do not leave open wounds exposed because they may get infected. Sometimes protruding bone ends fall back into place when the limb is placed in a "splintable position." However, it is not the EMT's responsibility to reduce a fracture in the field. (pp. 710–711)

26. (C) To ensure proper immobilization and increase patient comfort when using a rigid splint, pad the spaces between the body part and the splint. (pp. 710–711)

27. (B) The method of splinting is always dictated by the severity of the patient's condition and the priority decision. If the patient is a high priority for load-and-go transport, choose a fast method of splinting. If the patient is a low priority for transport, choose a slower-but-better splinting method. (p. 711)

28. (D) If the patient with a musculoskeletal injury is unstable, the EMT should care for life-threatening problems first, consider aligning the injuries to an anatomical position, and secure the entire body to a long spine board. In the case of a critical patient, consider using a long backboard as a total body splint and a lifting/spinal immobilization device. Do not take the time to apply two traction splints. (p. 711)

29. (D) Hazards of improper splinting include aggravation of a bone or joint injury, reduced distal circulation, and delay in transport of a patient with life-threatening injury. (p. 712)

30. (C) If the lower leg is cyanotic or lacks a pulse when a knee joint injury is assessed, the EMT should realign with gentle traction if no resistance is met. Call medical direction if you need some encouragement. An attempt at restoring a pulse must be made, otherwise the patient could lose the lower leg. (p. 724)

31. (B) Examples of a bipolar traction splint include Hare®, Fernotrac®, and Thomas Half-ring®. (pp. 735–737)

32. (B) The amount of traction the EMT should pull when applying a Sager® traction splint is about 10 percent of the body weight up to 15 pounds. (p. 737)

33. (B) The indications for a traction splint are a possible mid-shaft femur fracture with no joint or lower leg injury. (p. 723)

34. (B) Whenever possible, three rescuers should be used to apply a traction splint. This allows one rescuer to support the injury site when the limb is lifted to position the traction splint. (pp. 735–737)

35. (C) If the patient has multiple leg fractures and exhibits signs of shock, the EMT should apply the PASG as a splint. The patient will most likely be in shock, so the PASG will serve a dual purpose. Be sure to follow your local protocols because not all areas use the PASG. (p. 720)

36. (D) Signs and symptoms of a knee injury include pain and tenderness, swelling, and deformity. Discoloration to the thigh would be a sign of an injury to the mid-shaft femur. (p. 708)

37. (A) Elderly patients are more susceptible to hip fractures because of brittle bones or bones weakened by disease. (pp. 721–722)

38. (B) When a patient has a fractured hip, the injured limb may appear shorter than the uninjured leg. (pp. 721–722)

39. (C) When a patient who was involved in a serious fall has an unexplained sensation of having to empty his or her bladder, the patient may have sustained a pelvic fracture. (p. 719)

40. (D) When securing a patient who has a pelvic injury, you should not raise the lower legs. (pp. 719–720)

COMPLETE THE FOLLOWING

1. Signs and symptoms of a musculoskeletal injury include the following: (p. 708)
   A) Pain and tenderness
   B) Deformity or angulation
   C) Grating, or crepitus
   D) Swelling
   E) Bruising
   F) Exposed bone ends
   G) Joints locked into position
   H) Nerve and blood vessel compromise

2. The eight signs and symptoms of a hip fracture include the following: (p. 722)

   A) Localized pain

   B) Sensitivity to pressure on the lateral prominence of the hip

   C) Discoloration of surrounding tissues (delayed sign)

   D) Swelling

   E) Inability to move the limb while on the back

   F) Inability to stand

   G) Foot on the injured side is turned outward

   H) Injured limb may appear shorter

LABEL THE DIAGRAM (PP. 699–700)

1. Skull
2. Cervical vertebrae
3. Clavicle
4. Sternum
5. Ribs
6. Thoracic vertebrae
7. Lumbar vertebrae
8. Pubis
9. Tibia
10. Fibula
11. Tarsals
12. Metatarsals
13. Phalanges
14. Maxilla
15. Mandible
16. Scapula
17. Humerus
18. Ulna
19. Radius
20. Sacrum
21. Coccyx
22. Carpals
23. Metacarpals
24. Phalanges
25. Ischium
26. Femur
27. Patella

INSIDE/OUTSIDE (P. 717)

1. Patients who experience long bone fractures often experience shock in addition to the bone injury because the bones are vascular and bleed a significant amount over the first 2 hours.

2. The EMT should splint on the suspicion of a fracture rather than the confirmation of an actual fracture because it often takes an X-ray in the ED to confirm that the patient has a fracture. Some types of fractures do not have deformity but could be made worse if the patient was allowed to walk on them or bear his or her weight.

3. Swelling and inflammation are the body's natural response to injury.

STREET SCENES DISCUSSION

1. You would have observed an open cut or laceration with bleeding where the bone exited the skin.

2. Yes. To apply a splint to a grossly deformed long bone, it will be necessary to move the bone into a splintable (straight) position by using gentle traction on the extremity.

3. If the patient does not have a distal pulse, contact medical direction, who may allow you to manipulate the extremity once gently to try to restore the pulse.

4. If the patient's vital signs are stable and there is no evidence of multiple fractures, an ALS unit is probably not needed.

Chapter 31: Trauma to the Head, Neck, and Spine

MATCH TERMINOLOGY/ DEFINITIONS

1. (P) Autonomic nervous system—controls involuntary functions (p. 748)

2. (K) Central nervous system—the brain and spinal cord (p. 749)

3. (I) Cerebrospinal fluid (CSF)—the fluid that surrounds the brain and spinal cord (p. 748)

4. (B) Concussion—mild closed head injury without detectable damage to the brain; complete recovery is usually expected (p. 751)

5. (J) Contusion—in brain injuries, a bruised brain caused when the force of a blow is great enough to rupture blood vessels (pp. 751–752)

6. (H) Cranium—the bony structure making up the forehead and the top, back, and upper sides of the skull (p. 748)

7. (X) Dermatome—an area of the skin that is innervated by a single spinal nerve (p. 764)

8. (S) Foramen magnum—the opening at the base of the skull through which the spinal cord passes from the brain (p. 752)

9. (W) Hematoma—in a head injury, a collection of blood within the skull or brain (p. 752)

10. (V) Herniation—pushing of a portion of the brain through the foramen magnum as a result of increased intracranial pressure (p. 753)

11. (T) Intracranial pressure (ICP)—pressure inside the skull (p. 752)

12. (R) Laceration—in brain injuries, a cut to the brain (p. 752)

13. (D) Malar—the cheek bone; also called the zygomatic bone (p. 789)

14. (Q) Mandible—the lower jaw bone (p. 748)

15. (U) Maxillae—the two fused bones forming the upper jaw (p. 748)

16. (M) Nasal bones—the bones that form the upper third, or bridge, of the nose (p. 748)

17. (C) Nervous system—provides overall control of thought, sensation, and the voluntary and involuntary motor functions of the body; the major components are the brain and the spinal cord (p. 789)

18. (O) Neurogenic shock—a state of shock caused by nerve paralysis that is sometimes caused by spinal injuries. (p. 765)

19. (N) Orbits—the bony structures around the eyes; the eye sockets (p. 748)

20. (A) Peripheral nervous system—the nerves that enter and exit the spinal cord between the vertebrae and the 12 pairs of cranial nerves that travel between the brain and organs without passing through the spinal cord, and all of the body's other motor and sensory nerves (p. 748)

21. (E) Spinous process—the bony bump on a vertebra. (p. 749)

22. (L) Temporal bone—bone that forms part of the side of the skull and floor of the cranial cavity. There is a right and a left temporal bone. (p. 748)

23. (G) Temporomandibular joint—the movable joint formed between the mandible and the temporal bone; also called the TMJ. (p. 748)

24. (F) Vertebrae—the bones of the spinal column (singular is vertebra) (p. 749)

MULTIPLE-CHOICE REVIEW

1. (B) The function of the spinal column is to protect the spinal cord. (p. 749)

2. (C) The spine is made up of 33 vertebrae. (p. 749)

3. (C) When a patient has a scalp injury, expect profuse bleeding because the scalp is very vascular. Do not try to determine the wound depth or palpate the site with your fingertips because you may be exposed to bloodborne pathogens. (p. 750)

4. (C) A bruise behind the ear is called Battle sign. It usually takes a few hours to develop from a basilar skull fracture. (p. 755)

5. (B) Discoloration of the soft tissues under both eyes is called raccoon eyes. This sign is also associated with a basilar skull fracture. (p. 755)

6. (A) The signs and symptoms of a skull or traumatic brain injury include blood or fluid leakage from the ears and/or nose. (pp. 755–756)

7. (B) Skull or traumatic brain injury may result in altered mental status and unequal pupils. Difficulty moving below the waist is a sign of a spine injury. (pp. 755–756)

8. (A) Temperature increase is a late sign of skull injury or traumatic brain injury. It is due to inflammation, infection, or damage to temperature-regulating centers. (p. 756)

9. (C) Shock (hypoperfusion) from blood loss is generally *not* a sign of head injury, except in infants. There simply is not enough room within an adult's skull to permit enough bleeding to cause shock. If there is a head injury with shock, evaluate for blood loss occurring elsewhere. Neurogenic shock is possible with spinal injury accompanying head injury, though this type of shock is rarely seen in the field. (p. 756)

10. (B) The significance of an increase in carbon dioxide in the injured brain is that it causes brain tissue swelling. Hyperventilating the patient with supplemental oxygen at a rate of at least 25 ventilations per minute may reduce brain tissue swelling, but this is a controversial treatment and you should always follow your Medical Director's guidelines. (pp. 756–757)

11. (A) A patient with a GCS of less than 8 should be taken to a trauma center (if one is available in your region). (pp. 759–760)

12. (D) If an object has penetrated a patient's skull, stabilize the object with bulky dressings. This will minimize accidental movement of the object. Do not pull out an impaled object! (p. 757)

13. (B) The primary concern for emergency care of facial fractures or jaw injuries is the patient's airway. Such fractures create the potential for bleeding into the airway and difficulty maintaining a patent airway. (p. 757)

14. (D) The cervical and lumbar vertebrae are most frequently injured because they are not supported by other bony structures. (p. 762)

15. (C) Excessive pulling of the spine, which commonly occurs during a hanging, is called a distraction injury. (p. 762)

16. (C) On your size-up of an automobile collision, you notice that both sides of the windshield have a spider-web crack. It is wise to call for a backup ambulance because both the driver and the passenger will need to be treated for spinal injury. (pp. 762–763)

17. (D) A fall from *three* times the patient's height is considered a high index of suspicion for a spinal injury. The EMT should also maintain a high degree of suspicion for a spinal injury when the patient has been involved in a motor vehicle collision or a motorcycle crash, or has open fractures to the ankles that resulted from a fall. (pp. 762–763)

18. (D) Lateral bending injuries are caused by using improper lifting techniques. Diving accidents commonly cause flexion, extension, or compression injuries of the cervical spine. (p. 763)

19. (A) The unconscious trauma patient should be treated as if he has a spine injury. (p. 765)

20. (D) The most reliable sign of spinal-cord injury in the conscious patient is paralysis of the extremities. (pp. 765–766)

21. (B) A lack of spinal pain does not rule out the possibility of spinal-cord injury because other distracting and painful injuries may mask it. (pp. 765–766)

22. (A) When assessing a suspected spine-injured patient, you note a reversal of the normal breathing pattern. This is likely a result of damage to the nerves that control the rib cage. (pp. 765–766)

23. (D) A patient found on her back with arms extended above her head may have a cervical-spine injury. (pp. 765–766)

24. (A) If a patient is up and walking around at the scene of a high-speed collision, the EMT should assess for a potential spinal injury. (pp. 765–766)

25. (A) If a patient has the mechanism of injury for a spinal injury, do not assess for spinal pain by asking the patient to move. Keep the patient as still as possible, and assess for equality of strength and tingling in the extremities. (p. 765)

26. (A) After performing the primary assessment and rapid trauma exam on a spine-injured patient, your next step is to determine the patient's priority because this will be important in deciding how to immobilize him or her. (p. 768)

27. (B) If a patient complains of pain when you are attempting to place her or his head in a neutral in-line position, steady the head in the position found. (p. 767)

28. (B) When treating a patient with a spine injury, one EMT should maintain constant manual in-line stabilization until the patient is secured to a backboard. (p. 767)

29. (C) The cervical collar does not completely eliminate neck movement. All of the other answer choices are true. (pp. 767–769)

30. (C) If a stable patient is found in a sitting position on the ground and is complaining about back pain, the EMT should immobilize with a short spine board, KED®, or an extrication vest. This will immobilize the head, neck, and torso until the patient can be transferred to a long spine board. (p. 768)

31. (B) The rapid extrication procedure is *not* used for stable, low-priority patients. All of the other answer choices are true. (p. 768)

32. **(A)** When immobilizing a 6-year-old or younger child on a long backboard, provide padding beneath the shoulder blades. This eliminates the void behind the shoulders caused by the child's large head. (p. 778)

33. **(B)** If a helmet has a snug fit that allows little or no movement of the patient's head within the helmet, the helmet may be left in place. (pp. 782–783)

34. **(B)** The correct order of steps for applying a short spine immobilization device is as follows: position the device behind the patient, secure the device to the patient's torso, evaluate torso fixation and pad behind the neck as necessary, and secure the patient's head to the device. (pp. 770–771)

35. **(D)** Prior to and after immobilization, the EMT should assess distal circulation, sensation, and motor function in all extremities. (p. 767)

36. **(D)** The time it takes to develop the symptoms from an increased ICP depend on the rate of bleeding into the head, the location of the bleed, and the age of the patient. (pp. 752–753)

37. **(C)** The patient whose neck was slashed went into sudden cardiac arrest. Although it could have been due to massive blood loss, there is a high likelihood that he sustained an air embolism that went to the heart. (p. 761)

38. **(C)** Examples of findings that may lead you to consider a spine injury include all of the choices *except* an increase in the pulse rate because the signals from the brain to the adrenal glands to release epinephrine, which helps to increase the heart rate, would not likely occur due to the spinal-cord injury. (pp. 765–766)

INSIDE/OUTSIDE (P. 765)

1. If your 35-year-old male patient who was involved in a car crash sustains an injury to the third, fourth, or fifth cervical vertebrae, he may have an injury to the phrenic, which controls the movement of the diaphragm (the main muscle of breathing).

2. Refer to the patient in the answer for Inside/Outside question 1. At some point in the development of the patient's developing injury, he begins to exhibit hypotension. Loss of smooth muscle control allows the dilation of the blood vessels, especially in the periphery, which causes distal pooling of the blood and ultimately hypotension.

3. The patient's pulse rate does not increase, as would the pulse rate for most other patients who are in shock, because the messages from the brain to the adrenal gland, which secretes epinephrine to increase the heartbeat, travel through the spinal cord. In this instance, the spinal cord may be damaged or severed.

COMPLETE THE FOLLOWING

1. Signs of skull fracture or traumatic brain injury include the following: (any ten) (pp. 754–756)
   - Visible bone fragments
   - Altered mental status
   - Deep laceration or severe bruise or hematoma
   - Depressions or deformities of the skull
   - Severe pain at the site of a head injury

   - Battle sign
   - Raccoon eyes
   - One eye that appears to be sunken
   - Bleeding from the ears and/or nose
   - Clear fluid flowing from the ears and/or nose
   - Personality change, ranging from irritability to irrational behavior (a major sign)
   - Increase in blood pressure and decreased pulse rate (Cushing triad, also called Cushing reflex)
   - Irregular breathing patterns
   - Temperature increase (late sign due to inflammation, infection, or damage to temperature-regulating centers in the brain)
   - Blurred or multiple-image vision in one or both eyes
   - Impaired hearing or ringing in the ears
   - Equilibrium problems
   - Forceful or projectile vomiting
   - Posturing (decorticate or decerebrate)
   - Paralysis or disability on one side of the body
   - Seizures
   - Deteriorating vital signs

2. Four types of traumatic brain injury include the following: (pp. 751–752)
   A) Concussion
   B) Hematoma (subdural/epidural)
   C) Laceration
   D) Contusion

LABEL THE DIAGRAM (P. 750)

1. Cervical   4. Sacral
2. Thoracic   5. Coccyx
3. Lumbar

STREET SCENES DISCUSSION

1. The airway is always the highest priority for assessment and treatment.

2. The decision to immobilize him is based on the mechanism of injury, not on whether or not he has neck pain.

3. Serious head injuries are associated with irregular breathing patterns, high blood pressure, and a pulse rate under 60.

CASE STUDY: DEEP DIVE IN A SHALLOW POOL

1. You would want to know if the patient struck his head, where he entered the pool, if there was any loss of consciousness, exactly how he flipped over, and if the patient at any point had any movement or sensation in his arms or legs.

2. As long as the patient is floating with assistance and as long as manual stabilization of his head and neck is being maintained, you can float him to the shallow end of the pool, where it will be easier to apply a long backboard.

3. Equipment needed includes: a long backboard that floats, a rigid cervical collar, a head immobilizer, some padding, and straps or cravats.

4. Ask him if he remembers what happened, if he is having trouble breathing, and if he has feeling or sensation in his arms and legs. You should ask the OPQRST questions about his chief complaint.

5. Tell the patient that you are going to do everything you can to immobilize his spine properly and get him to the most appropriate hospital as quickly as possible.

6. Your partner should complete the initial assessment; take baseline vital signs; make sure the patient is securely immobilized; and reassess distal circulation, sensation, and motor function.

7. Many spine injury calls go to court, so make sure the prehospital care report (PCR) is very accurate. Be sure to document the actions of the bystander who was in the pool when you arrived and how the injury was reported to have occurred (MOI). Be very specific that the patient stated that he had no sensation or movement in his arms and legs prior to your arrival and that distal circulation, sensation, and motor function were checked and rechecked before and after immobilization.

Chapter 32: Multisystem Trauma

MATCH TERMINOLOGY/ DEFINITIONS

1. (C) Multiple trauma—more than one serious injury (p. 792)

2. (A) Multisystem trauma—one or more injuries that affect more than one body system (p. 792)

3. (B) Trauma score—a system of evaluating trauma patients according to a numerical rating system to determine the severity of the patient's trauma (p. 800)

MULTIPLE-CHOICE REVIEW

1. (B) The patient with a fractured right leg and a crushed pelvis is called a multiple-trauma patient. (p. 792)

2. (C) When a patient has an obvious angulated forearm and is unresponsive, your assessment and treatment priority is the airway. (p. 792)

3. (C) The multiple-trauma patient most likely will be stabilized in the surgical suite. (pp. 799–800)

4. (A) The three "Ts" involved in the management of a multiple-trauma patient are timing, transport, and team-work. (p. 792)

5. (B) The CDC's guidelines for trauma triage and transport consider physiological determinants, the MOI, and anatomic criteria. (pp. 794–795)

6. (B) When a trauma patient is making gurgling sounds as he breathes, you should suction his airway. (p. 799)

7. (D) Sometimes a long backboard can act as a full body splint when the critical patient must be immobilized quickly. (p. 799)

8. (D) When a patient has two fractured femurs, a crushed pelvis, and a possible abdominal injury, you should not apply a traction splint. Do consider applying a PASG (if local protocol allows), and request an ALS intercept en route to the hospital. (pp. 799–800)

9. (C) When trying to minimize the on-scene care of a multiple-trauma patient, do not take the time to bandage all lacerations. (p. 799)

10. (C) Even when you are trying to cut scene time for a multiple-trauma patient, the one thing you do not cut out is scene safety—no matter how serious the patient is. (pp. 799–800)

11. (B) The geriatric patient who fell and is on anticoagulant medications should be a higher priority due to the potential for serious life-threatening internal hemorrhaging. (p. 795)

12. (A) The scoring system for trauma patients also helps to allow the trauma centers to evaluate themselves as well as determine where the patient should be transported. (pp. 800–801)

INSIDE/OUTSIDE (P. 795)

1. When a patient is exhibiting an elevated pulse, respiratory distress, and diminished or absent lung sounds on the left side of his chest after being stabbed with an ice pick in the left chest, you should suspect that he has sustained a pneumothorax on the "inside."

2. If the patient has audible lung sounds on both sides of the chest but has distended neck veins, a narrowing pulse pressure, and increased pulse and respiration, you should suspect that he has a cardiac tamponade on the "inside."

COMPLETE THE FOLLOWING

1. Treatments that would be appropriate on the scene of a critical trauma patient include: (any five) (p. 799)
  - Suctioning the airway
  - Inserting an oral or nasal airway
  - Restoring a patent airway by sealing a sucking chest wound
  - Ventilating with a bag-valve mask
  - Administering high-concentration oxygen
  - Controlling bleeding
  - Immobilizing the patient with a cervical collar and a long backboard
  - Inflating a pneumatic antishock garment

STREET SCENES DISCUSSION

1. Yes, if you suspect supine hypotensive syndrome due to compression of the vena cava by the uterus.

2. You should consider turning the patient and backboard on the side to help clear the airway.

3. No, not with her other problems. Application of a traction splint would take too long.

4. Make sure additional units are responding and that all other patients are assessed and treated.

Chapter 33: Environmental Emergencies

MATCH TERMINOLOGY/ DEFINITIONS

▶ PART A

1. (C) Active rewarming—application of an external heat source to rewarm the body of a hypothermic patient (p. 809)

2. (J) Air embolism—gas bubble in the bloodstream; the more accurate term is arterial gas embolism (AGE) (p. 822)

3. (H) Central rewarming—application of heat to the lateral chest, neck, armpits, and groin of a hypothermic patient (p. 810)

4. **(F)** Conduction—the transfer of heat from one material to another through direct contact (p. 805)

5. **(D)** Convection—carrying away of heat by currents of air or water or other gases or liquids (p. 807)

6. **(G)** Decompression sickness—a condition resulting from nitrogen trapped in the body's tissues caused by coming up too quickly from a deep, prolonged dive. A symptom of decompression sickness is "the bends," or deep pain in the muscles and joints. (p. 822)

7. **(I)** Drowning—the process of experiencing respiratory impairment from submersion/immersion in liquid, which may result in death, morbidity (illness or adverse effects), or no morbidity (p. 818)

8. **(A)** Evaporation—the change from liquid to gas. When the body perspires or gets wet, evaporation of the perspiration or other liquid into the air has a cooling effect on the body (p. 807)

9. **(B)** Hyperthermia—an increase in body temperature above normal; life threatening in its extreme (p. 814)

10. **(E)** Hypothermia—generalized cooling that reduces body temperature below normal; life threatening in its extreme (p. 807)

▶ **PART B**

1. **(E)** Local cooling—cooling or freezing of particular (local) parts of the body (p. 811)

2. **(B)** Passive rewarming—covering a hypothermic patient and taking other steps to prevent further heat loss and help the body rewarm itself (p. 809)

3. **(C)** Radiation—sending out energy, such as heat, in waves into space (p. 807)

4. **(D)** Respiration—breathing; during breathing, body heat is lost as warm air is exhaled from the body (p. 806)

5. **(G)** Toxins—substances produced by animals or plants that are poisonous to humans (p. 826)

6. **(F)** Venom—a toxin (poison) produced by certain animals such as snakes, spiders, and some marine life forms (p. 826)

7. **(H)** Water chill—chilling caused by conduction of heat from the body when the body or clothing is wet (p. 805)

8. **(A)** Wind chill—chilling caused by convection of heat from the body in the presence of air currents (p. 807)

MULTIPLE-CHOICE REVIEW

1. **(A)** Water conducts heat away from the body 25 times faster than still air. (p. 806)

2. **(C)** The body loses heat from respiration, radiation, conduction, convection, and evaporation. Excretion is the elimination of solid wastes, and induction is to place something into the body. Condensation is the accumulation of moisture on an object. (pp. 805–806)

3. **(C)** When there is more wind, there is greater heat loss. (p. 806)

4. **(C)** Most radiant heat loss occurs from a person's head and neck. This is why one should always cover the head when going outside on a cold day. (p. 806)

5. **(D)** Having a headache does not predispose the patient to hypothermia. Predisposing factors to hypothermia include

burns, diabetes, and spinal-cord injuries. Other predisposing factors include shock, head injuries, generalized infection, and hypoglycemia. Also the elderly, infants, and young children are at risk. (p. 807)

6. **(D)** Infants and children do *not* have more body fat than adults. Infants and children are more prone to hypothermia because they have small muscle mass, they have large skin surface in relation to their total body mass, and they are unable to shiver effectively. (p. 807)

7. **(B)** You should consider hypothermia when a patient has been in a cold environment for a considerable length of time. (p. 808)

8. **(B)** When a patient's core body temperature drops below 90°F, the patient may no longer be shivering. (p. 807)

9. **(A)** Hypothermic patients do *not* have a high blood pressure and low pulse. Signs and symptoms of hypothermia include stiff or rigid posture, cool abdominal skin temperature, and loss of motor coordination. (pp. 808–809)

10. **(B)** Passive rewarming involves simply covering the patient. Administering heated oxygen and applying heat packs are part of active rewarming. Never massage the limbs of any hypothermic patient. (p. 809)

11. **(C)** Never give hot liquids to a hypothermic patient quickly. You can give warm liquids slowly. The treatment of the hypothermic patient includes removal of all of the patient's wet clothing, actively rewarming the patient during transport, providing care for shock, and providing oxygen. (p. 809)

12. **(A)** When actively rewarming a patient, apply heat to the chest, neck, armpits, and groin. Never give the person stimulants to drink. (p. 809)

13. **(A)** The reason why you should rewarm the body's core first is to prevent blood from collecting in the extremities due to vasodilation, which could cause a fatal form of shock. (p. 810)

14. **(C)** When transporting an alert patient with mild hypothermia, it is recommended that you keep the patient at rest and avoid unnecessary exercise. Because the blood is the coldest in the extremities, unnecessary movement could quickly circulate the cold blood and lower the core body temperature. The wet clothing must come off so the patient can be dried and warmed. (p. 809)

15. **(B)** In a heat emergency, EMT care of a patient with moist, pale, normal-to-cool skin includes placing the patient in an air-conditioned ambulance, elevating the patient's legs (if appropriate), and administering oxygen. It may also include cooling or fanning, but never so far as to cause the patient to shiver. (pp. 814–815)

16. **(C)** If in a heat emergency a patient with moist, pale, normal-to-cool skin is responsive and not nauseated, the EMT should have him or her drink water. (pp. 814–815)

17. **(C)** When treating an unresponsive hypothermia patient who is not responding appropriately, provide high-concentration oxygen that has been passed through a warm humidifier. If necessary, the oxygen that has been kept warm in the ambulance passenger compartment can be used. If there is no other choice, oxygen from a cold cylinder may be used. (p. 810)

18. **(B)** Because patients with extreme hypothermia may not reach biological death for over 30 minutes, the medical philosophy is "they are not dead until they're warm and dead." In other words, a patient is not considered dead

until after she is rewarmed and resuscitative measures are applied. (p. 810)

19. **(A)** A cold injury usually occurring to exposed areas of the body that is brought about by direct contact with a cold object or exposure to cold air is called an early local cold injury. This injury is commonly called frostnip. (p. 811)

20. **(A)** The skin color of a patient with a superficial local cold injury changes from red to white. (p. 811)

21. **(C)** If a superficial local cold injury is on an extremity, the EMT should not re-expose the injury to cold. Immersion in hot water will burn the injury. The extremity should be splinted, but it should be covered. (p. 811)

22. **(C)** Muscles, bones, deep blood vessels, and organ membranes that have become frozen form a type of injury called a deep local cold injury. (p. 812)

23. **(B)** In frostbite, the affected area first appears white and waxy. When the condition progresses to actual freezing, the skin turns mottled or blotchy and the color turns from white to grayish yellow and finally grayish blue. (p. 812)

24. **(C)** Do not allow the frostbite patient to drink alcohol or smoke because constriction of blood vessels and decreased circulation to the injured tissues may result. (p. 813)

25. **(A)** Active rewarming of a frozen part is seldom recommended in the field. Very hot water may burn the part; the patient's face should be left uncovered. (p. 813)

26. **(C)** When assessing a patient you suspect is in extreme hypothermia, check the carotid pulse for 30–45 seconds. (p. 810)

27. **(C)** The environment associated with hyperthermia includes heat and high humidity. (p. 814)

28. **(B)** The higher the humidity, the less your perspiration evaporates as a means of losing excessive body heat. (p. 814)

29. **(B)** The medical problems resulting from dry heat are often worse than those from moist heat because moist heat tires people before they can harm themselves through overexertion. Dry heat does not affect the respiratory system more quickly than humid heat. (p. 814)

30. **(D)** Fluid build-up in the lungs is related to *too much* salt in the body, not too little. When salts are lost by the body through sweating, the patient may have muscle cramps, weakness or exhaustion, and dizziness or periods of faintness. (p. 814)

31. **(B)** A patient with heat exhaustion presents with moist, pale, normal-to-cool skin. A rapid, strong pulse and lack of sweating are sometimes found with heat stroke. (p. 814)

32. **(B)** The signs and symptoms of a heat emergency in patients who have hot and dry or moist skin include seizures. Muscle cramps usually occur only in early heat exposure from salt loss. (p. 815)

33. **(C)** When responding to a water-related emergency, you should suspect, in addition to drowning, that substance abuse may be involved, the patient may have sustained an internal injury or fracture, and the patient may have struck his or her head or neck. Profuse perspiration is not a likely cause unless it is a hot tub. (pp. 817–818)

34. **(B)** Substance abuse is a large contributor to adolescent and adult drownings. Car crash immersions are rare. (p. 818)

35. **(C)** During a drowning incident, water flowing past the epiglottis causes a reflex spasm of the larynx. (p. 818)

36. **(B)** About 10 percent of drowning victims die from lack of air (suffocation). (p. 818)

37. **(A)** If you are not an experienced swimmer, you should never attempt to go into the water to do a rescue. You should wear a personal floatation device on the shore and the appropriate exposure suit if you are going into the water. Get qualified help immediately. (p. 817)

38. **(B)** If you suspect that a patient still in the pool has a possible spine injury, you should immobilize and apply a spineboard while he is still in the water. Expediting the removal from the water could complicate the injury. Do not encourage the patient to swim because swimming may further injure him. (p. 819)

39. **(C)** Two special medical problems seen in scuba-diving accidents are decompression sickness and air embolism. (p. 822)

40. **(A)** The risk of decompression sickness is increased by air travel within 12 hours of a dive. (p. 822)

41. **(C)** A toxin produced by some animals that is harmful to humans is called venom. (p. 826)

42. **(D)** Typical sources of injected poisons include spider, scorpion, and snake bites, and insect stings. (p. 826)

43. **(B)** While cleaning out the crawl space below the house, you experience blotchy skin, redness in your arm, weakness, and nausea. It is possible that you were bitten by a poisonous spider. (pp. 826–827)

44. **(A)** Lack of sensation on one side of the body is usually due to a head injury or cerebrovascular accident. Signs and symptoms of injected poisoning include puncture marks, muscle cramps, chest tightening, joint pain, excessive saliva formation, and profuse sweating. (pp. 827–828)

45. **(D)** Never transport a live snake in the ambulance. Arrange for separate transport of a live specimen. If you suspect that your patient has been bitten by a snake, you should call for medical direction; clean the injection site with soap and water; and remove rings, bracelets, or other constricting items on the bitten limb. (p. 830)

46. **(B)** The patient is not likely to have inability to move both legs unless he sustained a spine injury. (p. 830)

47. **(D)** If the patient has convulsions or a rapid lapse into unconsciousness leading to respiratory or cardiac arrest, you should suspect that he may have an air embolism (AGE). (pp. 822–823)

48. **(A)** If the patient has personality changes and fatigue, and in addition he is acting like he is intoxicated, although there is no way he could have taken anything, you should suspect decompression sickness. (pp. 822–823)

INSIDE/OUTSIDE (P. 817)

1. When the patient's skin is hot on the "outside" and the patient has a body temperature over 103°F, you should suspect that he has hyperthermia.

2. The patient who is cold and has hypothermia with an altered mental status on the "outside" most likely has a body temperature of 91.5°F on the "inside."

COMPLETE THE FOLLOWING

1. List six signs and symptoms of a heat emergency patient with moist, pale, and normal-to-cool skin: (p. 814)
   A) Muscular cramps, usually in the legs and abdomen
   B) Weakness or exhaustion, sometimes dizziness or periods of faintness
   C) Rapid, shallow breathing
   D) Weak pulse
   E) Heavy perspiration
   F) Loss of consciousness is possible, but it is usually brief if it occurs

2. List six signs and symptoms of a heat emergency patient with hot and dry or hot and moist skin: (any six) (p. 815)
   - Rapid, shallow breathing
   - Full and rapid pulse
   - Generalized weakness
   - Little or no perspiration
   - Loss of consciousness or altered mental status
   - Dilated pupils
   - Seizures may be seen; no muscle cramps

3. List 12 signs and symptoms of an injected poisoning (insect, spider, or scorpion): (any 12) (pp. 827–828)
   - Altered state of awareness
   - Noticeable stings or bites on the skin
   - Puncture marks (especially note the fingers, forearms, toes, and legs)
   - Blotchy skin (mottled skin)
   - Localized pain or itching
   - Numbness in a limb or body part
   - Burning sensations at the site followed by pain spreading throughout the limb
   - Redness
   - Swelling or blistering at the site
   - Weakness or collapse
   - Difficult breathing and abnormal pulse rate
   - Headache and dizziness
   - Chills
   - Fever
   - Nausea and vomiting
   - Muscle cramps, chest tightening, joint pain
   - Excessive saliva formation, profuse sweating
   - Anaphylaxis

4. List five signs and/or symptoms of snake bite: (any five) (p. 830)
   - Noticeable bite on the skin. This may appear as nothing more than a discoloration.
   - Pain and swelling in the area of the bite. This may be slow to develop, taking from 30 minutes to several hours.
   - Rapid pulse and labored breathing
   - Progressive general weakness
   - Vision problems (dim or blurred)
   - Nausea and vomiting
   - Seizures
   - Drowsiness or unconsciousness

STREET SCENES DISCUSSION

1. Active rewarming involves heat packs; hot air; blankets; and warmed, humidified oxygen. In the hospital environment, active rewarming may include warm fluids, dialysis, warm enemas, and bypass.

2. Yes, of course, and prepare to apply the AED.

3. In the early stages of hypothermia, the heartbeat may be rapid. In a later stage, it slows. In this patient's situation, he may have been in early-stage hypothermia or he may have had another problem, such as shock from internal bleeding.

CASE STUDY: TOO COLD FOR COMFORT

1. Mental status, ABCs, and ruling out trauma.

2. No. The parent is on the way, so you can begin to talk to the children and patient.

3. SAMPLE history and OPQRST of the chief complaint, which is altered mental status in this case.

4. Comfortable, lying supine, wrapped in blankets.

5. A mild case of hypothermia.

6. Yes, oxygen would be helpful via nonrebreather mask.

7. A slightly decreased temperature but not as low at 90°F, which is considered severe hypothermia.

8. She is a child, she is thin with little fat insulation, and she has been playing in cold water and the wind all afternoon.

9. Children love to swim and will do so all day long. Suggest that they have frequent breaks to warm up out of the water and wind.

Chapter 34: Obstetrics and Gynecology

MATCH TERMINOLOGY/ DEFINITIONS

▶ **PART A**

1. **(I)** Abortion—spontaneous (miscarriage) or induced termination of pregnancy (p. 868)

2. **(R)** Abruptio placentae—a condition in which the placenta separates from the uterine wall; a cause of prebirth bleeding (p. 867)

3. **(D)** Afterbirth—the placenta, umbilical cord, and some tissues from the lining of the uterus that are delivered after the birth of the baby (p. 843)

4. **(K)** Amniotic sac—the "bag of waters" that surrounds the developing fetus (p. 841)

5. **(M)** Breech presentation—when the buttocks or both legs of a baby deliver first during birth (p. 861)

6. **(A)** Cephalic presentation—when the baby appears head-first during birth (p. 846)

7. **(B)** Cervix—the neck of the uterus at the entrance to the birth canal (p. 840)

8. **(O)** Crowning—when part of the baby is visible through the vaginal opening (p. 846)

9. **(Q)** Eclampsia—a severe complication of pregnancy that produces seizures and coma (p. 868)

10. **(C)** Ectopic pregnancy—when implantation of the fertilized egg is not in the body of the uterus, occurring instead in the oviduct, the cervix, or the abdominopelvic cavity (p. 867)

11. **(E)** Fetus—the baby as he or she develops in the womb (p. 840)

©2012 Pearson Education, Inc.
Emergency Care, 12th Ed.

12. **(G)** Induced abortion—expulsion of a fetus as a result of deliberate actions taken to stop a pregnancy (p. 868)

13. **(J)** Labor—three stages of the delivery of a baby that begin with the contractions of the uterus and end with the expulsion of the placenta (p. 843)

14. **(H)** Lightening—the sensation of the fetus moving from high in the abdomen to low in the birth canal (p. 874)

15. **(N)** Limb presentation—when an infant's limb protrudes from the vagina before the appearance of any other body part (p. 862)

16. **(L)** Meconium staining—amniotic fluid that is greenish or brownish-yellow rather than clear as a result of fetal defecation; an indication of possible maternal or fetal distress during labor (p. 845)

17. **(F)** Miscarriage—spontaneous abortion (p. 868)

18. **(P)** Multiple birth—when more than one baby is born during a single delivery (p. 863)

▶ **Part B**

1. **(J)** Ovary—the female reproductive organ that produces ova (p. 839)

2. **(F)** Ovulation—the phase of the female reproductive cycle where an ovum is released from the ovary (p. 840)

3. **(D)** Oviduct—fallopian tube; tube that carries eggs from an ovary to the uterus (p. 839)

4. **(N)** Perineum—the surface area between the vagina and anus (p. 874)

5. **(O)** Placenta—the organ of pregnancy where exchange of oxygen, food, and waste occurs between a mother and her fetus (p. 841)

6. **(I)** Placenta previa—a condition in which the placenta is formed in an abnormal location (low in the uterus and close to or over the cervical opening) and will not allow for a normal delivery of the fetus; a cause of excessive prebirth bleeding (p. 867)

7. **(M)** Preeclampsia—a complication of pregnancy where the woman retains large amounts of fluid and has hypertension; she may also experience seizures and/or coma during birth, which is very dangerous to both mother and infant (p. 868)

8. **(C)** Premature infant—any newborn weighing less than 5½ pounds or born before the thirty-seventh week of pregnancy (p. 864)

9. **(A)** Prolapsed umbilical cord—when the umbilical cord presents first and is squeezed between the vaginal wall and the baby's head (p. 862)

10. **(L)** Spontaneous abortion—when the fetus and placenta deliver before the twenty-eighth week of pregnancy; commonly called a miscarriage (p. 868)

11. **(E)** Stillborn—born dead (p. 874)

12. **(B)** Supine hypotensive syndrome—dizziness and a drop in blood pressure caused when the mother is in a supine position and the weight of the uterus, infant, placenta, and amniotic fluid compress the inferior vena cava, reducing return of blood to the heart and cardiac output (p. 843)

13. **(G)** Umbilical cord—the fetal structure containing the blood vessels that carry blood to and from the placenta (p. 841)

14. **(K)** Uterus—the muscular abdominal organ where the fetus develops; the womb (p. 840)

15. **(H)** Vagina—the birth canal (p. 839)

MULTIPLE-CHOICE REVIEW

1. **(B)** The 9 months of pregnancy are divided into 3-month trimesters. During the second trimester, the uterus grows very rapidly while the woman's blood volume, cardiac output, and heart rate increase. (p. 841)

2. **(B)** The normal birth position is the head-first position and is called a cephalic birth. Breech is buttocks or feet-first birth. (p. 846)

3. **(C)** The first stage of labor starts with regular contractions of the uterus. This can occur earlier or later than 9 months. It ends with full dilatation of the cervix. (p. 844)

4. **(D)** The second stage of labor starts with the entry of the baby into the birth canal. (p. 844)

5. **(A)** The third stage of labor begins after the birth of the baby. (p. 844)

6. **(B)** The third stage of labor is complete when the afterbirth is expelled. Expulsion should occur within 20 minutes from the birth of the baby. (p. 845)

7. **(B)** The process by which the cervix gradually widens and thins out is called dilation. (p. 845)

8. **(A)** As the fetus moves downward and the cervix dilates, the amniotic sac normally breaks and fluid leaks out. If this fluid is greenish or brownish-yellow in color, it may indicate fetal or maternal distress. (p. 845)

9. **(C)** The greenish or brownish-yellow fluid expelled from the amniotic sac is called meconium staining and could indicate that the fetus is in distress and made a bowel movement. There is no such thing as amniotic bile. Bile is a chemical that helps break down fats during digestion. (p. 845)

10. **(C)** When a mother in labor states that she feels the need to move her bowels, the birth moment is nearing because the fetus is pressing on her bowel as it moves down the birth canal. This does not indicate that the baby is in distress. (p. 845)

11. **(B)** The contraction duration is timed from the beginning of the contraction to relaxation of the uterus. The contraction interval is defined in the answer for multiple-choice question 12. (pp. 844–845)

12. **(A)** The contraction interval, or frequency, is timed from the start of one contraction to the start of the next. The contraction duration is defined in the answer for multiple-choice question 11. (pp. 844–845)

13. **(B)** Delivery is imminent when the contractions last 30 seconds and are 2 to 3 minutes apart. (p. 845)

14. **(B)** The EMT's primary roles at a normal childbirth scene are to determine whether the delivery will occur at the scene and, if so, to assist the mother as she delivers the child. If delivery is imminent, do not delay it. There is no need to immobilize the patient during emergency childbirth. (p. 849)

15. **(C)** The sterile obstetrical kit does *not* contain heavy, flat twine to tie the cord. Occasionally, in an off-duty situation, you may be required to improvise using heavy, flat twine or new shoelaces to tie the cord. (p. 850)

16. **(B)** When evaluating the mother for a possible home delivery, the EMT should ask about the frequency and duration of contractions. It is normal if the mother feels the need to urinate, but if she has to move her bowels, this is a signal that the infant is moving down the birth canal. The father's blood type is not important to field care but would

be important to hospital care if a transfusion is necessary. (pp. 846–847)

17. **(A)** It is important to ask the mother if you can examine for crowning if the mother is straining during contractions. If she is, birth will probably occur too soon for transport. EMTs do not automatically examine every woman in her ninth month for crowning, and you would need the patient's permission to do so. (pp. 846–847)

18. **(C)** You should ask the mother if her water broke and prepare for a quiet ride to the hospital. This is her first pregnancy and only an 8-month term, so this may be false labor or just the beginning of labor. (p. 846)

19. **(A)** If you determine that the delivery is imminent based on the presence of crowning and other signs, you should contact medical direction or follow your local protocol. Do not ask the mother to go to the bathroom first, as the infant may be expelled into the toilet. Do not attempt to hold back a delivery by asking the mother to hold her legs closed. (p. 847)

20. **(B)** If a full-term pregnant woman in a supine position complains of dizziness and you note a drop in blood pressure, the woman could be suffering from supine hypotension syndrome (vena cava syndrome). This is a condition in which the heavy mass created by the weight of the uterus, coupled with the infant's weight, placenta, and amniotic fluid, compresses the inferior vena cava, reducing return of blood to the heart and reducing cardiac output, thus resulting in low blood pressure. Cushing reflex occurs in head injuries. (p. 843)

21. **(B)** To lessen the pressure of the uterus on the inferior vena cava, you should transport the patient on her left side. See the answer for multiple-choice question 20. (p. 843)

22. **(D)** During a delivery, the EMT needs infection control gear such as surgical gloves, a mask, and eye protection as well as a gown. A Tyvek suit is not needed for protection against blood spraying. (p. 849)

23. **(D)** During delivery, encourage the mother to breathe deeply through her mouth. She may feel better if she pants, although she should be discouraged from breathing rapidly and deeply enough to bring on hyperventilation. (p. 849)

24. **(A)** Do not pull on the baby's shoulders or any other part of the baby. When supporting the baby's head during a delivery, the EMT should apply gentle pressure to control the delivery, place one hand below the head, and spread fingers evenly around the baby's head. (p. 849)

25. **(B)** If the amniotic sac has not broken by the time the baby's head is delivered, use your finger to puncture the membrane. Then pull the membranes away from the baby's mouth and nose. (p. 851)

26. **(C)** If you cannot loosen or unwrap the umbilical cord from around the infant's neck, you should clamp the cord in two places and cut between the clamps. This way the child will not strangle, and the cord will not tear. (p. 851)

27. **(A)** Most babies are born face down and then rotate to either side. (p. 846)

28. **(B)** When suctioning a newborn, compress the syringe before placing it in the baby's mouth to avoid blowing fluids into the baby's airway. (p. 857)

29. **(B)** Once the baby's feet are delivered, lay the baby on her side with head slightly lower than her torso. This is done to allow blood, fluids, and mucus to drain from the mouth and nose. Remember, newborns are very slippery; **never** pick up a baby by the feet because you could drop the child. (p. 855)

30. **(D)** To assess the newborn, the EMT does not check the response to a sternal rub because it could injure the child. A general evaluation usually calls for noting ease of breathing, the heart rate, crying (vigorous crying is a good sign), movement (the more active, the better), skin color (blue coloration at the hands and feet may or may not disappear, but it should not spread to other parts of the body). (p. 854)

31. **(C)** It is necessary to suction the baby's mouth before the nose because suctioning the nose first may cause the baby to gasp or begin breathing and aspirate any meconium, blood, fluids, or mucus from the mouth into the lungs. (p. 866)

32. **(C)** If assessment of the infant's breathing reveals shallow, slow, or absent respirations, the EMT should provide artificial ventilations at 40 to 60 per minute. Do not use an oxygen mask. (p. 857)

33. **(A)** In a normal birth, the infant must be breathing on her own before you clamp and cut the cord. (p. 857)

34. **(D)** The first umbilical cord clamp should be placed about 10 inches from the baby. (p. 856)

35. **(C)** The second umbilical cord clamp should be placed about 7 inches from the baby. (p. 856)

36. **(D)** If the placenta does not deliver within 20 minutes of the baby's birth, transport the mother and baby to a medical facility without delay. (p. 859)

37. **(B)** It is not uncommon for the mother to tear part of the perineum during a delivery. If this occurs, apply a sanitary napkin and apply gentle pressure. Let the mother know that torn tissue is normal and that the problem will be cared for quickly at the medical facility. (p. 860)

38. **(D)** Initiate rapid transport on recognition of a breech presentation. Never pull on the baby's legs. Provide high-concentration oxygen. Place the mother in a head-down position with the pelvis elevated. (p. 861)

39. **(A)** If you see the umbilical cord presenting first, gently push up on the baby's head or buttocks to take pressure off the cord. This may be the only chance that the baby has for survival, so continue to push up on the baby until you are relieved by a physician. All patients with prolapsed cords require rapid transport! (pp. 862–863)

40. **(D)** When a baby's limb presents first, the EMT should begin rapid transport of the patient immediately. Do not try to replace the limb into the vagina. (p. 862)

41. **(B)** When assisting with the delivery of twins, clamp the cord of the first baby before the second baby is born. Labor contractions will continue after the first baby is born. (p. 864)

42. **(B)** Newly born infants lose heat rapidly. This heat loss affects their comfort and decreases their glucose level, which affects their ability to carry oxygen in their blood and increases their shivering. (p. 855)

43. **(B)** When oxygen is administered to an infant, it should be given by flowing it past the baby's face. Use humidified oxygen, if available, so it doesn't dry out the baby's respiratory tract. (pp. 857–858)

44. **(B)** If you suspect meconium staining when the infant is born, avoid stimulating the infant before suctioning the oropharynx. This reduces the risk of aspiration. (p. 845)

©2012 Pearson Education, Inc.
Emergency Care, 12th Ed.

45. (D) A condition in which the placenta is formed low in the uterus and close to the cervical opening, preventing the normal delivery of the fetus, is called placenta previa. (p. 867)

46. (D) Seizures in pregnancy are usually associated with extreme swelling of the extremities. In addition, the patient will have *elevated* blood pressure. Seizures tend to occur *late* in pregnancy and pose a threat to *both* the mother and unborn baby. (p. 868)

47. (C) Massive bleeding and shock are the gravest dangers associated with blunt trauma to the pregnant woman's abdomen or pelvis. Perform a patient assessment and treat her injuries as you would those of any trauma patient. (p. 869)

48. (A) Because of the physiology of a pregnant woman, her vital signs may be interpreted as suggestive of shock when they are actually normal. The pregnant woman has a pulse rate that is 10–15 beats per minute *faster* than her non-pregnant counterpart and a blood volume as much as 48 percent *higher* than her nonpregnant state. Shock is *more* difficult to assess in the pregnant patient, and it is the most likely cause of prehospital death from injury to the uterus. (p. 869)

49. (B) Unless a back or neck injury is suspected, all pregnant women who have suffered blunt trauma injury should be transported in the left lateral recumbent position. If you suspect neck or back injury, first secure the mother to a spine board, then tip the board and patient as a unit to the left to relieve pressure on the abdominal organs and vena cava. (p. 870)

50. (C) If vaginal bleeding is associated with abdominal pain, treat the patient as if she has a potentially life-threatening condition. The most serious complication of vaginal bleeding is hypovolemic shock due to blood loss. (p. 867)

COMPLETE THE FOLLOWING

1. When evaluating the woman in labor, the EMT should: (any seven) (p. 846)
   - Ask her name and age and expected due date.
   - Ask if this is her first pregnancy.
   - Ask her if she has seen a doctor regarding her pregnancy.
   - Ask her when the labor pains started and how often she is having pains.
   - Ask her if her "bag of waters" has broken and if she has had any bleeding or bloody show.
   - Ask her is she feels the urge to push or if she feels as though she needs to move her bowels.
   - Examine the mother for crowning.
   - Feel for uterine contractions.
   - Take vital signs at this time if they have not been taken yet.

2. Take the following steps when providing care for a woman who presents with a prolapsed cord: (p. 862)
   A) Position the mother with her head down and pelvis raised with a blanket or pillow, using gravity to lesson pressure on the birth canal.
   B) Provide the mother with high-concentration oxygen by way of a nonrebreather mask to increase the concentration carried to the infant.
   C) Check the cord for pulses and wrap the exposed cord, using a sterile towel from the obstetric kit. This cord must be kept warm.

D) Insert several fingers of your gloved hand into the mother's vagina so that you can gently push up on the baby's head or buttocks to keep pressure off the cord.
E) Keeping mother, child, and EMT as a unit, transport immediately to a medical facility. Be prepared to push up on the baby's head or buttocks until you reach the hospital.
F) All patients with prolapsed cords require rapid transport. Have your partner obtain vital signs while en route to the hospital if possible.

3. Complete the following (p. 854):
   A) Extremities blue, trunk pink
   B) >100
   C) No reaction
   D) Only slight activity (flexing extremities)
   E) Good breathing, strong cry

LABEL THE DIAGRAMS (P. 841)

1. Amniotic sac
2. Umbilical cord
3. Placenta
4. Uterus
5. Pubic bone
6. Cervix
7. Vagina

INSIDE/OUTSIDE (P. 842)

1. A pregnant woman who has a pink coloration to her skin "outside" has an increased blood volume on the "inside."

2. A pregnant woman who exhibits nausea, vomiting, and heartburn on the "outside" has a GI tract that has been displaced by the growing uterus on the "inside."

3. A woman in active labor has a contraction on the "inside;" the EMT observes regular pain with contraction and palpable hardening of the uterus with each contraction on the "outside."

4. If the fetus is not presenting in the head-first position into the birth canal on the "inside," the EMT may observe a limb presentation on the "outside."

STREET SCENES DISCUSSION

1. If the amniotic sac has not broken by the time the baby's head is delivered, use your finger to puncture the membrane. Then pull the membrane away from the baby's mouth and nose.

2. This is called meconium staining. Meconium-stained amniotic fluid is caused by fetal feces (waste) released during labor, usually because of maternal or fetal stress. If meconium is present, suction the infant immediately—first the mouth and then the nose. Maintain an open airway and be prepared to provide artificial ventilation or CPR if needed. Transport as soon as possible.

3. Be sure to put the mother on high-concentration oxygen via nonrebreather mask, keep her warm, elevate her legs, and massage her abdomen above the uterus. It may also be helpful to encourage the mother to nurse the infant because breastfeeding stimulates the uterus to contract.

MATCH TERMINOLOGY/DEFINITIONS

1. **(C)** Adolescent—child from 12 to 18 years of age (p. 884)

2. **(H)** Fontanelle—a soft spot on an infant's anterior scalp formed by the joining of not-yet-fused bones of the skull (p. 881)

3. **(G)** Newborn—child between birth and 1 year of age (p. 883)

4. **(F)** Pediatric—of or pertaining to a patient who has yet to reach puberty (p. 878)

5. **(A)** Preschooler—child from 3 to 6 years of age (p. 884)

6. **(B)** Retractions—pulling in of the skin and soft tissue between the ribs when breathing; typically a sign of respiratory distress in children (p. 890)

7. **(D)** School-aged child—child from 6 to 12 years of age (p. 884)

8. **(E)** Toddler—child from 1 to 3 years of age (p. 883)

MULTIPLE-CHOICE REVIEW

1. **(B)** A toddler is between 1 and 3 years old. (p. 883)

2. **(C)** A school-aged child is between 6 and 12 years old. (p. 884)

3. **(D)** When assessing the toddler, examine the head *last*, not first. Toddlers fear having their head or face touched by strangers. To build confidence, examine a toddler's heart and lungs first, then the head. (p. 883)

4. **(C)** Until about age 4 to 6, a child's head is proportionately larger and heavier than the adult's. This is why padding needs to be placed behind the shoulders when the child is immobilized. It is also the reason why children fly head first when involved in auto collisions or fall out of a window. (p. 899)

5. **(B)** The soft spot on an infant's anterior skull is called a fontanelle. (p. 881)

6. **(A)** A sunken fontanelle may indicate dehydration. See the answer for multiple-choice question 7. (p. 881)

7. **(B)** A bulging fontanelle may indicate elevated intracranial pressure. It is also a sign of meningitis. It may also bulge when the infant cries. (p. 881)

8. **(D)** Newborns usually breathe primarily through their noses. This is why secretions in and obstruction of the nasal passageways that are not resolved by the caregiver can cause breathing problems. (p. 881)

9. **(B)** In an infant, hyperextension of the neck may result in airway obstruction because hyperextension can kink the flexible trachea. (p. 881)

10. **(D)** Suctioning of a child's airway for longer than a few seconds at a time could lead to vagal stimulation, a very slow heart rate, and ultimately cardiac arrest. Suctioning temporarily cuts off the body's oxygen supply; if it is prolonged, it is especially dangerous to infants and children. (p. 899)

11. **(A)** The tongues of infants and children are more likely than an adult's to fall back into and block the airway because their tongues are proportionately larger than the adult's. (p. 881)

12. **(B)** The insertion procedure for an oropharyngeal airway (OPA) in an infant or child is done with the tip pointing toward the tongue and throat, which is the same position it will be in after insertion. Flipping it over the tongue may cause a tear in the soft palate. (p. 900)

13. **(A)** When assessing the capillary refill of a child 5 years old or younger, peripheral perfusion is considered satisfactory if the color returns in less than 2 seconds. (p. 906)

14. **(D)** Loss of consciousness is not a sign of a mild airway obstruction in an infant or child. It is a sign of severe respiratory distress. (p. 908)

15. **(C)** A child with a severe airway obstruction, or severe partial one, *cannot* cry and is moving very little air, and the cough becomes ineffective. (p. 902)

16. **(C)** The effects of hypoxia on an infant or a child are slowed heart rate and altered mental status. Hypoxia is the underlying reason for many of the most serious medical problems with children. (p. 908)

17. **(D)** Always use infection control barriers even when ventilating infants and children. Guidelines to use when ventilating the infant or child include avoid breathing too hard through the pocket face mask or using excessive bag pressure and volume, and use properly sized face masks to ensure a good mask seal. Also remember that, if ventilation is not successful in raising the patient's chest, perform procedures for clearing an obstructed airway, then try to ventilate again. (p. 904)

18. **(B)** The flow-restricted, oxygen-powered ventilation device is contraindicated in infants and children. Special units (pediatric automatic transport ventilators) are designed for pediatric patients; they require additional training, but they are not typically used in the field by EMTs. (p. 905)

19. **(B)** Common causes of shock in a child include infection, trauma, blood loss, and dehydration. (p. 905)

20. **(D)** Croup is not a cause of shock. Less common causes of shock in a child include allergic reactions, poisoning, and cardiac events (rare). (p. 910)

21. **(B)** The blood volume of infants and children is approximately 8 percent of the total body weight. (p. 906)

22. **(D)** Children decompensate very rapidly, *not* very slowly! When children are in shock, they compensate very well, appear better than they actually are, and "go sour quickly" once they decompensate. (p. 907)

23. **(C)** When a child is bleeding internally, the EMT should avoid waiting for signs of decompensated shock before treating for shock. At this point, the child has approximately 30 percent blood loss. (p. 907)

24. **(B)** Decreased urine output (less wet diapers) and absence of tears are signs of shock in infants and children. (p. 906)

25. **(B)** When treating a child in shock, the EMT should elevate the patient's legs unless there are injuries that would contraindicate it. (p. 907)

26. **(A)** Because children have a large skin surface area in proportion to their body mass, they can easily become victims of hypothermia. (p. 907)

27. **(B)** If a child has an airway respiratory disease, it is very important that the EMT *avoid* inserting a tongue blade into the mouth, which could stimulate a laryngospasm. Administering blow-by oxygen is an appropriate action. (p. 911)

28. **(A)** Stridor on inspiration is an upper airway problem. The signs of an airway disease in a child include breathing effort on exhalation, rapid breathing, and wheezing. (p. 911)

29. **(C)** A viral illness that causes inflammation of the upper airway and bronchi, and is often accompanied by a "seal bark" cough, is called croup. Epiglottitis is a bacterial infection that produces swelling of the epiglottis and usually develops in an older child; the patient exhibits with drooling due to the inability to swallow. (p. 911)

30. **(B)** The early signs of respiratory distress in a child include nasal flaring; retraction of the muscles above, below, and between the sternum and ribs; use of abdominal muscles; stridor; audible wheezing; grunting; and a breathing rate greater than 60. Slowing or irregular respiration is a late sign of respiratory distress in a child. (p. 909)

31. **(B)** Hypothermia does *not* cause fever. Causes of fever in children include upper respiratory and other types of infection. (p. 912)

32. **(A)** Rectal or oral thermometers generally are *not* used in the out-of-hospital setting unless permitted by local medical direction. (p. 912)

33. **(C)** When treating an infant or child with a high fever, monitor for shivering while cooling with tepid water. Do not use alcohol because it is a fire hazard and can be absorbed by the skin. Do not cover with a towel soaked in ice water, which can rapidly cause hypothermia. (p. 912)

34. **(B)** Infants are more susceptible to dehydration because, compared to adults, a greater percentage of their body is water. (p. 913)

35. **(C)** Fever is the *most common* cause of seizures in infants and children. While a fever is rarely life threatening in children who have one, a fever should be considered life threatening by the EMT. (p. 914)

36. **(B)** Severe aspirin poisoning does not cause dehydration; it can cause seizures, shock, and coma. (p. 915)

37. **(A)** A common cause of lead poisoning in children is ingesting chips of lead-based paint. Eating fish from freshwater lakes is generally not a problem unless the lake is polluted. (p. 916)

38. **(C)** If you are treating a child who accidentally ingested a handful of her mother's vitamin tablets, you should be concerned because many vitamin pills contain iron, which can be fatal to a child. (p. 916)

39. **(D)** The majority of meningitis cases occur between the ages of 1 month and 5 years. (p. 913)

40. **(D)** In cases of sudden infant death syndrome (SIDS), the EMT should provide resuscitation and transport to the hospital. He or she should avoid accusatory actions, such as looking for evidence of neglect, and instead be supportive because parents who lose a child to SIDS often suffer intense guilt feelings. (p. 904)

41. **(B)** The number one cause of death in infants and children is trauma. Much trauma to infants and children occurs because they are curious and learning about their environment. (p. 919)

42. **(C)** The child who has been struck by a vehicle may present with a triad of injuries (Waddell's triad) that include head injury, lower extremity injury (possibly a fractured femur), and abdominal injury (with possible internal bleeding and shock). (p. 918)

43. **(D)** The most frequent sign of head injury is altered mental status. Respiratory arrest is a common secondary effect. Head injury itself is seldom a cause of shock except in infants. Suspect internal injuries whenever a head-injured child presents with shock. (p. 918)

44. **(D)** The musculoskeletal structures of the chest are less developed in infants and children, so they are more likely to incur injury to structures beneath the ribs. (p. 920)

45. **(C)** Because the abdominal muscles of infants and small children are immature and very thin, they offer less protection for underlying organs. (p. 919)

46. **(D)** You must keep the infant or child covered to prevent a drop in body temperature. Burned patients who become hypothermic have a higher death rate. (p. 920)

47. **(D)** A parent's concern about the child's injuries is normal and to be expected. Indications that child abuse may be occurring include repeated responses to provide care for the same child or family, poorly healing wounds or improperly healed fractures, and indications of past injuries. (pp. 922–923)

48. **(C)** Torn clothing on the child is not necessarily an indication of child abuse because active children damage their clothing all the time. When you respond to the home of a person whom you suspect of child abuse, observe for a family member who has trouble controlling anger, indications of alcohol and drug abuse, and any adult who appears in a state of depression. (pp. 922–923)

49. **(C)** You should talk with the child separately about how an injury occurred, but it is not your role to ask the child if he or she has been abused. Always report your suspicions to the ED staff and in accordance with local policies. If you are a mandated reporter in your state, you may need to contact the hotline. (p. 924)

50. **(D)** When treating a child who you suspect is suffering from epiglottitis, it is important to transport the child immediately, not place anything in the child's mouth, and constantly monitor the respiratory status. (p. 911)

51. **(C)** The primary cause of cardiac arrest in children is a respiratory disorder that leads to respiratory failure. (p. 899)

52. **(A)** In assessing breathing, you should observe for chest expansion, the effort of breathing, and the sounds of breathing. (p. 899)

53. **(B)** There is appropriate MOI to do a spinal immobilization on this child. The BVM may be useful at some point, but this child is verbally responsive and will not take the OPA (perhaps an NPA would work?). Unless there is a history of asthma, the albuterol (Proventil® or Ventilin®) treatment is probably not appropriate, nor is the Epi-Pen®. (p. 918)

54. **(C)** This patient is a high priority based on the MOI, the altered mental status, and the potential for shock. (p. 919)

▌ INSIDE/OUTSIDE (P. 899)

1. Pad behind the 4-year-old child's shoulders to compensate for the proportionately larger head when immobilizing the neck of the child.

2. Place the 4-year-old child in the neutral or extended, but not hyperextended, position to open the airway. If you hyperextend, it is actually possible to kink the flexible trachea and partially close it.

INSIDE/OUTSIDE (P. 907)

1. When the body of a child who is losing blood starts to compensate, on the "inside" the heart beats faster, the blood vessels constrict, and the respiratory rate increases.

2. When the body of a child who is losing blood starts to compensate, on the "outside" the pulse rate is increased, the skin gets pale, the capillary refill is delayed, and the mental status becomes altered.

INSIDE/OUTSIDE (P. 908)

1. During respiratory distress, on the "inside," the child's heart rate increases and the blood vessels constrict.

2. During respiratory distress, on the "outside," the child's breathing gets difficult, and the respiratory rate and pulse rate both increase.

3. During respiratory failure, on the "inside," the child's compensation is overwhelmed, and he or she becomes hypoxic and begins to tire.

4. During respiratory failure, on the "outside," the child becomes cyanotic, with slow and irregular respirations and an altered mental status.

COMPLETE THE FOLLOWING

1. Signs of respiratory distress in a child include the following: (any ten) (p. 909)
   - Nasal flaring
   - Retraction of the muscles above, below, and between the sternum and ribs
   - Use of abdominal muscles
   - Stridor
   - Audible wheezing
   - Grunting
   - Breathing rate greater than 60
   - Cyanosis
   - Decreased muscle tone
   - Poor peripheral perfusion
   - Delayed capillary refill
   - Altered mental status
   - Decreased heart rate

COMPLETE THE CHART (P. 903)

1. 1 second
2. 1 second
3. 1 second
4. 10 to 12 breaths/minute
5. 12 to 20 breaths/minute
6. 12 to 20 breaths/minute

STREET SCENES DISCUSSION

1. The child may have had a seizure.

2. If the child's mental status did not improve and you suspected the child had a temperature as well as a rash, there may be an infectious disease involved. Be sure to use a face mask, eye shield, and disposable gloves.

3. Follow up in case there is an infectious disease to which you may have been exposed.

CASE STUDY: THE CASE OF THE POISONED JUICE

1. Use gloves, an eye shield, and a mask.

2. Find out exactly who drank the juice. Separate the healthy children from the juice drinkers to limit the "sympathy" sickness.

3. Dehydration.

4. A shunt is a tube to drain excess cerebrospinal fluid in the head into the abdomen. Shunts are used for children who are hydrocephalic.

5. Pulse of 90 to 140, respirations of 25 to 40; BP is usually not taken on a child under 3.

6. Pulse of 80 to 130, respirations of 20 to 30; BP is usually not taken on a child under 3.

7. Pulse of 80 to 120, respirations of 20 to 30, and BP of 99 systolic.

8. Have the caretaker hold the infant. Be sure to keep the infant warm; warm your stethoscope and hands prior to touching the child. Observe the breathing from a distance.

9. Have the caretaker hold the toddler. Assure the child that he was not bad. Remove an article of clothing, examine, and then replace the clothing. Examine in a trunk-to-head approach to build confidence.

10. Use a toy, let them help you, and approach from toes to head.

11. In a child safety car seat.

12. Ask the parent if this is how the infant normally reacts to this stimuli.

13. The juice can be analyzed to determine what organism caused the problem.

CASE STUDY: ABUSER OR LOVING PARENT?

1. At a motor vehicle collision scene, traffic is usually your greatest hazard.

2. Yes, because the limping driver could change his mind. You do not want to delay transporting the child in order to call for another ambulance later in the call.

3. Your initial concerns for the child are mental status and the status of his ABCs.

4. Yes, it is a significant finding. His mental status is probably deteriorating.

5. One way to determine a child's mental status is to ask the parent what is "normal" for the child.

6. The cracks are evidence that both of the patients' heads struck the windshield. This is a very significant mechanism of injury (MOI).

7. In addition to helping you determine what happened to the child, the mother's statement also tells you that the child is normally very active and expressive. He is not now.

8. Yes, and also evaluate the need for assisting ventilation.

9. Yes, request an ALS intercept. The patient may need to be intubated, and the extra hands would be helpful.

10. Just provide the facts. The mother may have broken at least two laws: She may have been driving while legally intoxicated and she did not use the proper restraints on the child. If she had followed the laws that are designed to protect children, the injuries probably would not have been so severe.

MATCH TERMINOLOGY/ DEFINITIONS

1. **(B)** Alzheimer's disease—chronic disorder resulting in dementia (p. 936)

2. **(E)** Aortic dissection—a separation of the layers of the artery described as a tearing sensation (p. 933)

3. **(C)** Pneumonia—an inflammation in the tissue of the lung (p. 933)

4. **(D)** Dysrhythmia—an abnormal heart rhythm (p. 933)

5. **(A)** Geriatric—elderly person, generally considered 65 years of age or older (p. 933)

MULTIPLE-CHOICE REVIEW

1. **(C)** Starting at age 30, our organ systems lose about 1 percent function each year. (pp. 934–935)

2. **(C)** Common causes of traumatic injuries in the older patient are car crashes or falls. (p. 940)

3. **(D)** Assessing the airway of an older patient is often difficult because of dentures and because of arthritic changes in the bones of the neck. (p. 977)

4. **(B)** Older patients are less likely to show severe symptoms in certain conditions, so it can be difficult to determine the patient's priority. (p. 937)

5. **(C)** The family tells you that the patient was wrong in some responses during your interview with the patient. These incorrect responses are sometimes the result of a neurological condition as well as taking multiple medications. (p. 940)

6. **(B)** Replacing lost circumstances with imaginary ones is known as confabulation. (p. 938)

7. **(D)** Patients have high, low, and decreased sensitivity to pain. (p. 938)

8. **(B)** As a person ages, the systolic blood pressure has a tendency to increase. (p. 933)

9. **(D)** Hip fractures are common in elderly patients, especially women, due to loss of calcium. (p. 939)

10. **(C)** An EMT should consider that any injury of an elderly person could be a sign of abuse or neglect. (pp. 944–945)

11. **(B)** Her symptoms are not those of an allergy; the excessive doses of the NSAIDs can cause GI distress and aggravate her ulcers, causing them to bleed (coffee-ground vomit), and also cause dizziness. (p. 940)

12. **(A)** If the patient is on anticonvulsant meds, she must take the right amount and not drop her dose or she will ultimately have a seizure. (p. 940)

INSIDE/OUTSIDE (P. 932)

1. The patient who has thinner, wrinkled skin on the "outside" has decreased collagen and elastin fiber in the skin, as well as the breakdown of the remaining fibers on the "inside."

2. The patient who has graying hair on the "outside" has a decreasing number of melanocytes (pigment-producing cells) on the "inside."

3. The patient who has a stooped posture and arthritic joint deformities on the "outside" has demineralization of the bones (loss of calcium) and accumulated wear and tear on the joints on the "inside."

4. The patient who has a loss of central nervous system neurons on the "inside" will likely exhibit a diminished sensitivity of the senses, slower cognitive processing (slower to answer questions), and slowed movement and reflexes on the "outside."

COMPLETE THE FOLLOWING

The Physiological Effects of Aging and Implications for Assessment (pp. 933–934)

1. Decreased delivery of oxygenated blood to the tissues; increased risk of heart attack, stroke, aortic aneurysm, and peripheral artery disease.

2. Reduced stroke volume and cardiac output may lead to orthostatic hypotension, decreased brain perfusion, and reduced tolerance for activity.

3. Decreased ability to increase oxygen intake when needed; increased risk of pneumonia.

4. Constipation, bowel obstruction, weight loss, malnutrition.

5. Increased risk of drug toxicity and drug interactions; increased edema; decreased blood clotting.

6. Decreased energy metabolism; problems with temperature regulation.

7. Fractures may occur with minimal force, and sometimes with little pain.

8. Patients may be prone to injury, wandering away, being taken advantage of, or abused; patients may neglect themselves.

9. May attempt suicide, or neglect self; elderly with sleep disorders are more likely to be physically abused.

10. Skin easily bruised and torn.

STREET SCENES DISCUSSION

1. If you decide that the patient's condition is serious enough to use the ambulance lights and siren, you probably should call for ALS.

2. Many elderly people are on fixed incomes. Some feel they cannot pay big heating bills, so they keep the temperature down and wear lots of clothing instead. Older people cannot regulate body temperature very well, and this could cause medical problems.

3. The elderly patient may be afraid of losing his independence, of being left in the care of strangers, or just going to the hospital where he has lost friends and loved ones. You can help ease this transition by treating the patient in a respectful, dignified manner; acknowledging his fears and concerns; and attempting to put the patient's fears in perspective.

MATCH TERMINOLOGY/ DEFINITIONS

1. **(O)** Autism spectrum disorders (ASD)—developmental disorders that affect, among other things, the ability to communicate, report medical conditions, self-regulate behaviors, and interact with others (p. 954)

2. **(D)** Automatic implanted cardiac defibrillator (AICD)—a device implanted under the skin that can detect life-threatening cardiac dysrhythmias and respond by delivering one or more high-energy shocks to correct the rhythm (p. 962)

3. **(P)** Bariatrics—the branch of medicine that deals with the causes, prevention, and treatment of obesity (p. 953)

4. **(J)** Central IV catheter—a catheter surgically inserted for long-term delivery of medications or fluids into the central circulation (p. 967)

5. **(L)** Continuous positive airway pressure (CPAP)—a device worn by a patient that blows oxygen or air under constant low pressure through a tube and mask to keep airway passages from collapsing at the end of a breath (p. 959)

6. **(I)** Dialysis—the process of filtering the blood to remove toxic or unwanted wastes and fluids (p. 966)

7. **(A)** Disability—a physical, emotional, behavioral, or cognitive condition that interferes with a person's ability to carry out everyday tasks, such as working or caring for oneself (p. 950)

8. **(E)** Feeding tube—a tube used to provide delivery of nutrients to the stomach; a nasogastric type is inserted through the nose and into the stomach; a gastric type is surgically implanted through the abdominal wall and into the stomach (p. 964)

9. **(C)** Left ventricular assist device (LVAD)—a battery-powered mechanical pump implanted in the body to assist a failing left ventricle in pumping blood to the body (p. 963)

10. **(M)** Obesity—a condition of having too much body fat, defined as a body mass index of 30 or greater (p. 953)

11. **(K)** Ostomy bag—an external pouch that collects fecal matter diverted from the colon or ileum through a surgical opening (colostomy or ileostomy) in the abdominal wall (p. 966)

12. **(N)** Pacemaker—a device implanted under the skin with wires implanted into the heart to modify the heart rate as needed to maintain an adequate heart rate (p. 962)

13. **(G)** Stoma—a surgically created opening into the body, as with a tracheostomy, colonostomy, or ileostomy (p. 960)

14. **(F)** Tracheostomy—a surgical opening in the neck into the trachea (p. 960)

15. **(H)** Urinary catheter—a tube inserted into the bladder through the urethra to drain urine from the bladder (p. 965)

16. **(B)** Ventilator—a device that breathes for a patient (p. 961)

MULTIPLE-CHOICE REVIEW

1. **(D)** To ensure proper care for the patient with special needs, the EMT must be able to recognize, understand, and evaluate the patient's specific special health care needs in addition to the chief complaint. (p. 956)

2. **(A)** The EMT may find patients with special care needs when responding to calls in any of the locations except the emergency department. (p. 950)

3. **(C)** One of the best resources to help you when confronted with a special needs patient who is on a specific device would be to use the family member, or caregiver, who is with the patient. (p. 957)

4. **(C)** A condition, such as a heart murmur, that is present at birth of the special needs patient is considered congenital. (p. 959)

5. **(B)** A device designed to keep the air passages from collapsing at the end of a breath is called a CPAP. These devices are often used by obese patients who have sleep apnea as well as by EMS providers for congestive heart failure. (p. 959)

6. **(D)** A patient who has a tracheostomy tube may need to be suctioned occasionally. This is especially common during times of distress, the first few weeks after the tube insertion, and if the patient has an infection. (p. 960)

7. **(C)** A device that is programmed to take over the functions of timing and rate of the patient's breathing is called a ventilator. (p. 961)

8. **(C)** If the patient on the device in multiple-choice question 7 has an electrical or battery failure, the EMT will need to begin bag-mask ventilation. (p. 961)

9. **(D)** A cardiac device that is occasionally implanted in the patient's left upper abdominal quadrant is called a pacemaker. (p. 962)

10. **(C)** A cardiac chamber that pumps blood through the aorta to the body is called a left ventricular assist device. (p. 963)

11. **(B)** A tube that is inserted into a patient who has lost the ability to regulate his urine is called a urinary catheter. (p. 965)

12. **(A)** When a patient tells you that he needs to go to the hospital or clinic for dialysis every other day, this dialysis is done to detoxify the blood. (p. 966)

13. **(C)** Examples of devices commercially available as a Groshong®, Hickman®, or a Broviac® would be called a central venous line. (p. 967)

14. **(D)** A special needle is required to access devices called an implanted port, Port-a-Cath®, and Mediport®. (p. 967)

15. **(C)** A major health risk that is on the rise in the United States is obesity, which will increase the occurrence of type 2 diabetes. (p. 953)

16. **(A)** If you suspect a hearing problem, the best way to communicate with the patient is to use a pad of paper and write questions. Not all patients can lip read, and screaming just distorts the sounds and is not effective. (p. 952)

17. **(C)** Cardiac patients whose AICD fires experience momentary pain. Most are told to call EMS if this happens two times or more in a 24-hour period, if they become dizzy or do not feel well, or if they develop chest pain. (p. 963)

18. **(D)** When dealing with an autistic patient who is having a "melt-down," the best strategy is to remember that calm creates calm. A show of force is scary, and commanding in a loud voice does not help the matter. (p. 955)

19. **(C)** The best strategy for interaction with the patient described in multiple-choice question 18 is to keep things as basic as possible (i.e., use less stuff, keep questions basic, and keep instructions simple and basic). Jumping right in to treat quickly does not help in this situation. (pp. 954–955)

STREET SCENES DISCUSSION

1. Amber has a respiratory infection that is getting worse and is affecting her ability to breathe.

2. When a patient has a trach tube, she cannot clear her throat by simply coughing or spitting. If it becomes partially obstructed with secretions, it is necessary to suction the tube to keep it clear.

3. Initially, when Amber was breathing, gurgling sounds could be heard. These sounds were due to the partial obstruction of the tube from secretions.

Chapter 38: EMS Operations

MATCH TERMINOLOGY/ DEFINITIONS

1. **(B)** Due regard—legal term, which appears in most states' driving laws, referring to the responsibility of the emergency vehicle operator to drive safely and keep the safety of all others in mind at all times (p. 984)

2. **(A)** EMD—Emergency Medical Dispatcher (p. 982)

3. **(D)** Landing zone (LZ)—large, flat area without aerial obstruction in which a helicopter can land to pick up a patient (p. 1002)

4. **(C)** True emergency—call in which the driver of the emergency vehicle responds with lights and siren because he or she is of the understanding that loss of life or limb may be possible (p. 984)

MULTIPLE-CHOICE REVIEW

1. **(C)** The federal agency that develops specifications for ambulance vehicle designs is the U.S. Department of Transportation. (p. 976)

2. **(B)** The purpose for carrying an EPA-registered, intermediate-level disinfectant on the ambulance is to destroy mycobacterium tuberculosis. (p. 978)

3. **(D)** The telemetry repeater is used in the ambulance to boost the radio signal. Equipment that should be in the portable first-in kit to be taken directly to a patient's side includes the suction unit, rigid cervical collar, and blood pressure cuff. (p. 395)

4. **(D)** The suction unit is used in the "A" (airway) step of the primary assessment of a trauma patient. Supplies used for the "C" (circulation) step include disposable gloves, occlusive dressings, and the AED. (pp. 976–977)

5. **(A)** The rubber bulb syringe is a supply used for childbirth. Equipment used to obtain vital signs includes an adult and a pediatric stethoscope, sphygmomanometer kit, and a penlight. (p. 977)

6. **(A)** A device used to carry patients over a long distance is called a Stokes basket. The scoop stretcher is used to lift and move patients without a spine injury through tight places. See the answer for multiple-choice question 7. (p. 977)

7. **(C)** A Reeves® stretcher is used for carrying a patient who must lie supine down stairs when a cot is too heavy or wide, *not* for spine injury. The Stokes basket, or basket stretcher, is used to carry patients in high-angle rescue. (p. 977)

8. **(D)** A typical fixed oxygen delivery system consists of a 3,000-liter reservoir, a two-stage regulator, and the necessary reducing valve and yokes. (p. 976)

9. **(C)** The automatic transport ventilator (ATV) is *not* an essential item to carry on the ambulance or EMS vehicle for prehospital respiratory care. (p. 976)

10. **(D)** The fixed suction unit in the ambulance should reach a vacuum of at least 300 mmHg within 4 seconds. It should provide an airflow of *30* liters per minute and should be usable by a person at the *head* of the patient. Oxygen tanks require periodic hydrostatic testing. (p. 976)

11. **(B)** The mechanical CPR compressor is a helpful device, but it is not essential for assisting with cardiopulmonary resuscitation. (pp. 976–977)

12. **(D)** Burn sheets are not used for immobilization. Equipment carried on an ambulance or EMS vehicle that is used for immobilization includes a Hare® traction splint, triangular bandages, and padded aluminum splints. (pp. 977–980)

13. **(A)** Chemical cold packs are carried on an ambulance or EMS vehicle primarily for use with musculoskeletal injuries. (pp. 977–980)

14. **(D)** The Hare® traction device is for splinting. Supplies used for wound care include sterile burn sheets, 5×9-inch combine dressings, and self-adhering roller bandages. (pp. 977–980)

15. **(B)** Sterilized aluminum foil is used to maintain body heat or as an occlusive dressing. Body parts should be wrapped in a plastic bag and kept cool. Use a paper cup over an avulsed eye. Never use aluminum foil to cover an injury directly because it can cut the patient. (pp. 977–980)

16. **(C)** Large safety pins are used with a sling. Supplies for childbirth include a rubber bulb syringe, sanitary napkins, and sterile surgical gloves. (pp. 977–980)

17. **(C)** Every shift, both you and your partner should complete the equipment checklist. Preventive maintenance, oil changes, and waxing the ambulance are done routinely but not on each shift. (p. 981)

18. **(B)** The battery is checked on the ambulance or EMS vehicle with the engine off. (p. 980)

19. **(D)** It is not the EMD's job to advise the caller that an ambulance is not needed. The responsibilities of the Emergency Medical Dispatcher (EMD) include dispatching and coordinating EMS resources, interrogating the caller, prioritizing the call, and coordinating with other public safety agencies. (pp. 982–984)

20. **(C)** When an EMD questions a patient or caller, he or she does not routinely ask if the patient has been in the hospital recently. This is part of the EMT's SAMPLE history taken at the scene. (pp. 982–984)

21. **(B)** The brand of vehicle is not important to EMS but would be for the police report. When speaking with a caller who is at the scene of a traffic collision, the EMD should ask if traffic is moving, how many lanes of traffic are open, and if any of the vehicles are on fire. (pp. 982–984)

22. **(D)** To be a safe ambulance operator, the EMT should be tolerant of other drivers, always wear glasses or contact lenses if required, and have a positive attitude about his or her ability as a driver. (p. 984)

23. **(D)** Most state statutes prohibit passing of a school bus that has its red lights blinking. Stop and wait for the bus driver to shut off the red lights, which signals that all the children

are in a safe position. Then proceed with caution. State statutes *do* allow emergency vehicle operators to do all of the following under certain conditions: park the vehicle anywhere as long as it does not damage personal property; proceed past red stop signals, flashing red stop signals, and stop signs; and exceed the posted speed limit as long as life and property are not endangered. (pp. 984–985)

24. **(A)** At the scene of a collision, you examine a patient and find that she is stable. This situation is no longer considered a true emergency; further use of lights and siren would be inappropriate. (pp. 985–986)

25. **(D)** Do not use the siren throughout the call. Use the siren sparingly. Never assume that all motorists will hear your signal, and be prepared for erratic movements of motorists. (pp. 985–986)

26. **(B)** The decision about the use of lights and sirens should always be made with the medical condition of the patient in mind. The continuous sound of a siren may cause a sick or an injured person to suffer increased fear and anxiety, and his or her condition may deteriorate as stress increases. (pp. 985–986)

27. **(B)** Escorts or multivehicle responses are a very dangerous means of response. Motorists often do not expect to see the second emergency vehicle and may collide with it. (p. 986)

28. **(D)** The type of emergency (except MCIs) does not affect ambulance response; factors that do affect ambulance response include time of the day, weather, and road maintenance and construction. See also the answer to Complete the Following question 2. (pp. 986–987)

29. **(B)** Park in front of the wreckage (upstream) if you are the first emergency vehicle on the scene so your flashing lights can warn approaching motorists until flares and other signals can be placed. Park 100 feet and uphill from a wreckage that involves fire. (p. 988)

30. **(B)** Packaging is the sequence of operations required to ready the patient to be moved and to combine the patient and the patient-carrying device into a unit ready for transfer. (p. 990)

31. **(A)** An unconscious patient who has no potential spine injury should be positioned in the ambulance in the recovery position, which promotes maintenance of an open airway and the drainage of fluids. (p. 990)

32. **(B)** Forming a general impression of the patient is done when you first see the patient, *not* en route to the hospital. En route, the EMT rechecks bandages and splints, provides reassessment, continues to monitor vital signs, and notifies the receiving facility of estimated time of arrival. (p. 993)

33. **(D)** If a patient develops cardiac arrest en route to the hospital, the EMT's first action should be to tell the operator to stop the vehicle. (p. 993)

34. **(B)** When delivering the patient to the hospital, the EMT should *never* move a patient onto the hospital stretcher and leave. This is considered abandonment. (p. 993)

35. **(C)** When approaching a helicopter, first wait for the pilot or medic to wave you in. Then approach from the front or side of the craft. All other approach directions could cause injury or death. Remember to always follow the directions of the flight crew. (p. 1003)

36. **(C)** Patients who are cardiac arrest victims are rarely candidates for helicopter transport. (p. 1002)

37. **(C)** The first-arriving EMS unit on the scene of a collision on a highway should park the vehicle in the upstream location. The ideal location for an ambulance is in the downstream location so it is safe to load the patient. (p. 988)

38. **(A)** The GPS unit should not be a substitute for an intimate knowledge of the response area you are assigned to. Do not let it be a distraction to the driver. (p. 987)

COMPLETE THE FOLLOWING

1. The seven questions an EMD should ask a caller reporting a medical emergency are as follows: (pp. 982–984)
   A) What is the exact location of the patient?
   B) What is your call-back number?
   C) What's the problem?
   D) How old is the patient?
   E) What's the patient's sex?
   F) Is the patient conscious?
   G) Is the patient breathing?

2. The seven factors that can affect ambulance response are the following: (pp. 986–987)
   A) Day of the week
   B) Time of the day
   C) Weather
   D) Road maintenance and construction
   E) Railroads
   F) Bridges and tunnels
   G) Schools and school buses

3. The four major ways the EMT on the scene of a collision should describe the landing zone to the air rescue service are as follows: (p. 1002)
   A) Terrain
   B) Major landmarks
   C) Estimated distance to nearest town
   D) Other pertinent information

LABEL THE PHOTOGRAPHS (P. 1000)

1. Low-level
2. Intermediate
3. High-level
4. Sterilization

STREET SCENES DISCUSSION

1. Notify the dispatcher, call the police, and ensure that there are no injuries caused by the collision. While waiting for the police to respond, ask the dispatcher to reassign the initial call to another unit.

2. The driver of the emergency vehicle would be at fault.

3. Because you cannot stop the ambulance fast enough if an unsuspecting motorist drives in front of you. Even with emergency lights and siren on, you cannot assume that other drivers will see you or hear you approach.

CASE STUDY: THE AMBULANCE COLLISION

1. Yes, the ambulance driver should have stopped before proceeding through the intersection.

2. Yes, by wearing a shoulder harness.

3. It was necessary to assign yet another ambulance to handle that call.

4. Do no harm.

5. The service may lose business. The EMS personnel may be ridiculed, and some patients may actually be afraid to get into your ambulance!

6. Because he is allowed to look into incidents of this nature with close scrutiny. This is especially true in the public sector, when injury has occurred.

7. Absolutely. Civilian motorists are not required to drive with "due regard for the safety of all others."

8. He does, unless his service is willing to assist him or unless he has some insurance or legal aid.

9. Yes, he could.

10. Proper driver screening and qualification, driver training, driving SOPs (which include always wearing a shoulder harness in the front of the vehicle, how to negotiate an intersection, and proper use of emergency lights and siren), retraining, keeping the emergency vehicles in good shape, and a good quality improvement program.

Chapter 39: Hazardous Materials, Multiple-Casualty Incidents, and Incident Management

MATCH TERMINOLOGY/ DEFINITIONS

1. **(O)** Cold zone—area in which the Incident Command post and support functions are located (p. 1010)

2. **(L)** Command—the first on the scene to establish order and initiate the Incident Command System (p. 1020)

3. **(V)** Decontamination—a chemical and/or physical process that reduces or prevents the spread of contamination from persons or equipment; the removal of hazardous substances from employees and their equipment to the extent necessary to preclude foreseeable health effects (p. 1015)

4. **(U)** Disaster plan—a predefined set of instructions for a community's emergency responders (p. 1020)

5. **(M)** Hazardous material—any substance or material in a form that poses an unreasonable risk to health, safety, and property when transported in commerce (p. 1007)

6. **(N)** Hot zone—area immediately surrounding a hazmat incident; extends far enough to prevent adverse effects outside the zone (p. 1010)

7. **(Q)** Incident Command—the person who assumes overall direction of an incident (p. 1022)

8. **(R)** Incident Command System—a subset of the National Incident Management System (NIMS) (p. 1020)

9. **(J)** Multiple-casualty incident (MCI)—any medical or trauma incident involving multiple patients (p. 1019)

10. **(K)** National Incident Management System (NIMS)—the management system used by federal, state, and local governments to manage emergencies in the United States (p. 1020)

11. **(P)** Single incident command—command organization in which a single agency controls all resources and operations (p. 1021)

12. **(H)** Staging area—the area where ambulances are parked and other resources are held until needed (p. 1031)

13. **(I)** Staging supervisor—person responsible for overseeing ambulances and ambulance personnel at a multiple-casualty incident (p. 1031)

14. **(G)** Transportation supervisor—person responsible for communicating with sector officers and hospitals to manage transportation of patients to hospitals from a multiple-casualty incident (p. 1031)

15. **(E)** Treatment area—the area in which patients are treated at a multiple-casualty incident (p. 1030)

16. **(F)** Treatment supervisor—person responsible for overseeing treatment of patients who have been triaged at a multiple-casualty incident (p. 1030)

17. **(C)** Triage—process of quickly assessing patients at a multiple-casualty incident and assigning each a priority for receiving treatment; from a French word meaning "to sort" (p. 1026)

18. **(B)** Triage area—the area where secondary triage takes place at a multiple-casualty incident (p. 1026)

19. **(D)** Triage supervisor—the person responsible for overseeing triage at a multiple-casualty incident (p. 1026)

20. **(A)** Triage tag—color-coded tag indicating the priority group to which a patient has been assigned (p. 1029)

21. **(T)** Unified command—command organization in which several agencies work independently but cooperatively (p. 1022)

22. **(S)** Warm zone—area where personnel and equipment decontamination and hot zone support take place; it includes control points for the access corridor and thus assists in reducing the spread of contamination (p. 1010)

MULTIPLE-CHOICE REVIEW

1. **(A)** Using the *Emergency Response Guidebook*, the EMT would find that ethyl acetate is a chemical that irritates the eyes and respiratory tract. See Table 39–1. (p. 1008)

2. **(B)** Using the *Emergency Response Guidebook*, the EMT would find that Benzene (benzol) is a chemical that has toxic vapors that can be absorbed through the skin. See Table 39–1. (p. 1008)

3. **(D)** The regulations that require training in hazardous materials for responders to hazmat incidents are found in the OSHA CFR 1910.120. (p. 1009)

4. **(B)** The level of training for those who initially respond to releases or potential releases of hazardous materials in order to protect people, property, and the environment is called First Responder Operations. (p. 1009)

5. **(A)** The level of training for those who are likely to witness or discover a hazardous substance release is called First Responder Awareness. (p. 1009)

6. **(C)** The standard that deals with competencies for EMS personnel at a hazardous materials incident is called NFPA 473. (p. 1015)

7. **(D)** Pet stores generally are not hazmat locations. Examples of potential hazardous materials locations include garden centers, chemical plants, and trucking terminals. (p. 1009)

8. **(C)** Unless EMS personnel are trained to the level of Hazardous Materials Technician, they must remain in the cold zone. (p. 1009)

9. **(C)** All victims leaving the hot zone should be considered contaminated until proven otherwise. (p. 1010)

10. (A) The primary concern at the scene of a hazardous materials incident is the safety of the EMT and crew, patients, and the public. Stabilizing the incident often takes a long time. Exposed patients need to be removed but this, too, does not happen quickly because of the need to identify the hazmat material and decontaminate the patients. (p. 1009)

11. (B) Upon arrival at a tanker truck crash where the vehicle has overturned and is rapidly leaking its contents onto the street, the EMT should isolate the area and call for the appropriate backup assistance. Do not try to stop or seal the leak because this would expose many rescuers to the chemical. Sending in the least senior EMT to assess the patient is not an appropriate move because it could sacrifice a rescuer. (p. 1010)

12. (B) The safe zone of a hazardous materials incident should be established in an upwind/same-level location. If it was established downwind, you would increase the chance of being exposed to the chemicals. Zones established downhill may be contaminated by hazardous runoff. (p. 1010)

13. (C) Initiating rescue attempts inside the hot zone is delayed until the product and proper protection needs are determined. The role of Command at a hazardous materials incident is to delegate responsibility for directing bystanders to a safe area, establishing a perimeter, and evacuating people if necessary. (pp. 1010–1011)

14. (A) A contaminated victim of a hazardous materials incident coming in contact with other people who are not contaminated is referred to as secondary contamination. (p. 1015)

15. (C) The designations on the sides of tanker trucks are called hazardous material placards. (p. 1012)

16. (B) The commonly used placard system for fixed facilities is called the NFPA 704 system. (p. 1011)

17. (B) All employers are required to post in an obvious spot the information about all the chemicals in the workplace on a form called a Material Safety Data Sheet (MSDS). (p. 1011)

18. (A) The NFPA rules are really only guidelines and do not detail how to manage an incident. Resources that the EMT should use at a hazardous materials incident include the local hazmat team, the *Emergency Response Guidebook,* and CHEM-TEL. (pp. 1012–1014)

19. (A) CHEMTREC is a 24-hour service for identifying hazardous materials. It also provides instructions for handling spills. (p. 1012)

20. (B) The responsibilities of EMS personnel at a hazardous materials incident are taking care of the injured and monitoring and rehabilitating hazmat team members. (p. 1014)

21. (A) The rehabilitation operations at a hazardous materials incident should be located in the cold zone, *not* the warm zone. It should also be protected from the weather, easily accessible to EMS, and free from exhaust fumes. (p. 1014)

22. (D) As soon as possible after a hazmat team member exits the hot zone, the EMT should reassess his vital signs. Remember that hazmat team members should have their baseline vitals taken while suiting up, and both preentry and exit vitals should be tracked on a flow sheet. (p. 1014)

23. (C) Always try to contain the runoff water when it is necessary to decontaminate a patient before hazmat specialists arrive. Flushing water down the nearest drain could contaminate the area's entire water supply. (p. 1018)

24. (D) A good local disaster plan is not generic; rather, it should be written to address the events that are conceivable for a particular location (e.g., Florida needs to plan for hurricanes, Kansas needs to plan for tornadoes). (p. 1020)

25. (D) Upon arrival of the first EMS unit at the scene of an MCI, the crew leader should assume command, conduct a scene walk-through, and call for backup. Do *not* begin patient treatment; even though this might save one or two lives, it would be at the expense of the majority of the patients because response would be delayed and disorganized. (p. 1022)

26. (C) Once units arrive at an MCI, as much face-to-face communication as possible should be used, especially between Command and area supervisors and between area supervisors and subordinates. This will help to reduce radio channel crowding. (p. 1023)

27. (C) If an MCI involves hazardous materials, a rehabilitation sector is needed. (p. 1026)

28. (A) The individual at an MCI who is responsible for the sorting and prioritizing of the patients is the triage supervisor. (p. 1026)

29. (A) Patients who are assessed to have decreased mental status at an MCI are considered Priority 1. Other examples of Priority 1 patients are those with airway and breathing difficulties, uncontrolled or severe bleeding, severe medical problems, shock, and severe burns. (p. 1028)

30. (A) Patients who are assessed to have shock at an MCI are considered Priority 1. See the answer for multiple-choice question 29. (p. 1029)

31. (B) Patients who are assessed to have multiple bone or joint injuries at an MCI are considered Priority 2 unless they show signs of impending shock. Other examples of Priority 2 patients are those with burns without airway problems and those with back injuries with or without spinal cord damage. (p. 1029)

32. (D) Patients who are assessed to have died at the MCI scene are considered Priority 4 (or zero). (p. 1029)

33. (C) The individual at an MCI who is responsible for maintaining a supply of vehicles and personnel at a location away from the incident site is the staging supervisor. (p. 1030)

34. (C) The individual at an MCI who is responsible for determining patient destinations and notifying the hospitals of the incoming patients is the transportation supervisor. (p. 1030)

35. (D) Patient transport decisions at an MCI are based upon priority, destination facilities, and transportation resources. The patient's family preferences are not a consideration in a disaster situation. (pp. 1030–1032)

36. (A) The rehabilitation area should not be located in the warm zone. (p. 1014)

37. (A) If the team member has a pulse rate over 110, it is recommended that his oral temperature be taken. If his oral temperature is over 100.6°F, he should stay in rehab (or go to the hospital as needed) but not go back into a suit. (p. 1014)

38. (D) During periods of extreme physical exertion, it is recommended that fluid be replaced at 1 quart per hour. Of course, there is some variability based on the person involved here. (p. 1014)

39. (D) If you want to offer fluids other than just water, consider a sports drink that is watered down 2:1 with water. (p. 1014)

40. (B) The first step in the START system is to announce over the PA system that those who can walk without becoming further injured go to a nearby specific location. This will separate the "walking wounded" from the rest of the patients. (pp. 1027–1028)

41. (D) The parameters of START are RPM: *r*espirations, *p*ulse or circulation, and *m*ental status. (pp. 1027–1028)

42. (B) Acceptable treatment while evaluating a patient for a START triage category includes opening an airway, inserting an OPA, and putting pressure on a bleeding wound to control bleeding. (pp. 1027–1028)

COMPLETE THE FOLLOWING

1. The information you should be prepared to give when you call for assistance from CHEMTREC includes the following (keep the line of communication open at all times): (p. 1014)
   - Give your name, your call-back number, and your FAX number.
   - Explain the nature and location of the problem.
   - Report the identification number(s) of the material(s) involved if there is a safe way for you to obtain this information.
   - Give the name of the carrier, shipper, manufacturer, consignee, and point of origin.
   - Describe the container type and size.
   - Report if the container is on railcar, in a truck, in open storage, or in housed storage.
   - Estimate the quantity of material transported and released.
   - Report local conditions (e.g., the weather, terrain, proximity to schools and/or hospitals).
   - Report injuries and exposures.
   - Report local emergency services that have been notified.

2. The characteristics of the rehabilitation operations at a hazardous materials incident must include the following: (any four) (p. 1014)
   - Located in the cold zone
   - Protection from the weather
   - Large enough to accommodate multiple rescue crews
   - Easily accessible to EMS units
   - Free from exhaust fumes
   - Location and setup allow for rapid reentry into the emergency operation

COMPLETE THE CHART (P. 1026)

1. EMS Staging Officer (Supervisor)
2. EMS Safety Officer (Supervisor)
3. Transportation Officer (Supervisor)
4. Triage Officer (Supervisor)
5. Rehabilitation Officer (Supervisor)
6. P-2 Tx Leader

STREET SCENES DISCUSSION

1. Yes, a helicopter would be appropriate, provided there is a nearby landing zone that will not keep ambulances from transporting patients.

2. With a short transport time, you could have the ambulances turn around and return to the scene to pick up additional patients.

3. Some EMS providers have used a school bus to transport low-priority patients to a hospital. If you ever use a bus for this purpose, medically clear each patient on the bus to ensure that they are low priority and arrange for medical personnel to travel with them on the bus to the hospital.

CASE STUDY: THE SCHOOL BUS MCI

1. Size up the situation, establish command, make contact with the fire and police command officers.

2. **(A)** You should don the Command vest. **(B)** Your responsibilities are the overall management of the medical aspects of the incident; working directly with the chief officers of the police and fire departments; ensuring the safety of all your personnel; and designating triage, treatment, transport, and staging area supervisors.

3. Triage supervisor.

4. Set up the triage area and begin tagging patients and classifying into priority for removal from the scene to the treatment area.

5. Respond three to the scene and seven to a staging area about a mile away with easy access to the scene. The ambulances responding to the scene help fill out the complement of command officers and provide personnel to triage patients.

6. The first crew leader at the staging area should be designated as the staging officer and be responsible for the release of ambulances and personnel to the scene as directed by command. If this is a lengthy operation, he or she should also attend to the human needs of the staging personnel by locating restrooms and food. He or she will need to be able to communicate with arriving mutual aid units, providing them with maps and directions to the scene and hospital as it becomes necessary.

7. Yes, but only upon direction of Command and/or the staging supervisor.

8. Transportation and treatment area supervisors would be helpful in managing the flow of patients.

9. On long backboards with rigid extrication collars applied.

10. Take the patients to the respective section of the treatment area depending on their triage tag priority.

11. Priority 2.

12. Priority 1.

13. Priority 4 (or zero).

14. Priority 1.

15. Allow one parent per child to assist and stay with the child in the treatment area if space permits.

16. Transportation area supervisor.

17. Do a roll call of the hospitals for bed availability and the number of patients of each priority they can handle.

18. Consider the use of a helicopter.

19. Priority 3 patients with minor injuries who are medically cleared. Medical personnel are still needed on the bus just in case a patient's status changes.

20. Appoint a Public Information Officer (PIO), plan for rehabilitation operations and a light meal after the incident, and consider setting up plans for critical incident stress management (CISM) for all personnel who were at the scene and who are interested in talking about what they saw and did.

Chapter 40: Highway Safety and Vehicle Extrication

MATCH TERMINOLOGY/ DEFINITIONS

1. **(H)** A Post—post in front of the driver's compartment that supports the roof and windshield (p. 1055)

2. **(A)** B Post—when moving toward the rear of the vehicle, the second post you see, which supports the roof (p. 1055)

3. **(G)** Complex access—access that requires tools or special equipment to reach the patient (p. 1056)

4. **(J)** Cribbing—blocks of hardwood, usually 4 × 4 × 18-inch or 2 × 4 × 18-inch, used to stabilize a vehicle (p. 1054)

5. **(D)** Disentanglement—three-part procedure used by rescue personnel to free a patient trapped in a vehicle (p. 1058)

6. **(E)** Entrapment—when a patient is pinned and requires assistance, sometimes mechanical, to free him (p. 1043)

7. **(K)** Extrication—process by which entrapped patients are rescued from vehicles, buildings, tunnels, or other places (p. 1044)

8. **(I)** Laminated glass—safety glass used in automobile windshields; made of two sheets of plate glass bonded to a sheet of tough plastic (p. 1056)

9. **(C)** Nader pin—named after a well-known consumer advocate, this case-hardened pin is held by the cams of an automobile's door-locking system (p. 1056)

10. **(F)** Stabilization—to crib or block a vehicle or structure to prevent further unintended, uncontrolled movement (p. 1053)

11. **(B)** Tempered glass—glass used in an automobile's side and rear windows designed to break into small, rounded pieces rather than sharp fragments (p. 1056)

MULTIPLE-CHOICE REVIEW

1. **(B)** The correct term is specialty rescue teams. Such teams may be provided by a variety of agencies, such as EMS, fire, police, industrial, or commercial services. (p. 1038)

2. **(B)** Defining patient care is not a phase of extrication. The phases of extrication encompass ten steps that include gaining access to the patient, disentangling the patient, and sizing up the situation. See also the answer for Complete the Following question 1. (pp. 1041–1042)

3. **(A)** An important part of a rescue scene size-up is determining the extent of entrapment. Starting IVs on the patient is not part of the size-up and is a paramedic skill. Removing shattered glass, if needed, should be done as far away from the patient as possible. Informing the patient about the extent of vehicle damage will make him more anxious. Don't lie if asked, but focus on treating the patient. (p. 1043)

4. **(C)** During size-up of a collision, you must be able to "read" a collision and develop an action plan based on your knowledge of rescue operations and estimate of the patient's condition and priority. Knowledge includes previous experience. Remember: you were called to rescue the patient, not the vehicle! (p. 1043)

5. **(B)** When developing an action plan for patient extrication, always keep in mind that time is important to the critical trauma patient's management. The cost of vehicle damage or the type of vehicle is less relevant to the extrication as is the presence of bystanders, although they should not interfere with your operations. (p. 1043)

6. **(C)** If a vehicle has an airbag that deployed, the manufacturer recommends lifting the bag and examining the steering wheel and dash. If either is damaged, it is likely that the patient's chest is damaged, which would mean great potential for internal injury. The use of a HEPA mask is not required; gloves and eye protection are recommended. (p. 1048)

7. **(B)** The unsafe act that contributes most to collision scene injuries is failure to wear protective gear during rescue operations. (p. 1044)

8. **(D)** By limiting the inner circle to rescuers who are in protective gear, you help to *decrease* potential injuries. Factors that may contribute to injuries of rescuers at a collision include a careless attitude toward personal safety, a lack of skill in tool use, and physical problems that impede strenuous effort. (p. 1044)

9. **(D)** Plastic "bump caps" do not provide adequate protection; use quality headgear. Good protective gear at the scene of a collision includes fire-resistant trousers or turnout pants; steel toe, high-top work shoes; and firefighter or leather gloves. (p. 1046)

10. **(A)** To ensure eye protection at the collision scene, the EMT should wear safety goggles with a soft vinyl frame and cover the patient with an aluminized blanket. Safety glasses can be worn, but they must have *large* lenses and side shields. Thermal masks are cold-weather gear. A hinged plastic helmet shield allows particles to enter from under the shield. Paper blankets, light tarps, and wool blankets simply hide the patient's view of the glass or metal about to strike him or her. (p. 1046)

11. **(C)** An aluminized rescue blanket may be used to protect your patient from poor weather and flying particles. The rescuer should be properly attired for cold weather conditions. (p. 1047)

12. **(A)** The EMT should watch for spilled fuel or other combustibles prior to igniting flares. Do not throw flares out of the moving vehicle or use them as a traffic wand. Never turn your back on traffic; walk toward the traffic so you can observe oncoming vehicles. (pp. 1042, 1047–1048)

13. **(C)** When there is an electrical hazard, such as a broken utility pole, the safe zone should be far enough away to ensure that an arcing wire does not cause injury. If you feel a ground gradient, you are already too close to the electricity. (pp. 1048–1050)

14. **(C)** The federal highway standards require emergency responders to wear ANSI safety vests when working in highway operations. (p. 1044)

15. **(B)** If a vehicle collides with a broken utility pole and the utility wires are down, you should tell the vehicle's occupants to stay in the vehicle until the power company arrives. (p. 1049)

16. (B) In wet weather, a phenomenon known as a ground gradient may provide your first clue that a wire is down. (p. 1049)

17. (A) If you feel a tingling sensation in your legs and lower torso, you should turn 180 degrees and shuffle with both feet together (or hop on one foot) to safety. Either technique helps prevent your body from completing a circuit with the energized ground, which can cause electrocution. Hopping is much more dangerous because of the likelihood of falling, which may complete the circuit. (p. 1049)

18. (D) Do *not* apply a short spine board to the driver because this is the time for a quick removal. If there is a fire in the car's engine compartment and people are trapped within the vehicle, you should quickly and carefully remove the patient, ensure that the fire department has been called, don protective gear, and use your fire extinguisher. (pp. 1050–1051)

19. (C) When a vehicle's hood is closed and there is an engine fire, you should *not* attempt to open the hood because this will fuel the fire with oxygen and the fire will flare up. (pp. 1050–1051)

20. (A) When a vehicle rolls off the roadway into dried grass in a field, it is possible that a fire may occur from the catalytic converter. The catalytic converter is under the car, and its temperature can reach over 1,200°F. (p. 1052)

21. (C) "Try Before You Pry" is the foundation for the simple access procedure. Disentanglement is removing the vehicle from around the patient who is entrapped. Stabilization is ensuring that the vehicle is less likely to roll or move during extrication efforts. (p. 1056)

22. (D) Once a vehicle is stabilized and an entry point is gained, do *not* pull a patient out of an access hole prior to spinal immobilization. (p. 1056)

23. (C) If an unconscious patient is in a sitting position behind the wheel with legs pinned by the vehicle, the best approach to disentanglement is to cut the roof, displace the doors, and then displace the dash. This allows for plenty of room to work and for vertical rapid extrication if the patient's condition deteriorates. (p. 1056)

24. (D) Removing the roof of a vehicle does *not* stabilize a vehicle. (pp. 1056–1057)

25. (C) When an extrication involves displacing the dash or steering wheel but the airbag has not yet deployed, disconnect the battery cable. Be aware that the airbag can still deploy until the battery cable is disconnected. (p. 1058)

COMPLETE THE FOLLOWING

1. The ten phases of the extrication or rescue process are as follows: (pp. 1041–1042)
   A) Preparing for the rescue
   B) Sizing up the situation
   C) Recognizing and managing hazards
   D) Stabilizing the vehicle prior to entering
   E) Gaining access to the patient
   F) Providing initial patient assessment and rapid trauma exam
   G) Disentangling the patient
   H) Immobilizing and extricating the patient from the vehicle
   I) Providing a detailed physical exam, ongoing assessment, treatment, and transporting to the most appropriate hospital
   J) Terminating the rescue

2. The personal protective equipment (PPE) that you should be wearing when in the inner circle at a vehicle extrication includes the following: (pp. 1044–1047)
   A) Hand protection—leather gloves
   B) Body protection—turnout gear
   C) Eye protection—full goggles with sides on them
   D) Head protection—a helmet

LABEL THE PHOTOGRAPHS (P. 1051)

1. Markings to identify proper extinguisher.

2. Extinguishing a fire in the engine compartment when the hood is fully open.

3. Extinguishing a fire in the engine compartment when the hood is partially open.

4. Extinguishing a fire under the dash. Care must be taken not to fill the vehicle's interior with a cloud of agent.

5. Extinguishing fuel burning under a vehicle. Flames are swept away from the vehicle.

STREET SCENES DISCUSSION

1. The strategy depends on the abilities and training of the rescuers and the equipment available to them. However, taking the roof off first has an advantage: If the patient takes a turn for the worse, he or she can be removed through the roof on a long backboard.

2. This is a serious mechanism of injury (MOI). The patient should be transported to a trauma center.

3. ALS should be requested right away because of the mechanism of injury (MOI) and the patient's unresponsiveness.

Chapter 41: EMS Response to Terrorism

MATCH TERMINOLOGY/ DEFINITIONS

1. **(I)** Contamination—contact with a material that is present where it does not belong and that is somehow harmful to persons, animals, or the environment (p. 1073)

2. **(C)** Dissemination—spreading (p. 1076)

3. **(A)** Domestic terrorism—terrorism directed against the government or population without foreign direction (p. 1065)

4. **(D)** Exposure—the dose or concentration of an agent multiplied by the time, or duration (p. 1072)

5. **(H)** International terrorism—terrorism that is foreign-based or directed (p. 1065)

6. **(E)** Permeation—the movement of a substance through a surface or, on a molecular level, through intact materials (p. 1073)

7. **(B)** Rem—roentgen equivalent (in) humans; a measure of radiation dosage (p. 1087)

8. **(F)** Routes of entry—pathways into the body, generally by absorption, ingestion, injection, or inhalation (p. 1072)

9. **(G)** Secondary devices—destructive devices, such as bombs, placed to be activated after an initial attack and timed to injure emergency responders who rush in to help care for those targeted by an initial attack (p. 1067)

10. **(O)** Strategies—broad general plans designed to achieve desired outcomes (p. 1090)

11. **(M)** Tactics—specific operational actions to accomplish assigned tasks (p. 1090)

12. **(K)** Terrorism—the unlawful use of force or violence against persons or property to intimidate or coerce a government, the civilian population, or any segment thereof, in furtherance of political or social objectives (p. 1064)

13. **(J)** Weaponization—packaging or producing a material, such as a chemical, biological, or radiological agent, so that it can be used as a weapon, for example, by dissemination in a bomb detonation or as an aerosol sprayed over an area or introduced into a ventilation system (p. 1077)

14. **(L)** Weapons of mass destruction (WMD)—weapons, devices, or agents intended to cause widespread harm and/or fear among a population (p. 1066)

15. **(N)** Zoonotic—able to move through the animal–human barrier; transmissible from animals to humans (p. 1082)

16. **(P)** Miosis—abnormal constriction of the pupil (p. 1078)

MULTIPLE-CHOICE REVIEW

1. **(B)** CBRNE is used to remember the types of terrorism attacks. (p. 1070)

2. **(C)** Environmental terrorists, survivalists, militias, and racial-hate groups are examples of domestic terrorists. (p. 1065)

3. **(D)** Clues of a suspicious incident can be remembered using OTTO. (p. ???1067)

4. **(D)** Controversial businesses, infrastructure systems, and public buildings are potential high-risk targets. (p. 1068)

5. **(B)** April 19 is the anniversary of the Alfred P. Murrah building bombing in Oklahoma City. (p. 1069)

6. **(A)** Car crashes involving more than two patients with serious traumatic injuries is the exception. Unexplained symptoms of skin or eye irritation; unexplained vapor clouds, mists, and plumes; and unexplained signs of airway irritation are all examples of signs that EMTs may be dealing with a suspicious incident. (p. 1069)

7. **(C)** The E in TRACEM-P stands for "etiological/biological." (p. 1070)

8. **(B)** Alpha particles, beta particles, and gamma rays can cause radiological harm. (p. 1069)

9. **(C)** Osmosis is not considered a way that a WMD would enter the body. (p. 1072)

10. **(D)** Radiological or nuclear incidents can cause psychological, mechanical, and thermal harm. (p. 1087)

11. **(B)** The primary harm from a nuclear explosion is mechanical. (p. 1087)

12. **(B)** Standard Precautions are not designed to protect from a radiological incident. (p. 1087)

13. **(C)** Inhalation is the most likely route for anthrax. (p. 1080)

14. **(A)** The dermal route of exposure is very effective with vesicants, (p. 1078)

15. **(D)** A biological agent's use as a weapon is influenced by infectivity, virulence, toxicity, incubation period, transmissibility, and lethality. (pp. 1079–1081)

16. **(C)** Virulence is the quality of being poisonous. (p. 1080)

17. **(C)** Lethality of an agent is the relative ease with which the agent causes death in a susceptible population. (p. 1081)

18. **(D)** Smallpox was declared eradicated by the World Health Organization (WHO) in 1980. (p. 1086)

19. **(A)** Demulsification is not a common mechanism for performing decontamination. (p. 1093)

20. **(C)** Dilution is the process that reduces the concentration of a contaminant. (p. 1093)

21. **(C)** Explosive incidents often cause mechanical harm, thermal harm, and chemical hazards. (p. 1095)

22. **(B)** After a building collapse, the dust that is inhaled often contains asbestos particles. (p. 1091)

23. **(C)** Ricin is designed to interrupt the body's protein manufacturing process at the cellular level by altering the RNA needed for proper proteins. (p. 1082)

24. **(D)** Bleeding capillaries in the eyes that are not due to trauma and a fever are indications of a viral hemorrhagic fever. (p. 1082)

INSIDE/OUTSIDE (P. 1078)

1. When a nerve agent acts on the parasympathetic nervous system, the enzyme that is usually inhibited is called acetylcholinesterase.

2. The seven most common signs and symptoms that occur due to overstimulation of the parasympathetic nervous system are the following:
   A) Salivation   E) GI upset
   B) Lacrimation   F) Emesis
   C) Urination   G) Miosis
   D) Defecation

COMPLETE THE FOLLOWING

1. The four major routes of entry of poisons into the body are as follows: (p. 1072)
   A) Absorption   C) Injection
   B) Ingestion   D) Inhalation

2. Four broad classifications of chemical weapons are as follows: (p. 1078)
   A) Choking agents   C) Cyanides
   B) Vesicating agents   D) Nerve agents

STREET SCENES DISCUSSION

1. This organization could be a potential threat to emergency service personnel because of the trouble in the world and America's position in the Middle East. Regardless of your personal opinion on this issue, it is clear that there are people who have strong feelings and who would go to great lengths to hurt those they believe have opposing views. Always be very careful when responding to any incident of this nature.

2. It is extremely unusual to find a motor vehicle collision in an isolated location such as an alleyway with no one around and with the vehicle completely on fire. This "smells" of an arson job or a potential setup.

3. It is always acceptable practice to stop and not proceed if the emergency services personnel feel they are in imminent danger. The first priority is always your safety and that of your crew!

4. Examples of groups or types of domestic terrorists that have been identified include environmental terrorists; survivalists; militias; racial-hate groups; and groups with extreme political, religious, or other philosophies or beliefs.

Interim Exam 3

1. (B) The circulation of blood throughout the body, filling the capillaries and supplying the cells and tissues with oxygen and nutrients, is called perfusion. Physiology is the study of how the body functions. Metabolism is the process of all the physical and chemical changes within the body that are necessary for life. (pp. 617–619, 102)

2. (B) When a trauma patient is making gurgling sounds as he breathes, you should suction his airway. (pp. 188–192)

3. (D) Sometimes a long backboard can act as a full body splint when the critical patient must be immobilized quickly. (p. 797)

4. (D) When a patient has two fractured femurs, a crushed pelvis, and a possible abdominal injury, you should not apply a traction splint. Do consider applying the PASG (if local protocol allows), and request ALS intercept en route to the hospital. (pp. 718–724)

5. (C) When trying to minimize the on-scene care of a multiple-trauma patient, do not take the time to bandage all lacerations. (p. 792)

6. (C) Even when you are trying to cut scene time for a multiple-trauma patient, the one thing you do not cut out is scene safety—no matter how serious the patient is. (pp. 792–794)

7. (A) Because internal bleeding is not visible, the EMT must base severity of blood loss on signs and symptoms exhibited. Mechanism of injury may also be a good clue to internal injury. What the patient tells you does not reveal how much blood has been lost. (pp. 630–632)

8. (D) The patient's history of diabetes is *not* significant in determining bleeding severity. The factors on which severity of bleeding depends are the rate of bleeding and the amount of blood loss, the patient's age and weight, and the ability of the patient's body to respond and defend against blood loss. (pp. 630–632)

9. (B) Blood that oozes and is dark red is most likely from a capillary. Venous bleeding will be a steady flow of dark red or maroon blood. Arteries spurt and their blood is usually bright red. (pp. 620–621)

10. (C) You are treating a patient who has a slashed wrist, which is spurting bright red blood. After trying direct pressure and elevation to control the bleeding, the next step would be to press on the brachial artery. (pp. 620–621)

11. (D) When all other methods have failed to control bleeding, the EMT should apply a tourniquet to an extremity. (pp. 622–629)

12. (C) Vomiting bile is usually not a sign of internal bleeding. Signs of internal bleeding include painful, swollen, or deformed extremities; a tender, rigid abdomen; and bruising. (p. 632)

13. (C) A fall from a height will usually produce a blunt injury, unless the patient falls onto something that penetrates, such as a fence. Examples of penetrating trauma include handgun bullet wounds, carving-knife wounds, and screwdriver stab wounds. (pp. 652–659)

14. (C) Gunshot wounds are considered penetrating trauma. Examples of blunt trauma include blast injuries, auto-pedestrian collisions, and falls. (pp. 690–692)

15. (A) The signs and symptoms of internal bleeding are the same as those of shock. Patients with these signs are difficult to stabilize in the field. (pp. 630–632)

16. (B) Hypovolemic, cardiogenic, and neurogenic are all types of shock. Hydrophobia is another name for rabies. (p. 633)

17. (C) At a point when the body can no longer compensate for the low blood volume, decompensated shock begins. Anaphylactic shock is a severe allergic reaction with respiratory distress and hypotension. (pp. 632–634)

18. (C) The brain and spinal cord are the major components of the central nervous system. The peripheral nerves branch out from the spinal cord. (pp. 747–750)

19. (D) The nervous system is divided into the central, peripheral, and autonomic nervous systems. Voluntary is a type of skeletal muscle that allows movement. (pp. 747–750)

20. (D) The cranium consists of the forehead and the top, back, and upper sides of the skull. The maxilla is the upper jaw, and the mandible is the lower jaw. (pp. 747–750)

21. (A) The bones forming the face include the zygomatic, mandible, and maxillae. Vertebrae are bones of the spine. (pp. 747–750)

22. (A) The brain and spinal cord are bathed in cerebrospinal fluid. Lymphatic fluid is responsible for maintaining our immune system. Synovial fluid lubricates the joints. (pp. 747–750)

23. (B) The spine is divided into sections called vertebrae. Coccygeal is the name of one section of the vertebrae. (pp. 747–750)

24. (B) The lumbar area of the spine includes five vertebrae. (pp. 747–750)

25. (D) Cholera is a bacterial disease that could be used in an act of biological terrorism to inflict serious illness, severe diarrhea, dehydration, and electrolyte imbalances in its victims. (pp. 1079–1087)

26. (B) When a patient strikes her head and states she feels groggy and has a headache, she most likely has a concussion. (pp. 750–759)

27. (D) While the patient most likely has a concussion, any altered mental status after striking the head, such as "just sitting there staring off into space for a few minutes," can be an early indication of a contusion, a concussion, or a coup injury. An attention deficit is not usually injury induced. (pp. 750–759)

28. (B) Memory loss after a head injury is referred to as amnesia. (pp. 750–759)

29. (C) Bruising of the brain on the side of the injury is referred to as a coup injury. Bruising on the opposite side of the injury is called contrecoup. A hematoma is a collection of blood within tissue. A hematoma in the cranium is usually named by its location, such as epidural (outside the dura), subdural (below the dura), or intracerebral (within the brain). (pp. 750–759)

30. (D) A collection of blood within the skull or the brain is called a subdural, epidural, and intracerebral hematoma, depending on the specific location. (pp. 750–759)

31. **(D)** Decreased respiration does *not* lead to increased cellular perfusion; rather, it decreases perfusion. Head injury is made worse by limited room for expansion inside the skull. As pressure in the skull increases, it becomes more difficult for blood to flow into the head. This leads to an increased level of carbon dioxide in the brain. (pp. 750–759)

32. **(B)** An assessment strategy used to check an extremity for injury or paralysis in the conscious patient is assessing equality of strength by checking hand grip or pushing against the patient's hands and feet. (pp. 754–757)

33. **(B)** Incubation period is the time between exposure and appearance of symptoms. (pp. 1079–1087)

34. **(D)** If a patient has a traumatic brain injury with skull fracture, the patient's pupils tend to be unequal. (pp. 754–757)

35. **(D)** The vitals of a patient with a traumatic brain injury are increased blood pressure, decreased pulse. (pp. 754–757)

36. **(A)** Consider the possibility of a cranial fracture whenever you note deep lacerations or severe bruises to the scalp or forehead. (pp. 754–757)

37. **(B)** The spinal column is made up of 33 irregularly shaped bones. (pp. 747–750)

38. **(B)** Any blunt trauma above the clavicles may damage the *cervical* vertebrae. (pp. 761–765)

39. **(A)** Priapism is a persistent erection of the penis. (pp. 761–765)

40. **(B)** The patient with a cervical spine injury in a supine position often has his arms stretched out above his head. (pp. 761–765)

41. **(C)** Injuries to an elderly person should be considered as possibly due to abuse or neglect. (pp. 944–945)

42. **(C)** Geriatric patients have decreased elasticity of the lungs and decreased activity of cilia, both of which result in decreased ability to clear foreign substances from the lungs. (pp. 931–934)

43. **(D)** As a normal process of aging, geriatric patients lose skin elasticity and sweat glands shrink. This results in thin, dry, wrinkled skin. (pp. 931–934)

44. **(B)** Geriatric patients usually have diminished function of the thyroid gland, which results in decreased energy and decreased tolerance of heat and cold. (pp. 931–934)

45. **(C)** A fall in an elderly patient may indicate a more serious problem, such as abnormal heart rhythm, which may cause a diminished cardiac output. (pp. 940–944)

46. **(C)** An unstable object impaled in the cheek wall should be pulled out if easily done. This minimizes the potential for bleeding into the airway. (pp. 652–659)

47. **(A)** If possible, a patient with facial fractures should be transported on a long spine board in the supine position. Then the patient and board can be rotated to the side to ensure drainage from the patient's mouth. (pp. 757–759)

48. **(D)** The pressure point for controlling bleeding from the leg is the femoral artery. (pp. 622–629)

49. **(A)** Do *not* pick embedded particles out of the cut. Care for an open wound includes controlling bleeding, bandaging the dressing in place, and cleaning the wound surface. (pp. 622–629)

50. **(B)** The best method for control of nasal bleeding is pinching the nostrils together. (pp. 622–629)

51. **(C)** The first step in caring for possible internal bleeding after ensuring respiration and circulation and controlling life-threatening external bleeding is treating for shock. Do not place the patient in a sitting position if you suspect shock. (pp. 630–632)

52. **(D)** A razor blade cut is an example of a laceration. The term *incision* was used in the old training curriculum. (pp. 646–652)

53. **(D)** The condition in which flaps of skin are torn loose or pulled off completely is called avulsion. (pp. 646–652)

54. **(C)** After the control of profuse bleeding in a patient who has an object impaled in the forearm, you should stabilize the object. Do not remove the object. (pp. 652–659)

55. **(D)** Pale, cool, clammy skin is a sign of shock. (p. 634)

56. **(A)** An object impaled in the eye should be stabilized with gauze and protected with a disposable cup. It is also important to cover the other eye to limit movement of the eyes. (pp. 652–659)

57. **(C)** A lacerated eyelid or injury to the eyeball should be covered with folded 4 × 4s to carefully hold the eyelid or eyball in place. (pp. 652–659)

58. **(A)** All open wounds to the chest should be considered life-threatening. (pp. 646–652)

59. **(C)** Before moving a supine patient with possible spinal injuries onto a long spine board, you should always apply a rigid collar. A KED is not needed for a supine patient. (pp. 754–757)

60. **(A)** The initial effort to control bleeding from a severed neck artery should be direct pressure or pinching. Then apply the occlusive dressing. Remember Standard Precautions. (pp. 622–629)

61. **(B)** The most reliable sign of spinal-cord injury in conscious patients is paralysis of extremities. Tenderness along the spine may indicate injury to the bones or muscles. (pp. 754–757)

62. **(D)** When caring for an open abdominal wound with evisceration, do not replace the organ but cover with a moistened dressing. (pp. 690–692)

63. **(C)** A patient in acute abdominal distress without vomiting should be transported face up with the knees bent to relieve the pressure on the abdominal muscles. (pp. 871–873)

64. **(C)** When a joint is locked into position, the EMT should splint it in the position found. Do not apply force to move a joint. (pp. 709–712)

65. **(A)** A splint properly applied to an extremity should prevent an open bone injury, motion of bone fragments, and damage to muscles and blood vessels. It should *not* impede circulation. (pp. 712–716)

66. **(B)** A fracture to the humerus shaft is best cared for by immobilizing with a rigid splint or sling and swathe, which limits movement in all directions. (pp. 709–712)

67. **(D)** A fracture to the proximal end of the humerus is best cared for by immobilizing with a sling and swathe. (p. 730)

68. **(B)** The best way to immobilize a fractured elbow when the arm is found in the bent position and there is a distal pulse is to keep the arm in its found position and apply a short, paddled splint. Do not straighten fractured joints that have pulses. (p. 731)

69. **(B)** When splinting, if a severe deformity exists or distal circulation is compromised, you should align to the anatomical position with gentle traction. (p. 711)

70. **(C)** The first step in immobilizing a fractured wrist with distal pulse is to place the broken hand in its position of function. (p. 712)

71. **(A)** A patient with a fractured pelvis should be immobilized on an orthopedic stretcher or long spine board with legs bound together with wide cravats. The PASG could be applied if local protocols permit. In many localities, application requires an order from a physician. (pp. 718–720)

72. **(D)** A fractured femur is best immobilized with a traction splint. (pp. 723–724)

73. **(A)** Before immobilizing a fractured knee, assess for distal circulation and sensory and motor function. If there is no pulse, you may need to manipulate the extremity. (p. 738)

74. **(C)** The best method for immobilizing a suspected ankle fracture is a pillow splint. (pp. 726–727)

75. **(B)** A sprain is an injury in which ligaments are torn. (p. 706)

76. **(C)** Definitive care for open extremity injuries is *not* provided in the prehospital setting. All other choices are true. (p. 706)

77. **(D)** Muscle is attached to bone by tendons. (pp. 696–702)

78. **(B)** A partial thickness burn involves the epidermis and dermis. (pp. 660–665)

79. **(A)** The entire back of an adult patient's right upper extremity is 4.5 percent (the entire arm is 9, so half is 4.5 percent) and her entire chest is 9 percent; therefore 9 + 4.5 = 13.5 percent. (pp. 660–665)

80. **(C)** A moderate burn involves superficial burns covering more than 50 percent of the body surface. (pp. 660–665)

81. **(A)** Partial thickness burns cause swelling and blistering. (pp. 660–665)

82. **(D)** A patient suffering chemical burns to the skin caused by dry lime should be treated by first brushing away the lime. Also, if you look up the chemical, you would note that it should not be mixed with water or phenol. (pp. 666–670)

83. **(D)** Acid burns to the eyes should be flooded with water for at least 20 minutes. (pp. 666–670)

84. **(A)** A method for estimating the extent of a burn is the rule of nines. (pp. 660–665)

85. **(D)** If a woman is having her first baby, the first stage of labor will usually last an average of 16 hours. (pp. 843–845)

86. **(B)** During the most active stage of labor, the uterus usually contracts every 2 to 3 minutes (with contractions commonly lasting 30 seconds to 1 minute). (pp. 843–845)

87. **(C)** If the amniotic sac does not break during delivery, the EMT should puncture it with a finger, then remove the membranes from the baby's nose and mouth. (pp. 847–848)

88. **(B)** To assist the mother in delivering the baby's upper shoulder, gently support the baby's head. Do not pull on the infant. (pp. 849–853)

89. **(B)** After delivery, first position the newborn on his side, then suction the baby's nose and mouth before clamping the cord. Do not slap infants on their buttocks because this may injure them, or worse, you may drop the slippery child. (pp. 849–853)

90. **(C)** If spontaneous respiration does not begin after suctioning the baby's mouth and nose, the EMT should vigorously rub the baby's back; then consider mechanical ventilatory assistance. (pp. 857–858)

91. **(D)** Do not pull the patient out the side windows. To assist with patient access, the EMT should initially try opening each car doors, roll down windows, and ask the patient to unlock the doors. (p. 1056)

92. **(A)** Requirements for speed of removal dictate the specific technique used for spinal immobilization of a patient at a collision scene. (pp. 1050–1060)

93. **(D)** The steps should be (1) sizing up the situation, (2) stabilizing the vehicle, (3) gaining the access, (4) disentangling the patient. (pp. 1041–1043)

94. **(D)** The number of ambulances in the region is *not* a consideration unless this is an MCI. Considerations for size-up of a collision include potential hazards, need for additional EMS units, and the number of patients involved. (pp. 1043–1044)

95. **(C)** To minimize injuries at a collision, EMTs should wear highly visible clothing so they do not get hit by a car while attending to their patient. Use the proper tools for the task and do not deactivate the safety guards on tools or you will be injured. It is not always feasible to wait until the police arrive on the scene. (pp. 1040–1041)

96. **(B)** The vehicle's catalytic converter can be a source of ignition at a collision because it is often over 1,200°F. (p. 1052)

97. **(A)** The three-step process of disentanglement described in the text includes creating exitways by displacing doors and roof posts, disentangling occupants by displacing the front end, and gaining access by disposing of the roof. Opening the trunk and disconnecting the battery cable are not priority tasks. (pp. 1056–1058)

98. **(B)** If a vehicle's electrical system must be disrupted, disconnect the ground cable from the battery. (p. 1052)

99. **(D)** When positioning flares, use a formula that includes the stopping distance for the posted speed plus the margin of safety. (p. 1042)

100. **(C)** Once the vehicle has been stabilized, the next part of an extrication procedure for patient rescue is to displace doors and roof posts. (p. 1043)

101. **(A)** The Emergency Medical Dispatcher (EMD) has told you the exact location of a collision, how many and what kinds of vehicles are involved, and any known hazards. Other information that would be helpful from the EMD concerning this collision would be how many persons are injured. (p. 982)

102. **(C)** The EMD does not need to ask the person's name. All other questions are pertinent. (p. 982)

103. **(A)** When operating a siren, be aware that the continuous sound of a siren could worsen a patient's condition. All motorists will *not* hear and honor your signal. If you use the siren continuously, there should be a valid reason for doing so. The noise from the siren can damage your ears over a period of time. (p. 985)

104. **(D)** Factors that affect an ambulance's response to a scene include day of the week, time of the day, and detours. Danger zones usually cannot be planned for. (pp. 985–986)

105. **(B)** If a patient develops cardiac arrest during transport, have the operator of the ambulance stop the ambulance so you can begin defibrillation. Also alert the hospital about the cardiac arrest. (pp. 496–497)

106. **(C)** When transferring a nonemergency patient to the emergency department personnel, you should check to see what is to be done with the patient. (pp. 989–991)

107. **(C)** The last step when transferring a patient is to obtain your release, which often takes the form of a thank-you for the information provided. (pp. 993–995)

108. **(C)** At the hospital, as soon as you are free from patient-care activities, you should prepare the prehospital care report. (pp. 995–997)

109. **(D)** Suction catheters, contaminated dressings, and blood-soaked linens are considered biohazards; unopened gauze bandages are not. (pp. 995–1001)

110. **(D)** Completeness and operability of equipment is *not* always ensured in the EMS/hospital equipment exchange program. Always inspect it; if you find parts that are broken or incomplete, notify someone in authority so the device can be repaired or replaced. (pp. 995–1001)

111. **(D)** Vigorous cleaning of the ambulance while parked at the hospital is prevented or restricted by time, equipment, and space. There is, however, no law against it. (pp. 995–1001)

112. **(C)** The first clamp placed on the umbilical cord should be about 10 inches from the baby. (pp. 847–848)

113. **(A)** If bleeding continues from the umbilical cord after clamping and cutting, the EMT should clamp the cord again, close to the original clamp. (pp. 847–848)

114. **(A)** The maximum amount of time to wait for the placenta to be delivered before transporting is 20 minutes. (pp. 858–860)

115. **(A)** Delivery of the placenta is usually accompanied by the loss of no more than 500 cc of blood. (pp. 858–860)

116. **(B)** The first step to control vaginal bleeding after birth is to place a sanitary napkin over the vaginal opening. Do not pack the vagina. Consider massaging the uterus if bleeding persists. Allow the mother to nurse the baby, which will control bleeding by stimulating contraction of the uterus. (pp. 858–860)

117. **(B)** Along with physical and mental fitness, ambulance operators should be able to perform under stress. (pp. 35–36)

118. **(D)** When driving an ambulance, you should realize that there are no state laws that grant the absolute right of way. (pp. 984–985)

119. **(B)** If upon viewing the vaginal area, you see the umbilical cord presenting first (a prolapsed cord delivery), you should gently push up on the baby's head or buttocks to keep pressure off the cord. Do not cut the cord because it is the infant's blood supply. Never attempt to push the cord back into the vagina. (pp. 862–863)

120. **(C)** If an arm presentation without a prolapsed cord is noted, the EMT should transport immediately, providing high-concentration oxygen. (p. 862)

121. **(C)** A baby is considered premature if the baby weighs less than 5 pounds or is born before the thirty-seventh week. (pp. 838–840)

122. **(D)** Airway passages *do* swell when a child has airway disease. All other signs listed are indications of a respiratory disease. (pp. 909–912)

123. **(C)** The soft spot on top of an infant's head is called the fontanelle. (pp. 878–882)

124. **(C)** After calming a snake-bite victim and treating for shock, locate the fang marks. Next, you should cleanse the wound site with soap and water. (pp. 828–830)

125. **(A)** When a patient who was working in a hot environment complains of severe muscle cramps in the legs and feels faint, you should move the patient to a cool place and begin care by administering oxygen by nonrebreather. (pp. 814–816)

126. **(D)** In cases of sudden infant death syndrome, the EMT should provide resuscitation and transport to the hospital. (p. 917)

127. **(C)** Injuries to the center of the back and upper arms might lead you to consider child abuse. Multiple skinned knees and sprained ankles are common in children. (pp. 921–924)

128. **(D)** With frostbite, the affected area feels frozen, but only on the surface. (pp. 807–809)

129. **(A)** The initial sign of hypothermia is shivering. (pp. 808–809)

130. **(A)** Extreme hypothermia is characterized by unconsciousness and absence of discernible vital signs. If there is shivering, numbness, and drowsiness, the patient is not yet in severe hypothermia. (pp. 808–809)

131. **(C)** Common causes of shock in children include infection, trauma, blood loss, and dehydration. (pp. 905–907)

132. **(C)** A sunken fontanelle may indicate dehydration. (pp. 905–907)

133. **(A)** Flowing oxygen over the face of a small child so it will be inhaled is referred to as the blow-by technique. (pp. 899–905)

134. **(B)** A complication of a rapidly rising temperature in a child is often a seizure. (pp. 914–915)

135. **(D)** A group of viral illnesses that cause inflammation of the larynx, trachea, and bronchi is called croup. (pp. 910–912)

136. **(D)** The strong, white, fibrous material covering the bones is called the periosteum. (pp. 699–704)

137. **(C)** The coming apart of a joint is referred to as a dislocation. (pp. 699–704)

138. **(A)** Overstretching or overexertion of a muscle is called a strain. (p. 706)

139. **(B)** A patient with hot and dry or hot and moist skin is experiencing a true emergency that requires rapid cooling and immediate transport. (pp. 814–816)

140. **(A)** As frostbite progresses and exposure continues, the skin turns from white and waxy to blotchy and grayish yellow and finally to grayish blue. (pp. 810–813)

141. **(C)** To treat a patient with deep frostbite, cover the frostbitten area, handle it as gently as possible, and transport the patient. Do not rub the area or apply cold. Do not rewarm the area unless you can ensure that it will not refreeze. (pp. 810–813)

142. **(C)** The indications for a traction splint are painful, swollen, and deformed mid-thigh with no joint or lower leg injury. (pp. 723–724)

143. **(C)** The Hazardous Materials Technician actually plugs, patches, or stops the release of a hazardous material. First Responder Awareness rescuers are trained only to recognize the problem and initiate a response from the proper organizations. First Responder Operations rescuers are trained to initially respond to releases or potential releases of hazardous materials in order to protect people, property, and the environment. The most advanced level of training is for the Hazardous Materials Specialist; this level of rescuer is expected to have advanced knowledge and skills and to command and support activities at the incident site. (pp. 1008–1009)

144. **(C)** The "safe zone" should be established on the same level as and upwind from the hazardous materials accident site. This positioning prevents flowing liquids or burning gases from spreading into the "safe zone." (pp. 1009–1010)

145. **(B)** A resource that must be maintained at the work site by the employer and that must be available to all employees working with hazardous materials is called the Material Safety Data Sheet. This sheet generally names the substance, its physical properties, fire and explosion hazard information, health hazard information, and emergency first-aid treatment. (pp. 1011–1012)

146. (B) EMS personnel at a hazmat incident are responsible for caring for the injured and monitoring and rehabilitating the hazmat team members. (pp. 1009–1014)

147. (D) Categorizing a patient as Priority 1 at an MCI means the patient has treatable life-threatening illness or injuries. (pp. 1026–1031)

148. (A) The MCI officer responsible for communicating with each treatment area to determine the number and priority of the patients in that sector is called the staging supervisor. (pp. 1019–1020)

149. (C) A Priority 2 patient at an MCI would be color-coded yellow. Priority 1 patients would be red, Priority 3 would be green, and Priority 4 would be black or gray. (pp. 1026–1031)

150. (C) Patients at an MCI who are assessed to have minor injuries are categorized as Priority 3. See the answer for multiple-choice question 149. (pp. 1026–1031)

Appendix A Basic Cardiac Life Support Review

MATCH TERMINOLOGY/ DEFINITIONS

1. (G) Biological death—when brain cells die (p. 1124)

2. (K) Brachial pulse—pulse measured by feeling the major artery of the arm; the absence of this pulse is used as a sign, in infants, that heartbeat has stopped and CPR should begin. (p. 1131)

3. (L) Cardiopulmonary resuscitation—actions you take to revive a person (or at least temporarily prevent biological death) by keeping the person's heart and lungs working (p. 1124)

4. (D) Carotid pulse—pulse felt between the groove of the Adam's apple and the muscles located along the side of the neck (p. 1130)

5. (C) Clinical death—when breathing and heartbeat stop (p. 1124)

6. (E) 50:50 rule—requirement that the amount of time you spend compressing the patient's chest should be the same as the time spent for release (p. 1132)

7. (F) Gastric distention—bulging of the stomach that may be caused by forcing air into the patient's stomach during rescue breathing (p. 1128)

8. (J) Head-tilt, chin-lift maneuver—maneuver that provides for maximum opening of the airway (p. 1126)

9. (B) Abdominal thrusts—manual thrusts to the abdomen used to dislodge an airway obstruction (p. 1137)

10. (M) Jaw-thrust maneuver—maneuver used to open the airway of a patient with a suspected spine injury (p. 1127)

11. (H) Line of lividity—red or purple skin discoloration that occurs when gravity causes the blood to sink to the lowest parts of the body and collect there (p. 1136)

12. (I) Recovery position—lying the patient on the side to allow for drainage from the mouth and to prevent the tongue from falling backward (p. 1130)

13. (A) Rescue breathing—providing artificial ventilations to a person who has stopped breathing or whose breathing is inadequate (p. 1128)

MULTIPLE-CHOICE REVIEW

1. (B) When a patient's breathing and heartbeat stop, the *brain* cells will begin to die after 4 to 6 minutes. Heart, liver, and kidney cells begin to die after about 1 hour. (p. 1124)

2. (D) Once clinical death occurs, brain cells begin to die within 4 to 6 minutes. However, it usually takes 10 minutes for biological death to occur. (p. 1124)

3. (C) In the CAB method of cardiopulmonary resuscitation, the A stands for "airway." (p. 1125)

4. (C) In the CAB method of cardiopulmonary resuscitation, the C stands for "circulation." (p. 1125)

5. (D) To determine if an adult or child is pulseless, the EMT should check for a pulse at the carotid artery. (p. 1125)

6. (A) To determine pulselessness in an infant, the EMT should use the brachial artery because the carotid pulse is difficult to determine in an infant. (p. 1125)

7. (B) If you are alone and you have determined unresponsiveness in an adult, the next thing you should do before starting CPR is to activate EMS. (p. 1126)

8. (C) When an unconscious patient's head flexes forward, the *tongue* could cause an airway obstruction. (p. 1126)

9. (C) One of the best ways way to relieve an airway obstruction due to the positioning of the patient's tongue is the head-tilt, chin-lift maneuver. The jaw-thrust maneuver is used on a trauma patient. (p. 1126)

10. (C) The head-tilt, chin-lift maneuver should not be used on a diving accident victim due to the potential for cervical-spine injury. The jaw-thrust is taught only to health care providers. (p. 1126)

11. (A) The recommended maneuver for opening the airway of a patient with possible cervical-spine injury is the jaw-thrust maneuver. (p. 1127)

12. (B) After opening the airway in a patient who requires rescue breathing, the EMT should inflate the patient's lung with two breaths, 1 second each. (p. 1127)

13. (C) Initial ventilations did not result in chest rise. Your next step is to perform the steps of CPR. (p. 1128)

14. (B) A common problem in the resuscitation of infants and children caused by improper head position or too quick ventilations is gastric distention. (p. 1128)

15. (B) In adult rescue breathing, the EMT provides 10–12 breaths every minute. (p. 1128)

16. (A) Infants should be ventilated at the rate of one breath every 3 seconds (60 seconds/20 breaths per minute = 3 seconds). Keep it on the high side of the range listed in Table B-2 in the text. (p. 1128)

17. (C) When a patient has a distended abdomen due to air being forced into the stomach, the EMT should be prepared to suction should the patient vomit. Do not decrease the oxygen concentration; pressing on the abdomen would produce vomiting. (pp. 1128–1130)

18. (A) The recovery position is used because it protects the airway and allows for drainage from the mouth. It also prevents the tongue from blocking the airway. (p. 1130)

19. (C) When delivering chest compressions during CPR, avoid using a stabbing motion to deliver compressions. Use a rhythmic 50 percent compression–50 percent relaxation motion. (p. 1132)

20. **(D)** The adult CPR compression point is located on the middle of the sternum, centered from side to side. (p. 1132)

21. **(A)** Before beginning CPR, the health care provider should assess the patient's pulse for a maximum of 10 seconds. (p. 1130)

22. **(D)** For an adult, the one-rescuer compression-to-ventilations ratio is 30:2. (p. 1133)

23. **(C)** The adult CPR compression rate in one-rescuer CPR is at least 100 times a minute. (p. 1133)

24. **(B)** The adult CPR compression rate in two-rescuer CPR is at least 100 times a minute when an advanced airway is in place. (p. 1133)

25. **(B)** The compression depth for an adult or older child (beyond puberty) should be at least 2 inches in the middle of the chest, between the nipples, and at least 100 times a minute. (p. 1133)

26. **(C)** The compression depth for an infant should be one-third to one-half the depth of the chest at a rate of at least 100 times a minute. (p. 1135)

27. **(B)** The compression-to-ventilation ratio for a young child or infant when there are two rescuers should be 15:2. This provides additional ventilation, with the presumption that the arrest may have been a primary respiratory event. With adults, the arrest is usually due to an electrical event (VF/pulseless VT). Note that the two-person CPR procedure is not taught to citizens, only to health care providers. (p. 1135)

28. **(C)** The compression-to-ventilation ratio for a young child or infant when there is only one rescuer doing the CPR is 30:2. This is the ratio taught in all the citizen courses and, as such, it is the universal compression-to-ventilation ratio because only health care courses address two-rescuer CPR. (p. 1135)

29. **(D)** The compression rate when performing CPR on an infant is at least 100 times a minute. (p. 1135)

30. **(C)** When opening the airway of an infant, use a slight head-tilt. Full hyperextension of the neck can cause the airway to close. (p. 1133)

31. **(B)** With effective CPR, the patient's pupils may constrict. Dilation occurs when the patient is hypoxic. (p. 1134)

32. **(D)** CPR compressions are delivered to children with the heel of one hand. The fingertips are used to deliver compressions for infants. (p. 1133)

33. **(A)** With the exceptions of defibrillation and advanced cardiac life support measures being initiated, CPR should not be interrupted for more than 10 seconds. (p. 1135)

34. **(B)** If you are treating a patient with a partial airway obstruction, poor air exchange, and gray skin, you should treat the patient for a complete airway obstruction. (p. 1137)

35. **(B)** Complete airway obstruction in a conscious patient is indicated by an inability to speak. Crowing, gurgling, and snoring are all sounds of partial airway obstruction. (p. 1137)

36. **(C)** When you have recognized complete airway obstruction in a conscious adult patient, you should deliver manual abdominal thrusts until the obstruction is relieved. Only unconscious patients are placed in a supine position when ventilations are attempted. (p. 1137)

37. **(D)** To deliver chest thrusts to an unconscious patient, place the patient in the supine position. (p. 1138)

38. **(D)** You are treating an unresponsive adult patient with a complete airway obstruction. You have been unsuccessful in your initial two attempts to ventilate the patient. You should continue with chest compressions, look in mouth, ventilations. (p. 1138)

39. **(C)** When treating an 8-month-pregnant female who has a complete airway obstruction, the EMT should use chest thrusts. (p. 1138)

40. **(B)** If a patient has a partial airway obstruction and is able to speak and cough forcefully, you should carefully watch the patient. Do not interfere with the patient's attempts to expel the foreign body. However, be prepared to provide help if the partial airway obstruction becomes a complete obstruction. (p. 1137)

41. **(B)** The major difference between the adult and infant procedures for foreign body airway obstruction when you suspect a severe or complete obstruction is that infants receive a combination of back slaps and chest compressions. Adults do not receive the back slaps, only the chest compressions. For all ages, the rescuer should look in the mouth but not automatically sweep it out unless an obstruction is actually seen. (p. 1138)

42. **(A)** While you are trying to clear an obstructed airway in an adult, the patient loses consciousness. You open the airway, look in the mouth, and attempt to ventilate. If this fails, begin CPR compressions. (p. 1138)

43. **(B)** You have been unsuccessful in initially ventilating an unconscious infant. You reposition the head and attempt to ventilate again but are unsuccessful. Your next step is to perform back blows and chest thrusts. (p. 1139)

44. **(D)** Signs of choking in an infant are *lack* of a strong cry, ineffective cough, agitation, wheezing, blue color, and breathing difficulty. (p. 1139)

45. **(B)** In health care provider CPR training, infants are up to 1 year of age, children are from 1 year to puberty, and adults are from puberty till death. Remember that citizen CPR courses do not teach this distinction and still define a child as age 1 to 8. (p. 1138)

COMPLETE THE FOLLOWING

1. The special circumstances in which the EMT should not initiate CPR even though the patient is pulseless include: (any four) (pp. 1135–1136)
   - A line of lividity
   - Obvious decomposition
   - Obvious mortal wounds
   - Rigor mortis
   - Stillbirth

2. Situations in which the EMT may stop CPR include: (any four) (p. 1136)
   - Spontaneous circulation occurs (then provide rescue breathing as needed)
   - Spontaneous circulation and breathing occur
   - Another trained rescuer can take over for you
   - You turn care of the patient over to a person with a higher level of training
   - You receive a "no CPR" order from a physician or other authority per local protocols
   - You are too exhausted to continue

3. List the information missing from the following chart. (p. 1135)
   - **A)** At least 2 inches
   - **B)** At least 100/minute
   - **C)** 1-second duration
   - **D)** Carotid artery (throat)
   - **E)** 30:2
   - **F)** 30:2
   - **G)** 15:2